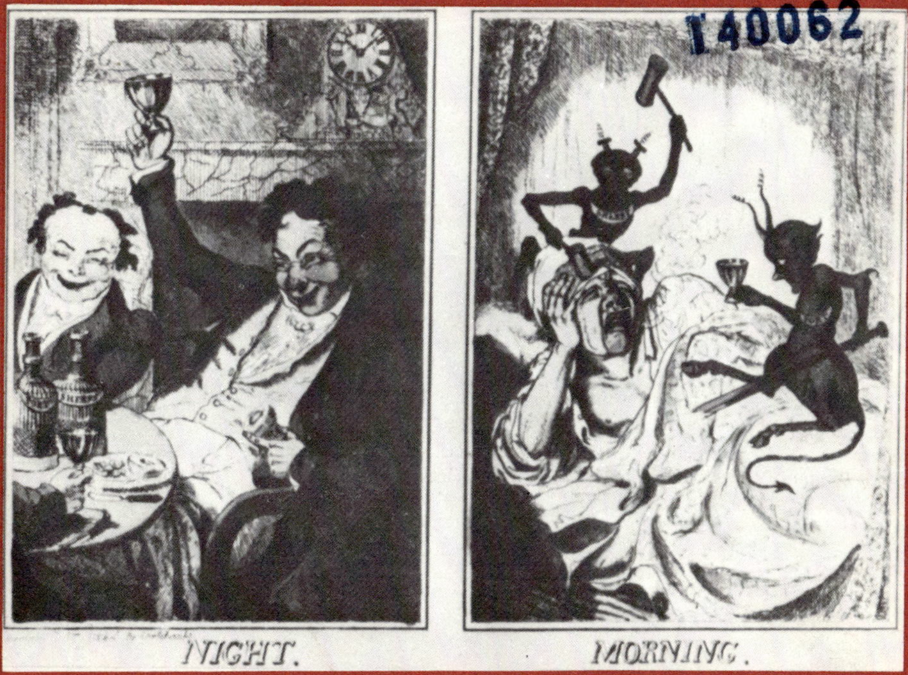

THE INTERNATIONAL JOURNAL OF THE Addictions

Volume 9 Number 1 1974

THE INTERNATIONAL JOURNAL OF THE ADDICTIONS

See inside back cover

The International Journal of the Addictions, February 1974

Published six times annually—February, April, June, August, October, and December—by Marcel Dekker, Inc., 270 Madison Avenue, New York, N. Y. 10016. The subscription rate for Volume 9 (1974), containing 6 issues, is $40.00 (*prepaid*). All subscribers outside the United States add $5.10 for postage. Back volume prices will be sent on request. *Please mail payment with order* to the following address: Marcel Dekker Journals, P. O. Box 11305, Church Street Station, New York, New York 10249. Second-class postage paid at New York, N. Y. and at additional mailing offices.

Printed in the U. S. A.

Contributions to This Journal Are Published Free of Charge

The International Journal of the Addictions, 9(1), pp. 1–23, 1974

British Opiate Users: I. People Approaching London Drug Treatment Centres

Herbert H. Blumberg, Ph.D.

S. Daryl Cohen, M.B., B.Ch.

B. Elizabeth Dronfield, B.A., Dip. Crim.

Elizabeth A. Mordecai, B.A.

J. Colin Roberts, B.A., Dip. Soc. Admin.

David Hawks, Ph.D.

Addiction Research Unit
Institute of Psychiatry
University of London
London, England

As part of a long-term study of opiate users, people approaching the drug treatment centers ("clinics") in Greater London during 1971 were interviewed approximately at the time of their first clinic appointments. The present paper is devoted to descriptive material regarding the sample as a whole. The differences between people given an opiate script and those not given one were also examined; these differences are not referred to in this paper as they are the subject of a second paper.

Bransby (1971) has described distributions for several basic variables—with results similar to some of those in the present paper—for people notified to the Department of Health and Social Security prior to March 1970. In the few instances where the present results differ from those of Bransby (e.g., greater incidence in our present sample of methadone as first opiate used), recent reports from Bransby and his colleagues confirm the historical changes.

Treatment centers (commonly called drug clinics) for people using opiates and/or cocaine were opened in 1968 following the Second Brain Report and the implementation of its recommendations by the Dangerous Drugs Act, 1967, and subsequent regulations—in particular that (apart from treatment to relieve pain due to organic disease) only doctors licensed to do so may write prescriptions for drugs named in the regulations (heroin and cocaine) and that they may do so only in certain settings.

SAMPLE

Sixteen London drug clinics are in operation at the moment for out-patient treatment, and these account for the large majority of people seen at all out-patient drug clinics (and their equivalents) throughout Great Britain.

Our sample consists basically of people approaching any out-patient drug clinic in Greater London between mid-November 1970 and mid-November 1971. Three further requirements had to be met before a person was considered to be within our sample: (1) he/she had to have *fixed* (i.e., injected intravenously in a nonmedical context) any drug at some time in the past (virtually all respondents had fixed opiates), (2) he/she had to be seen by a doctor at the clinic*, and (3) he/she must not have received an opiate script or scripts, on an out-patient basis, covering more than seven consecutive days before mid-November 1970 from any of the clinics in the UK since their founding in 1968.

* During the year about 150 people, at least, had merely requested an appointment but for one reason or another never got to the point of actually consulting with a doctor. At one clinic, moreover, assessments are carried out by the nursing and social-work staff in cooperation with the doctor, but the person does not get to see the doctor at this stage. Such people have not been included in the sample during the first year of the study if they did not finally speak with the doctor.

We wanted our sample to consist of people coming to a clinic for the first time. It was discovered during piloting of the survey that a small number of people had been to a clinic before, but only briefly; some of these people had been refused a prescription for an opiate and some had even received a prescription but clearly felt that this had not constituted a treatment program since they had not had their prescription renewed for a second week and had ceased attendance. So, in addition to those who had never been to a clinic before the commencement of interviewing (November 1970), we included those who had been but were given no prescription and that small number who were given an initial prescription (to cover an evaluation period) which was not renewed after the first week. We felt, then, that in effect all our respondents were coming newly to a clinic.

In order ultimately to be able to measure the effects, on respondents, of the interviews themselves, we have refrained at least temporarily from interviewing every fourth person out of the 307 eligible subjects (thus forming an "uninterviewed control group"). As a result, there were 230 people whom we wanted to interview, of whom we actually interviewed 210, giving a response rate of over 90%.*

METHOD

Our intention has been to carry out a prospective study by interviewing people as early, in terms of their interactions with the clinics, as feasible and then to reinterview them annually (hopefully for 5 years).†

To find out about new subjects, a member of our office staff would make a weekly telephone call to each clinic, inquiring about new patients who had been seen during the preceding week or had made appointments for the coming week. We have also had frequent occasion to be at the clinics in order to arrange for interviews. The sampling for the first 6 months has been checked by a member of our staff comparing our list of respondents with the list of names notified to the Home Office.

All interviews have been voluntary, and it has been stressed at the beginning of each interview that individual responses are confidential and

* In fact, interviews have also recently been secured with some of the 20 people who are counted as nonrespondents in the present report.

† As part of our research program we are continuing to interview one-fourth of new patients arriving at clinics after 1971 (an extended sample, beyond the end date defining the sample dealt with in the present paper), as well as reinterviewing the original sample at the anniversaries of their first interview.

can have no direct effect on the treatment a respondent might receive from the clinic. Respondents received a nominal payment of £1 to cover expenses.

The interviews were highly structured and lasted approximately 45 to 90 min. The areas covered were (1) family and demographic background; (2) current life style—attitudes, general social activities, illegal acts, friends, accommodation, use of social agencies, and ratings made by the interviewer concerning appearance and demeanor; and (3) drugs—early use, current use, periods of abstention, and physical complications resulting from use. Many of the questions were derived from the survey carried out by Stimson and Ogborne (1970). Additional information was derived from clinic notes and from forms filled out by the doctors at the clinics. This additional information also provides checks on the validity of some of the answers given by respondents.

Because we wished to ask more than could be included in an interview with any one respondent, six different forms of the interview were compiled and used in rotation by each interviewer. Key items were asked of all respondents, but additional material was included on only some of the forms (in such a way that every variable could be compared with every other variable for at least a representative subsample).

In general, *identical* data analyses have been carried out *separately* for the 112 "*odd-numbered*" and 98 "*even-numbered*" respondents.* The "odd" group has been used to test hypotheses, to form descriptions, and discover which items were related to particular key variables. The "even" group was used to attempt to replicate the findings. Most of the findings reported in this paper have been thus replicated, but for a few of the analyses it was decided in advance to include all respondents together, in order to have a sample of adequate size for those particular analyses. Except where they are described as "trends" or "tendencies," all of the findings reported in this paper were statistically significant, at least at the 5% level, in *both* groups (or in the single combined group, for those few analyses that were carried out only once). The factorial structure of

* If one adds to the 210 total the 20 nonrespondents whom we wanted to interview and the 77 people in the uninterviewed Control Group, the overall total is 307. Every person number evenly divisible by 4 was allocated to the uninterviewed Control Group; otherwise, when the middle digit of a person number was odd, the respondent was allocated to the odd subsample; when the middle digit was even, the respondent was in the even subsample. Thus in every cycle of 20 person numbers, 5 were assigned to the Control Group, 8 were in the odd subsample, and 7 in the even subsample. This cycle has nothing to do with the six different forms of the schedule, which each interviewer used in his/her individual rotation.

the variables is, in fact, such that very few of the significant differences in the "odd" group were not replicated in the "even" group.

The sections which follow are devoted to the main results and discussion of the data analyses.

PROCEDURAL VARIABLES

A few variables provide checks on sample homogeneity across time and clinics. Sequential respondent number (higher numbers being allocated as the year proceeded) had no consistent significant relationship with any other variables. This suggests that clinic treatment policy and the characteristics of people approaching clinics did not change systematically over the course of the year.

It should also be pointed out that current opiate use could influence respondents' answers to survey questions; however, "amount of time since last fix" and interviewer's rating of subject's sleepiness did not correlate significantly with any of the major variables in the present study.

PERSONAL BACKGROUND

Some of the background characteristics of the sample are summarized in Table 1.

Family and Demographic Variables

Sex Differences. There were 167 male respondents and 43 females. The female respondents worked fewer weeks in the 12 months prior to

Table 1
Background Characteristics of the Sample

Item	Description
Sex	167 male, 43 female
Age	26% late teens, 72% 20–29 years of age, 2% 30 years or more
Birthplace	Over 90% United Kingdom (majority in or near London)
Education	Approximately similar to British norms
Employment	39% full time, 4% part time, 50% unemployed, 7% housewife, student, miscellaneous
Personality	Low on authoritarianism, "normal" on anxiety and extraversion

interview, had fewer court convictions, and were more likely to be married or "going with" someone than the males. Among married respondents, women were more likely to fix with their spouses than men were. Female respondents were also a little more likely to tell us that they had underestimated their use of methadone while talking with the doctor. d'Orban (1970) reported that female heroin addicts who had been admitted to one British women's prison showed more severe psychiatric abnormality than do male heroin addicts. However, in our own findings, sex did not appear to be related to any "psychiatric" variables.

Age and Place of Birth. Approximately 26% of the respondents were in their late teenage years, 72% were in their 20s, and 2% were 30 years of age or older. Median present age was 21.7 years. Age was not significantly related to any other important variables except that younger respondents were more extraverted (General Survey, adapted from Couch, 1960). Although age was positively correlated with age of first fix, this was to be expected simply because older respondents had had more of a chance to have their first fixes at a later age.

More than 90% of the respondents were born in the United Kingdom and grew up there; however, clinics do not generally provide even initial appointments for anyone not eligible to be under the National Health Service. Of all respondents, 46% were born in Greater London, 20% in another major city, 29% were born in a town or suburb (including suburbs of Greater London), and 5% in rural areas. Thus the majority of those approaching London drug clinics have grown up in or near London.

A number of respondents complained that they have had to come to London—or been unable to leave—because clinic facilities, or their equivalent, elsewhere in Britain are often inadequate, characterized by discourtesy, or lacking altogether.

Upbringing. Incidence of parental death appears to be no higher in the present population than in samples of psychiatric patients or normal controls (cf. Birtchnell, 1969, 1970). The parents of 20% of the sample were (alive and) living apart from each other.

About 33% of the respondents had been separated from one or both parents for more than a year before the age of 15 (22% had been away from both parents, 9% from just their fathers, and 2% from just their mothers; cf. Bowlby, 1970). Just under 74% of all the respondents were brought up by their natural parents, 17% by one parent or other family member, 4% by adopted parents, and 5% institutionally.

On average, respondents had between two and three siblings. Out of the approximately 180 respondents who had at least one sibling, 20 reported that one or more sibs had fixed, 70 said that one or more sibs had smoked cannabis, and 55 had at least one sib who had been convicted of something.

Education and Employment

Respondents were asked about the highest examination they had completed; 59% had not completed any, 22% had at least one "0" Level or Certificate of Secondary Education, 4% a vocational exam, 10% at least one "A" Level, 3% had entered a degree or diploma program, and the remaining 2% had at least a first degree or teaching diploma. The sample does not appear to differ markedly in this respect from the national averages for Great Britain (Central Statistics Office, 1971). As might be expected in any population, the more educated respondents were less likely to have court convictions and were rated by the interviewer as being especially cooperative.

At the time of interview, about 39% of all respondents were working full time, 4% part time, 50% were unemployed, and 7% were housewives, students, and miscellaneous. The rate unemployed would be lower if the present sample were completely comparable to those used in most previous studies—i.e., which excluded people who approach clinics without being "taken on" (this latter group have a relatively high rate of unemployment—see the second paper in the present series, Blumberg et al., in press). The several indices of employment were in general significantly intercorrelated: present work status (interview), present work status (clinic notes), amount of employment (number of weeks worked in the past year), and the doctor's rating of how much he expected the respondent to be employed "in the near future."

Amount of employment was significantly related to only a few variables: frequency of seeing one's father in the previous 12 months (negative correlation), frequency of drinking alcohol in the 4 weeks prior to interview (positive correlation), and the respondent's rating of how much he/she "needs" heroin (negative correlation).

Respondents were asked where their money had come from in the 4 weeks preceding the interview. Out of 205 respondents (each of whom was specifically asked about every alternative), 66% indicated at least some money from own (or spouse's) earnings, 49% borrowing from (or sharing with) friends, 38% money from relatives, 37% selling things (except drugs), 34% social security, 32% selling drugs, and 22% stealing.

Respondents seemed about equally divided into those who thought that "in general" fixing helped their efficiency at work, those who felt it made no difference, and those who thought it hindered (respondents were not prompted with the alternatives, which were coded from answers to a general question about how fixing affected work efficiency).

Out of 206 respondents, 76 answered "yes" to whether they had ever lost a job because of their drugs use. When asked for a possible explanation, respondents less often cited (1) the mere fact of being discovered as a person who used drugs than (2) other reasons, such as poor performance (with or without discovery of drug use). However, it is at least possible that even if they had not been using drugs, the respondents might have had a similar overall job-loss rate.

Personality and Attitude

Respondents appeared to score low on trusting and authoritarianism (cf. Kohn and Mercer, 1971) and to have normal scores on anxiety and extraversion (four scales adapted from the General Survey; Couch, 1960).* Extraversion and neuroticism scores were in a normal range as measured on a short version of the Eysenck Personality Inventroy (EPI); this is in keeping with previous findings cited by Mott (1972), and may in part be due to drug use.

CURRENT LIFE STYLE (APART FROM DRUGS)

Social Agencies, Friends, and Residence

Of the 100 respondents who were asked about the amount of contact they had ever had with various social agencies, 81 had had some contact with the Ministry of Social Security, 70 with the probation service (includes probation reports), 63 with a solicitor or legal advice people, 27 with various forms of local authority social-work assistance, 23 with Release (an advisory service), 18 with various day-centers (Chelsea Centre, St. Martin's-in-the-Field, etc.), 16 with BIT (information service), and eight with a drug hostel (a surprisingly low number, perhaps).

As a rough index of their involvement with other people using opiates,

* This finding is, however, based on American norms since we have not yet compiled British ones, but it is encouraging to note that the factor structure of the test does appear to come out properly in the present data, and that scores were not due to acquiescence (cf. Blumberg, 1973).

respondents were asked, "About how many people do you know now to say hello to who have probably fixed at least once?" (Stimson and Ogborne, 1970). Those who know more people also had higher scores on the following: anxiety (EPI), aggression (General Survey), number of arrests in the 12 months prior to interview, sum of admitted illegal activities (in the 3 months prior to interview), doctor's rating of continued employment in the near future as being *unlikely* (but there was no actual relationship with other employment indices), importance of "altering perception of sights and sounds" as a reason for smoking cannabis, and having less wish to come off fixing completely.

Few respondents had had more than three addresses in the course of the preceding 12 months. A number of questions were asked about the place which was occupied *longest* during the preceding year: 48% of the respondents lived with their families (with or without cohabitee and/or others), 28% with spouse/cohabitee (with or without nonrelatives), 16% with nonrelatives only, and 10% alone. The average number of other people living with the respondent was 2.5; and for one-third of the sample other people in the place were fixing, besides themselves.

At the time of interview, 20% of the respondents were married and living with their spouses, 19% lived with their steady boy/girlfriends, 25% had steady boy/girlfriends with whom they were not living, leaving 34% who said they had no such liaisons.

Illegal Activities

Four selected indices of illegal activities were all found to be rather closely intercorrelated: number of convictions prior to the previous 12 months, number of different admitted illegal activities in the past 3 months (whether charged or not), convictions (as recorded in the clinic notes), and doctor's estimate of whether the respondent "is likely to go to prison" in the near future. Examination of various data indicates that very few of the respondents had ever carried out any violent crimes—indeed, very few of the crimes committed would be likely to be regarded as serious.

The following are all *percentages of the 208 people* who were asked questions about court convictions. There were 80% who had had at least one conviction; 46% had had a conviction in the 12 months prior to interview; and 69% had had one prior to that. There were 52% who had been convicted of at least one *drug* offense; 28% in the year prior to interview, and 37% before that. There were 59% who had been convicted of at least one *nondrug* offense; 25% during the year prior to interview, 52% prior to that.

Of 103 people who were asked how many convictions they had had *prior* to their first fix, 47% had had at least one. Only 13% of the 103 people had been convicted of a nondrug offense during the year prior to interview without having had any convictions prior to their first fix.

While it is useful to know these figures when one is considering the within-sample findings presently to be described, it is difficult to draw valid inferences from these distributions alone. The number of charges and convictions may be as large as it is for a number of reasons, including the fact that the sample may well constitute a group who are watched especially closely by the police. A number of investigators (Cicourel, 1968; Erickson, 1971; Shur, 1970; Skolnick, 1966) have indicated that most self-reported offenses—in various general populations—are never detected and that the rate of detection will vary with circumstance. In the present samples of opiate users, although the median number of arrests in the 12 months prior to interview was 0.6, the median reported number of "times searched" was 4.0 (the most frequent site being in the street) and 11% (of 102 respondents who were asked) report having been "planted" with a drug by the police in this 12-month period. As will be seen below, 95% of the respondents do admit to having been in illegal possession of drugs in the course of the 3 months prior to interview. In cases of "planting," however, respondents indicate either that they did not have any drugs on that occasion or else that they had disposed of them very quickly.

As noted earlier, those with more education had fewer convictions prior to the year before interview, and women had fewer convictions than men during the year prior to interview.

A description of the admitted illegal activities (all of which related to the 3 months prior to interview, whether the respondent was charged or not) is as follows: 95% of the respondents had been (not surprisingly) in illegal possession of drugs, 50% had sold drugs, 41% had received goods knowing them to have been stolen, 33% had stolen things from a shop, and 22% had obtained something by false pretenses. These items were asked as a checklist to which the interviewee was asked to respond "yes" or "no." Perhaps surprisingly (though in keeping with some of the studies based on general populations), there were very few abstentions and little apparent reluctance on the part of the respondents to volunteer information (cf. Belson and Hood, undated). No broad norms could be located for "admitted crimes whether or not charged."

Those who had engaged in more illegal activities reported a higher frequency of "being on the street after midnight." The doctor rated them as more likely to be unemployed in the near future even though, perhaps surprisingly, their employment records did not differ substantially from those of respondents with fewer admitted illegal activiities.

Self-reported illegal activities were also positively related to various drug items: having more friends who fix, being more likely to ask the doctor for drugs, having more hospitalizations related to drug use (in the past, including the year prior to interview), being more likely to admit to swapping or lending prescribed drugs, using a larger number of different drugs, disliking to fix sleepers, and being more likely to agree with a statement that "to improve sexual experience" is at least one reason why they use cannabis.

DRUG USE AND RELATED ISSUES

Early Use

The decision to start using a drug or to start fixing must be subject to social, personality and motivational, and (although often overlooked) cognitive considerations. Once the drug is tried, these considerations would still be relevant to continued use, but added to them would be further mechanisms of conditioning and possibly physiological addiction.

Social considerations are perhaps best thought of largely in terms of diffusion of innovation (cf. Katz, Levin, and Hamilton, 1963) and role acquisition. One would expect that mass media might provide a person with generally relevant information but that the actual decision to use or not use a drug would be more a matter of personal contact with users who might permit one to consider the possibility of use. Before starting to fix, respondents in the present study knew (fairly well) a median of about nine people who had fixed. Only about 2% of the respondents had not known *any* such people. It is *not* the case that respondents have commonly been turned on to fixing by "pushers" whom they hardly knew.

As regards motivation, a number of needs and drives would appear to be particularly relevant to initial drug use—among them, curiosity drive (for new experiences) (Cofer and Appley, 1964—a factor without clear contradiction or confirmation in the present study), the need for anxiety reduction (substantiated in our findings in that low anxiety related to number of times an opiate had to be on hand before being fixed—see below), and, particularly where use is related to one's social context, affiliative needs (this, too, seemed to be substantiated in our analyses—see the relationship between older siblings and various other factors). Weil (1972) describes a specific normal drive to experience altered states of consciousness. Not only might initial drug use follow from these specific needs and drives, but also one might suggest that opiates provide *generalized* need reduction and that withdrawal symptoms represent in part a return of the needs which have been eased.

Social factors are especially relevant in determining whether one *encounters* opiates. Once opiates are present, social factors are still relevant but only insofar as they interact with one's needs, one's personality, and other individual factors. The *number* of occasions that an opiate and syringe are both on hand before a person actually first fixes the opiate would seem to provide at least one reasonably useful index of these individual factors—that is, an index of personal readiness to try opiates. What is of relevance here are the large individual differences on this index among our respondents.

For 60% of the respondents, an opiate and syringe had been on hand fewer than 10 times before they fixed the opiate (in the majority of these cases this fix took place on the very first occasion); for 13% the materials had been on hand between 10 and about 100 times; and for 27% of the sample, use did not occur until the material had been on hand for at least about 100 times (or else continually for periods summing to at least 100 days).

The number of times an opiate and syringe were on hand (before fixing) was found to be related to only three other variables—all three of the correlations being positive and small but statistically significant (in both the odd and even subsamples): low aggression, low anxiety, and number of older siblings. These last two relationships call to mind Schachter's (1959) experiments on affiliation, in which he found that—only in an anxiety-provoking situation—those subjects who had no older siblings were more likely to prefer the company of other people (indicating a need for affiliation). If one argues that this need might be met, not only by "being in the company of other people," but also by an opiate itself, or indeed by conforming to the patterns of behavior of one's company in order to achieve a sort of solidarity with them, then our figures arguably confirm Schachter's model as well as help to explain the dynamics of first opiate use. Cottrell (1972, pp. 230–231) provides further discussion of "drive due to social facilitation" being especially high when there is anxiety and/or when one is an oldest or an only child.

Cognitive factors and conscious decision clearly have some part in determining whether or not a person would try opiates. A small sample (30 respondents) were asked whether their first opiate fix was planned in advance: 18 described it as "unplanned" (but that is not to say it was unexpected), eight more said it was unplanned but they were "seeking an occasion," and for four it was planned in advance. Thus a clear minority had *anticipated* their first opiate fix. Moreover, as regards their willingness to try it when the occasion of their first opiate fix did arise, all but three of the 30 respondents described themselves as "willing" and the remaining three were uncertain (but not unwilling). This is in accord with the findings of Chein (1954, and cf. Rathod, 1972) regarding "initiation on a convivial basis."

The relative importances of social, personality, and cognitive factors plainly will vary with the time and place of a particular situation. For instance, in parts of some American cities, at present, social contact probably accounts for a reasonably large amount of the variance regarding whether or not a person tries heroin. In our own data, once an opiate is available, there is considerable variance in the number of times an opiate

Table 2
Median Ages of Various Drug Events[a]

Event	Median age (years)
1. First smoked straight cigarettes daily (for over a week)	14.0
2. First smoked cannabis	16.1
3. Alcohol: first drank regularly once a week	16.6
4. First tried LSD	19.1
5. First fix (interview data)	18.2
6. First fix (clinic notes)	18.0
7. First fix of heroin or methadone (interview data)	18.3
8. First fix of heroin or methadone (clinic notes)	18.5
9. First fixed daily for at least 7 days	19.8
10. (Present age)	21.7

[a] Differences of less than about 0.5 year are not significant. For about 48% of the sample the first substance fixed was heroin or methadone. The semi-interquartile range for each event extends from about 1 year under the median (2 years under, in the case of present age) to about 2 years over it. Included above the medians are the 4% of the sample who had never smoked straight cigarettes daily, the 15% who had never drunk regularly, and the 15% who had never tried LSD.

must be on hand before a given person will try it. However, only a small part of this variance seems to be accounted for on the basis of the stable personality traits or other variables surveyed, the remainder possibly being related in part to chance-like factors, some examples of which might be the momentary state of anxiety or curiosity.

Once opiates are tried, *further* use would be partly a function of learning (both classical and operant) and, possibly later on, of physiological addiction. However, one should not assume that anyone who fixes once or twice will inevitably continue to do so, nor that irregular opiate use necessarily leads to regular use. A drug, once tried, may become viewed as "available" for continued future use according to the needs of the person and the supply of the drug. The median ages of first use of a variety of substances are listed in Table 2, and the persistent presence of many of these drugs in the lives of people (who approach drug clinics) follows this notion of "availability." There is unlikely to be any direct causal connection in the *sequence* of drugs, which has previously been shown to depend on background variables and social context (Weppner and Agar, 1971).

Recent Use

For each of a variety of drugs and classes of drugs, respondents were asked about: frequency of use, liking, need, ease of obtainability, source, and intent for future use. The main results are given in Table 3. There were also questions about friends' drug use.

Frequency of Use. Most of the respondents had at the very least *tried* most of the drugs and drug classes that were asked about—over 90% had tried cannabis, oral amphetamines, English heroin, methadone ampoules, other opiates, and oral sleepers and tranquilizers. About 89% had at least tried powdered ("Chinese") heroin and 83% had fixed sleepers—high prevalences indicating a sizable black market in Chinese heroin, and a matter of concern given the rate of physical complications among people fixing adulterated substances and sleepers.

About 87% of the respondents had tried psychedelics, 76% fixing amphetamines, 75% methedrine ampules, and 56% cocaine.

Apart from tobacco and coffee or tea, the drugs most frequently used by respondents were in fact heroin and methadone, followed by alcohol and cannabis (for both of which the average use was just under weekly in the month prior to coming to clinic). Hardly any respondents had been using methadone linctus or tablets.

Table 3
Characteristics of Drug Use[a]

Substance	Frequency	Liking	Need	Obtainability	Intent
Cannabis	2.3	3.5	1.3	4.4	3.0
Amphetamines[b]	1.2	2.4	1.2	4.1	2.4
Heroin[c]	2.7	4.7	2.8	4.1	2.5
Methadone[d]	3.8	4.0	2.9	4.6	2.2
Other opiates	1.9	3.6	2.0	3.0	2.2
Cocaine	1.3	4.2	1.5	1.7	2.6
Tobacco	5.0	4.3	3.3	—	2.7
Methedrine	1.0	3.8	1.3	1.3	2.6
Alcohol	2.6	2.9	1.3	—	3.0
Sleepers[e]	1.4	2.0	1.4	4.6	2.0
Sniffing	1.0	2.1	1.0	—	1.8
Psychedelics	1.1	2.9	1.2	3.9	2.6
Coffee/tea	4.9	4.6	2.7	—	—

[a] Respondents who had never tried a particular drug are excluded from all means for that drug. Entries are mean figures for those respondents who were given an opiate script by the clinic. In several cases the means for those not given an opiate script differ from the figures in this table (see Table 3 of the second paper in the present series), but the overall pattern of the present table would not be very much changed by taking these differences into account. The numerical scales are not strictly linear but can reasonably be used for rough comparisons within columns (the standard error of the mean is between 0.2 and 0.4 for most of the entries). Frequency was measured on a scale ranging from 1 (not taken in the past 4 weeks) to 5 (taken daily). Liking was measured on a scale ranging from 1 (dislike) to 5 (like a lot). Need was measured on a scale ranging from 1 (no need) to 4 (strong need). Obtainability was measured on a scale ranging from 1 (very difficult to obtain) to 5 (very easy to obtain). Intent was measured on a scale ranging from 1 (trying to get off completely) to 5 (trying to increase).

[b] The means refer to oral amphetamines. Figures for injected amphetamines are similar.

[c] The means refer to English heroin but the figures for Chinese heroin are similar.

[d] Means refer to methadone ampules.

[e] Means refer to injected sleepers and tranquilizers, oral use being more frequent and disliked less.

On average, respondents indicated that they were using about the same amount of heroin and methadone as 1 year prior to being interviewed, though there was some tendency for use to be greater at the time of interview. Median estimated daily use of heroin was about 50 mg, with 25% of the sample claiming to use over 100 mg. Mostly, this was Chinese heroin, which (being in powder form) is open to adulteration. Consequently, estimates of weight are subject to inaccuracy. Median estimated daily use of methadone ampules was about 10 mg, with nearly half of the respondents (included below the median) not using any, and 25% reporting use of more than about 40 mg.

Liking, Need, Obtainability, and Intent. As the fixing of sleepers and tranquilizers is significantly correlated with the incidence of abcesses (in the present data), and these in turn would contribute to an increased rate of septicaemia (although our sample was not large enough to confirm this), it is reassuring to note that respondents do not express much liking or need for fixing them (in contrast with their higher liking and need for heroin and methadone). The figures in the last column of Table 3 suggest that respondents are trying to cut down on their use of opiates as well as of sleepers and tranquilizers. It is of interest to note that two drugs which have been very infrequently prescribed in the past year or two, namely cocaine and methedrine ampules, were both rated as relatively difficult to obtain. This is evidence that concomitant increase in illicit supply does not inevitably occur, but one must be careful about extrapolating from such observations to other drugs or to some point in the future.

One must keep in mind that the figures in Table 2 are *means.* For example, mean need was as high for tobacco as for heroin partly because of a "ceiling effect" (the upper endpoint of the rating scale was used frequently in both cases) and partly because more respondents had been abstaining from heroin than from tobacco (using methadone in some cases), but obviously there are some respondents who need heroin much more than they need tobacco.

Friends' Drug Use. Respondents were also asked various questions about their three "closest friends" (whom they identified by initials or other anonymous symbols). For 56% of the respondents, all three of these friends had taken drugs orally at least (excluding cannabis and alcohol and drugs taken as prescribed), and for 80% two, at least, of the three friends had done so. For 60% of the respondents, all three closest friends had tried cannabis, and, for 81% at least two of the three had done so. For 80% at least one of the three friends had fixed.

Abstention

Respondents were asked how many periods of abstention from fixing and oral methadone (lasting at least a fortnight) they had had since they first started fixing regularly (that is, daily for 7 days or more). About 37% of the respondents had had no such abstentions, 30% had had one or two, 17% three or four, 10% five or six, and 6% had had seven or more abstentions. Only 16% of the respondents had had one or more abstentions commencing in hospital, and for most of these there was only one. About 24% had had one or more abstentions in prison, and for most of these this was on only one occasion. Of those respondents who had had at least one abstention, the longest abstention for the majority of them lasted no more than about 10 weeks, but for 23% it had lasted at least about 1 year.

There were 77 respondents (33% of the sample) who reported at least one period of abstention from opiates in the *12 months prior to being interviewed.* These respondents were asked a number of questions about their most recent abstentions. Of those who explained the circumstances, in 44 cases the most recent abstention resulted from their own decision, and in only a further six cases was it due to "no means of obtaining supplies." In six cases the abstention was initiated by being in hospital, and in seven by being in prison (but these figures might be overly high because a recent hospitalization or court referral in some cases led to a respondent coming to clinic and, therefore, to being interviewed as part of the sample).

About two-thirds of the abstentions were effected by stopping quickly, and one-third by stopping gradually. Respondents were asked, "If you wanted to stop fixing completely, which of the following could be effective for you *in the long run*?" While the answers may in part reflect liking for the particular method suggested, it is still noteworthy that procedures in which the respondent would stop on his/her own decision or in which the doctor would slowly reduce overall script size were the most likely to be endorsed; those involving various forms of compulsory treatment were least endorsed.

Physical Complications

A number of questions dealt with the frequencies of various physical complications. Since there are some large differences between those given an opiate script and those not given one (most of the incidences are higher for those *not* given one), the discussion of this important topic is postponed to the second paper in this series (see Table 4 of Blumberg et al., in press, and the accompanying discussion).

CONTACT WITH CLINIC

A series of questions was asked separately of the respondent and the doctor about the initial consultations up until the time the doctor conveyed to the respondent a final decision about his/her preparedness, or otherwise, to prescribe opiates or other drugs. The data from these series are internally and mutually consistent but, with some notable exceptions, are not related to major external variables. In the information given by the doctors, the main cluster* of significantly intercorrelated items consisted of the following: certainty that the patient should be taken on by the clinic, lack of open dispute about the amount or kind of drugs to be prescribed, a rating that the patient appeared to be truthful, and description of the overall relationship with the patient as being a good one. This last item was, in turn, related to (1) a positive response to a question about liking the patient, (2) a feeling that the patient was unlikely to break off treatment against advice in the near future, and (3) a respondent's being more likely to be given a regular opiate script than to be among those who (asked for drugs but) were not given any regular opiate script.

There is substantial agreement between the respondent and the doctor as to whether the respondent asked for drugs before the script decision. And there is also substantial agreement as to whether there was a good relationship between the doctor and respondent. The respondent's rating of a good relationship is, in turn, part of a significantly intercorrelated cluster which also contains the following items: respondent feels that the doctor liked him/her, that the doctor acted openly, that the doctor believed what he/she (the respondent) said, and that he/she (the respondent) acted in a friendly manner.

Several of the interviewer's ratings were significantly correlated among themselves: respondent's cooperativeness, credibility, wakefulness, consistency, and lack of hostility. These ratings were not, however, significantly related to any other variables, except that respondents rated as more cooperative had had more education and were also more likely to be thought of by the doctor as unlikely to go to prison "in the near future."

* "Cluster" here has the following meaning: it is a subgroup of items such that most of the correlations between items within the subgroup are significantly greater than zero, while most of the correlations between (1) items in the subgroup and (2) other items in the group are not of significant magnitude.

The *lack* of significant relationships between interviewer ratings and treatment variables at least suggests that our results are not greatly affected by differential respondent cooperativeness or interviewer bias.

In addition to being asked how many of their acquaintances had had occasion to fix drugs, respondents were also asked how many of these had come to a clinic and why the others had not. The median of the figures given for number of acquaintances known (who had fixed) was compared with the median of the figures given for the number who had come to a clinic. The ratio of these two medians was approximately 2:1—i.e., half of the people who had fixed had come to a clinic.* Nevertheless, there are some respondents who have had most of their acquaintances come to a clinic, while some respondents claim to know upward of 100 people who have fixed opiates, few of whom had come to a clinic. The main reasons respondents gave to an open question as to why they themselves had come were either that their drug use had become too expensive in the absence of a legal supply or that they wanted to cut down or stop using. The main reason given as to why some of their acquaintances had *not* come to a clinic was that they did not use frequently enough to merit wanting treatment, but another reason commonly cited seemed to amount to not wanting involvement with the clinic and/or official bodies (cf. O'Malley et al., 1972).

CONCLUSIONS

A survey involving 210 people who have fixed and a questionnaire which on average took approximately 1 hour to administer yielded much information, of which only some is reported here. The requirements of statistical significance and independent replication achieved a certain economy in the presentation of results. Even so, there is much that is reported here that is not readily interpretable. It is the intention to consider, in this section, some of the broad issues suggested by the results reported.

* One must be cautious about concluding that, out of the overall number of people in Britain who have used opiates, about half have come to a clinic. However, one would have to be equally cautious about estimates of the nonclinic opiate-using population made in more traditional ways (proportion of clinic patients among opiate users admitted to hospital or prison—cf. Holahan, 1972, pp. 285–288), since—compared with people given an opiate script at clinic—rates of illegal activities, physical complications, and probably mortality appear to be *higher* among those refused an opiate script by a clinic (see Blumberg et al., 1974) and may well be *lower* (but perhaps higher per injection!) among casual users who do not approach a clinic at all.

Reticence in Approaching the Drug Treatment Centres

The data indicate that at least 50% of those who approach a clinic had first injected an opiate 3 years (or more) previously. At least half of the sample had injected opiates "daily for at least 7 days" 2 years before they approached a clinic, and 37% (of those who had ever fixed daily for a week) used opiates without any abstentions of over a fortnight. Enquiries made of respondents regarding their associates who had fixed suggested that perhaps one-half of the latter were not registered with clinics.

These items of information together suggest that at any one time a considerable number of people are using opiates, possibly on at least a fairly frequent basis, without being known to the drug treatment centers. Statistics compiled on the basis of the numbers attending these centers are likely, therefore, to considerably underestimate the numbers using opiates in the population. Added to the number who are at any one time not known to the clinics are those who, having approached clinics, are not prescribed opiates and whose contact therefore is likely to be extremely tenuous. A preliminary follow-up (of early respondents) about 8 months after the initial interview indicated that of 20 who had been given at least an initial opiate script, 12 were still coming to clinic regularly, whereas of 14 who were *not* given such a script, only one was still coming to clinic ($\chi^2 = 7.62$, $p < .01$). To the extent that a number of those not given prescriptions might not, in fact, be using opiates (a negative urine was associated with the decision not to offer a prescription), the number "actually using opiates but not in touch with clinics" will be diminished. However, it is notable that the majority of those refused scripts and having a negative urine at least claimed to have been using opiates in the immediate past.

The reasons given for not approaching clinics were various but included the statement that opiate need or use was insufficient to warrant this, reluctance to be notified to official bodies, and the feeling that little advantage could be achieved since the majority registered with clinics were not prescribed heroin anyway.

Implications for Treatment Policy

One must consider the possibility—although it is in no way proven by the present data—that reluctance on the part of opiate users to approach the clinics is partly due to the tendency for clinics to prescribe only small quantities of injectable methadone even initially, or to prescribe methadone linctus, or to refuse opiate prescriptions altogether. This is likely to be especially the case when the supply of powdered heroin on the black market is such that there is little net advantage in resorting to the clinics for supplies of opiates. Certainly our data suggest that powdered heroin was readily available. This is not to deny, of course, that a proportion of addicts do approach clinics in order to come off drugs, or that there may be some price advantage in getting opiates on prescription, or that people prescribed opiates by clinics may suffer fewer complications, or that they may receive less attention from the police.

To suggest, however, that the black market would be curtailed if more heroin were prescribed by the clinics is simplistic since other considerations than the availability of clinic-prescribed heroin dictate the activities of this market. It is not completely clear that increased prescriptions of English heroin would lead to a decrease in the amount of Chinese heroin on the black market nor that a sufficient supply of prescribed English heroin and injectable methadone to users would appreciably diminish the overall black market. However, given that there may be more than an element of truth in the assertion that a policy of diminishing prescription of heroin may have contributed to an expansion of the black market in powdered heroin, it would be unfortunate if a similar parsimony in the prescription of methadone had a comparable effect on powdered heroin. The retrospective analysis of a historical development, however accurate, does not necessarily lead logically to a recommendation for future policy since the situation itself has changed in the meantime.

SUMMARY

Interviews were secured with over 90% of a sample of 230 people, all of whom had *fixed* drugs, had approached any outpatient drug treatment center in Greater London during the 1-year period commencing mid-November 1970, and had no significant previous clinic contact. Results include descriptions of family and demographic background, current life styles, illegal activities, initial and current drug use, periods of abstention, and physical complications.

Males constituted 80% of the sample. Most of the respondents were between 18 and 25 years of age. About half of the respondents held full-time employment at the time of interview. About 25% of the sample had been convicted of at least one nondrug offense in the previous year, but the majority of these respondents also had had at least one conviction prior to their first fix. Eleven percent of respondents report having been "planted" in the 12-month period prior to interview. Most respondents had at least tried a wide variety of drugs, including the injection of sedatives and of Chinese heroin. From the time of first fix of heroin or methadone, there was a median interval of about 1 year before respondents "first fixed daily for 7 days," and a further interval of about 2 years before approaching a drug clinic—but this is subject to considerable variability. On average about half of respondents' acquaintances who had fixed also have come to clinics. The main reason given as to why the remainder did not do so was simply that they did not use enough opiates to warrant it.

ACKNOWLEDGMENTS

We express our gratitude to the Medical Research Council and the Department of Health and Social Security for their joint funding of this completely independent research. We are extremely grateful to the clinic staffs, who somehow found the time to help fully with the research, and to the following consultants and deputies who have kindly permitted us access to our sample: Doctors T. H. Bewley, H. Dale Beckett, P. Boyd, J. Buchanan, P. H. Connell, E. Curry, P. J. Dally, S. Das Gupta, J. Denham, G. Garmany, M. M. Glatt, F. P. Haldane, D. E. N. Hassall, J. Hinton, L. K. V. Howell, K. H. Lotinga, J. Lyon, J. W. Mack, W. Massey, M. Mitcheson, G. B. Oppenheim, J. L. Reed, M. Tripp, J. G. Weir, and J. H. Willis. We also wish to thank the respondents for their kind cooperation; the staff of the University College Computer Centre; and the office staff—Nadine Butler, Christine Guest, Marion Horton, and Sue Rees—who have helped with the difficult job of maintaining contact with all of the clinics, coordinating our records, and ensuring that someone would be available at the correct times and places for interviewing respondents. We appreciate the comments of Griffith Edwards and Iain Crow, who read a draft of these papers.

REFERENCES

BELSON, W., and HOOD, R. *The Research Potential of the Case Records of Approved School Boys. Part I. Aims, Methods, Findings.* London: Survey Research Center, London School of Economics and Political Science.

BIRTCHNELL, J. Parent death in relation to age and parental age at birth in psychiatric patients and general population controls. *Brit. J. Preventive and Social Med.* 23: 244–250, 1969.

BIRTCHNELL, J. Early parent death and mental illness. *British J. Psychiat.* 116: 281–282, 1970.

BLUMBERG, H. H. Specificity of acquiescence. *J. Personality Assessment* 37: 479–485, 1973.

BLUMBERG, H. H., COHEN, S. D., DRONFIELD, B. E., MORDECAI, E. A., ROBERTS, J. C., and HAWKS, D. British opiate users: II. Differences between those given an opiate script and those not given one. *Intern. J. Addictions* 9: 205–220, 1974.

BOWLBY, J. Disruption of affectional bonds and its effects on behavior. *J. Contemp. Psycho.* 2: 75–86, 1970.

BRANSBY, E. R. A study of patients notified by hospitals as addicted to drugs: first report. *Health Trends* 3: 75–78, November 1971.

CENTRAL STATISTICS OFFICE. *Annual Abstract of Statistics.* London: HMSO, 1971.

CHEIN, I., et al. *Narcotics, Delinquency and Social Policy: The Road to H.* London: Tavistock Publication, 1954.

CICOUREL, A. V. *The Social Organization of Juvenile Justice.* New York: Wiley, 1968.

COFER, C. N., and APPLEY, M. A. *Motivation: theory and research.* New York: Wiley, 1964.

COTTRELL, N. B. Social facilitation. In C. G. McClintock (ed.) *Experimental Social Psychology.* New York: Holt, Rinehart, and Winston, 1972, p. 185–236.

COUCH, A. S. *Psychological Determinants of Interpersonal Behavior.* Unpublished doctoral dissertation, Harvard Univ., 1960.

ERICKSON, M. L. The group context of delinquent behavior. *Social Problems* 19: 114–129, 1971.

HOLAHAN, J. F. The economics of heroin. In *Dealing with Drug Abuse: A Report to the Ford Foundation.* London: Macmillan, 1972, p. 255–299.

KATZ, E., LEVIN, M. L., and HAMILTON, H. Traditions of research on the diffusion of innovation. *Amer. Sociol. Rev.* 28: 237–252, 1963.

KOHN, P. M., and MERCER, G. W. Drug use, drug-use attitudes, and the authoritarianism-rebellion dimension. *J. Health Social Behavior* 12: 125–131, 1971.

MOTT, J. The psychological basis of drug dependence: the intellectual and personality characteristics of opiate users. *Brit. J. Addictions.* 67: 88–99, 1972.

O'MALLEY, J. E., ANDERSON, W. H., and LAZARE, A. Failure of outpatient treatment of drug abuse: I. heroin. *Amer. J. Psychiat.* 128: 865–872, 1972.

d'ORBAN, P. T. Heroin dependency and delinquency in women—a study of heroin addicts in Holloway Prison. *Brit. J. Addictions.* 65: 67–78, 1970.

RATHOD, N. H. The use of heroin and methadone by injection in a New Town. *Brit. J. Addictions,* 67: 113–121, 1972.

SCHACTER, S. *The Psychology of Affiliation.* Palo Alto, California: Stanford Univ. Press, 1959.

SHUR, E. M. *The Social and Legal Sources of Crime in America.* Englewood, New Jersey: Spectrum Books, 1970.

SKOLNICK, J. K. *Justice without Trial.* New York: Wiley, 1966.

STIMSON, G. V., and OGBORNE, A. C. A survey of a representative sample of addicts prescribed heroin at London Clinics. *Bull. Narcotics* 22(4): 13–22, 1970.

WEIL, A. T. Altered states of consciousness. In *Dealing with Drug Abuse: A Report to the Ford Foundation.* London: Macmillan, 1972, pp. 329–344.

WEPPNER, R. S., and AGAR, M. H. Immediate precursors to heroin addiction. *J. Health Social Behavior* 12: 10–18, 1971.

The International Journal of the Addictions, 9(1), pp. 25–40, 1974

Effects of the Vietnam Experience on Subsequent Drug Use Among Servicemen

Michael Rohrbaugh, Ph.D.*
University of North Dakota, Grand Forks, North Dakota

Gerald Eads, M.S.
Fort Riley, Kansas

Samuel Press, M.D.
Albany Medical College, Albany, New York

Abstract

Data from three samples of active duty servicemen (total n = 1743) surveyed in 1971 at a midwestern military installation provided only limited evidence that service in Southeast Asia

* This research was conducted while the authors were members of the Department of Psychiatry, Irwin Army Hospital, Fort Riley, Kansas, (Dr. Rohrbaugh, Dr. Press), and the Drug and Alcohol Abuse Control Program, Fort Riley, Kansas (Mr. Eads). Reprint requests should be sent to Michael Rohrbaugh, Department of Psychology, University of North Dakota, Grand Forks, North Dakota 58201. The views expressed in this paper are those of the authors and should not be construed as an official Department of the Army or Department of Defense position.

affected subsequent drug use. Reported incidence of opiate use in the presurvey month was higher for Vietnam returnees than for nonreturnee controls from the same units on only one of three surveys. Results suggest that stateside use of at least the nonopiate drugs is as endemic to the general military population as it is to the special population of combat-zone returnees.

As United States military involvement in Southeast Asia decreases, troubling questions remain as to the impact which involvement there has had domestically. Of particular concern is the problem of drug use among servicemen, and most pertinent is the question of whether (or to what extent) the nation's increasing drug abuse epidemic has been affected by the return of veterans who were involved with drugs while serving in Vietnam.

It is well known that illegal drugs, particularly opiate and cannabis derivatives, are readily available in Southeast Asia. Reports of widespread use among GIs serving there have proliferated in the news media, as well as in technical and professional publications (e.g., Postel, 1968; Sapol and Roffman, 1970; Colbach, 1971; Stanton, 1972). Anecdotal reports of Vietnam "addicts" who carried their habits to the streets of American cities and towns have also appeared, and a number of veterans have participated in rehabilitation programs at United States military bases and VA hospitals. Nevertheless, there have been few empirical studies of the general impact of serving in Vietnam on subsequent patterns of drug use. This paper addresses the question of whether Vietnam returnees serving at stateside military installations in 1971 were more likely to be recent drug users than other soldiers who had not been to Southeast Asia. Data are drawn from a series of surveys conducted at a midwestern Army installation, and include systematic comparisons of questionnaire responses from Vietnam returnees and nonreturnee "controls."

METHOD

The data presented were collected in February, September, and December 1971 in the course of the Fort Riley, Kansas, Drug Abuse and Morale Monitoring System (DAMMS) project.* The DAMMS project

* Fort Riley's Drug and Alcohol Abuse Control Program assists in the rehabilitation of servicemen with drug or alcohol-related problems. Participants enter the program through self or command referral, or are identified as potentially drug dependent through the DOD urine testing procedures. Facilities include Rap Center, Detoxification, Halfway House, and Alcoholism Units, as well as an Education/Prevention section.

involved periodic (quarterly) surveys of a representative sample of the post active duty population, and was designed to provide local commanders with up-to-date information on troop drug use and morale-related attitudes and perceptions. Consequently, the survey instruments were rather lengthy and broad in scope, and yielded considerable additional data which will not be discussed here.

An "enlisted form" questionnaire, which varied slightly in make-up from survey to survey, incorporated questions on extent of drug use: (1) in the month prior to the survey (recent use); (2) prior to entering the military (civilian use), and (3) in one's lifetime (i.e., "Have you *ever* used. . . ?"). Vietnam veterans participating in the September and December surveys were also asked about their drug use *in* Southeast Asia. Major drug categories (opiates, amphetamines, hallucinogens, barbiturates, cocaine, marijuana, and alcohol) were listed with appropriate slang labels included in parentheses, and respondents were asked to indicate how often they had used each drug by checking alternatives ranging from "never" to "more than twice daily."

Questionnaires were administered to enlisted men (Grade E5 and below) from a sample of platoon-sized units, selected at random but representative of the post population at the time of each survey. Units in the sample were different for each survey, and stratification of the sample was consistent with the breakdown of major and subordinate units and associated troop strengths. From two-thirds to three-fourths of each sample was drawn from the First Infantry Division (Mech) which resides at Fort Riley. Thus a good number of the respondents who had served in Vietnam were infantrymen. The total numbers of questionnaires analyzed in the February, September, and December surveys were 782, 480, and 481, respectively.

Questionnaires were administered in the unit area with command personnel (officers and NCOs) absent from the testing room. The surveys were introduced in an informal manner by drug center or medical personnel dressed in civilian clothes, and every attempt was made to insure anonymity and confidentiality. Our impression was that these efforts were generally successful in developing a relaxed and trusting atmosphere in the testing situation.

A certain proportion of the questionnaires returned were excluded from data analyses for technical reasons which included: (1) missing or incomplete data, (2) inconsistent responding, and (3) respondents indicating on a control question that their answers were not entirely truthful. The questionnaires eliminated included 6.1% of those collected in February, 5.1% of those from September, and 9.2% from December. There were no indications in any survey of differential rejection rates for returnee and nonreturnee subjects.

COMPOSITION OF THE SAMPLES

Respondents were asked whether or not they had served in Southeast Asia, and if so, how many months had elapsed since their return. In the February questionnaire the question used to identify returnees and nonreturnee controls referred to service in a combat zone (i.e., Vietnam *or* Korea), whereas the corresponding items for the September and December surveys asked explicitly about experience in Southeast Asia (and not Korea). Thus the somewhat lower proportion of returnees in the September (35.2%) and December (35.2%) samples, compared to the February sample (49.4%), is due in part to differing definitions, but probably also reflects a generally decreasing incidence of combat veterans in the lower enlisted grades due to troop withdrawals.

Of the combat zone veterans in the February sample, 47.7% had been returned for less than 6 months, and 20.2% had been in the United States at least 1 year. Returnees back less than 6 months included 66.0 and 35.6% of the September and December veteran samples, respectively; and comparable proportions of those returned longer than 1 year were 21.1 and 24.7% is September and December, respectively. Thus the September sample included proportionately more recent returnees than the February and December samples.

In examining reported current drug use as a function of whether or not enlisted personnel had served in a combat area, it was also important to determine whether the returnee and nonreturnee groups differed with respect to other variables. Table 1 shows some demographic characteristics of the returnee and nonreturnee samples from each of the three surveys. As would be expected, the soldiers who had not been in Vietnam tended to be younger and of lower grade (rank) than the veteran group. Returnees were distinctly more prone to report having AWOLs, Articles 15 (nonjudicial punishment), and courts-martial on their records; but in view of the relative comparability of the groups in reported *civilian* arrests, the discrepant rates of military offenses may be largely explained by the fact that veterans had spent more time in the Army. Table 1 also shows that more Vietnam veterans than nonveterans: (1) enlisted (i.e., were not drafted into military service); (2) reenlisted; and (3) intended to make the military their career. Minority group membership, if anything, was slightly higher among the returnees.

Table 1
Profile of Returnee and Nonreturnee Samples

	February 1971		September 1971		December 1971	
	Returnees (n = 396) %	Controls (n = 386) %	Returnees (n = 169) %	Controls (n = 311) %	Returnees (n = 169) %	Controls (n = 312) %
Age 20 or below	17.4	32.4	23.7	57.2	18.2	49.6
Grade E4 or below	61.0	91.7	68.6	92.0	58.0	90.2
Nonwhite	21.7	16.1	23.1	19.9	18.1	13.8
High school graduate, GED, or more	86.9	89.7	89.3	87.5	84.1	85.6
Have been AWOL	19.9	12.7	24.9	16.4	31.8	19.8
Have had:						
Civilian arrest	18.9	22.0	24.3	18.6	23.9	21.7
Article 15	37.4	24.6	40.8	19.6	48.3	27.2
Court martial	6.8	3.1	6 5	1.3	6.8	4.3
Drafted into Army	31.1	57.3	34.3	67.5	26.1	56.6
Have reenlisted	—	—	29.6	4.5	43.8	9.8
Intend to make service a career	7.3	2.3	10.1	1.6	10.8	2.8

The important point is that the samples did differ demographically, and this necessarily confounds an attempt to isolate the effects of combat-zone experience on subsequent drug use. The extent to which sample differences on variables such as age influenced differences observed between returnees and nonreturnees on the drug use measures is discussed in greater detail below.

RESULTS

Drug Use in Southeast Asia

Table 2 shows percentages of the returnee samples reporting at least one drug experience during the Vietnam tour. Incidence data are available only from the September and December surveys, since the February questionnaire did not provide for analysis of Vietnam use by type of drug. Approximately one-fourth of the returnee group admitted using heroin or other opiates at least once in Vietnam, and the greater proportion of these users (51.1% in September sample and 65.9% in the December sample) said that they had used opiates as often as once or twice daily. A number of subjects also reported cocaine use; however, cocaine

Table 2
Proportion of Returnees Reporting at Least One Drug Experience During Tour in Southeast Asia

	September 1971 survey (n = 169)		December 1971 survey (n = 169)	
	No.	%	No.	%
Opiates	45	26.6	41	24 2
Amphetamines	36	21.3	35	20.7
Barbiturates	32	18.9	26	15.4
Hallucinogens	23	13.6	23	13.6
Cocaine	26	15.4	21	12.4
Marijuana	107	63.2	85	50.2
Alcohol	141	83.3	135	79.8

Table 3
Proportion of Returnee Drug Users Who First Used Drugs in Southeast Asia

	September 1971 survey (n = 169)		December 1971 survey (n = 169)	
	No. who ever used drug	Percent who first used drug in Southeast Asia	No. who ever used drug	Percent who first used drug in Southeast Asia
Opiates	45	71.1	42	81.0
Amphetamines	45	26.7	47	23.4
Barbiturates	42	28.6	41	19.5
Hallucinogens	49	14.3	44	9.1
Cocaine	31	45.2	36	36.1
Marijuana	103	39.8	100	48.0
Alcohol	146	2.7	153	5.2

per se has not been found in Southeast Asia, and it is likely that substances found there called "cocaine" are actually heroin (Fisher, Nelson, and Panzarella, 1972). Over half of the returnees indicated that they had used marijuana (or hashish) in Vietnam, and of those users, 43.0 and 47.1%, respectively, admitted to having used cannabis at least daily. Other types of drug use were also evident; Vietnam amphetamine use, for example, was reported by over 20% of both returnee samples.

In general, the incidence figures presented here are somewhat higher than those obtained in Stanton's (1972) survey of Army personnel leaving Vietnam in November 1969, but are fairly consistent (at least as regards heroin use) with data collected from returning veterans by Nelson and

Panzarella (1971). However, there cannot be complete assurance that the present samples are truly representative of the general population of Vietnam veterans, inasmuch as veterans discharged from the military soon after their return to the United States are not well represented.

Table 3 shows percentage figures representing veterans who were first introduced to drug use while serving in Vietnam. Entries in the table are based only on veterans who admitted having used each drug at some time in their lives. It is striking that the clear majority of the men who had *ever* used opiates first did so in Southeast Asia. Initiation to marijuana use in Vietnam also seemed to occur relatively more often than introduction to amphetamine, barbiturate, hallucinogen, or alcohol use.

Recent Stateside Drug Use Among Vietnam Returnees and Controls

The main question of interest in this report is whether combat-zone returnees differ in their patterns of stateside drug use from other soldiers who have not served in Vietnam. Table 4 shows percent figures for incidence of recent drug use as reported by the returnee and nonreturnee control samples, where "recent use" is defined as at least one experience with a given drug in the month prior to the survey. Also included are similar data for premilitary (civilian) use, which provide a rough baseline for evaluating between-group differences in recent use. The civilian figures show the proportion of subjects reporting at least one drug experience *at any time* prior to their entry into the Army; hence the percentages tend to be higher than those for recent use because they are based on a time period longer than a month.

Chi-square (χ^2) tests revealed no differences between the groups on overall measures of recent use: The proportion of returnees reporting use of *any* illegal drug in the presurvey month was roughly comparable to the like figure for controls on each of the three surveys.

With regard to recent usage of specific drugs, the only statistically significant differences in the direction of greater use by Vietnam veterans occurred for opiates on the September survey ($\chi^2 = 6.02$, $p < .02$). Incidence of opiate use was also slightly higher for returnees in the December sample, but the difference fell short of acceptable confidence levels ($\chi^2 = 2.40$, $p < .20$). Returnee vs control comparisons for drugs other than opiates were either nonsignificant or significant in the direction of greater use by the controls. In view of the level of use reported *in* Vietnam, it is perhaps surprising that a higher proportion of nonreturnees reported current marijuana use in the February survey ($\chi^2 = 9.70$, $p <$

Table 4
Incidence of Recent and Premilitary Drug Use Among Returnees and Nonreturnee Controls[a]

	Current use		Premilitary use	
	Returnees	Controls	Returnees	Controls
February Survey (396 returnees and 386 controls)				
Opiates	2.1	2.9	4.5	6.5
Amphetamines	10.4	13.9	15.7	21.0
Barbiturates	7.5	6.7	12.4	13.7
Hallucinogens	11.9	14.3	11.4	18.7**
Cocaine	2.6	4.7	7.1	9.1
Marijuana	25.2	35.5**	28.5	39.1**
Alcohol	78.0	81.6	87.9	87.6
Use of *any* illegal drug	33.7	38.6	—	—
September Survey (169 returnees and 311 controls)				
Opiates	11.2	5.1*	7.7	4.5
Amphetamines	21.3	19.9	14.8	19.6
Barbiturates	11.2	13.8	14.8	15.1
Hallucinogens	24.3	18.0	15.4	16.4
Cocaine	10.1	9.0	10.1	8.4
Marijuana	43.2	44.4	38.5	42.1
Alcohol	84.0	85.5	84.0	86.2
Use of *any* illegal drug	46.7	47.3	—	—
December Survey (169 returnees and 312 controls)				
Opiates	10.3	6.4	8.0	6.1
Amphetamines	17.8	21.1	16.1	23.2
Barbiturates	17.2	19.6	12.6	18.7
Hallucinogens	15.5	20.5	12.6	19.9*
Cocaine	6.9	10.4	9.2	11.9
Marijuana	36.8	45.6	28.2	42.2**
Alcohol	78.7	82.3	79.9	83.2
Use of *any* illegal drug	40.0	48.0	—	—

[a] Entries represent proportion of samples reporting at least one drug experience in the presurvey month (Recent use) and prior to entry into the Army (Premilitary use).

* Two-tailed chi-square test, $p < .05$.

** Two-tailed chi-square test, $p < .01$.

.01), and tended also to do so in the December survey ($\chi^2 = 3.69, p < .10$). However, the control subjects also showed a higher incidence of premilitary use (February: $\chi^2 = 9.79$, $p < .01$; December: $\chi^2 = 9.73$, $p < .01$), which itself could account for differences in current use.

The marijuana comparisons highlight the importance of taking premilitary use patterns into account in evaluating differences between veterans and nonveterans on measures of recent stateside use. Other potentially confounding variables should also be considered. As has been noted above (Table 1), for example, returnees in the veteran samples were older than the nonveterans. Since greater drug use might be expected among younger GIs, it is possible that confounding effects of age have also served to mask or exaggerate between-group differences in recent drug use attributable (or not attributable) to the Vietnam experience. It is therefore pertinent to ask how the relationships (or correlations) between recent use and prior service in Southeast Asia would be affected if the veteran and nonveteran samples were matched according to age and premilitary use, or if variance attributable to those variables was in some way controlled or "partialed out."

Because matching would necessarily involve eliminating data, we attempted to control the confounding variables a posteriori by applying partial correlation procedures (McNemar, 1962). The general problem was to determine how the correlations between drug use and Vietnam experience change if age and premilitary use are statistically held constant. To this end, the relationships (or lack thereof) shown in Table 4 between returnee vs nonreturnee status and recent use vs no use of the various drugs were converted to correlation coefficients (phi, r) following standard procedures for correlating dichotomous variables (McNemar, 1962). The dichotomies were ordered such that positive values of r reflect tendencies toward greater proportionate drug use among returnees than controls. As would be expected, the "significance" decisions based on the phi correlations (Table 5) closely approximate those obtained from chi-square tests (Table 4). Point-biserial correlation coefficients were similarly computed to index the relationships between veteran status and age, and between current and premilitary drug use and age. Consistent with Table 1, the correlations between age and having served in Southeast Asia were positive and significant ($r = .19$, $.34$, and $.31$; p's $< .01$) for each of the three surveys. Correlations of age and drug use also confirmed the hypothesis that younger soldiers were more likely to report recent and premilitary drug experiences. Parenthetically, age was most clearly associated with marijuana, amphetamine, and hallucinogen use, and least associated with opiate, cocaine, and alcohol use.

Table 5
Correlations of Recent Use and Vietnam Experience with Age and Premilitary Use Controlled[a]

	Unadjusted r			Partial r with age and premilitary use constant		
	February	September	December	February	September	December
Opiates	−.03	.11*	.07	−.01	.11*	.07
Amphetamines	−.06	.02	−.04	−.01	.11*	.03
Barbiturates	.02	−.04	−.03	.04	−.00	.06
Hallucinogens	−.04	.07	−.06	.03	.13**	.00
Cocaine	−.06	.02	−.05	−.04	.01	−.04
Marijuana	−.11**	−.01	−.09	−.03	.06	.04
Alcohol	−.05	−.02	−.05	−.07	.03	−.03
Use of *any* illegal drug	−.05	−.07	−.08	−.02	−.04	−.04

[a] Correlations are phi coefficients with dichotomies ordered such that positive values of r represent proportionately more use among returnees than controls.
* Correlation significant (two-tailed test), $p < .05$.
** Correlation significant (two-tailed test), $p < .01$.

Table 5 presents the main results of the partial correlation analyses. The left column in each panel shows the correlations between recent stateside use and Vietnam experience, which correspond to the percentage comparisons in Table 4. Figures in the right columns represent partial correlation coefficients adjusted for the effects of age and premilitary drug use. In general, controlling age and premilitary use moves the adjusted correlations between Vietnam experience and recent drug use in a positive direction, but more so for some drugs than for others. The tendency for controls to report more recent marijuana use (February and December surveys) is substantially reduced, suggesting that differential rates of current marijuana use simply reflect the fact that nonreturnees in our samples were younger and more likely to have been involved in the expanding drug scene before entering the military.

The only significant relationships remaining after the partial correlation analyses appear in the September data, where there is marginal evidence of an effect of the Vietnam experience on subsequent use of opiates, amphetamines, and hallucinogens. Interestingly, differences between Vietnam veterans and controls in reported opiate use were increased by the age correction, but decreased by controlling for variation in premilitary use. Hence, the correlations were little affected by the correction procedures. There continues to be only limited evidence that Vietnam returnees constitute a special risk group with regard to subsequent opiate use.

The emergence of significant correlations for hallucinogens and amphetamines on the September survey is difficult to explain because similar relationships were not even approximated in the data from February and December. While amphetamines were rather commonly used *in* Vietnam (Table 2), the fact that hallucinogens were the *least* used drugs does little to clarify the September relationship between combat-zone experience and recent psychedelic use.

A final concern is that the preceding analyses are based only on total proportions of self-admitted drug users; no attention is given to variations in extent of frequency of use. Consequently, it is also important to ask whether returnees who did use drugs in the presurvey month were more prone to "heavy" use than nonveteran users. To check this possibility, *t* tests were performed for each drug category on each survey, comparing returnee and control users on the rate or frequency of their reported current use. Nonusers in each category were excluded from the analyses. While means were more often than not in the direction of more frequent use by the veterans, all comparisons were statistically nonsignificant. Hence there is no substantial evidence that returnees who did use drugs after their return to the States did so with greater frequency than users who had not been to Southeast Asia.

Drug Use and Time Returned from Southeast Asia

The fact that recently returned veterans were not differentiated from those who had been back for longer periods of time may also have influenced the relationships between Vietnam experience and the measures of recent drug use. Perhaps returnees were more prone to drug use shortly after their return to the United States; if so, the inclusion of personnel returned for longer periods may have reduced the incidence rates for the total veteran group.

Accordingly, reported drug use was tabulated separately for returnees in each survey sample who had been returned from Southeast Asia: (1) less than 6 months; (2) 6 months to 1 year; and (3) longer than 1 year. Comparisons of these groups revealed no systematic changes in incidence of drug use attributable to time returned from the combat zone, and there was no evidence that use of any drug was more likely to occur within the first 6 months following an individual's return to the United States than at a later date.

Relationship Between Drug Use in Southeast Asia and Recent Use in the United States

Of additional interest is the relationship between drug use in Southeast Asia and recent use stateside. Did returnees who admitted recent use at Fort Riley also report having used the same drugs in Vietnam? Conversely, did subjects who admitted use in Vietnam also tend to report recent use? Data pertinent to these questions appear in Table 6, which shows for each drug use category: (1) the proportion of returnees who were recent users and who also used the drug in Southeast Asia; and (2) the proportion of returnees who used in Vietnam and also used in the presurvey month. Note that again "use" is broadly defined to include one or more experiences with a drug in the month prior to the survey (recent use) or in one's entire combat-zone tour (RVN use).

Most returnees who reported recent use also indicated that they used the same drugs in Vietnam. This relationship is most evident among users of opiates and marijuana, the drugs most available and most commonly used in Southeast Asia (Table 2). RVN use among stateside using veterans occurred to the least extent for hallucinogens and barbiturates, the drugs least commonly used in Vietnam. However, recent use figures for veterans who used in Vietnam do not fit this pattern. Here, RVN users of opiates and cocaine reported the *lowest* incidences of recent use, suggesting that the proportion of opiate users who discontinue their use

Table 6
Relationships Between Recent Drug Use and Use in Vietnam[a]

	RVN users who use currently				Recent users who also used in RVN			
	No. using in RVN		% Using in presurvey month		No. using in presurvey month		% using in RVN	
	September	December	September	December	September	December	September	December
Opiates	45	41	42.2	43.9	19	19	100.0	94.7
Amphetamines	36	35	80.6	68.6	36	30	80.6	80.0
Barbiturates	32	26	37.5	69.2	19	31	63.2	58.1
Hallucinogens	23	23	82.6	65.2	41	25	46.3	60.0
Cocaine	26	21	46.2	33.3	17	12	70.6	58.3
Marijuana	107	85	64.5	65.9	73	62	94.5	90.3
Alcohol	141	135	93.7	91.1	143	135	93.0	91.1
Any illegal drug	110	88	66.4	68.2	78	66	93.6	90.9

[a] Based only on samples of Vietnam returnees.

after returning to the United States was high relative to discontinuance rates for other drugs. This may indicate that opiate use among servicemen in Vietnam differs in important ways from stateside use, or that factors which encourage and maintain heroin use in Southeast Asia are operative to a much lesser extent domestically.

It is also striking that relatively few of the September veterans discontinued their use of hallucinogens and amphetamines after returning to the United States. This contrasts somewhat with the December data, but appears to be consistent with partial correlation analyses (September, above), showing a relationship between prior service in Vietnam and recent use of those drugs.

COMMENT

To summarize, data from three stateside surveys provide only limited evidence that service in Southeast Asia affected subsequent drug use. Reported incidence of recent opiate use was higher for returnee than for nonreturnee servicemen on only one of three surveys. Similar differences in recent use of amphetamines and hallucinogens appeared on a single survey, but only when age and premilitary use patterns were statistically controlled. Soldiers who had not served in Vietnam tended to report more marijuana use in the presurvey month than the veteran group, but the difference was attributable to the fact that the controls were younger and more likely to have used drugs before entering the military. Further analyses revealed no systematic relationships between recent drug use and time returned from Southeast Asia.

In view of the addictive potential of the opiate drugs and the many anecdotal reports of "addicted" Vietnam returnees, the absence of a more striking correlation between Vietnam experience and later opiate use is somewhat surprising. It may be important, however, that "casualties" of Vietnam drug use were not well represented in the population from which our samples were drawn. It is difficult to estimate how many Vietnam veterans *would* have been in the survey samples had they not been: (1) previously separated from the military for problems associated with drug use, (2) AWOL, or (3) actively participating in an in-patient rehabilitation program. It should be noted, however, that drug-related separations at Fort Riley have included at least as many nonreturnees as returnees. Nevertheless, the possibility of sampling bias in the present study resulting from underrepresentation of Vietnam drug abuse "casualties" cannot be completely ruled out.

While this may have influenced the data on current opiate use, it is more difficult to apply a sampling bias argument to the failure to observe current use differences for other types of drug use which produce many fewer "casulaties." For example, over half of the returnees sampled reported at least experimental use of marijuana in Vietnam, yet there were no detectable residual effects of the Vietnam experience on subsequent use of that drug. This appears to have less to do with discontinuance of marijuana use by returning veterans (about 65% of the RVN "pot" users reported "current" use in the presurvey month) than with the fact that marijuana consumption has risen to a high level in the entire population of young servicemen.

Several other methodological problems deserve comment: First, self-report data obviously need not correlate perfectly with actual behavior. It could be, for example, that subjects in the present samples were more likely to admit past than recent drug use. Second, it must be assumed that errors or distortions of self-report were equally distributed in the veteran and nonveteran populations. Because greater attention may have been given to identifying drug users in Vietnam than at stateside installations during the years 1970 and 1971, it is possible that returnees were somewhat more apprehensive about admitting their drug use.

The self-report data suggest that opiates, despite their addictive characteristics, were among the drugs most likely to be discontinued by returning veterans. This is consistent with other reports (Zinberg, 1972; Ingraham, 1972) that Vietnam heroin use differs in important respects from stateside use. For example, Zinberg has pointed out that GI users commonly smoked or inhaled heroin in Southeast Asia and usually used the drug in a social context (i.e., in groups). Stateside addicts, by contrast, typically inject (mainline) their heroin, and usually do so alone. Opiate users in the military are also from different and more varied backgrounds, they often do not show a history of chronic drug use, and some are able to function effectively while continuing their use. This is not to mention the relative availability, quality, and lower cost of heroin and opium in Southeast Asia: Relative to the Vietnamese variety, domestic heroin is much more expensive, difficult to obtain, and heavily adulterated.

Further evidence along those lines has been discussed by Ingraham (1972), who interviewed 78 Army enlisted men identified as opiate users by urinalysis testing conducted prior to their departure from Vietnam. As a group, the opiate-positive subjects did not differ demographically from nonusing (opiate-negative) returnees, and the vast majority of users emphatically denied both the need and the desire for rehabilitation beyond initial detoxification. Ingraham suggests that understanding the Vietnam drug epidemic requires understanding of the social system (i.e., the "head" system) which supports drug use in Southeast Asia—a social system which arose in part from the unique set of frustrations associated with the fighting there. He also notes that "heads," even those habituated to heroin, did not consider themselves "addicts" or "junkies" in the usual sense of the word. In fact, they abhorred behavior patterns associated with the civilian stereotype (e.g., crime, chronic drug use, dereliction), and "heads" who exhibited these characteristics were excluded from the social system. Thus there may have been good reason for veterans to discontinue opiate use after returning home: The game must be played by different rules—and the new rules require behavior which is incompatible with the "head" self-concept.

Finally, it should be emphasized that the data presented here in no way bear on the more general question of whether United States military involvement in Southeast Asia was responsible for the general rise in societal drug abuse evidenced in recent years. It does appear, however, that the perceived public health menace embodied in the returning serviceman "addict" may in some respects have been overexaggerated. Our drug problems are probably at least as much of domestic origin as they are imported.

The views expressed in this paper are those of the authors and should not be construed as an official Department of the Army or Department of Defense position.

ACKNOWLEDGMENTS

This research was conducted in conjunction with the Drug and Alcohol Abuse Control Program, Fort Riley, Kansas, and could not have been completed without the continuing support and encouragement of Major General Edward M. Flanagan, Colonel John B. Moring, Colonel Harley F. Mooney, Lieutenant Colonel Larry R. Atkinson, Major James N. James, and Major Howard J. Frase. Thanks are also due to Captain William Roberts, who coordinated administration of the surveys, and to Specialist Five Thomas Hogan, who performed many of the statistical analyses.

REFERENCES

COLBACH, E. Marijuana use by GIs in Vietnam. *Amer. J. Psychiat.* 128: 204–207, 1971.

FISHER, A. H., NELSON, K. E., and PANZARELLA, J. Patterns of Drug Usage Among Vietnam Veterans. HumRRO Professional Paper 12–72, May 1972.

INGRAHAM, L. H. The Vietnam Epidemic: A descriptive profile of the Army returnee and his treatment in Army detection and detoxification centers. Paper presented at the Third Annual Psychology in the Air Force Symposium, USAF Academy, Colorado Springs, April 1972.

NcNEMAR, Q. *Psychological Statistics*. New York: Wiley, 1962.

NELSON, K. E., and PANZARELLA, J. Preliminary findings—Prevalence of drug use, enlisted Vietnam returnees processing for ETS separation, Oakland Overseas Processing Center. Report for Department of the Army (Department of Neuropsychiatry, Letterman General Hospital, Presidio, San Francisco), March 1971.

POSTEL, W. B. Marihuana use in Vietnam: a preliminary report. *USARV Med. Bull.* 11: 56–59, 1968.

SAPOL, E., and ROFFMAN, R. A. Marihuana in Vietnam. *Intern. J. Addictions* 5: 1–42, 1970.

STANTON, M. D. Drug use in Vietnam. *Arch. Gen. Psychiat.* 26: 279–286, 1972.

ZINBERG, N. W. Heroin use in Vietnam and the United States. *Arch. Gen. Psychiat.* 26: 486–488, 1972.

The International Journal of the Addictions, 9(1), pp. 41–55, 1974

Rehabilitation of Drug and Alcohol Abusers in the U.S. Army

Harvey L. Ruben,* M.D., M.P.H.

Yale University School of Medicine, New Haven, Connecticut

INTRODUCTION

Rehabilitation may be defined as the use of therapy and education to restore the handicapped or delinquent to a useful life, including former rank, privileges, or rights (Baker, 1971). The United States Army Alcohol and Drug Abuse Prevention and Control Program has been discussed in a number of papers (Ruben, 1972; Baker, 1971, 1972). Rehabilitation is an essential aspect of that program. Although rehabilitation can be defined as above, it is a difficult concept with which to deal operationally. One way to grasp rehabilitation is to determine when it has been successfully accomplished. The United States Army Program guidelines define successful rehabilitation as having been accomplished when the drug or alcohol abusing soldier has been assigned to his unit for 60 days or more during rehabilitation and is functioning effectively at full duty at the end of that period (DA Circular 600–85, 1972). In addition, the drug abuser must have had 8 consecutive weeks of negative urine tests, and the al-

* Formarly Psychiatry Consultant, Alcohol and Drug Policies Office, Office of The Surgeon General, Department of the Army, Washington, D.C., 20314. Present address: Assessment and Acute Treatment Service, Connecticut Mental Health Center, New Haven, Connecticut 06519.

coholic must apparently be free from any significant problem with alcohol during the period of rehabilitation. Such a definition of success is ultimately somewhat arbitrary. The drug or alcohol abuser may suffer setbacks during the course of his rehabilitation which do not detract from its overall success. Moreover, the program guidelines do stipulate that the assessment of success or failure is a command decision, based on consideration of all aspects of the individual's functioning, in conjunction with advice of concerned rehabilitation team members.

Defining rehabilitation and outlining criteria for success allow one to recognize it once it has occurred. This does not elucidate how to go about the process of rehabilitation, however. That question caused great difficulty for both the framers of the army program and for the professionals and para-professionals who joined the treatment teams. One of the basic conceptual difficulties was to determine the scope and extent of rehabilitation which would be offered by the army program. According to the public health model, rehabilitation is tertiary prevention: the identification and treatment of chronic cases of a disease in order to limit its effects and to decrease its incidence and prevalence. The army program is aimed mainly at primary and secondary prevention: the identification of causative agents and the treatment of early cases. (Military medicine is generally involved in primary and secondary prevention, while the Veterans Administration has its mission in areas of tertiary prevention.)

Thus an initial decision confronting the army was to what extent to be involved in long-term rehabilitation of the chronic drug or alcohol abuser. One argument was that the mission of the army is not rehabilitation, that the army can identify and offer initial treatment, but then must refer to the Veterans Administration after appropriately separating the individual from the service. The counter-argument noted President Nixon's mandate to the military in June 1971 that drug and alcohol abusers be treated and rehabilitated as adequately as possible in the army prior to discharge. An apparent compromise was established, whereby from 30 to 60 days of rehabilitative efforts were extended to all drug abusers to determine whether further rehabilitative efforts were warranted in that particular case. It was believed that during this period, those motivated to change would evidence some success within the rehabilitation process. These soldiers would be continued in a long-term rehabilitation program integrated with their military duties. Those who showed an inability to respond to the military program would be referred to the Veterans Administration for rehabilitation in a civilian setting and separated from the army with an honorable discharge.

After solving the problems of the definition and the length of successful rehabilitation, the army was still confronted with deciding who should attempt to rehabilitate the drug and alcohol abuser and how to go about it. The decision was made to establish alcohol and drug abuse prevention and control teams to undertake rehabilitative efforts with command direction. The team would consist of military and civilian personnel in accordance with local requirements. Included in the team were military spaces for a physician (a psychiatrist if one was available), a chaplain, and two enlisted para-professionals. Also, the team was authorized civilian members to include a social worker, a psychologist, and eight para-professional drug and alcohol counsellors with appropriate aptitude, training, or experience. Clerical support brought the authorized number of team members to 15 (Table 1). Given this staffing mission, local commanders started hiring necessary civilian personnel (Table 2). However, few of the military or the civilian team members had much experience with drug or alcohol rehabilitation. Consequently, an immediate worldwide training effort was begun.

At the time of President Nixon's original mandate to the military, he also appointed Dr. Jerome Jaffee to head a Special Action Office for Drug Abuse Prevention to deal with this problem in the civilian community. At Dr. Jaffee's direction, the National Institutes of Mental Health established a number of drug and alcohol abuse training courses at various medical schools throughout the United States. These courses

Table 1
Drug and Alcohol Counseling Team Organization
(Composition of the 81 teams deployed around the world)

Position	Number	Status
Psychiatrists	1	Military
Psychologists	1	Civilian
Social workers	2	Civilian
Social work technicians (counsellors)	4	Civilian
Psychology technicians (counsellors)	2	Civilian
Psychiatric technicians (counsellors)	3	Military
Chaplain	1	Military
Chaplain's assistant	1	Military
TOTAL	15	6 Military, 9 Civilian × 81 = 1215 worldwide

Table 2
Criteria for Civilian Drug and Alcohol Counseling Team Members

Position	GS Rating	Education	Experience
Psychologist	11–12	Doctoral degree	PHD-GS-11 + 1 year experience-GS-12
Social worker	9–11	Master's degree	GS rating proportionate to experience in the field
Social work technician (counsellor including ex-addict)	5–7	High school diploma Bachelor's degree	GS rating proportionate to experience in the field
Psychology technician (counsellor, including ex-addict)	5–7	High school diploma Bachelor's degree	GS rating proportionate to experience in the field

were available to personnel from both civilian and military programs who were involved in this nationwide effort. At approximately the same time, the National Institute of Alcoholism and Alcohol Abuse (NIAAA) was established under Dr. Maurice Chafitz. The NIAAA was established specifically to combat the alcohol problem throughout the United States. It, too, arranged for courses in alcoholism counseling to be established at various medical centers throughout the country. The army program started using these governmentally sponsored training programs to train the rehabilitation teams in appropriate methods of functioning. At the same time, the army developed training programs of its own, utilizing consultation from the civilian training programs.

By the end of the first year of operation, it became evident that while the teams were essentially well trained in medical principles of treatment and rehabilitation, they needed greater sensitivity to problems of human adjustment, interaction, and relations. Consequently, the Surgeon General of the Army contracted with the Institute for Applied Behavioral Sciences of the National Training Laboratories to offer a basic human interactions laboratory and sensitivity training to 100 of the team members from around the world. Of these 100, 30 were chosen for additional advanced training in human relations, so that they would be qualified to train other team members in these techniques.

The problem of how the rehabilitation teams should function was the most difficult. The training in the civilian and the in-house courses was initially aimed at educating the team members to the psychological and pharmacological properties of drug and alcohol abuse. In addition, an attempt was made to sensitize them to some of the social precursors which lead to such abuse, to help them bridge the attitudinal gap traditionally existing between rehabilitation personnel and drug and alcohol abusers.

The problem of what to do was still confronting the army. In one recent book on drug abuse rehabilitation, the two authors discussed some eight different approaches which can be used in the rehabilitation of drug abusers (Brill and Lieberman, 1969). These include the punitive approach, the medical-psychiatric approach, the communal approach, the community-based approach, the religious approach, the chemotherapy approach (with cyclazocine or methadone maintenance), and the rational authority approach. Although many different rehabilitation techniques had been developed, none had proved so efficacious that it was clearly the modality of choice. Considering approaches to alcoholism rehabilitation, there was a narrower field of choice. The two approaches with which the civilian community had had the most success were originally Alcoholics Anonymous, and more recently aversive conditioning programs. Having become familiar with these various approaches, the military teams were in a position to choose those elements and principles of rehabilitation which were most applicable for military purposes.

THE ARMY MODEL

A review of some of the directions outlined in the Army Guidelines is useful at this point (DA Circular 600–85, 1972). The goal of rehabilitation as stated in the directive is to return the soldier to full, effective duty with short-term rehabilitative efforts or to provide continuity of care if he is to be separated from the military. For rehabilitation to succeed, the soldier must find a constructive way of life more attractive than drug abuse. The army's commitment to short-term rehabilitation puts pressure on the soldier to face the implications of his drug abuse. The guidelines direct that each program develop a modality most effective for its particular locale. The time frame during which rehabilitation must be carried out is a minimum of 30 days to a maximum of 60 days of inpatient and halfway house rehabilitation. The guidelines do stress that while alcohol and drug abuse have medical and psychological elements, they are primarily social problems. Thus army rehabilitation efforts are centered in the unit, rather than in the hospital or the stockade, to enable the soldier to cope with the realities of his military environment. Following inpatient medical detoxification as necessary, the individual is managed in the halfway house or rap center setting by the rehabilitation team. In this status, although the individual is involved in a medical program, he is not considered an inpatient nor is he carried on hospital rolls.

The rehabilitation program is the responsibility of the post commander. The rehabilitation team functions in the halfway house and the rap center as directed by the commander in order to provide group therapy, individual counseling, or other appropriate therapeutic interventions. Additionally, they work closely with the soldier's unit and advise his commanders in order to ease his return to full duty. It is hoped that by involving the individual's commander in the rehabilitation process, the transition to duty will be facilitated. If a soldier is clinically determined to be a drug abuser, he is given a temporary medical profile which signifies that he has known emotional and attitudinal problems which may compromise his judgment or reliability. When he is considered a success as defined above, his profile may be revised to indicate that he has no emotional difficulties and is medically qualified for full duty. This status will not preclude his further participation in the rehabilitation program.

Following detoxification if needed, the army model stresses early reintegration into the unit for both alcohol and drug abusers. Thus, whenever possible, thc soldier should maintain contact with his unit throughout the rehabilitation process. If he is to be assigned to a new unit, he should be contacted by a representative of his new unit while he is still in the detoxification phase. Upon completion of detoxification, rehabilitation may be carried out directly in the unit or during a transitional period at the halfway house. These individuals are, in most cases, drug abusers who have been identified by urinalysis screening or by voluntary self-referral. While many of these soldiers require inpatient detoxification, there are a number whose drug problems are so minimal that they may not require detoxification. If they do, they can be assigned immediately following detoxification to their new unit or returned to their previous unit without the need of a transitional period in the halfway house. In such cases the guidelines direct that the individual be involved in follow-up outpatient rehabilitation to ensure that adequate restoration to full duty can be accomplished within 2 to 4 weeks. The drug abuser must be maintained under biochemical survellance during this phase of his rehabilitation.

Some individuals need a more structured environment following detoxification and thus will benefit from living in the halfway house. Since the soldier is attempting to return to duty, the atmosphere of the halfway house should be appropriately military. Some soldiers will require the maximal structure of living-in full time for a short period (usually

Table 3
Rehabilitation Modalities

Psychological techniques	Psychotherapy	Individual therapy Couple and family therapy Group therapy Psychodrama
	Behavior modification	Contingency programs Aversive conditioning programs
	Modified therapeutic community	Confrontation groups Counsellors, ex-addicts
Medical techniques	Drug antagonists	Antabuse, used frequently Cyclazozine, used rarely
	Stabilizing medication	Tranquilizers, used frequently Methadone, used rarely
Religious techniques	Pastoral counseling "Jesus people" and other evangelical youth groups	
Self-help techniques	Alcoholics Anonymous	Alanon Alateen
	Transcendental meditation	

not more than 2 weeks). Others are able to immediately begin working with their duty units during the day, although they live at the halfway house when off duty. The halfway house allows a more gradual reintegration. It gives the soldier closer supervision and a more structured environment in which to begin rehabilitation.

The guidelines review a number of rehabilitation modalities which can be adequately utilized within the halfway house (Table 3). These include various forms of psychotherapy such as individual, couple, or group therapy, behavioral modification techniques utilizing principles of aversive conditioning, and therapeutic community techniques based on highly structured live-in treatment programs where intense interpersonal confrontations are established in a supportive setting. Many civilian therapeutic communities maintain the rehabilatee in a live-in setting for many months to years to insure success. While this has proven effective, such extended treatment is not appropriate for use within the active duty army environment.

Other modalities such as pastoral counseling or involvement with "Jesus people" are based on appeal to religious beliefs. "Jesus people" is an informal name for youth groups which testify that a personal religious conversion has revitalized them and turned them on to God and off alcohol and drugs. Such groups are replete with teenage missionaries who are idealistic and frequently persuasive to a significant proportion of the younger soldiers. Adjunctive medical therapy includes the use of antagonists such as disulfram. In addition, psychotropic agents (transquilizers) are used to make the stresses of the military environment more tolerable during the rehabilitation period. Methadone maintenance is generally believed unsuitable in the military setting, since the need for constant maintenance on the drug is incompatible with the realities of military life which may require sudden moves or long absences in the field, disrupting the program. In addition, the efficacy of methadone maintenance has yet to be entirely substantiated within the civilian programs which utilize it.

Alcoholics Anonymous (AA) is the self-help method which has proven most sucessful of all modalities for dealing with the rehabilitation of alcoholics. Alcoholics Anonymous is a fellowship of men and women who share their experience, strength, and hope in order to solve their common problems and help others recover from alcoholism. The only requirement for membership is an explicit desire to stop drinking. Alcoholics Anonymous groups are now found at almost all army installations. In addition to dealing with the alcoholic himself, AA offers support to family members through affiliated organizations such as Alanon and Alateen groups.

Another self-help method mentioned in the army guidelines is transcendental meditation, a technique derived from Indian philosophies, aimed at improving an individual's mental state by tapping levels of mental energy ordinarily unavailable. Although this approach is yet to be fully understood, a number of abusers assert that the urge to drink alcohol or take drugs subsides with achieving this "natural high."

Finally, the role of the chaplain is central to an adequate rehabilitative effort. Individuals involved in drug and alcohol abuse frequently are searching for lasting values and patterns of meaning which they can accept. The chaplain may be able to provide significant and practical help with that search, often succeeding where other attempts at rehabilitation fail. Since many abusers ultimately turn to religion, it is appropriate for the chaplain to be available to the rehabilitation teams. In addition, there are many times when troubled people will turn to their minister before turning to a health professional. It is also appropriate that the chaplain work closely with local AA groups, which also stress religious aspects of rehabilitation. Having contracts with various schools, churches, and religious groups, the chaplain can make significant contributions to the educational aspects of the preventive effort.

EVALUATION EFFORTS

In order to evaluate the efficacy of the program, the guidelines directed that a two-pronged evaluation effort be mounted both by command elements and representatives of the Surgeon General. The command and the medical evaluation and assistance teams visited every program on a regular basis, at least once a year. In addition, to further aid in evaluation, various reporting procedures were set up to gather data about the numbers and types of participants in the programs and their degree of success or failure. Individual definitions of successful program participation have been delineated above. Criteria for total program success or failure were also devised. During site visits, teams of behavioral scientists rated each program in relation to a list of 20 variables which were believed to comprise a successful program. In that fashion an overall evaluation of the program's efficacy could be derived. These variables included such items as operations of the detoxification unit, record keeping, confidentiality, command support, cooperation between the alcohol and drug programs, staff initiative, educational programs, patient follow-up, urinalysis monitoring, relationship with law inforcement personnel, percentage of civilians hired, and referral to civilian and VA programs. After the first year's operation, most of the programs were found to be functioning adequately with only a few being either outstanding or substandard. Based on this evaluation, various program adjustments were made to enhance the functioning of the program.

EXISTING DRUG PROGRAMS

Notwithstanding the rehabilitation guidelines reviewed above, the experience of our counseling teams in the last year and a half has been exceedingly variable. Some were able to create effective rehabilitation programs almost immediately and have continued their success. In almost all instances these programs were most rigorously supported by local command elements and given carte blanche to develop as they saw fit. In other instances the rehabilitation teams met with more resistance

Table 4
Drug and Alcohol Programs as of January 1, 1973
(with a breakdown of modalities used)

Place	Number	Modalities used in the 56 programs
Continental United States	36	1. All programs include drug abuse and alcoholism services
Europe	10	2. All programs include various types of individual and group psychotherapies, rap centers, pastoral counseling, Alcoholics Anonymous groups, antabuse and tranquilizers therapy.
Alaska	2	3. Residential halfway houses, 31
Thailand	2	4. Behavior modification techniques, 3
Korea	2	5. Jesus people groups, 7
Hawaii	2	6. Transendental meditation, 5
Canal Zone	2	
TOTAL	56	

on the part of local commanders and found it difficult to develop adequate programs. Table 4 gives a breakdown of the number and type of programs at army installations around the world.

From their inception the teams had to deal with thc attitudinal differences of the drug abusers and the team member. Some programs assumed a nonmilitary attitude, having the team members dressed in civilian clothes, growing beards, and wearing beads. These programs have invariably proven less successful than programs in which appropriate military demeanor was maintained. By assuming this overly permissive stance, the rehabilitation team was rarely able to assist the soldier to return successfully to his unit.

Certain programs initially attempted to utilize some form of methadone maintenance, but this was invariably found ineffectual because the drug abuser continued to abuse methadone as he had the opiates.

Other programs attempted to rely most heavily on individual counseling and psychotherapy which, as in the civilian community, did not prove to be exceedingly effective. The army programs with the most success combined a modified therapeutic community approach with the psychological counseling model and coordinated this with an active liaison to the man's commander. These programs offered the best of available modalities, while reintegrating the man into his actual military frame of reference. One innovative program, authorized on an experimental basis, established an on-going consultative relationship with a well-established civilian therapeutic community. Ex-addict counsellors from the civilian program came to work in the military program, while civilian professional consultants helped to adapt this therapeutic community setting to the military halfway house environment. This therapeutic community was voluntary and required members to be highly motivated to participate. (The rehabilitation team also offered other forms of individual and group psychotherapy for patients not motivated to participate in the therapeutic community). Participants in the community lived in the halfway house for 2 months, during which time they formed a work unit with specific duties on the post as directed by the post commander. Active liaison was maintained with a man's unit of origin. Following this 2-month period, the man returned to his unit but maintained continued out-patient rehabilitation contact with the rehabilitation team. The program also established a rap center, manned by ex-addicts and program participants, to provide information on drug abuse and to recruit potential members.

EXISTING ALCOHOL ABUSE PROGRAMS

In the military the attempt to rehabilitate alcoholics has proven equally or more difficult than to rehabilitate chronic drug abusers. This is related to several factors. Military and civilian communities have attempted a broader range of efforts and prototypes for handling drug abuse problems and amassed more varied experience in this area. Moreover, the alcohol-abusing individual in the military is frequently of senior enlisted or officer rank, with considerable time in and commitment to the service. As a result, it has been more difficult for command to confront and deal with the alcoholic. The archetypal drug abuser is usually anti-establishment, an admirer of the counterculture, and openly attempting to subvert the system. It is much easier for command to confront and challenge this behavior. Thus, whereas the drug abuse program has been functioning vigorously since the summer of 1971, the alcohol abuse program, born simultaneously and located at the same installations as the drug abuse programs, has really only gained momentum within the last year at most installations (Table 4).

The programs which have envolved have drawn heavily on civilian experience, especially the AA approach discussed above. General medical experience in the United States has been that the individual psychotherapeutic approach to alcoholism has proven far less effective than the group and supportive self-help approaches favored by AA. Halfway house facilities for alcoholics have generally been separate from the drug abuse halfway houses, due to the seeming incompatability of the two populations. The same principles of command involvement have been stressed in these programs as in the drug abuse programs. Here, in particular, education of commanders to the early signs of problem drinking has proved useful in effecting early referrals. When the alcholic is surfaced early, treatment can be instituted before physical or psychosocial problems have become irreversible. Utilization of civilian training programs by para-professional rehabilitation team members has allowed many of them to be certified as alcoholism counsellors by the National Institutes of Mental Health. Disulfram is used regularly by most military programs to provide assurance to the alcoholic that he will not be able to drink and subvert his rehabilitative efforts should he have the urge to do so.

Several other innovative approaches have been used by alcohol abuse programs. One has been to help the post commander establish an anti-alcohol abuse educational program. He may take care not to foster alcohol abuse through cut-rate liquor prices at the officers' clubs. Another approach has been to coordinate efforts with local military police units who refer all offenders for driving while intoxicated to the alcoholism program for mandatory treatment. Currently, a nationwide program is being established by the Army Military Police Corps in conjunction with the Alcohol Safety Action Program of the Department of Transportation, whereby military members who are stopped by civilian authorities and found to be driving under the influence of alcohol are referred to the nearest military alcoholism program for mandatory treatment. Finally, currently underway is the institution of aversive conditioning programs at two major military hospitals to utilize techniques developed by several civilian alcoholism treatment centers. This approach will be utilized for recalcitrant cases and for those individuals whose job sensitivity and security clearance make rehabilitation at the local setting difficult.

CONCLUSION

Alcohol and drug abuse rehabilitation is underway in the United States Army, and success is being realized. It has been a hard-fought battle, and there are many objectives yet to be obtained. The army has been forced to innovate and improvise and to repeat the same mistakes at many different locations because the limited scope of knowledge and expertise available precluded the clear preference for certain types of programs. Much has been learned which is believed to be mandatory for the successful implementation of a program.

Perhaps the primary lesson learned is that the program cannot function adequately and successfully without full command support and direction. Where command lacks responsibility, it continues to view drug and alcohol problems as medical concerns and tries literally to discharge the problem rather than to deal with it. Another essential lesson is that education of all involved parties is of the utmost importance. This education must include factual information about pharmacology and psychosocial consequences for the potential abuser, as well as for the commander. The commander must be educated to view drug and alcohol abuse problems as symptoms of underlying social unrest, rather than merely as character defects, or forms of illegal, sociopathic "acting-out." In line with this education, command must be made aware that social precursors of drug abuse include such entities as racial problems, demoralization (based on low self-esteem and self-worth), job dissatisfaction, dissent (based on perceiving an arbitrary, inhumane authority structure), and discipline problems. Through educating command to these social precursors, effective preventive and remedial actions can be devised and instituted.

Along with command involvement and educational efforts, the army experience has shown the effectiveness of a combination of the modified therapeutic community (in a halfway house setting) with psychological counseling and with continual contact with the military environment to which man must return. For the more casual abusers, the rap center model has proven an effective bridge between the abuser and the rehabilitation team.

Considering the actual nature of the interventions being suggested, the underlying assumption is that the rehabilitation team functions as a facilitator between the alienated, disenfranchised members of the military community and the command structure. This point holds the key to an effective alcohol and drug abuse program. The abusing individual is "acting-out" his underlying emotional difficulties. It is easier within the military than the civilian structure to identify those disturbing factors which form the substrate for the symptom's development. Thus, in the military especially, the approach to rehabilitation must lie in establishing quality channels of communication between command and cadre and thereby dispelling the need for such dysfunctional expressions of individual malcontent.

In the last year and a half, much attention has been given to the Army Alcohol and Drug Abuse Program by the various news media. Many of the comments have been favorable, others have been unfavorable. Likewise, members of Congress have at times criticized various aspects of the Army Program, sometimes justifiably, other times unfairly. There are obviously going to be major problems in the development and implementation of any health program of such massive proportions within a bureaucratic setting (Ruben, 1973). Considering the sensitive nature of a program dealing with drug and alcohol abuse, where such issues as confidentiality, relation to the rest of the military community, and command support are of such importance, the experience of the army in setting up this program has been surprisingly good.

The unjustified comments have frequently been based on an inadequate perception of the intent and scope of the program, perhaps due to poor public relations on the part of the army. The warranted criticisms have helped the army to enhance the effectiveness of the program. Especially in the areas of confidentiality and adequacy of urinalysis testing, the impetus for needed reform came from pressures by the media and Congress. The fact that the worldwide positive rate for urinalysis screening had dropped from 4 to 5% in 1971 to 1 to 2% by the end of 1972, and the fact that far fewer soldiers were turning themselves in for drug abuse treatment while an increasing number was seeking help for problems with alcohol during the same period, support the overall success of the army program. Even though the program has been successful, much room for improvement still exists, and program revision and redevelopment continues. The drug and alcohol problem in the military community is not totally analogous to that existing in the civilian community, but enough parallels exist that civilian programs should be able to gain some benefit from a careful review of the experience gained in the military.

SUMMARY

Since the inception of the United States Army Alcohol and Drug Abuse Prevention and Control Program in July 1971, the army has been intensively involved in developing rehabilitation programs for alcohol and drugs abusers. The author first reviews the guidelines developed by the army for the establishment of such rehabilitation efforts, and methods for program evaluation. He then discusses the various types of programs which have actually developed and comments on which have proved most workable. He concludes that civilian programs can gain some insights by reviewing the army's experience, for in spite of various difficulties, the programs on the whole have been successful.

REFERENCES

BAKER, S. L. Rehabilitation. Presented at the Army Worldwide Drug Abuse Conference, Ft. McNair, Washington, D.C., September 1971.

BAKER, S. L., The U.S. Army heroin abuse identification program in Vietnam: implications for methadone program. *Amer. J. Public. Health* 62: 857–860, 1972.

BRILL, L., and LIEBERMAN, L. *Authority and Addiction.* Boston: Little, Brown, 1969.

DEPARTMENT Of ARMY. Circular 600–85. Alcohol and drug abuse prevention program, June 1972.

RUBEN, H. L., The United States Army alcohol and drug abuse prevention and control program: one year later. Presented at the Mexican Army Medical Conference, Mexico City, November 1972.

RUBEN, H. L. Military psychiatry: a paradigm of a complete third party system. Presented at American Psychiatric Association Annual Meeting, Honolulu, Hawaii, May 1973.

The International Journal of the Addictions, 9(1), pp. 57–80, 1974

Values, Expectations, and Drug Use Among High School Students in a Rural Community

Roderick S. Carman, Ph.D.

Department of Psychology
University of Wyoming
Laramie, Wyoming

Abstract

Rotter's Social Learning Theory of Personality was used to investigate relationships among values for certain goals, expectations for achieving these goals, and self-reported drug use among high school students. It was hypothesized that students with low "freedom of movement" in important goal areas (low expectations and high values) would report (1) heavier drug usage, (2) more frequent periods of intoxication, and (3) more drug-related social complications. Support for the hypothesis was found. Low freedom of movement in the goal area of recognition-achievement did correlate with drug use in the predicted fashion, especially in the case of barbiturate and hallucinogen use.

In a previous report, evidence suggesting a relationship between personal values and drug use among high school students was presented (Carman, 1973). Questionnaire data collected from 327 high school students in a rural community revealed a slight but statistically significant trend for drug use to be associated with higher values placed on independence and autonomy. At the same time, a slight negative correlation was found between drug use and higher values placed on giving and receiving affection from peers and the achievement of close, intimate interpersonal relationships. Although it was tentatively concluded that such differences in personal values might be important in an adolescent's decision to engage in some form of drug use, the data did not bear directly on the question of development of particular *forms* of drug use. In order to explore this question, and in particular the possiblity that some forms of drug use might be related to failures in satisfying important needs or in achieving important goals, additional data were analyzed and this hypothesis tested.

Seeman (1959) has described a state of personal alienation and sense of powerlessness which may be important in the development of more pernicious forms of drug use. When, through a series of failure experiences, a person learns that highly valued goals are inaccessible and that his own behavior is not effective in determining the occurrence of rewards, one might expect a resultant fading of constructive efforts toward reaching important goals and the building of pressures toward the escape and tension reduction provided by heavy and frequent use of drugs. Unlike much drug use which is perhaps engaged in primarily for purposes of social conviviality or to provide a pleasant but not essential adjunct to social interactions, this more problem-oriented use might be expected to be characterized by higher frequency of usage, the use of harder drugs, and a higher rate of social complications resulting from the use of drugs. In addition to legal sanctions and social disapproval from the larger community, this form of drug use might well elicit negative reactions from other persons within a drug subculture where more moderate use is tolerated. Thus fruitful insights concerning the etiology of different forms of drug use might flow from making a distinction between drug use which develops in the service of ameliorating frustration and that use which is more social or convivial in nature.

THEORETICAL RATIONALE

In order to operationalize and examine the concepts of personal alienation and powerlessness and their possible relationship to the more destructive forms of drug use, a social learning theory of personality espoused by Rotter (1954) was employed in the present study. According to Rotter, low "freedom of movement," referring to the unavailability of positive satisfactions and low generalized expectations for success, would imply the presence of frustration and a pressure toward "irreal" or avoidant behavior. Such avoidant behavior would constitute a problem-solving mechanism and would offer the possibility of relief from unpleasant feelings associated with failure and frustration. At the same time, such avoidant tactics typically prove ultimately maladaptive because of additional problems generated by destructive and injurious outcomes. As with neurotic symptoms, drinking problems, and a host of other psychological and behavioral pathologies, problem-oriented drug use would be defined by Rotter as irreal or avoidant in nature, and would, therefore, be expected to be associated with low freedom of movement according to his theory.

Previous investigations of alcohol use among college students and military servicemen have supported a similar hypothesis, particularly in regard to problem drinking and low freedom of movement in the areas of academic achievement and job performance (Jessor, Carman, and Grossman, 1968; Carman, 1971).

HYPOTHESIS

It was specifically hypothesized that among drug-using high school students in a rural community, those who manifest low freedom of movement as characterized by low expectations for achieving valued goals would be more likely to report: (1) heavier drug usage, (2) more frequent periods of intoxication, and (3) greater social complications from drug use.

METHOD

As previously reported (Carman, 1973), subjects studied were 327 students in Grades 9 through 12 who attend a public school serving approximately 739 students in a rural community of about 12,000.

Questionnaires were administered to the students during their study hall periods.* First, the students were asked to list 10 goals they would like to accomplish or have happen to them in the foreseeable future. Next, scales were provided for each goal they had listed so that numerical

* See sample of questionnaries pages 64–79.

values could be assigned. Numerical values ranging from 0 to 100 were placed on the scales so that for each goal listed, a student could indicate a quantified estimate of the value he placed on that goal. An example is:

```
0                                                                100
!     !     !     !     !     !     !     !     !     !     !
_____________________________________________________________________
NEITHER LIKE              LIKE                          LIKE VERY
NOR DISLIKE                                             MUCH
```

Subjects were then asked to rate each goal in terms of how strongly they expected these goals to be realized. Again, a rating scale was provided and a check mark requested to show the subjective probability each student attached to the achievement of goals previously mentioned. An example is:

```
0                                                                100
!     !     !     !     !     !     !     !     !     !     !
_____________________________________________________________________
SURE IT WILL               EVEN CHANCE                  SURE IT
NOT HAPPEN                 "FIFTY-FIFTY"                WILL HAPPEN
```

Each goal item was scored in terms of *value* ratings and *expectation* ratings assigned by the subject from 0 to 100. Then, in cases where stated values exceeded expectations for a given goal, a numerical difference score was calculated. These difference or *disjunction* scores were then summed and averaged for each goal area to provide an index of freedom of movement. A high disjunction score signified low freedom of movement. Although all subjects were encouraged to list 10 goals, some gave a fewer number so that the average number of goals listed by all subjects was 8.7.

Finally, a drug-use questionnaire was administered which asked what drugs the students have used or use now; how often and how much they use marijuana; amphetamines (speed), hallucinogens (LSD, mescaline), barbiturates; how many times they have gotten "high" during the past year; and how often they have experienced trouble with family, friends, or authorities because of drugs.

Drug-use items were scored simply by assigning numerical values to responses in such a way that numerical scores increased with quantity and frequency of drug use, number of times "high" in the past year, and number of social complications reported. Product-moment correlations were then calculated between freedom of movement measures (average disjunctions for each goal area) and drug-use scores. As in previous studies which have used similar methods, internal consistency, expected theoretical relationships, and a low incidence of incomplete or obviously distorted responses tended to lend support for the validity of the questionnaire data (Hager, Vener, and Stewart, 1971; Clark and Tifft, 1966; Carman, 1968). Cases where important data were missing were dropped from the sample.

RESULTS AND DISCUSSION

Goals having to do with needs for recognition and achievement were most frequently mentioned (34% of toal) and were given the highest values. Next in order of frequency were goals related to peer affection and social relationships (15%), general experiential needs such as finding happiness (14%), desires for environmental and ecological improvement (10%), material possessions (9%), and independence (4%). For a more complete description of these values and their relationship to drug use in general, see Carman (1973).

With the exception of recognition-achievement goals, very high correlations were found between stated values and expectations (*r*'s between .83 and .87). That is, when students placed high values on certain goals, they also reported high expectations for achieving those goals. Similarly, when low values were reported, low expectations were also given. This suggests that for most of the goals listed, value-expectations disjunctions or low freedom of movement tended to be infrequent or nonexistent.

However, in the case of goals for recognition-achievement, values and expectations correlated less strongly ($r = .55$). Perhaps when such achievements as getting a good job, doing well in school, succeeding in sports, and developing demonstrable skills are considered, success or failure becomes more objective and obvious, and expectations more realistic. In any case, there did seem to be substantially greater liklihood for low freedom of movement to be present when goals of this type were considered. Therefore, it was decided to test the hypothesis concerning the relationship between low freedom of movement and problem-oriented drug use in terms of value-expectation disjunctions in the area of recognition-achievement.

Correlations which provide a test of the hypothesis are presented in Table 1. The number cases for each correlation varies since only cases involving reported use of each drug were considered. Also, a few cases were omitted because of missing data.

It appears that low freedom of movement in the area of recognition-achievement, as indicated by value-expectation disjunctions, is related

Table 1
Correlations between Average Value-Expection Disjunctions for Achievement and Drug Use

Drug use measure	r	N
Quantity-frequency of marijuana use	.28**	113
Quantity-frequency of hallucinogen use	.35**	67
Quantity-frequency of amphetamines use	.08	62
Quantity-frequency of barbiturate use	.41**	44
Times "high" during past year	.21*	119
Social complications related to drug use	.20*	119

* $p < .05$; ** $p < .01$; two-tail tests.

to problem-oriented drug use in a fashion consistent with the hypothesis. All correlations were in the predicted direction, and all but one were statistically significant.

Although marijuana was the most frequently used drug, the strongest relationships with freedom of movement were found in the case of hallucinogen use ($r = .35$) and barbiturate use ($r = .41$) Amphetamine use was not significantly related to freedom of movement, however. Thus the choice of a particular drug might be based on the purpose of its use, and it may be that definitions of drug use establish normative "prescriptions" regarding the various drugs. For assuaging frustration resulting from failure to achieve recognition goals, barbiturates and hallucinogens seem to be the popular choice among the students studied. A previous study of drinking among college students (Carman, 1965) revealed similar preferences for particular beverages dependent on the nature of drinking motivations present. Clearly, additional work is needed to determine the presence and nature of such discriminations.

Although much of the variance in reported drug use was not accounted for in the present study, evidence was found for a relationship between low freedom of movement in the area of recognition-achievement and a form of drug use which might be considered problem-oriented. *No* significant differences in freedom of movement were found between drug users and nondrug users in general, and freedom of movement did not seem to be an important factor in drug use except in regard to recognition and achievement goals. Thus freedom of movement as measured in this study seems to be primarily related to differences *among* drug users in terms of drugs used, amount of use, and nature of outcomes.

One might speculate then that adolescents who tend to value and seek greater independence and autonomy are also more inclined to experiment to some extent with drugs and subject themselves to some of the risks which attend an activity which is illegal and for the most part socially disapproved. In addition, the data seem to suggest that these rather more independent-minded young people see themselves in general as able to achieve the sort of freedom from interference that they prize. Given, however, a repertoire of drug using behavior which might have arisen largely in the context of strivings for independence *and* given the presence of significant failures in achievement and recognition in competition with peers, then one might expect a shift in the form of drug use toward that which has been previously described as problem-oriented. Should further study confirm such speculation, implications for counseling and treatment programs should be forthcoming. In the meantime, it would seem desirable to consider certain forms of drug use in the context of personal attitudes toward the accessibility of particular goals, and the objective opportunities available for satisfying important needs.

PERSONAL VALUES QUESTIONNAIRE

We're interested in learning something about the kinds of things people like or consider important. List below the ten things you would like to accomplish or have happen to you in the foreseeable future. We are sincerely interested in your goals and desires. We want to know how you really feel about your future. Try to be realistic and at the same time describe what you really want for yourself.

1. ______________________________

____

2. ______________________________

____

3. ______________________________

____

4. ______________________________

____

5. ______________________________

____

6. ______________________________

____

7. ______________________________

____

8. ______________________________

____

9. ______________________________

____

10. ______________________________

____

What we want to know is how strongly you like or want the things you listed before. How strongly you like something can be shown by putting a check mark somewhere along a line that runs from NEITHER LIKE NOR DISLIKE, at one end, to LIKE VERY MUCH, at the other end.

```
0                                                  100
!    !    !     !     !    !     !    !    !    !    !
------------------------------------------------------
NEITHER LIKE           LIKE                 LIKE VERY
NOR DISLIKE                                 MUCH
```

When you like something very much, you can show this by making a check ( ) in one of the spaces toward the end that says LIKE VERY MUCH. If you don't care about something, one way or the other, you can show that by marking a check in one of the spaces toward the other end. If you feel somewhere in between about something, put your check somewhere toward the middle of the line. Your check can be in any of the spaces along the line, depending on how you really feel.

Let's take an example:

How strongly do I like:

To have other people ask me to help organize a new club?

```
0                                                  100
!    !    !     !     !    !     !    !    !    !    !
------------------------------------------------------
NEITHER LIKE           LIKE                 LIKE VERY
NOR DISLIKE                                 MUCH
```

If you think about this for a minute, you can see that some persons would like this very much; some persons wouldn't care one way or the other, and some persons would be in between. Think about the way you feel. Now put your check mark in one of the spaces along the line that best shows how strongly you like this.

On this questionnaire we're not asking about what actually does happen to you, or what you expect to happen. We want to know how much you would like these different things to happen.

Each question should be answered by itself. Don't worry about how you have answered the others.

REMEMBER!

There are no right or wrong answers. Fill in each blank with the things you mentioned on Page 1. Place a check on the corresponding graph to show how strongly you really like each thing.

1. How strongly do I like:

____

0 ... 100

! ! ! ! ! ! ! ! ! ! !

NEITHER LIKE NOR DISLIKE — LIKE — LIKE VERY MUCH

2. How strongly do I like:

____

0 ... 100

! ! ! ! ! ! ! ! ! ! !

NEITHER LIKE NOR DISLIKE — LIKE — LIKE VERY MUCH

3. How strongly do I like:

____

0 ... 100

! ! ! ! ! ! ! ! ! ! !

NEITHER LIKE NOR DISLIKE — LIKE — LIKE VERY MUCH

4. How strongly do I like:

____

0 ... 100

! ! ! ! ! ! ! ! ! ! !

NEITHER LIKE NOR DISLIKE — LIKE — LIKE VERY MUCH

5. How strongly do I like:

____

0 ... 100

! ! ! ! ! ! ! ! ! ! !

NEITHER LIKE NOR DISLIKE — LIKE — LIKE VERY MUCH

6. How strongly do I like:

____

0 100

! ! ! ! ! ! ! ! ! ! !

NEITHER LIKE NOR DISLIKE — LIKE — LIKE VERY MUCH

7. How strongly do I like:

____

0 100

! ! ! ! ! ! ! ! ! ! !

NEITHER LIKE NOR DISLIKE — LIKE — LIKE VERY MUCH

8. How strongly do I like:

____

0 100

! ! ! ! ! ! ! ! ! ! !

NEITHER LIKE NOR DISLIKE — LIKE — LIKE VERY MUCH

9. How strongly do I like:

____

0 100

! ! ! ! ! ! ! ! ! ! !

NEITHER LIKE NOR DISLIKE — LIKE — LIKE VERY MUCH

10. How strongly do I like:

____

0 100

! ! ! ! ! ! ! ! ! ! !

PERSONAL EXPECTATIONS QUESTIONNAIRE

Now, what we want to know is how strongly you expect the things you listed to happen. How strongly you expect something can be shown by putting a check mark somewhere along a line that runs from SURE IT WILL HAPPEN, at one end, to SURE IT WILL NOT HAPPEN, at the other end.

0										100
!	!	!	!	!	!	!	!	!	!	!
SURE IT WILL NOT HAPPEN				EVEN CHANCE "FIFTY-FIFTY"					SURE IT WILL HAPPEN	

When you are very sure something will happen, you can show this by marking a check ( ) in one of the spaces toward the end that says SURE IT WILL HAPPEN. When you don't expect something to happen, you can show that by making acheck in one of the spaces toward the other end, SURE IT WILL NOT HAPPEN. If you think the chances are about even, put your check somewhere toward the middle of the line. Your check can be in any of the spaces along the line, depending on what you really expect.

Let's take an example:

How strongly do I expect:

To have other people ask me to help organize a new club?

0										100
!	!	!	!	!	!	!	!	!	!	!
SURE IT WILL NOT HAPPEN				EVEN CHANCE "FIFTY-FIFTY"					SURE IT WILL HAPPEN	

If you think about this for a minute, you can see that some persons would expect this very strongly, some persons wouldn't expect this at all, and some persons would be in between. Think about what you expect. Now put your check mark in one of the spaces along the line that best shows how strongly you expect this to happen.

On this questionnaire we're not asking about what you would like to have happen. Answer each question in terms of what you really expect. We want you to be as realistic as possible.

Each question should be answered by itself. Don't worry about how you have answered the others.

REMEMBER!

There are no right or wrong answers. Fill in each blank with the things you mentioned on Page one. Place a check on the corresponding graph to show how strongly you really expect each thing.

1. How strongly do I expect:

____

0										100
!	!	!	!	!	!	!	!	!	!	!

SURE IT WILL NOT HAPPEN — EVEN CHANCE "FIFTY-FIFTY" — SURE IT WILL HAPPEN

2. How strongly do I expect:

____

0										100
!	!	!	!	!	!	!	!	!	!	!

SURE IT WILL NOT HAPPEN — EVEN CHANCE "FIFTY-FIFTY" — SURE IT WILL HAPPEN

3. How strongly do I expect:

____

0										100
!	!	!	!	!	!	!	!	!	!	!

SURE IT WILL NOT HAPPEN — EVEN CHANCE "FIFTY-FIFTY" — SURE IT WILL HAPPEN

4. How strongly do I expect:

____

0										100
!	!	!	!	!	!	!	!	!	!	!

SURE IT WILL NOT HAPPEN — EVEN CHANCE "FIFTY-FIFTY" — SURE IT WILL HAPPEN

5. How strongly do I expect:

____

0										100
!	!	!	!	!	!	!	!	!	!	!

SURE IT WILL NOT HAPPEN — EVEN CHANCE "FIFTY-FIFTY" — SURE IT WILL HAPPEN

6. How strongly do I expect:

____

0 100

! ! ! ! ! ! ! ! ! ! !

SURE IT WILL NOT HAPPEN — EVEN CHANCE "FIFTY-FIFTY" — SURE IT WILL HAPPEN

7. How strongly do I expect:

____

0 100

! ! ! ! ! ! ! ! ! ! !

SURE IT WILL NOT HAPPEN — EVEN CHANCE "FIFTY-FIFTY" — SURE IT WILL HAPPEN

8. How strongly do I expect:

____

0 100

! ! ! ! ! ! ! ! ! ! !

SURE IT WILL NOT HAPPEN — EVEN CHANCE "FIFTY-FIFTY" — SURE IT WILL HAPPEN

9. How strongly do I expect:

____

0 100

! ! ! ! ! ! ! ! ! ! !

SURE IT WILL NOT HAPPEN — EVEN CHANCE "FIFTY-FIFTY" — SURE IT WILL HAPPEN

10. How strongly do I expect:

____

0 100

! ! ! ! ! ! ! ! ! ! !

SURE IT WILL NOT HAPPEN — EVEN CHANCE "FIFTY-FIFTY" — SURE IT WILL HAPPEN

DRUG USE QUESTIONNAIRE

In this questionnaire, we are interested in learning something about the use of marijuana, amphetamines (speed), barbiturates, hallucinogens (LSD, mescaline, etc.) and other drugs by high school students. Many social researchers are interested in drug use patterns and have been studying drug use in various settings (schools, armed forces, organizations) among diverse groups of people all over the country.

We wish to learn about your own experiences, if any, with drugs. Some of the questions we ask may seem funny to you, but we have you will answer seriously and carefully. Do not put your names on the questionnaire. This will insure that your identity will remain unknown.

It is important for this study that your answers be accurate and honest. For each question, you will be asked either to circle a letter or number. Everyone should answer every question.

1. Which of the following drugs have you used or do use now?

   a. Hallucinogens (LSD, mescaline, psilocybin)

   b. Marijuana (weed, grass, pot, hashhish)

   c. Heroin

   d. Amphetamines (Bennies, pep pills, etc.)

   e. Barbiturates (red birds, yellow jackets, reds, etc.)

   f. Cocaine

   g. Codeine

   h. Methamphetamines (spped, crystal, meth)

   i. Morphine

   j. None

2. How often do you usually smoke marijuana? (Circle one)

   a. Never
   b. Less than 1 time a year
   c. At least 1 time a year
   d. About 1 or 2 times a month
   e. About 1 or 2 times a week
   f. About 3 or 4 times a week
   g. 1 or 2 times a day

3. When you smoke marijuana, how much do you usually smoke at one time? (Circle one)

   a. Never smoke marijuana
   b. Part of a joint
   c. 1 joint
   d. 2 joints
   e. 3 or 4 joints
   f. 5 or more joints

4. How often do you usually take amphetamines (speed)? (Circle one)

   a. Never
   b. Less than 1 time a year
   c. At least one time a year
   d. About 1 or 2 times a month
   e. About 1 or 2 times a week
   f. About 3 or 4 times a week
   g. 1 or 2 times a day

5. When you take amphetamines (speed), how much do you usually take at once. (Circle one)

   a. Never take speed

   b. Part of one hit

   c. 1 hit

   d. 2 hits

   e. 3 or 4 hits

   f. 5 or more hits

6. How often do you usually take an hallucinogen (LSD, mescaline, etc.)? (Circle one)

   a. Never

   b. Less than 1 time a year

   c. At least 1 time a year

   d. About 1 or 2 times a month

   e. About 1 or 2 times a week

   f. 3 or 4 times a week

   g. 1 or 2 times a day

7. When you take an hallucinogen, how much do you usually take at one time? (Circle one)

   a. Never take an hallucinogen

   b. Part of one hit

   c. 1 hit

   d. 2 hits

   e. 3 or 4 hits

   f. 5 or more hits

8. How often do you usually take a barbiturate? (Circle one)

a. Never

b. less than 1 time a year

c. At least 1 time a year

d. About 1 or 2 times a month

e. About 1 or 2 times a week

f. About 3 or 4 times a week

g. 1 or 2 times a day

9. When you take a barbiturate, how much do you usually take at one time? (Circle one)

a. Never take a barbiturate

b. Part of one hit

c. 1 hit

d. 2 hits

e. 3 or 4 hits

f. 5 or more hits

10. How many times have you gotten really high in the last year? (Circle one)

a. Never

b. 1 time

c. 2 or 3 times

d. 4 or 5 times

e. 6 or 7 times

f. 8 or 9 times

g. 10 or more times

11. How many times have you gotten into trouble with your family because of drugs? (Circle one)

a. Never

b. Once or twice

c. Several times

12. How many times have you driven when you've been high on drugs? (Circle one)

a. Never

b. Once or twice

c. Several times

13. How many times have you gone to school high or taken drugs while at school? (Circle one)

a. Never

b. Once or twice

c. Several times

14. How many times have you left school early or not gone at all because you were high on drugs? (Circle one)

a. Never

b. Once or twice

c. Several times

15. How many times have your friends ever criticized you because of your using drugs? (Circle one)

a. Never

b. Once or twice

c. Several times

16. How many times have you had automobile accidents because of drugs? (Circle <u>one</u>)

    a. Never

    b. Once or twice

    c. Several times

17. How many times have you been called before some authority because of drugs? (Circle <u>one</u>)

    a. Never

    b. Once or twice

    c. Several times

18. How many times have you damaged property because of drugs? (Circle <u>one</u>)

    a. Never

    b. Once or twice

    c. Several times

19. How many times have you been injured or gotten ill as a result of your use of drugs? (Circle <u>one</u>)

    a. Never

    b. Once or twice

    c. Several times

20. How many times have you failed to get your date home in time because of drugs? (Circle <u>one</u>)

    a. Never

    b. Once or twice

    c. Several times

21. How many times have you ever felt that a friendship was damaged or lost because of your use of drugs? (Circle one)

    a. Never

    b. Once or twice

    c. Several times

22. How many times have you ever injured others because of your use of drugs? (Circle one)

    a. Never

    b. Once or twice

    c. Several times

23. How many times have you missed an appointment because of your use of drugs? (Circle one)

    a. Never

    b. Once or twice

    c. Several times

REFERENCES

CARMAN, R. S. Personality and drinking among college students. Unpublished M.A. thesis, University of Colorado, 1965.

CARMAN, R. S. Drinking behavior as related to personality and socio-cultural factors. Unpublished Ph.D. thesis, University of Colorado, 1968.

CARMAN, R. S. Expectations and socialization experiences related to drinking among U.S. servicemen. *Quart. J. Studies Alc.* 32: 1040–1047, 1971.

CARMAN, R. S. Drug use and personal values of high school students. *Intern. J. Addictions* 8(4): 733–739, 1973.

CLARK, J., and TIFFT, L. Polygraph and interview validation of self-reported deviant behavior. *Amer. Sociol. Rev.* 31: 516–523, 1966.

HAGER, D. L., VENER, A. M., and STEWART, C. S. Patterns of adolescent drug use in middle America. *J. Counseling Psychol.* 18: 292–297, 1971.

JESSOR, R., CARMAN, R. S., and GROSSMAN, P. Expectations for need satisfaction and patterns of alcohol use in college. *Quart. J. Studies Alc.* 29: 101–116, 1968.

ROTTER, J. B. *Social Learning and Clinical Psychology.* New York: Prentice-Hall, 1954.

SEEMAN, M. On the meaning of alienation. *Amer. Sociol. Rev.* 24: 783–791, 1959.

The International Journal of the Addictions, 9(1), pp. 81–99, 1974

Drug Abuse Training and Education: The Physician*

Stanley Einstein, Ph.D.†

Departments of Public Health, Community Medicine, and Psychiatry
New Jersey College of Medicine and Dentistry
Newark, New Jersey

Drug abuse training and education both past and present has been many things in the United States. A misnomer, an anachronism, a form of political expediency, a format for hustling, a focus of religiosity, etc. It has rarely ever been defined in terms of content, goals, or who is to be responsible for its development, maintenance, and evaluation. And because of the confusion, it has tended to grow arithmetically as the use of drugs for recreation has seemingly grown geometrically. Within this context the physician, his professional organizations, and the medical school are now being asked, and pushed, to intervene effectively.

This paper will attempt to explore those issues that relate to:

1. Why a given institutional structure, such as medicine, seeks to establish a drug training or educational program.
2. The consequences of our definitions of drugs, drug addicts, and drug addiction on such efforts.

* Delivered at 18th Annual AMA Conference of State Mental Health Representatives, April 13–15, 1972, Scottsdale, Arizona.

† Present address: Institute for the Study of Drug Misuse, New York, New York.

3. What the content of that program has been and what it should be.
4. The possible roles available to the medical arena in drug abuse intervention.

CRITICAL DEFINITIONS

All drug abuse training and education programs are contingent upon a series of definitions that a society makes concerning:

1. What is a drug?
2. What is a dangerous drug?
3. What drugs, taken in what way, by themselves or in combination with other drugs, and for what conscious or unconscious reasons, are to be condemned or condoned?
4. Whether the nonmedical use of drugs is a disease or a condition with medical facets.
5. Who is a drug user, a drug abuser, or a drug addict?
6. What is the format of training and what are its goals?
7. What is the format of education and what are its goals?
8. What are the roles and responsibilities of all those involved in an educational or training program—the student, the educational representative, and the general community?
9. What are the roles and responsibilities of all those involved in a drug educational or training program—the abstinent student, the nonabstinent student, the nondangerous drug using educational representative, and the abstinent and nonabstinent general community?
10. What is the content and process of drug-related delivery of care?
11. Who is to define this process and who is to be responsible for its success as well as its failure?
12. Thc agrccd upon techniques for attempting to change man's appetites; medical, legal, social, religious, etc.
13. The style of life and the value of life that is both experienced and aspired to.

DRUG RELATED DEFINITIONS

Drugs have been defined in terms of four sources: social-religious, medical, legal, and scientific (Table 1).

Table 1

Definitions and Sources of Definitions of Drugs

Social-Religious	Medical	Legal	Scientific
Imputed status: aid to ritualization	Medicine	Dangerous substance for individual and/or community	Any substance that by its chemical nature alters the structure or functioning of a living organism
Social rituals:	Prevent illness	Control of:	
Holidays	Maintain health	Growth	
Festivals	Treat illness	Manufacture	
Birthdays	Relieve pain	Distribution	
Special occasions		Importation	
Rites of passage		Use	
Religious rituals:		Possession	
The mass			
Greeting of sabbath			
Mescaline rites			

The oldest source of definition has been the social-religious. This source has historically taught us that a variety of substances, irrespective of their medical, psychiatric, or social consequences, are permitted for use if they fit into the social value structure or religious-ritual structure of a given community at a given point in time. As long as the user of the substance adhered to the social and religious rituals of his group, he was not given a deviant status.

From this perspective drugs were not considered dangerous or not dangerous. The critical definition became and indeed still is approved social or religious use or disapproved social or religious use.

Thus whereas alcohol has traditionally had sacramental value, and peyote has for members of the Native American Church, LSD is not given this status, notwithstanding its association with the League for Spiritual Discovery.

Thus notwithstanding alcohol's toxic effects, its devastating effect on an estimated 9,000,000 Americans and 130,000 American servicemen, we still honor it as a social beverage.

The most immediate consequence of religious-social definitions is that decisions to reinforce or inhibit the use of particular drugs are not related to the imputed dangers of drug effects but to the arbitrariness of human decision making.

An immediate concern for the physician is how he can get across the following notions to a patient or any one else that he is relating to that:

1. Certain substances are not to be used, or used in certain ways for certain reasons, simply because we don't want them to be.
2. His concern about the nonmedical use of drugs goes beyond disease and health concepts, and embraces the notion of maximizing human adaptation and functioning.

The medical field has by definition suggested that drug use is a problem when a substance is generally used for nonmedical reasons, outside of the authority of the physician and other specific health professionals (i.e., nurse and pharmacist), and specifically when the goal of such use is recreation, pleasure, and imputed self-exploration. By ambiguity and specious reasoning, the medical world has foisted upon the community the notion that nonmedical drug use is a medical problem to be handled by the medical profession. It is only a short step to also conclude that any type of intervention, be it treatment, education, or whatever, is the province of the physician.

A number of immediate consequences arise from this.

1. By training most physicians perceive behavior in terms of pathology and disease concepts which may limit them in being able to explore the varied meanings and ramifications of drug use or to introduce a new concept-social pharmacology.
2. By training most physicians assume that treatment and/or education should continue in the traditional medical model or pyramidal structure for lines of authority and decision making. Given this type of structure, the biggest constituency for drug education, the community, is given only a passive role for decision making and an active role for funding.
3. By status and imputed knowledge, the physician is asked to become active in a variety of drug educational roles which are often not commensurate with his training or interest. These include developing school drug abuse curriculum; serving on the traditional school program panel of physician, pharmacist, teacher, religious leader, policeman, ex-addict, and politician; talking to the PTA; allaying the anxiety of parents concerned about their children's possible drug use; developing and supervising student drug surveys; defining for the general community who is the drug abuser and there-in what is drug abuse, both in the school and the

business world; defining what the content and process of treatment programs should be; as well as what should go into legal control.

It becomes patently clear that consequences of the medical definition of drugs go far beyond the boundaries of the medical world.

Legal definitions of drugs and drug use are perhaps the most ambiguous because of their apparent clarity. Legally, at any point in time anywhere in the world, drugs are generally defined as substances which are considered to be dangerous either to the individual or to his community. This apparently simple definition leads to intervention through controlling growth, manufacture, distribution, sale, and possession as well as use.

This type of definition results in a number of immediate consequences for the medical world.

1. By training, most law enforcement representatives perceive changing or controlling man's appetites in terms of legal controls not withstanding the lack of data to substantiate that this is at all possible. Increasingly, the physician is turned to to reinforce the legal controls. What is his responsibility when he indicates that a youngster is a drug addict on the bases of eye dilation or track marks, or when he says a person isn't motivated for treatment, when none of these have anything to do with science? "Drug addict" at best connotes something about a person's drug behavior and not who he is. Motivation, at best, is a retrospective concept rather than a predictive one.
2. One of the consequences of legal definitions of drugs and drug use is the perception of drug related behavior in terms of deviant-criminal concepts. The effect of this, and the associated harrassment that physicians have experienced or anticipated in treating the drug addict and user, may have served to limit them in being able to explore the valid-achievable roles that he may and/or should play in contemporary social pharmacology as well as recreational drug use. The key issue for the physician is being able to pinpoint and evaluate the specific needs of the drug user that can best be met by him, as well as referring the drug user on to others who can better meet certain of these needs.
3. Given the relative absence of involvement by physicians in drug education in the United States in the past, law enforcement has

reinforced as facts a number of dangerous myths. These include:

3.1. Dangerous drugs should be the focus of our intervention efforts. By implication, certain drugs are not dangerous, and thus do not deserve being covered in drug education. There are no undangerous drugs!

3.2. Drugs can be categorized as *soft* and *hard.* By implication, educational efforts should focus on preventing participants in such programs from going on to hard drugs. The soft-hard drug typology is scientifically meaningless. On a very simplistic level it may put an intervention program in the awkward position of attacking heroin use and saying little about barbiturates, amphetamines, alcohol, etc., when our concern should be the development of nondrug options to the problems and pleasures of living and not to the relative toxicity of chemicals.

3.3. Drug use is a critical factor in determining and/or escalating criminal behavior in a given community. By implication, were drug use to disappear, crime, by type, incidence, and prevalence, should be dramatically lowered. Thus drug intervention is given the additional imputed task of changing the criminal nature of a given community. There is little hard data to substantiate the contention that this goal is achievable in this manner.

3.4. Removing blatant drug offending individuals from the mainstream of living in their community will serve a double function: helping them to become more conventional and less drug-oriented, and serving as a warning to latent offenders. Again there is little hard data to substantiate this.

If defining drugs legally has consequences that go beyond the legal system, and often impinge upon the delivery of health services, what role is there for the physician, as professional and citizen, in effecting these consequences?

Clearly the physician should use the knowledge and imputed status he already has, and gain the knowledge he still needs to see to it that effective drug-related intervention is based on facts and not fantasies, that policy making is based on the health needs of the patient and the community at large and not on expediency or the vested interests of parochial groups, and that he becomes a source of hope rather than one of harrassment.

It should be clear by now that drug definitions are not simply semantic games for the physician. From a scientific perspective a drug is any substance which through its chemical activity alters the structure and/or functioning of a living organism. As valid as this is, this definition is presently almost meaningless for our society. Our nation has decided not to be concerned about coffee, tea, tobacco, food, etc. And this has resulted in problems and confusion for the physician.

But this definition does raise an important issue for our consideration. Physicians can help communities acknowledge that they have a drug problem, not when certain people are using certain drugs, but when an increasing part of the population turns to things, to substances, to meet their legitimate and illegitimate needs rather than to people.

Pragmatically this is so because social institutions cannot continue for long if individuals isolate themselves from others, are involved in parallel play, or relate to others as objects rather than sources of humanness. And should this occur, the role of the physician, and the meaning of health illness and medicine, will significantly change.

All of this is a long way of saying that drug intervention efforts should utilize scientific definitions of drugs in order to define what entails a drug problem, and the physician can and should play an important role in this process.

DRUG ABUSE

Drug abuse has come to be one of those terms that everyone understands but no one apparently knows what to do with or about. One of the most frequently asked questions for the physician these days is: What are the alternatives to drug abuse? While the most immediate answers are treatment and education, the most immediate sensation is that of being overwhelmed. This is understandable when we acknowledge that the question is so huge in terms of what it actually and potentially encompasses. From an intervention point of view the possible alternatives to drug abuse, and the roles that we can play in these alternatives, become more obvious when we begin to pinpoint what drug abuse is or may be.

Drug abuse is not a single entity nor a unitary concept. Indeed, there are at least three sources of definitions for drug abuse. These are:

1. *Abusing drug laws and rituals.* This encompasses the breaking of drug-related laws, mores, and rituals by particular people, using particular drugs in particular ways and for particular reasons.

2. *Self-abuse.* The direct or indirect consequences resulting from the use of drugs for other than medically and/or socially approved reasons to the person taking them.
3. *Abuse of others.* The direct or indirect consequences of the use of drugs for other than medically and/or socially approved reasons to people other than the drug user. Developing meaningful and workable alternatives to drug abuse, and delineating the physician's role in this process, begins to be possible only if we note the type of drug abuse that we are considering at a given point in time.

The physician must be helped to understand what viable roles and actions are possible for him for each type of drug abuse. This again is not simply a semantic issue.

CONTINUOUS EDUCATION FOR THE PHYSICIAN

At the present time there are a limited number of techniques being used for the continuing education of the physician. Generically they can be divided into dependence upon conferences, symposia, workshops, lectures, etc.; journals, newsletters, and other printed materials; and the use of tapes.

All of these techniques are based on two assumptions that must be critically reviewed generally, and specifically done so they relate to the nonmedical use of drugs.

The first assumption is that the physician is indeed involved in a continuous drug-related information dissemination process, and second, that this is education. It might be fairer to acknowledge from the onset that since most medical students have learned little about the many facets of the nonmedical use of drugs, that at best what they receive is fragmented, rather than continuous. Second, it may not even be education. Much confusion continues to exist in distinguishing between education and training. In simplistic terms, education is a process by which a heterogeneous group becomes the focus of certain goals and techniques and terminates this process as a heterogeneous group.

Training on the other hand is a process by which a heterogeneous group is aided in becoming a homogeneous one for specific skills, abilities, attitudes, values, etc.

This distinction is no minor one as physicians attempt to reinforce certain patterns of drug use and inhibit others. Do we need heterogeneous or homogeneous groups of physicians to effectively intervene in the nonmedical use of drugs? Do we need drug expert physicians or simply capable physicians? What criteria should be developed, if any, to screen in and screen out physicians from drug-related continuous education programs as well as treatment programs of any type? These are some of the issues that must be confronted when we begin to consider drug-related continuous education programs for physicians.

FROM DEFINITIONS TO EDUCATION-TRAINING TO INTERVENTION

Just as many of the younger generation are now attempting to live a life that goes beyond drugs, we must go beyond definitions to key issues and toward tentative decisions and conclusions.

The failure of most physician drug education-training intervention is due to the fact that evaluation of what is needed is almost nonexistent, goal setting for the program is most often a myth, the roles of the constituents of the program are not clearly thought out or are confusing, the actual site of drug abuse education is rarely considered in the planning stages of a program, the modalities and materials being used may have little relevance to the initial evaluation or goals, there is little if any ongoing evaluation during the process, and follow up is a myth and prevention as a concept most often has little to do with offering the participants and the people they serve viable alternatives and life styles to the pressures and pleasures that they experience.

Obviously there are different models of drug education that are possible, each one having its own associated set of processes and consequences. It is suggested, however, that there are common denominators to most drug education programs and that continuing education for the physician will not and should not be significantly different from other programs.

Planning and carrying out a drug abuse continuing education program should include the following steps:

1. *Determination of the scope of the program* in terms of the types of drugs to be focused upon, the patterns of drug use to be included, and the specificity of the audience that is to be reached. The greater the heterogeneity of the group, the greater the possibility of coming to terms with the various options and roles

Table 2
Developing a Drug Abuse Continuing Education Curriculum
A Schematic Checklist

		Goals	Content: Facts	Content: Attitudes	Content: Skills	Roles	Process techniques	Resources
Student	Strengths							
	Weaknesses							
	Needs							
Teaching community	Strengths							
	Weaknesses							
	Needs							
General community	Strengths							
	Weaknesses							
	Needs							

that are available for intervention, including the problems associated with them, and the less likely that participants will go back to their offices and hospitals continuing to feel isolated. A heterogeneous group should be better able to focus on issues rather than dogma, which should result in openness rather than parochialism.

2. *Development of base line data* relevant to the incidence and prevalence of drug use and misuse, and attitudes about drugs, drug misuse, and drug misusers. Without this type of data, the program may get bogged down in concepts and theories that have little to do with the drug-related health needs of a given community or being able to anticipate them for the near future.
3. *Agreement upon data* that relates to the state of knowledge about what drugs do and don't do, and what people can do and can't do. Continuous education is not meant to reinforce mythology or dysfunctional ritualistic intervention.
4. *Development of a program goal system* that pinpoints the various levels of acceptable program-related behavioral alternatives to drug misuse. The goal system should meet the minimal criteria of being meaningful, achievable, and acceptable to those being educated, and acceptable to the educator and the general community. Selection of goals should be related to the value systems of a given constituency, their actual and imputed roles and status,

and their needs in the present and the immediate future. A program without clearly delineated goals is not a program; at best it is systematized activity. A program which does not include in its format the concepts of roles, consequences, continuity of intervention, and responsibility for the physician is a tax-exempt meeting and not an educational experience.

5. *Relating continuous drug education to formal and informal education* which prepares those being educated to a life of people-oriented issues and daily decision making that focuses on alternatives and values rather than to a life of drug-oriented issues that focuses only on certain types of people and drugs and dangers.
6. *Role definition* for all the participants in the drug education program so that each one knows what is expected of him, and what his boundaries and limitations are to be. Concepts such as continuity of education and continuity of responsibility are associated with this step.
7. *Determination of the techniques, modalities, and materials to be used* so that a coordinated effort is assured, the program's limitations can be made manageable, its strengths maintained or reinforced, and its outcome can be evaluated. This should be done in relation to the goals of the program and the strengths, weaknesses, and roles of the participants.
8. *Selection of the appropriate site of education* so that the choice is related to the initial evaluation, goal selection, role definitions, and the techniques and materials being used rather than based on the notions of availability, captive audiences, postgraduate credit issues, and vacation needs.
9. *Ongoing reevaluation* in order to assess whether the program should be continued, modified, or terminated; goals maintained or changed; roles changed or maintained; techniques shifted or maintained; materials revised, maintained, or dropped; site of the educational program shifted or maintained; and whether the resources necessary for effective continuing education are present and being utilized, are absent and are needed, or are adequate.
10. *Follow-up evaluation* at specific intervals after the program has been completed in order to determine the effects of the program.

All of the aforementioned is contingent upon our acknowledging that there is no such thing as the continuing drug education program, and that all such programs are effected by temporal and geographical considerations. A program for here and now may be inappropriate for here and tomorrow, or for that matter anywhere else tomorrow. Obviously, since programs are man-made, they must be man-tailored rather than viewed as being the oracles of Delphi, or indeed the Lord's design.

A FRAMEWORK FOR THE DEVELOPMENT OF A CONTINUING DRUG EDUCATION PROGRAM

The initial practical decision that has to be made in developing a drug education program has to do with the type of drug abuse we are most concerned about, or if we are concerned about all three types (abuse of laws and mores, self-abuse, abuse of others), giving priorities to each one.

The next step is to decide upon the focus of intervention. We have the choice of focusing our efforts on:

1. Drugs themselves.
2. Abstainers, be they individuals who have never used or misused drugs generally or specific drugs, or those who have ceased their misuse.
3. Active drug misusers.
4. Intervention agents and programs be they individuals doing treatment, teachers, school administrators, clergy, law enforcement representatives, media representatives, parents, peers, medical or nonmedical programs.
5. The general community.

The next decision facing us has to do with the content of the possible intervention (Table 3). Now that we have decided upon the type of drug abuse we wish to effect and what our primary focus is to be, we can come to terms with the direction of our efforts. Acknowledging that the direction or content areas that we select are arbitrary ones, we nevertheless should consider the following potential areas:

1. Physiological Health
2. Psychological Health
3. Social Health
4. Physical-Chemical Adaptation
5. Spatial Adaptation
6. Temporal Adaptation

Table 3

Alternatives to Drug Abuse by Type, Focus of Intervention, and Areas of Adaptation

		Physiological Health	Psychological Health	Social Health	Physical-Chemical Adaptation	Spatial Adaptation
Abuse of Drug Laws, Mores, Rituals	Drugs Abstainers Active Drug Users Intervention Agents General Community					
Self-Abuse	Drugs Abstainers Active Drug Users Intervention Agents General Community					
Abuse of Others	Drugs Abstainers Active Drug Users Intervention Agents General Community					

		Temporal Adaptation	Cultural Adaptation	Religious Adaptation	Political Adaptation	Economic Adaptation
Abuse of Drug Laws, Mores, Rituals	Drugs Abstainers Active Drug Users Intervention Agents General Community					
Self-Abuse	Drugs Abstainers Active Drug Users Intervention Agents General Community					
Abuse of Others	Drugs Abstainers Active Drug Users Intervention Agents General Community					

7. Cultural Adaptation
8. Religious Adaptation
9. Political Adaptation
10. Economic Adaptation

These ten content areas serve to remind us that all of us must somehow come to terms with our physio-psycho-social selves and needs, as well as a physical-chemical world, space and time, and the pressures of cultural, religious, political, and economic considerations.

The table that is created by this type of consideration permits us to consider what we can and can't do as we attempt to effect man's appetites and thereby effect his modes of adaptation. It also permits us to consider what our responsibilities and limitations are for each cell, so that we don't get bogged down by the enormity of the initial task and then do the most current thing—turn to the drug expert.

An analysis of this table allows us to understand that none of these 10 content areas have inherent high priority attached to them. Rather, by choosing any of them we are serving notice that this is our arbitrary choice as we seek to create meaningful alternatives to drug abuse. But oncc we have chosen a particular area, based on careful thought rather than as a panacea or total solution, we should have better results with it than has been our general experience.

For example, what program planning is necessary and possible, if our concern is an individual's or group's social health, while focusing upon active drug misusers, as we attempt to limit or eradicate drug-related self-abuse. Obviously one possibility is learning how to challenge the active drug user's ability to achieve those values or goals that are important to him through drugs only. It is the rare goal or value that can be achieved and/or experienced only through the use of drugs.

If a program can't come up with the content or the faculty for a particular cell, then we should plan to focus on areas or cells which permit us to effectively utilize the available expertise, time, and energy that is at hand. The rule of thumb is not that something is better than nothing. Nothing is nothing! This type of analysis of a continuous education program of drug abuse for physicians is no more than a suggested approach. It obviously is not a guide to the do's and don't's of drug abuse intervention. Rather it offers the physician and his professional societies a framework to which we can add or delete while permitting us to decide what role such education can and may play in a contemporary problem area which continues to be colored by ambiguities and hysteria.

DRUG TRAINING PROGRAMS AS PART OF CONTINUING EDUCATION

Returning to the operational definition that training assumes the changing of a heterogeneous group into a homogeneous one in terms of knowledge, attitudes, skills, etc., one has to consider that there are three major groups that can become the focus of drug-related training. These are the active drug user, intervention agents, and the general community. The physician may and should play a role with all of them.

THE ACTIVE DRUG USER

Traditionally, the kind of information given to the drug user has concerned itself with either the dangers associated with drug use in general, the use of specific drugs, or the legal consequences related to drug use.

Given that many people may continue to use drugs for nonmedical reasons, irrespective of the community's intervention, drug training may impart other kinds of knowledge and skills.

These include information concerning: (1) the kinds of private and community resources available in a specific area, and how to utilize them; (2) when drugs have been adulterated with poisonous materials, (3) what entails a proper and effective referral, and (4) the rights one has, particularly in terms of protecting oneself from becoming jeopardized (i.e., urine testing, drug related eye tests, civil commitment). Surely the physician's traditional role encompasses each of these issues. He should be helped to delineate other issues by which he can be of significant help to the drug user.

INTERVENTION AGENTS

More often than not the knowledge imparted to the intervention agent has tended to reinforce the notion that there is a specific type of person known as a drug addict; that certain drugs are dangerous and, implicity, others are less so; that a drug problem in a given community simply consists of certain people using certain drugs; and that the three avenues open for effective intervention are treatment, education, and the law, and that any of these interventions are inherently logical and good and their failure should be attributed to the drug user (Table 4). The training of intervention agents who are to be permitted to work in the field of drug abuse should go beyond the content areas of *drugs* (type, frequency, pat-

Table 4
Treating the Drug Abuser: A Schema for Training

Process	Purposes	Content
Standardized evaluation	Assess person's present strengths	Individual diagnosis
	Assess person's present weaknesses	
	Assess person's use of resources	System diagnosis
	Possible registration	
Goal setting	Meaningful for person	Developing heterogeneous goal systems
	Achievable by person	
	Acceptable to person	
	Flexible	
	Acceptable to treatment agent	
	Acceptable to community	
Role definition	Person's role defined	Systems of intervention and their role consequences
	Treatment agent's role defined	
	General community's role defined	
Treatment modalities	Appropriate for person	Ongoing diagnosis
	Appropriate to treatment agent's training	Specific skills
	Appropriate to treatment agent's availability	Shared programs
	Appropriate to community's needs	Community life style diagnosis
	Acute intervention	Techniques
	Chronic intervention	Techniques
	Continuity of care	Models of care
	Continuity of responsibility	Models of care
	Central case manager	Models of care
	Site of treatment	Relevance to goals and roles
Reevaluation	Assess status of condition	Health definitions, health criteria
	Goal assessment	Evaluation techniques
	Treatment modality assessment	Evaluation techniques
	Referral and/or termination	Individual diagnosis, system diagnosis
Follow-up	Status of condition	Adaptational criteria
	Assessment of treatment efforts	Role and technique evaluation
	Assessment of resources	Criteria and techniques
Early case finding	Signs and symptoms	Diagnosis
	Possible registration	Techniques and meaning
	Responsibilities and roles	Systems
	Consequences	Individual and community roles
Prevention	Nondrug alternatives	Life style systems

terns, meaning), *characteristics* of the drug user, and *consequences* of drug use, to include a base level of knowledge of the following areas:

1. Research
   1.1 Theories of Drug Use
   1.2 Theories of Drug Action
   1.3 Theories of Treatment
   1.4 Classification of Drugs
   1.5 Classification of Drug Users
   1.6 Classification of Nondrug Users
2. Treatment
   2.1 Types of Programs
   2.2 Evaluation Procedures
   2.3 Goal Systems
   2.4 Available Treatment Modalities
   2.5 Evaluation
   2.6 Policies and Procedures Effecting Treatment
   2.7 Professional Roles
   2.8 Criteria for Treatment Agents
   2.9 Drug Misuser Roles
   2.10 Follow-up Systems
3. Attitudes and Values Toward Drug Use, Misuse, and the Drug User
   3.1 Intervention Staff
   3.2 General Community
4. Public Policy Relating to Intervention
   4.1 Laws
   4.2 Policies
   4.3 Procedures
5. Economics of Drug Use
   5.1 Licit Factors
   5.2 Illicit Factors
6. The Politics of Drug Use Intervention
7. Education
   7.1 Nondrug Related Alternatives
   7.2 Drug Related Alternatives
   7.3 Decision Making
   7.4 Respect for People
   7.5 Respect for Drugs
   7.6 Respect for Feelings
   7.7 Built in Inequities of Living

8. Philosophy
   8.1 Nondrug Related Alternatives
   8.2 Drug Related Alternatives
9. Religion
   9.1 Nondrug Related Rituals
   9.2 Drug Related Rituals
10. Culture
   10.1 Drug and Nondrug Related and Oriented Literature
   10.2 Drug and Nondrug Related and Oriented Music and Songs
11. Patterns of Adaptation
   11.1 Roles
   11.2 Meanings
   11.3 Decision Making Factors
   11.4 Consequences
12. Mass Media
   12.1 People-Oriented Patterns of Living
   12.2 Drug-Oriented Patterns of Living
13. Other Intervention
   13.1 Early Case Finding
   13.2 Prevention
   13.3 Registration Systems

These areas should not only be covered in terms of hard facts relating each of them to the issue of drug use, but should also include the generic issues of roles, responsibilities, consequences, and meanings. The major outcome of this type of training is to be the creation of a cadre of intervention agents who know why they are doing what they are doing to whom, under what circumstances, and who have a realistic idea as to the kinds of outcomes, and what options are available if their original intervention is not successful. After the physician has himself been adequately trained in each of these facets, he can begin to take an active role as a source of information dissemination based on his areas of actual strengths and not based on his imputed strengths and status.

THE GENERAL COMMUNITY

The general community has all too often been led to believe that drug abuse is a unique behavior which is best left to the physician or ex-addict whose efforts the community must fund. Aside from receiving training similar to the intervention agent, the general community must be helped to understand:

1. In what ways does a community reinforce the use and misuse of drugs?
2. In what ways does a community inhibit the use and misuse of drugs?
3. What are the viable roles, and their associated consequences and limitations, open to a community as a whole as well as to its individual constituents, for a given type of quality of life style?
4. What are the gaps in resources and services as well as what duplication of effort exists in a community?

In a sense the training for the general community should lead to one major conclusion: The community deserves the type of adaptation that it permits. The end result of such training should be a coming to terms with social pharmacology as well as drug abuse by defining and giving priorities to role definitions for all concerned, and various intervention efforts.

The physician and his professional societies as well as medical schools have an obligation to take an active role in these activities because they owe it to the community at large. If for no other reasons, this debt is based upon the tax funds that are used in training the medical student and physician, in the tax-exempt status of medical societies, and the social responsibility that goes with status and power.

This paper has been an attempt at presenting a schema for reacting to continuous drug education and training efforts rather than a blueprint for the selection of a specific program.

The International Journal of the Addictions, 9(1), pp. 101–126, 1974

Psychological Effects, Personality and Behavioral Changes Attributed to Marihuana Use

Gary Fisher, Ph.D.

Department of Psychiatry
Cedars-Sinai Medical Center
Los Angeles, California

Allan Steckler, Dr.P.H.

Department of Health Sciences
California State University
Northridge, California

Abstract

Data from 530 marihuana users on the psychological effects, personality and behavioral changes attributed to their marihuana use are presented. Age, sex, marital status, and educational level are reported. Data were analyzed according to five use patterns: (1) trial users, (2) past users, (3) occasional users, (4) regular users, and (5) daily users. *S*s reported on the occurrence of 33 psychological effects of marihuana, changes in 14 behavioral and personality variables, effect on alcohol and tobacco consumption, effect on sexual orientation, and reasons for marihuana use.

> Results are consistent in that as marihuana use increases, there is an increase in pleasurable effects and beneficial results in personality and behavioral realms and a decrease in negative and untoward sequelae. Trial users report the least pleasant effects and the greatest untoward effects, and past users report considerably less benefits than current users.

The recent volume *Marihuana: A Signal of Misunderstanding* (Shafer et al., 1972), the official report of the National Commission on Marihuana and Drug Abuse, has increased the already widespread interest in the marihuana phenomenon. Until the past 6 or 7 years, most reports of the effects of marihuana were either anecdotal in style or based on poorly designed studies from abroad. More recently there have been laboratory studies on the physiological effects of marihuana (e.g., Isbell, 1967; Weil, Zinberg, and Nelsen, 1968); effect on human performance (e.g., Clarke, 1971; Crancer, 1969; Jones and Stone, 1969; Kiplinger, 1971); and clinical reports on adverse reactions such as feelings of confusion and disorientation (e.g., Smith and Mehl, 1970); depression, panic, and depersonalization (e.g., Keeler, 1967); anxiety and paranoia (e.g., Durham, 1968); and psychotic reactions (e.g., Hekimian and Gershon, 1968). Especially among social scientists there is a trend away from an attempt to relate marihuana use to specific behavioral effects, such as opiate addiction or criminal activity, and to explore the complexity of factors which determine functional use or abuse of marihuana (e.g., Blum, 1969; Blumer, 1967; Fisher and Strantz, 1972; Goode, 1970; Kaplan, 1970; McGlothlin and West, 1968; Smith and Mehl, 1970). The Canadian Commission of Inquiry into the Non-Medical Use of Drugs (Canadian Interim Report, 1970) has concluded, "... the psychological effects of cannabis vary greatly with a number of factors and are often difficult to predict... (and) depend to a considerable degree on the personality of the user, his past experience with cannabis or other drugs, his attitudes and the setting in which the drug is used."

The present study reports on the natural use of marihuana and presents data on the reported psychological effects of marihuana, the personality and behavioral changes attributed to marihuana use, and the reasons given for use. These data are self-report data and contain all the limitations inherent in such a study.

THE SAMPLE

The sample consists of 530 *S*s. Each *S* completed a 220-item questionnaire. The data were collected in 1969–1970 and sampling was conducted using two methods: The social network method and random sampling utilizing voter registration lists. The locale was predominantly Southern California. For the social network method, questionnaires were distributed to acquaintances of the researchers who were asked to enlist the cooperation of their marihuana-using friends. A cover letter explaining the research as well as a stamped, return-addressed envelope accompanied the questionnaire. Anonymity of respondents was assured. Since we were primarily interested in an adult middle to upper class sample, an attempt was made to restrict social networks to this population. However, college and university students were included in these networks. In order to broaden the base of sampling, random sampling, from voter registration lists from Los Angeles County, was conducted. Precincts that were predominantly middle-upper to upper class were utilized. The return rate from the mail-out questionnaire was 35%. Of those 525 usable returned questionnaires, 98 were from *S*s who had used or were currently using marihuana. Thus the user rate from this sample was 18.7%. Of the total 530 users studies, 98 (18.5%) were from the random mail-out sample.

For analysis the sample was categorized according to marihuana use pattern. The following categories were established: (1) *Trial users*: N = 47 (*S*s who had only used marihuana from one to three times); (2) *past users*: N = 79 (*S*s who had used marihuana in the past but who currently considered themselves nonusers); (3) *occasional users*: N = 147 (*S*s whose current use was less than once per week); (4) *regular users*: N = 200 (*S*s who use at least once per week to those who use up to 6 days a week); (5) *daily users*: N = 57 (*S*s who use at least once every day).

DEMOGRAPHIC CHARACTERISTICS OF SAMPLE

Age

Age distribution by marihuana use group is given in Table 1. The

Table 1
Age Distribution by Marihuana Use Groups

	Trial users		Past users		Occasional users		Regular users		Daily users	
Age	%	N	%	N	%	N	%	N	%	N
20 and under	21.7	(10)	17.9	(14)	12.4	(18)	31.2	(62)	28.6	(16)
21–30	47.8	(22)	57.7	(45)	57.2	(83)	57.8	(115)	58.9	(33)
31–40	17.4	(8)	12.8	(10)	17.9	(26)	8.0	(16)	8.9	(5)
Over 40	13.0	(6)	11.5	(9)	12.4	(18)	3.0	(6)	3.6	(2)

majority of users in all use groups are in the 21 to 30 year age bracket. The range in age was from 16 to 66 years. The sample is essentially of adults with a tendency for the more frequent users to be younger.

Sex

Sex distribution by marihuana use groups is given in Table 2. The sample consisted of 300 males and 224 females. There was a tendency for the more frequent users to be male and for the occasional users to be female. Trial and past use groups did not differ in sex composition.

Table 2
Sex Distribution by Marihuana Use Group

	Trial users		Past users		Occasional users		Regular users		Daily users	
Sex	%	*N*	%	*N*	%	*N*	%	*N*	%	*N*
Male	47.8	(22)	47.4	(37)	61.4	(89)	59.3	(118)	60.7	(34)
Female	52.2	(24)	52.6	(41)	38.6	(56)	40.7	(81)	39.3	(22)

Marital Status

Marital status by marihuana use group is shown in Table 3. The majority of respondents in all categories are single. The regular and daily users have the highest percentage of single respondents, and part of this is undoubtedly due to their being a younger group. About 10% of *S*s in all use categories are divorced or separated.

Table 3
Marital Status by Marihuana Use Group

	Trial users		Past users		Occasional users		Regular users		Daily users	
Marital status	%	*N*	%	*N*	%	*N*	%	*N*	%	*N*
Single	50.0	(23)	55.3	(42)	54.6	(77)	70.9	(139)	64.3	(36)
Married	41.3	(19)	35.5	(27)	33.3	(47)	17.9	(35)	25 0	(14)
Divorced/ separated	8.7	(4)	9.2	(7)	9.9	(14)	10.2	(20)	10.7	(6)
Widowed	0	(0)	0	(0)	2.1	(3)	1.0	(2)	0	(0)

Educational Level

Educational level by marihuana use group is shown in Table 4. The sample is fairly well educated with only a small percentage of *S*s having less than some college education. Occasional users are the best educated—64.4% having baccalaureate or graduate degrees, and the trial users the least educated—13.3% having less than some college education.

Table 4
Educational Level by Marihuana Use Groups

	Trial users		Past users		Occasional users		Regular users		Daily users	
Education	%	*N*	%	*N*	%	*N*	%	*N*	%	*N*
Less than high school	2.2	(1)	0	(0)	0.7	(1)	1.5	(3)	5.4	(3)
High school graduate	11.1	(5)	6.3	(5)	2.7	(4)	4.1	(8)	1.8	(1)
Some college	51.1	(23)	46.8	(37)	32.2	(47)	60.4	(119)	57.1	(32)
College graduate	17.8	(8)	22.8	(18)	24.7	(36)	15.2	(30)	23.2	(13)
Graduate or professional degree	17.8	(8)	24.1	(19)	39.7	(58)	18.8	(37)	12.5	(7)

PSYCHOLOGICAL EFFECTS OF MARIHUANA

Respondents were asked about the feelings and experiences that occur to them when using marihuana. The question was asked "Check the following words which you would use to describe the feelings and experiences *you* have with marihuana." Table 5 shows the results of this question. The phenomena are listed from the most frequently checked to the least frequently checked for the total group. It is readily apparent that *S*s use marihuana because they have more pleasant than unpleasant experiences. Of the 33 phenomena studied, 14 can be considered desirable, 12 undesirable, and seven neutral, depending on a *S*'s reaction to the phenomenon (e.g., distortion of time sense, altered depth perception, openness to suggestion). Of the 16 top ranked occurring phenomena, 10 are positively valued, six neutrally valued, and none negatively valued. Among the 10 lowest ranked occurring phenomena, eight are negatively valued, one neutrally valued, and one positively valued.

Over half of all *S*s experience tranquility (73.3%), increased sensory awareness (69.3%), hunger (68.9%), giggles (64.8%), distortion of time sense (63.3%), and drowsiness (56.3%). Over 40% of all *S*s experience euphoria (49.6%), introspectiveness (45.8%), difficulty with concentration (43.2%), love for fellow man (40.7%), and psychological insight (40.7%). About one-third of all *S*s report experiencing eroticism (39.6%), openness

Table 5

Marihuana-Induced Phenomena Experienced by Subjects by Use Pattern Groups

Item	Rank frequency	Total *Ss* reporting % N	Trial users % N	Past users % N	Occasional users % N	Regular users % N	Daily users % N
Tranquility	1	73. 3 (387)	40. 4 (19)	53. 8 (42)	77. 0 (114)	81. 4 (162)	89. 3 (50)
Increased sensory awareness	2	69. 3 (366)	31. 9 (15)	53. 8 (42)	67. 6 (100)	81. 9 (163)	82. 1 (46)
Hunger	3	68. 9 (364)	25. 5 (12)	64. 1 (50)	59. 5 (88)	82. 4 (164)	89. 3 (50)
Giggles	4	64. 8 (342)	34. 0 (16)	57. 7 (45)	66. 2 (98)	73. 9 (147)	64. 3 (36)
Distortion of time sense	5	63. 3 (334)	36. 2 (17)	57. 7 (45)	60. 8 (90)	72. 9 (145)	66. 1 (37)
Drowsiness	6	56. 3 (297)	17. 0 (8)	61. 5 (48)	58. 1 (86)	63. 3 (126)	51. 8 (29)
Euphoria	7	49. 6 (262)	23. 4 (11)	32. 1 (25)	48. 0 (71)	59. 3 (118)	66. 1 (37)
Introspectiveness	8	45. 8 (242)	12. 8 (6)	30. 8 (24)	41. 9 (62)	57. 8 (115)	62 5 (35)
Difficulty with concentration	9	43. 2 (228)	21. 3 (10)	55. 1 (43)	31. 8 (47)	53. 3 (106)	39. 3 (22)
Love for fellow man	10. 5	40. 7 (215)	12. 8 (6)	32. 1 (25)	35. 1 (52)	50. 8 (101)	55. 4 (31)
Psychological insight	10. 5	40. 7 (215)	6. 4 (3)	24. 5 (23)	27. 7 (41)	58. 8 (117)	55. 4 (31)
Eroticism	12	39. 6 (209)	12. 8 (6)	33. 3 (26)	39. 9 (59)	48. 2 (96)	39. 3 (22)
Openness to suggestion	13	36. 2 (191)	10. 6 (5)	33. 3 (26)	25. 0 (37)	44. 7 (89)	60. 7 (34)
Heightened creativity	14	32. 8 (173)	6. 4 (3)	17. 9 (14)	25. 0 (37)	43. 7 (87)	57. 1 (32)
Greater honesty	15	30. 5 (161)	6. 4 (3)	21. 8 (17)	25. 7 (38)	36. 2 (72)	55. 4 (31)
Altered depth perception	16	25. 6 (135)	21. 3 (10)	26. 9 (21)	21. 6 (32)	30. 7 (61)	19. 6 (11)
Depression	17	23. 7 (125)	14. 9 (7)	33. 3 (26)	16. 9 (25)	29. 1 (58)	16. 1 (9)
Fear	18	23. 3 (123)	19. 1 (9)	25. 6 (20)	19. 6 (29)	26. 6 (53)	21. 4 (12)
Synesthesia	19	22. 5 (119)	4. 3 (2)	19. 2 (15)	19. 6 (29)	27. 1 (54)	33. 9 (19)
Greater ability to concentrate	20	22. 2 (117)	12. 8 (6)	3. 9 (3)	22. 3 (33)	25. 6 (51)	42. 9 (24)

Sadness	21	21.2 (112)	14.9 (7)	23.1 (18)	19.6 (29)	22.1 (44)	25.0 (14)
Self-consciousness or embarrassment	22	18.6 (98)	10.6 (5)	19.2 (15)	9.5 (14)	25.1 (50)	25.0 (14)
Religious or mystical feelings	23	18.0 (95)	2.1 (1)	14.1 (11)	13.5 (20)	22.1 (44)	33.9 (19)
Hallucinations	24	17.2 (91)	8.5 (4)	15.4 (12)	12.8 (19)	19.1 (38)	32.1 (18)
Hyperactivity	25	15.5 (82)	6.4 (3)	11.5 (9)	10.1 (15)	20.1 (40)	26.8 (15)
Better judgment	26	13.4 (71)	2.1 (1)	5.1 (4)	6.8 (10)	19.1 (38)	32.1 (18)
Telepathy	27.5	12.5 (66)	6.4 (3)	10.3 (8)	7.4 (11)	16.1 (32)	21.4 (12)
Poor judgment	27.5	12.5 (66)	8.5 (4)	24.4 (19)	8.1 (12)	12.6 (25)	10.7 (6)
Headaches	29	11.4 (60)	14.9 (7)	14.1 (11)	8.1 (12)	10.6 (21)	16.1 (9)
Grandeur or feeling of omnipotence	30	8.5 (45)	2.1 (1)	11.5 (9)	7.4 (11)	7.5 (15)	16.1 (9)
Nausea	31	7.4 (39)	4.3 (2)	14.1 (11)	8.1 (12)	4.0 (8)	10.7 (6)
Anger	32	4.2 (22)	0.0 (0)	2.6 (2)	5.4 (8)	4.5 (9)	5.4 (3)
Less honesty	33	2.8 (15)	2.1 (1)	5.1 (4)	.7 (1)	3.0 (6)	5.4 (3)

to suggestion (36.2%), heightened creativity (32.8%), and greater honesty (30.5%). Fewer than 10% of all *S*s experienced grandeur or feelings of omnipotence (8.5%), nausea (7.4%), anger (4.2%), and being less honest (2.8%). The most frequently reported negatively valued phenomena are depression and fear, and these two reactions are reported by 23.7 and 23.3% of *S*s, respectively.

Consequently, *S*s using marihuana report experiencing considerably more pleasant than unpleasant phenomena, and what we have conservatively called neutral phenomena (e.g., openness to suggestion, altered depth perception) are probably experienced more as a pleasant effect rather than as a negative effect.

Table 6 is generated from the data in Table 5 and reports the ranked frequency of reported phenomena by use pattern group. An attempt was made to determine if there was a difference in reported effects by *S*s with differing use patterns. As use increases there is an increase in the reported frequency of the varying phenomena. This is understandable in that the more one uses marihuana, the more likely the occurrence of a variety of psychic effects. There are marked differences among use pattern groups in the frequency of the occurrence of certain phenomena. As use increases, there is an increase in the reporting of positively valued phenomena. Trial users report the least pleasant experience and the most unpleasant experiences. This would undoubtedly relate to their not becoming marihuana users in that their experiences were not that pleasant. For example, of the 13 most frequently reported phenomena for trial users, only four are positively valued, four negatively valued, and five neutrally valued whereas for daily users, of the 13 most frequently reported phenomena, nine are positively valued, none are negatively valued, and four are neutrally valued. In addition, what we have called "neutrally" valued probably become positively valued as marihuana use increases. It is of interest that characteristic but unusual phenomena which might be distressing to the novice is less prominent to the habitual user. For example, *altered depth perception* is ranked seventh by trial users, fifteenth by past users, seventeenth by occasional users, sixteenth by regular users, and twenty-sixth by daily users. Obviously, adaptation to this characteristic phenomenon occurs with increased use, and it becomes less prominent in the consciousness of the user. This same phenomenon apparently applies to *difficulty with concentration*, which is ranked seventh by trial users, fifth by past users, eleventh by occasional users, tenth by regular users, and fifteenth by daily users. *Distortion of time sense*, another characteristic phenomenon, apparently does not "adapt" in the same fashion, as this phenomenon is ranked high by all groups: second by trial users, third by past users, fourth by occasional users, fifth by regular users, and fourth by daily users. *Hunger* is also among the top five ranked phenomena by all use pattern groups.

It is interesting to observe the difference among groups in reported *drowsiness*. Trial users rank it tenth, past users second, occasional and regular users sixth, and daily users thirteenth. Although it is somewhat pretentious to speculate on the dynamics of these differences, it may be that trial users did not relax enough to get the drowsiness sensation, past users had it so frequently so as to make the experience uninteresting, occasional and regular users experience it as part of the total marihuana experience, and daily users have integrated use into their life style to such an extent that marihuana ceases to dull the consciousness as it does in less frequent users.

Post-marihuana *depression* is a sometimes complaint of marihuana users. Past users rank depression ninth and trial users rank it twelfth, whereas occasional users rank it twenty-one, regular users seventeenth, and daily users twenty-eighth. Consequently there is a large difference in the occurrence of depression among use pattern groups with past users reporting the greatest, and daily users the least prominence of this phenomenon in their marihuana experience.

Great differences also occur among use pattern groups in the prominence of other negatively valued phenomenon: *fear* is ranked ninth by trial users, sixteenth by past users, and twenty-fourth by daily users; *headaches* are ranked twelfth by trial users, and twenty-seventh, twenty-ninth, and twenty-eighth by occasional, regular, and daily users, respectively; *sadness* is ranked twelfth by trial users and twenty-second by regular and daily users.

The greatest differences among use pattern groups appear to be in the prominence and frequency of positively valued phenomena. Positive psychologically oriented phenomena are reported more frequently as use increases. For example, *heightened creativity* is ranked ninth by daily users (57.1%), fourteenth by regular users (43.7%), fourteenth by occasional users (25.0%), twenty-second by past users (17.9%), and twenty-fourth by trial users (6.4%). *Greater honesty* is ranked eleventh by daily users (55.4%), fifteenth by regular users (36.2%), thirteenth by occasional users (25.7%), nineteenth by past users (21.8%), and twenty-fourth by trial users (6.4%). *Introspectiveness* is ranked seventh by daily users (62.5%), ninth by regular users (57.8%), thirteenth by past users (30.8%), and fifteenth by trial users (12.8%). *Euphoria* is ranked fourth by daily

Table 6

Rank	Trial users	Percentage of *S*s reporting	Rank	Past users	Percentage of *S*s reporting	Rank	Occasional users	Percentage of *S*s reporting
1	Tranquility	(40. 4)	1	Hunger	(64. 1)	1	Tranquility	(77. 0)
2	Distortion of time sense	(36. 2)	2	Drowsiness	(61. 5)	2	Increased sensory awareness	(67. 6)
3	Giggles	(34. 0)	3. 5	Giggles	(57 7)	3	Giggles	(66. 2)
4	Increased sensory awareness	(31. 9)	3. 5	Distortion of time sense	(57. 7)	4	Distortion of time sense	(60. 8)
5	Hunger	(25. 5)	5	Difficulty with concentration	(55. 1)	5	Hunger	(59. 5)
6	Euphoria	(23. 4)	6. 5	Tranquility	(53. 8)	6	Drowsiness	(58. 1)
7. 5	Altered depth perception	(21. 3)	6. 5	Increased sensory awareness	(53. 8)	7	Euphoria	(48. 0)
7. 5	Difficulty with concentration	(21. 3)	9	Eroticism	(33. 3)	8	Introspectiveness	(41. 9)
9	Fear	(19. 1)	9	Depression	(33. 3)	9	Eroticism	(39. 9)
10	Drowsiness	(17. 0)	9	Openness to suggestion	(33. 3)	10	Love for fellow man	(35. 1)
12	Headaches	(14. 9)	11. 5	Euphoria	(32. 1)	11	Difficulty with concentration	(31. 8)
12	Sadness	(14. 9)	11. 5	Love for fellow man	(32. 1)	12	Psychological insight	(27. 7)
12	Depression	(14. 9)	13	Introspectiveness	(30. 8)	13	Greater honesty	(25. 7)
15. 5	Introspectiveness	(12. 8)	14	Psychological insight	(29. 5)	14. 5	Openness to suggestion	(25. 0)
15. 5	Love for fellow man	(12. 8)	15	Altered depth perception	(26. 9)	14. 5	Heightened creativity	(25. 0)
15. 5	Eroticism	(12. 8)	16	Fear	(25. 6)	16	Greater ability to concentrate	(22. 3)
15. 5	Greater ability to concentrate	(12. 8)	17	Poor judgment	(24. 4)	17	Altered depth perception	(21. 6)

Rank Order of Marihuana-Induced Experiences by Use Pattern Groups

Rank	Regular users	Percentage of *S*s reporting	Rank	Daily users	Percentage of *S*s reporting
1	Hunger	(82.4)	1.5	Tranquility	(89.3)
2	Increased sensory awareness	(81.9)	1.5	Hunger	(89.3)
3	Tranquility	(81.4)	3	Increased sensory awareness	(82.1)
4	Giggles	(73.9)	4.5	Distortion of time sense	(66.1)
5	Distortion of time sense	(72.9)	4.5	Euphoria	(66.1)
6	Drowsiness	(63.3)	6	Giggles	(64.3)
7	Euphoria	(59.3)	7	Introspectiveness	(62.5)
8	Psychological insight	(58.8)	8	Openness to suggestion	(60.7)
9	Introspectiveness	(57.8)	9	Heightened creativity	(57.1)
10	Difficulty with concentration	(53.3)	11	Greater honesty	(55.4)
11	Love for fellow man	(50.8)	11	Love for fellow man	(55.4)
12	Eroticism	(48.2)	11	Psychological insight	(55.4)
13	Openness to suggestion	(44.7)	13	Drowsiness	(51.8)
14	Heightened creativity	(43.7)	14	Greater ability to concentrate	(42.9)
15	Greater honesty	(36.2)	15.5	Difficulty with concentration	(39.3)
16	Altered depth perception	(30.7)	15.5	Eroticism	(39.3)
17	Depression	(29.1)	17.5	Synesthesia	(33.9)

(*continued*)

Table 6

Rank	Trial users	Percentage of *S*s reporting	Rank	Past users	Percentage of *S*s reporting	Rank	Occasional users	Percentage of *S*s reporting
18. 5	Self-consciousness or embarrassment	(10. 6)	18	Sadness	(23. 1)	19	Sadness	(19. 6)
18. 5	Openness to suggestion	(10. 6)	19	Greater honesty	(21. 8)	19	Fear	(19. 6)
20. 5	Poor judgment	(8. 5)	20. 5	Synesthesia	(19. 2)	19	Synesthesia	(19. 6)
20. 5	Hallucinations	(8. 5)	20. 5	Self-consciousness or embarrassment	(19. 2)	21	Depression	(16. 9)
24	Psychological insight	(6. 4)	22	Heightened creativity	(17. 9)	22	Religious or mystical feelings	(13. 5)
24	Heightened creativity	(6. 4)	23	Hallucinations	(15. 4)	23	Hallucinations	(12. 8)
24	Greater honesty	(6. 4)	25	Nausea	(14. 1)	24	Hyperactivity	(10. 1)
24	Telepathy	(6. 4)	25	Headaches	(14. 1)	25	Self-consciousness or embarrassment	(9. 5)
24	Hyperactivity	(6. 4)	25	Religious or mystical feelings	(14. 1)	27	Headaches	(8. 1)
27. 5	Nausea	(4. 3)	27. 5	Hyperactivity	(11. 5)	27	Poor judgment	(8. 1)
27. 5	Synesthesia	(4. 3)	27. 5	Grandeur or feelings of omnipotence	(11. 5)	27	Nausea	(8. 1)
30. 5	Less honesty	(2. 1)	29	Telepathy	(10. 3)	29. 5	Grandeur or feelings of omnipotence	(7. 4)
30. 5	Better judgment	(2. 1)	30. 5	Better judgment	(5. 1)	29. 5	Telepathy	(7. 4)
30. 5	Religious or mystical feelings	(2. 1)	30. 5	Less honesty	(5. 1)	31	Better judgment	(6. 8)
30. 5	Grandeur or feelings of omnipotence	(2. 1)	32	Greater ability to concentrate	(3. 9)	32	Anger	(5. 4)
33	Anger	(0. 0)	33	Anger	(2. 6)	33	Less honesty	(0. 7)

(continued)

Rank	Regular users	Percentage of *S*s reporting	Rank	Daily users	Percentage of *S*s reporting
18	Synesthesia	(27. 1)	17. 5	Religious or mystical feelings	(33. 9)
19	Fear	(26. 6)	19. 5	Better judgment	(32. 1)
20	Greater ability to concentrate	(25. 6)	19. 5	Hallucinations	(32. 1)
21	Self-consciousness or embarrassment	(25. 1)	21	Hyperactivity	(26. 8)
22. 5	Sadness	(22. 1)	22. 5	Sadness	(25. 0)
22. 5	Religious or mystical feelings	(22. 1)	22. 5	Self-consciousness or embarrassment	(25. 0)
24	Hyperactivity	(20. 1)	24. 5	Telepathy	(21. 4)
25. 5	Better judgment	(19. 1)	24. 5	Fear	(21. 4)
25. 5	Hallucinations	(19. 1)	26	Altered depth perception	(19. 6)
27	Telepathy	(16. 1)	28	Headaches	(16. 1)
28	Poor judgment	(12. 6)	28	Depression	(16. 1)
29	Headaches	(10. 6)	28	Grandeur or feelings of omnipotence	(16. 1)
30	Grandeur or feelings of omnipotence	(7. 4)	30. 5	Nausea	(10. 7)
31	Anger	(4. 5)	30. 5	Poor judgment	(10. 7)
32	Nausea	(4. 0)	32. 5	Anger	(5. 4)
33	Less honesty	(3. 0)	32. 5	Less honesty	(5. 4)

users (66.1%), seventh by regular users (59.3%), and eleventh by past users (32.1%). It is of interest to note that *greater ability to concentrate* is reported by 42.9% of daily users and ranked fourteenth, whereas only 3.9% of past users reported this phenomenon and ranked it thirty-second. It is also of interest that *eroticism* is ranked highest (ninth) by occasional (39.9%) and past users (33.3%), followed by regular users (48.2%) who rank it twelfth, and ranked equally low (fifteenth) by trial (12.8%) and daily users (39.3%). Thus eroticism appears to be of less prominence for daily and regular users than for less frequent users, and this may be because eroticism is less integrated for less frequent users than for more frequent users. Worth comment is the fact that few *S*s report feelings of *anger* with marihuana. Anger is ranked thirtieth by daily, thirty-first by regular, thirty-second by occasional, and thirty-third by past and trial users. *Less honesty* is another infrequently reported phenomenon by all groups: ranked last by daily, regular, and occasional users, and thirtieth by past and trial users. *Poor judgment* is ranked low by current users: thirtieth by daily, twenty-eighth by regular, and twenty-seventh by occasional users, but ranked considerably higher (seventeenth) by past users and twentieth by trial users. *Hallucinations*, a supposedly common phenomenon with marihuana use, is ranked relatively low by all groups: twentieth by trial, twenty-third by past and occasional, twenty-fifth by regular, and nineteenth by daily users.

Thus the differences in experienced phenomena by use pattern groups are fairly clear: those who use it most report the greatest frequency of the most favorable phenomena and the least relative occurrence of negatively valued phenomenon, whereas past users and trial users, respectively, report the highest relative occurrence of negatively valued phenomena and the lowest relative occurrence of positively valued phenomena.

CHANGE IN SEXUAL ORIENTATION, AND ALCOHOL AND TOBACCO CONSUMPTION AS AN EFFECT OF MARIHUANA USE

Respondents were asked if the use of marihuana had altered their sexual orientation. Of the 495 *S*s answering this item, 88.3% answered that marihuana use had no effect on their sexual orientation whereas 11.7% stated it had had some effect. Four *S*s (0.9%) (one past user, two occasional users, and one daily user) stated their sexual orientation had changed in the direction of homosexuality; 24 *S*s (4.9%) (two past users, three occasional users, 15 regular users, and four daily users) stated their sexual orientation had changed in the direction of heterosexuality; and 30 *S*s (6.1 %) (one trial user, one past user, five occasional users, 17 regular users, and six daily users) stated their sexual orientation had changed in the direction of bisexuality. For this latter category, we have no data indicating what percentage of *S*s who were tending toward a bisexual orientation were previously exclusively heterosexual and what percentage had previously been exclusively homosexual. Thus the most frequent change (6.1 %) in sexual orientation is toward bisexuality, followed by a change (4.9 %) toward heterosexuality, with few *S*s (0.9 %) changing toward homosexuality. These data do not support the contention that marihuana use causes marked changes in sexual orientation.

Respondents were asked if marihuana had altered their use of alcohol. Table 7 shows the results of this question by use pattern group. As marihuana use increases, there is a decrease in the use of alcohol. Very few *S*s (total of 13) report an increase in alcohol consumption. The percentage of *S*s reporting a decrease in alcohol consumption rises sharply as marihuana use increases. These data tend to support the contention that marihuana replaces alcohol use. Other data available indicate that when *S*s were asked their use of alcohol, current users reported more use of alcohol than nonusers or past users. Thus it is not that marihuana users use less alcohol than nonusers, but that the more they use marihuana, the less they use alcohol. A confounding factor in these data, however, is that wine consumption was not separated out from use of hard liquor. It is apparently a very common practice that wine and marihuana are used simultaneously. Consequently marihuana users reported usage of alcohol may be highly determined by their use of wine rather than hard liquor. When *S*s were asked if the reasons for their use of marihuana

Table 7

Effect of Marihuana in Changing Use of Alcohol by Use Pattern Group

Change in alcohol use	Use pattern group: Trial users %	N	Past users %	N	Occasional users %	N	Regular users %	N	Daily users %	N
Alcohol increased	3.0	(1)	1.3	(1)	0.7	(1)	4.7	(9)	1.8	(1)
Alcohol decreased	6.1	(2)	14.7	(11)	27.5	(39)	41.7	(80)	60.0	(33)
No change	90.1	(30)	84.0	(63)	71.8	(102)	53.6	(103)	38.2	(21)
		(33)		(75)		(142)		(192)		(55)

Table 8

Effect of Marihuana Use on Tobacco Use by Use Pattern Group

Change in tobacco use	Use pattern group							
	Past users		Occasional users		Regular users		Daily users	
	%	N	%	N	%	N	%	N
Tobacco increase	5.4	(4)	2.9	(4)	10.5	(20)	10.9	(6)
Tobacco decrease	12.2	(9)	5.0	(7)	12.1	(23)	29.1	(16)
No change	82.4	(61)	92.1	(129)	77.4	(147)	60.0	(33)
		(74)		(140)		(190)		(55)

paralleled most peoples use of alcohol, among the current users there was an inverse relationship between answering this question positively and frequency of marihuana use. That is, 66.9% of occasional users, 42.7% of regular users, and 34.6% of daily users answered "yes," i.e., that their *reasons* for using marihuana were the same as most peoples' *reasons* for using alcohol. Thus it appears that as an individual's marihuana use increases, his use of alcohol declines, that the heavier the use of marihuana, the less likely is the individual to judgc the reason for his use of marihuana parallels other peoples' reason for using alcohol, but that in frequency of use, the heavier the use of marihuana, the heavier the use of alcohol. This last fact, however, might be highly contaminated by the use of wine by marihuana users rather than hard liquor, though we have no data on this factor.

Respondents were asked if their marihuana use had increased, decreased, or had no effect on their use of tobacco. Table 8 shows the results of this question by use pattern group. The majority of respondents in all use groups state that marihuana use has had no effect on their tobacco consumption. Very few respondents (from 2.9 to 10.9%) state their tobacco use has increased as a function of their marihuana use. Twice as many daily users (29.1%) than any other use group state that their tobacco consumption has *decreased* as a function of their marihuana use. Consequently marihuana use does not appear to affect tobacco consumption with the exception of daily marihuana users, 29.1% of whom state their tobacco consumption decreased as a function of marihuana use.

CHANGES IN ATTRIBUTES OF SELF AS A FUNCTION OF MARIHUANA USE

Respondents were asked if they attributed any change in themselves in a number of areas in their life as a function of their use of marihuana. Table 9 shows the results of this question.

Table 9
Changes in Attributes of Self as a Function of Marihuana Use by Use Pattern Group

	Use pattern group							
	Past users		Occasional users		Regular users		Daily users	
	%	*N*	%	*N*	%	*N*	%	*N*
Self-knowledge								
Increased	30.4	(21)	34.3	(48)	59.3	(115)	70.9	(39)
Decreased	1.5	(1)	0.0	(0)	0.0	(0)	0.0	(0)
No change	47.8	(33)	54.3	(76)	32 5	(63)	20.0	(11)
Doesn't apply	20.3	(14)	11.4	(16)	8.3	(16)	9.1	(5)
Self-approval								
Increased	8.7	(6)	21.4	(30)	35.9	(69)	56.4	(31)
Decreased	13.0	(9)	2.1	(3)	2.1	(4)	1.8	(1)
No change	56.5	(39)	64.3	(90)	47.9	(92)	30.9	(17)
Doesn't apply	21.7	(15)	12.1	(17)	14.1	(27)	10.9	(6)
Sexual pleasure								
Increased	25.4	(17)	33.6	(47)	57.5	(111)	69.8	(37)
Decreased	1.5	(1)	0.7	(1)	1.0	(2)	0.0	(0)
No change	53.7	(36)	56.4	(79)	34.2	(66)	26.4	(14)
Doesn't apply	19.4	(13)	9.3	(13)	7.3	(14)	3.8	(2)
Enjoyment of music, movies, paintings, TV								
Increased	36.2	(25)	55.4	(77)	81.4	(158)	83.3	(45)
Decreased	0.0	(0)	0.7	(1)	0.0	(0)	0.0	(0)
No change	43.5	(30)	37.4	(52)	16.0	(31)	14.8	(8)
Doesn't apply	20.3	(14)	6.5	(9)	2.6	(5)	1.9	(1)
Enjoyment of nature								
Increased	34.8	(24)	46.7	(64)	75.5	(145)	75.9	(41)
Decreased	1.5	(1)	0.7	(1)	0.0	(0)	0.0	(0)
No change	46.4	(32)	46.7	(64)	20.3	(39)	22.2	(12)
Doesn't apply	17.4	(12)	5.8	(8)	4.1	(8)	1.9	(1)
Ability to communicate with others								
Increased	18.6	(13)	25.0	(35)	47.1	(89)	63.5	(33)
Decreased	5.7	(4)	0.7	(1)	2.7	(5)	1.9	(1)
No change	58.6	(41)	62.9	(88)	40.7	(77)	30.8	(16)
Doesn't apply	17.1	(12)	11.4	(16)	9.5	(18)	3.9	(2)
Ability to think through problems								
Increased	10.3	(7)	12.1	(17)	22.4	(43)	39.6	(21)
Decreased	11.8	(8)	3.6	(5)	7.3	(14)	3.8	(2)
No change	58.8	(40)	73.6	(103)	62.0	(119)	54.7	(29)
Doesn't apply	19.1	(13)	10.7	(15)	8.3	(16)	1.9	(1)

(continued)

Table 9 (continued)

	Use pattern group			
	Past users	Occasional users	Regular users	Daily users
	% N	% N	% N	% N
Creativity, imagination				
Increased	10.3 (7)	23.0 (32)	49.0 (94)	63.0 (34)
Decreased	7.4 (5)	0.7 (1)	0.5 (1)	1.9 (1)
No change	61.8 (42)	66.2 (92)	44.8 (86)	33.3 (18)
Doesn't apply	20.6 (14)	10.1 (14)	5.7 (11)	1.9 (1)
Memory				
Increased	3.0 (2)	2.9 (4)	6.8 (13)	15.1 (8)
Decreased	16.4 (11)	7.9 (11)	20.4 (39)	20.8 (11)
No change	59.7 (40)	77.0 (107)	67.0 (128)	62.3 (33)
Doesn't apply	20.9 (14)	12.2 (17)	5.8 (11)	1.9 (1)
Mystical interest				
Increased	19.4 (13)	23.0 (32)	43.0 (83)	52.8 (28)
Decreased	1.5 (1)	1.4 (2)	1.0 (2)	1.9 (1)
No change	55.2 (37)	59.7 (83)	44.0 (85)	41.5 (22)
Doesn't apply	23.9 (16)	15.8 (22)	11.9 (23)	3.8 (2)
Sense of responsibility				
Increased	4.4 (3)	6.4 (9)	10.4 (20)	18.9 (10)
Decreased	15.9 (11)	3.6 (5)	12.5 (24)	9.4 (5)
No change	60.9 (42)	73.6 (103)	66.1 (127)	66.0 (35)
Doesn't apply	18.8 (13)	16.4 (23)	10.9 (21)	5.7 (3)
Acceptance of conventional values				
Increased	5.9 (4)	0.7 (1)	3.6 (7)	5.6 (3)
Decreased	32.4 (22)	37.7 (52)	58.0 (112)	61.1 (33)
No change	41.2 (28)	51.4 (71)	26.9 (52)	24.1 (13)
Doesn't apply	20.6 (14)	10.1 (14)	11.4 (22)	9.3 (5)
Conformity to conventional modes of behavior				
Increased	0.0 (0)	0.7 (1)	2.1 (4)	1.9 (1)
Decreased	25.4 (17)	34.8 (48)	56.5 (109)	64.8 (35)
No change	56.7 (38)	55.1 (76)	32.6 (63)	31.5 (17)
Doesn't apply	17.9 (12)	9.4 (13)	8.8 (17)	1.9 (1)
Conventional religious interest				
Increased	4.4 (3)	3.6 (5)	4.7 (9)	7.6 (4)
Decreased	10.3 (7)	8.0 (11)	18.8 (36)	24.5 (13)
No change	64.7 (44)	70.3 (97)	57.1 (109)	49.1 (26)
Doesn't apply	20.6 (14)	18.1 (25)	19.4 (37)	18.9 (10)

Self-Knowledge and Self-Approval. As marihuana use increases, there is an increase in self-knowledge and self-approval. Among daily users, 70.9% reported an increase of self-knowledge, and only one *S* of the total group reported a decrease in self-knowledge. Daily users also reported the highest increase, 56.4%, in self-approval, and past users reported the highest decrease, 13.0%, in self-approval. Consequently, the more one uses, the greater the probability of his reporting an increase in self-knowledge and self-approval, with no current users reporting a decrease in self-knowledge and a minimum number reporting a decrease in self-approval.

Enjoyment of Nature, Music, Movies, Sexual Pleasures, etc. As marihuana use increases, there is an increase in sexual pleasure. Daily users report the highest increase in sexual pleasure, 69.8%, and past users report the least amount of increase, 25.4%. Only three *S*s of the total group report a decrease in sexual pleasure. As use increases, there is an increase in the enjoyment of music, movies, painting, TV, etc. A high percentage of regular and daily users, 81.4 and 83.3% respectively, report an increase in enjoyment in these areas. Only one *S* of the total group reported a decrease of enjoyment in these areas. Again, past users report the least increase, 36.2%. As use increases, there is an increase in the enjoyment of nature. Only two *S*s of the total group report a decrease in this area. A high percentage of regular and daily users, 75.5 and 75.9%, respectively, report an increase in enjoyment of nature.

Ability to Communicate, Think Through Problems, and to be Creative and Imaginative. As marihuana use increases, there is an increase in the ability to communicate with others, to think through problems, and to be creative and imaginative. Only seven current users (about 1%) report a decrease in the ability to communicate, and three report a decrease in the ability to be creative and imaginative. A larger, but still negligible percentage (about 5%), report a decrease in the ability to think through problems. Daily users again report the greatest increase, 63.5%, in ability to communicate and the greatest increase, 63.0%, in creativity and imagination. Past users report the smallest percentage of increase and the largest percentage of decrease in all three areas.

Memory. Among all use groups, the majority of *S*s report no change in memory. However, 20% of both regular and daily users report a decrease in memory whereas 16% of past users and 8% of occasional users report such a decrease. It is of interest to note that 15% of daily users report an increase in memory function whereas only 7, 3, and 3% of the other use groups report such an increase. Consequently, the majority of *S*s report no change in memory with about 20% of regular and daily users reporting a decrease and 15% of daily users an increase.

Mystical Interest and Conventional Religious Interest. As use increases, there is an increase in mystical interest and a decrease in conventional religious interest. Except for daily users, the majority of users report no change in their interest in conventional religion. Very few *S*s report an increase in conventional religious interest and few *S*s report a decrease in mystical interest. Daily users report the highest increase, 52.8%, in mystical interest and the highest decrease, 24.5%, in conventional religious interest.

Sense of Responsibility. The majority of all *S*s in all use groups report no change in sense of responsibility. As use increases, there is an increase in sense of responsibility, with 18.9% of daily users reporting such an increase. Past users report the highest decrease, 15.9%, in sense of responsibility whereas 12.5% of regular users report a decrease, and 9.4% of daily and 3.6% of occasional users report such a decrease. Consequently, most *S*s report no change in sense of responsibility with past users reporting the highest decrease (15.9%) and daily users reporting the highest increase (18.9%).

Conformity to Conventional Modes of Behavior and Acceptance of Conventional Values. As use increases, there is a decrease in acceptance of conventional values and a decrease in conformity to conventional modes of behavior. Very few *S*s report an increase in either area. Past users report the least change and daily users the greatest changes in these two areas. There is a greater change for all groups in their value system than there is in their conformity to conventional modes of behavior. Consequently, behavior changes appear more slowly than value changes.

The results of these aspects of attributes of self as a function of marihuana use are not surprising. The greater the use of marihuana, the more favorable the reporting of the consequences of that use. Past users report the least favorable results and the greatest negative results, whereas daily users generally report the greatest favorable results and the least negative results. It is of interest that a very high percentage of users reported favorable results in almost all areas and a negligible number of users reported unfavorable results. The only exception to this is in the area of memory, where one-fifth of daily and regular users report decreases in memory function. This phenomenon is certainly not new and is part of the marihuana folklore.

REASONS FOR USING MARIHUANA

Respondents were asked "How frequently do you take marihuana for the following reasons" and the *S*s marked "never," "occasionally," "frequently," or "always" to 16 listed reasons. Table 10 shows the results to this question by use pattern group with the reasons listed in order from the most to least frequent given reason for using as "frequently" or "always."

As use increases, there is an increase in the frequency of using marihuana for a variety of reasons. Daily users use marihuana for a greater variety of reasons more often than do regular users, and they, in turn, use for a greater variety of reasons more often than do occasional users. For example, 44.4% of daily users report "frequent or always" use of marihuana for "developing inner life" whereas 16.7% of regular users and 5.8% of occasional users report using marihuana with that frequency for that reason. Again 29.1% of daily users report "frequent or always" use of marinhuana for introspective psychological purposes whereas 15.4% of regular and 9.2% of occasional users report using that often for that purpose. Among daily users, 34.5% report "frequent or always" use for "facilitating creative abilities" whereas 13.9% of regular and 5.8% of occasional users report using marihuana that frequently for that endeavor. This pattern is seen throughout the data and consistently applies to all motivations—the more one uses, the more varied are the reasons for use. Consequently, the greater the use of marihuana, the greater the effects of the drug and the more varied the experiences with the drug. This confirms other data in the study.

The primary reason for using marihuana is "to have fun," supporting the notion that marihuana, regardless of the plethora of reasons for use, is a pleasure-recreational drug. Of note is that this reason is given almost twice as frequently as the second most popular reason. The second most popular reason, like the first, is to increase and sustain pleasure. The third most frequent reason is again in the service of pleasure, i.e., to be relieved of boredom, monotony, and dullness. The fourth ranked reason is of a different quality, that of inducing relaxation by relieving tension. The fifth ranked reason is again in the service of pleasure, specifically sexual pleasure. The next four reasons given are in the area of psychological introspectiveness, creativity, and sociability. Relatively few *S*s (about 5%) state that they "frequently or always" use marihuana out of a compulsion or something they feel they have to have. Thus it appears that few *S*s

Table 10

Rank order	No. *S*s reporting frequent or always	Reason	Occasional users: Never %	N	Occasionally %	N	Frequent or always %	N
1	280	To have fun	10.6	(15)	25.5	(36)	63.8	(90)
2	147	To make a good mood last longer or to make a fine feeling into an even better one	30.7	(43)	45.0	(63)	24.3	(34)
3	81	To relieve boredom, e.g., break up monotony or a dull period	45.8	(65)	44.4	(63)	9.9	(14)
4	75	To relieve tension or nervousness	45.8	(65)	44.4	(63)	9.9	(14)
5	72	To improve your sexual appetite or sensitivity or to improve your sexual capacities	46.1	(65)	39.7	(56)	14.2	(20)
6	64	To develop inner life	74.8	(104)	19.4	(27)	5.8	(8)
7	60	To make you more friendly or extroverted, to enhance sociability	52.5	(73)	36.7	(51)	10.8	(15)
8	59	To find out more about yourself, e.g., about your personality, your inner problems, or your human potentials	62.4	(88)	28.4	(40)	9.2	(13)
9	54	To facilitate creative abilities	76.8	(106)	17.4	(24)	5.8	(8)
10	31	To make you feel less depressed or sad	74.6	(106)	23.2	(33)	2.1	(3)
11	26	To have a religious or mystical feeling or to come close to God	85.2	(121)	13.4	(19)	1.4	(2)
12.5	17	To relieve or counteract anger or irritability	84.3	(118)	15.0	(21)	0.7	(1)
12.5	17	To satisfy a strong craving or compulsion, something you just *had* to have	90.8	(129)	6.3	(9)	2.8	(4)
14.5	10	To make you feel less afraid or more courageous	90.8	(128)	7.8	(11)	1.4	(2)
14.5	10	To make you smarter or improve your ability to learn or remember things	95.7	(135)	4.3	(6)	0.0	(0)
16	1	To reduce sexual desires or sexual activities	97.1	(135)	2.9	(4)	0.0	(0)

Reasons for Using Marihuana by Use Pattern Group

Regular users			Daily users		
Never	Occasionally	Frequent or always	Never	Occasionally	Frequent or always
% N	% N	% N	% N	% N	% N
4.1 (8)	23.2 (45)	72.7 (141)	1.8 (1)	10.7 (6)	87.5 (49)
14.9 (29)	40.2 (78)	44.8 (87)	13.0 (7)	38.9 (21)	33.8 (26)
25.4 (50)	50.8 (100)	23.9 (47)	12.5 (7)	51.8 (29)	35.7 (20)
28.4 (55)	50.0 (97)	21.6 (42)	13.5 (7)	50.0 (26)	36.5 (19)
41.8 (82)	40.8 (80)	17.3 (34)	20.4 (11)	46.3 (25)	33.3 (18)
57.8 (111)	25.5 (49)	16.7 (32)	33.3 (18)	22.2 (12)	44.4 (24)
40.7 (79)	42.8 (83)	16.5 (32)	34.5 (19)	41.8 (23)	23.6 (13)
49.2 (96)	35.4 (69)	15.4 (30)	34.5 (19)	36.4 (20)	29.1 (16)
53.6 (104)	32.5 (63)	13.9 (27)	30.9 (17)	34.5 (19)	34.5 (19)
51.0 (98)	39.1 (75)	9.9 (19)	18.9 (10)	64.2 (34)	17.0 (9)
75.9 (148)	17.9 (35)	6.2 (12)	60.0 (33)	18.2 (10)	21.8 (12)
72.3 (141)	23.6 (46)	4.1 (8)	37.0 (20)	48.1 (26)	14.8 (8)
78.1 (153)	17.9 (35)	4.1 (8)	64.3 (35)	25.9 (14)	9.3 (5)
84.5 (164)	14.9 (29)	0.5 (1)	72.2 (39)	24.1 (13)	3.7 (2)
91.2 (176)	6.7 (13)	2.1 (4)	74.5 (41)	14.5 (8)	10.9 (6)
96.9 (186)	3.1 (6)	0.0 (0)	92.6 (50)	5.6 (3)	1.9 (1)

feel they are addicted or habituated to marihuana use. Marihuana is seldom used to make one feel less afraid and more courageous, a concept that heretofore has been much proposed by opponents of marihuana.

Summarily, the more one uses marihuana, the more varied the effects and the greater the breadth of reasons for use. Marihuana is used primarily for pleasure-recreational purposes and, secondly, for psychological introspective purposes. A sizeable number of daily users also use the drug to induce a religion-mystical consciousness. Few *S*s consistently use marihunana for any other reasons.

IMPLICATION FOR DRUG EDUCATION

Among our *S*s, there was a relationship between frequency of use and reported effects—the more frequent the use, the more varied the effects, the more pleasant and beneficial the effects, and the fewer the unpleasant and untoward effects. Those *S*s who had more unpleasant than pleasant effects either did not continue to use after trial experimentation or else they quit after some period of use. For those continuing to use, beneficial results far outweigh negatively valued results. In a previous paper (Fisher and Strantz, 1972) we have said, "... in approaching a project aimed at the ameliorating of drug abuse it behooves the change agent... (to) analyze whether use or abuse is occurring. He must first of all determine if the user... considers his drug use to be functional (usage) or dysfunctional (abusage), i.e., whether or not he sees his drug use as an integral part of his whole life style in that it enhances and enables him to meet needs and achieve goals, within his system, that he deems of value. If in fact, he evaluates his drug use as an enabling phenomenon within his total value orientation, it is highly unlikely that an external change agent is going to have much success in changing the user's *evaluation* of his drug experience.... If the user evaluates his drug usage as basically dysfunctional, i.e., not positively contributing to a realization of his value system, then the change agent has some entree into the user's psychological world." In a program with youthful drug offenders, Blumer (1967) sought to establish a core of prestigious youth leaders, who would be won over to a position of nonusage, and that these youths would by their opinion leadership position be influential in convincing other youths to give up drug usage. Blumer stated, "We found rather early we were not having any success in developing a form of collective abstinence. It became clear that the youths were well anchored in their drug use and well fortified in their belief against all the 'dangers' of drug use... we would invite any group of educators, scientists, welfare workers or police officials to try to meet effectively the well-buttressed arguments, based on personal experience and observation, that our youthful drug users present in frank, open and uncowed discussion. In sum, we learned that youthful drug users are just not interested in abstaining from drug use."

The results of this study would suggest that it would be highly unlikely that these marihuana users would give up their usage as they overwhelmingly report positive, rather than negative, results from their usage. If the dominant culture evaluates such drug usage to be dysfunctional, whereas the user judges such usage to be functional, what position and action can agents of the dominant culture take? The current position in America is to imprison the breaker of the cultural mores. An alternative would be to let the individual be his own judge as to the effective-ineffective use of the drug. A third alternative, the success of which rests upon the ingenuity of the establishment's change agent, is the ecological approach. Based on the assumption that for any one individual there exists a complex of interrelated variables relative to his drug use, and that it is the individual's evaluation of his drug use differential to each of these variables within his total system, we have earlier suggested, ". . . the only position the change agent can take is to induce a change in the *evaluation* by the user of his drug experience by changing the ecosystem of which that drug experience is but one part. The only entree the change agent has is through manipulating other variables in the ecosystem of the user. In manipulating and changing the character of the user's ecosystem lies the possibilities of changing the evaluation by the user of his drug usage" (Fisher and Strantz, 1972, p. 1409). We await with interest the reporting of research and treatment programs which successfully implement changes in the marihuana habituee's ecosystem which appreciably reduces his use of the drug.

ACKNOWLEDGMENTS

This study was conducted while both authors were at the University of California, Los Angeles, and was supported, in part, by NIMH Grant #5-T41 MH 10301. Computing assistance was obtained from the UCLA Health Sciences Computing Facility, sponsored by NIH Special Research Resources Grant RR–3.

REFERENCES

BLUM, R. H. *Society and Drugs*. San Francisco: Jossey-Bass, 1969.

BLUMER, H. The world of youthful drug abuse. *ADD Center Project*. Berkeley, California: Univ. California, 1967.

CANADIAN INTERIM REPORT. *Canadian Commission of Inquiry into the Non-Medical Use of Drugs*. Ottawa: Queen's Printer for Canada, 1970.

CLARKE, L. In Work with marihuana, I. Effects (S. H. Synder, ed.) *Psychol. Today* 4: 37–41 1971.

CRANCER, A. J., et al. Comparison of the effects of marihuana and alcohol on simulated driving performance. *Science* 164: 851–854 1969.

DURHAM, B. The marijuana psychosis (1968). In J. Kaplan (ed.) *Marihuana—The New Prohibition*. Cleveland: World, 1970.

FISHER, G., and STRANTZ, I. An ecosystems approach to the study of dangerous drug use and abuse with special reference to the marihuana issue, *Amer. J. Public Health* 62: 1407–1414, 1972.

GOODE, E. *The Marijuana Smokers*. New York: Basic Books, 1970.

HEKIMIAN, L. J., and GERSHON, S. Characteristics of drug abuses admitted to a psychiatric hospital. *J. Amer. Med. Assoc.* 205: 125–130, 1968.

ISBELL, H., et al. Effects of tetrahydrocannabinal in man. *Psychopharmacologia*, 11: 184–188, 1967.

JONES, R. T., and STONE, G. C. Psychological studies of marihuana and alcohol in man. Paper read at American Psychiatric Association Meeting, Bal Harbour, Florida, 1969.

KAPLAN, J. *Marijuana—The New Prohibition*. Cleveland: World, 1970.

KEELER, M. H. Adverse reactions to marijuana. *Amer. J. Psychiat.* 124: 128–131, 1967.

KIPLINGER, G. In Work with marihuana, I. Effects (S. H. Snyder, ed.) *Psychol. Today* 4: 37–41, 1971.

McGLOTHLIN, W. H., and WEST, L. J. The marihuana problem: an overview. *Amer. J. Psychiat.* 125: 126–134, 1968.

SHAFER, R. P. *Marihuana: A Signal of Misunderstanding*. New York: New American Library, 1972.

SMITH, D. E., and MEHL, C. An analysis of marijuana toxicity. In D. Smith (ed.) *Marihuana: The New Social Drug*. Englewood Cliffs, New Jersey: Prentice-Hall, 1970.

WEIL, A. T., ZINBERG, N. E., and NELSEN, J. Clinical and psychological effects of marijuana in man. *Science* 162: 1234–1242, 1968.

The International Journal of the Addictions, 9(1), pp. 127–136, 1974

Value Structure as a Predictor of Type of Discharge Among Residential Addicts

Jerome S. Miller, Ph.D.

NIDA Clinical Research Center
Lexington, Kentucky

John Sensenig, Ph.D.

University of Kentucky
Lexington, Kentucky

Jonathan S. Raymond, M.S.

NIDA Clinical Research Center
Lexington, Kentucky

Ever since Thomas and Znaniecki (1918) first suggested that the study of attitudes should be the central problem of social psychology, researchers in the area have placed a great deal of emphasis on the theory and measurement of attitude and attitude change. This concentration on attitudes was especially facilitated by a rapid development of methods for measuring attitudes and attitude change. As a result of the availability of measurement techniques and this concentration of emphasis and effort, social psychologists have provided, and are continuing to provide, a large body of literature concerning both attitudes and opinions.

While investigations into the nature of attitudes flourished, theoretical interest in values lagged behind. According to Rokeach (1971), one reason for this state of affairs was a lack of consensus and "a certain vagueness of understanding" about what was meant by values and how they differed from attitudes or opinions. A second reason was that simple and economical methods of measuring values had remained undeveloped. In the past, approaches to the measurement of values by Morris (1956), Kluckhohn and Stodtbeck (1961), Allport, Vernon, and Lindzey (1960), and others have been either too complex, too lengthy and time consuming, too general, or severely limited in the number of values employed.

Though a main focus of contemporary social psychology still centers on the study of attitudes and attitude change, some recent theoretical and empirical interest in values and value change has been aroused. This shift of interest toward values is due primarily to several emerging advantages of studying values, and is derived from the conceptual clarification of the differences between values and attitudes. While an attitude represents "an organization of interrelated beliefs that are all focussed on a specific object or situation. . . a value refers to desirable end states of existence (terminal value) or desirable modes of behavior (instrumental value)" (Rokeach, 1970, p. 2). A value is broader, more general, and probably more enduring than an attitude. A person conceivably may engage several thousands of attitudes, but be guided by only several dozen values at most. In short, values are more central, more dynamic, more economical, and more fundamental components of a person's social or personal identity.

Thus, as defined above, values are conceived to be partial determinants of both attitudes and behavior. By understanding how an individual preferentially orders his values, one may be able to understand and predict his social judgments, preferences, and behaviors. A value analysis approach might also be especially fruitful in the understanding of deviant behavior, i.e., drug addiction.

Prior research utilizing a value analysis approach to the study of addict behavior has proved to be particularly appropriate and valuable. Miller, Sensenig, and Reed (1972) used Stoner's (1968) value ranking instrument to study risky and cautious choice behavior in drug addicts. Using the Rokeach value ranking instrument (Rokeach, 1970), a later study by Miller, Sensenig, Stocker, and Campbell (1973) attempted a more comprehensive analysis of the value systems of drug addicts making comparisons, within their sample, between race and sex. This study revealed a number of meaningful distinctions among addicts' value systems and challenged the stereotype of homogeneity across addict samples. Further value studies were suggested by these findings.

Of special interest to the present study are two questions. How do stated values by addicts relate to their selection into a treatment population, and how do addicts' value structures correspond to treatment continuation or rejection? Employing the Rokeach value ranking instrument (Rokeach, 1970), the present study analyzes addicts' value systems with comparisons made according to the addicts' acceptance, continuation, and completion of treatment as well as their referral to a posttreatment program.

METHOD

Rokeach and his colleagues have developed and improved upon a value ranking instrument which has been administered to a number of diverse subject populations, including a national sample, analyzed by income, education, and race (Rokeach and Parker, 1970), political preference (Rokeach, 1970), religious beliefs (Rokeach, 1969), and extent of involvement with law enforcement (Rokeach, Miller, and Snyder, 1971).

According to Rokeach (1970), the value ranking instrument "is in many ways an ideal instrument. In a matter of 10 or 20 minutes it yields reasonably reliable measures of a respondent's 36 values; it is simple in design, easy to administer to individuals or groups and easy to understand regardless of educational level." The value instrument consists of one set of 18 *terminal* values which concern desirable end states of existence such as: "A world at peace," "Personal happiness," and "Inner harmony," and one set of *instrumental* values concerned with desirable modes of behavior such as: "Ambitious," "Loving," and "Polite." Each subject's task consists of ranking each of the two sets of values in relation to their order of importance to the subject as guiding principles in his or her life.

Due to the broad range of comparative data available from related research, and because of the relative ease with which it can be administered, the Rokeach Value Survey was employed in a prior study (Miller et al., 1973) to investigate value differences as to race and sex among narcotic addicts. The same large pool of data that had been used in the Miller et al. study was utilized in the present investigation. These data were obtained by administering the Value Survey to a cohort of 291 consecutive admissions to the NIMH Clinical Research Center as one of a number of procedures required for admission. All data were, thus, obtained prior to the assignment of subjects to treatment categories. The plan was to make comparisons between groups on the four major subgroup categories into which addicts fell during their hospital stay: addicts not suitable for treatment (NST), elopees (EL), addicts not suitable for aftercare (NSAC), and aftercare addicts (AC). NST addicts ($n = 125$) were screened out of the program during the initial screening procedure that immediately follows admission. ELs ($n = 28$) were addicts who independently chose to leave the program. Half, or 14, chose to elope during the evaluation-for-treatment phase; the other half left after having been adjudged suitable for treatment but prior to completion of their in-residence program. NSAC addicts ($n = 49$) were accepted into the residential program, but later were rejected before reaching the aftercare stage. AC addicts ($n = 89$) successfully completed the program and were referred to an aftercare program in the addict's home locality.

RESULTS AND DISCUSSION

By testing the median splits of combined ranking distributions with a chi-square analysis, several significant differences were found to exist between various pairs of groups on specific values. Table 1 shows the combined median, chi-square value, and level of significance for those values which did differ significantly.

Initial Selection

A major question with which the present study is concerned is: How do stated values of addicts relate to selection vs nonselection into a treatment population? This question may be answered by comparing the NST group with the other three groups under study (EL, NSAC, AC).

NST–AC Comparison. Table 1 shows that the largest number of significantly differing values occurred between the NST and the AC groups, and that these differences tended to show a greater degree of statistical significance. Significantly more NST addicts than AC addicts ranked the following values above the combined medians: the instrumental values "Obedient" ($p < .01$), "Polite" ($p < 0.5$), and "Clean" ($p < .05$); the terminal values "Pleasure" ($p < .025$) and "Exciting life" ($p < .025$). Significantly more AC addicts than NST addicts ranked the terminal values "A sense of accomplishment" ($p < .005$), "Wisdom" ($p < .005$), and "Inner harmony" ($p < .01$) above the combined medians.

In general, the AC group reports more concern with values expressive of self-understanding, inner direction, and task orientation. The value

Table 1
Combined Medians, Chi-Square Values, and Levels of Significant Differences Between the NST Group (n = 125) and AC (n = 49), and EL (n = 28) Groups

Groups[a]	Combined median	Chi-square	Significance level
NST–AC			
NST Higher-AC Lower			
Obedient (I)	14.50	6.94	.01
Pleasure (T)	11 83	6.26	.025
Exciting life (T)	12.18	6.03	.025
Polite (I)	13.06	4.24	.05
Clean (I)	7.97	3.98	.05
NST Lower-AC Higher			
Accomplishment (T)	8.57	9.17	.005
Wisdom (T)	4.94	8.58	.005
NST-EL			
NST Higher-EL Lower			
Pleasure (T)	11.62	7.91	.005
Capable (I)	7.94	5.03	.025
Imaginative (I)	13.11	5.03	.025
NST Lower-EL Higher			
Beauty (T)	13.62	4.87	.05
True friendship (T)	9.40	3.90	.05
NST-NSAC	No significant differences		

[a] (I), Instrumental value; (T), terminal value.

of "A sense of accomplishment" plus the terminal values of "Wisdom" and "Inner harmony" suggest an intrinsic motivation in AC addicts which might help explain their success in getting into and through treatment successfully. The NST group, on the other hand, appears to be more concerned with values which may be seen as only superficially related to treatment ("Polite," "Clean," "Obedient")—three values which distinguish the poor from the rich (Rokeach and Parker, 1970). The terminal values "Pleasure" and "An exciting life" suggest that the NST group may actually fit the common stereotype of the addict better than the AC group. Moreover, these terminal values may be significant of a greater attraction to the "street life" and actually genuine disinterest in treatment or acceptance into treatment.

NST–NSAC Comparison. As Table 1 shows, there is no noted difference between the NST and NSAC groups. The only value which approached significance was "Equality," and it was only marginally reliable ($p < .10$).

NST–EL Comparison. Table 1 shows significantly more NST than EL addicts to have ranked the terminal value "Pleasure" ($p < .005$) and the instrumental values "Capable" ($p < .025$) and "Imaginative" ($p < .025$) above the combined medians for the two groups. Significantly more EL than NST addicts ranked the terminal values of "A world of beauty" ($p < .05$) and "True friendship" ($p < .05$) above the combined median.

The NST group appears to be more concerned with obtaining pleasure as the ultimate goal in life. This may well be a carryover from drug experiences, and indicates that the NST group continues to value this orientation even though under treatment. The greater emphasis by NST addicts on the instrumental values of "Capable" and "Imaginative" suggests the intriguing possibility that an NST addict may be more characteristically the "hustler" type. The relationship between these instrumental values and the terminal value "Pleasure" is consistent with the notion that the NST group may be relatively concerned with being daring and creative, and that their needs for competence may well be seen as instrumental in assuring continued hedonic satisfaction.

The EL group appears to be more interested than the NST group in the interpersonal value "True friendship," which might indicate that they are less self-oriented than and more other-directed than the NST group. They also appear to be more aesthetic ("A world of beauty") than the NST addicts.

Continuation or Rejection

The second major question with which the present study is concerned is: How do addicts' value structures correspond to treatment continuation or rejection? This question may be answered by comparing the AC group with two groups of addicts who were either eliminated from further treatment (NSAC) or who eliminated themselves (EL).

AC–EL Comparison. As shown in Table 2, significantly more AC than EL addicts ranked the instrumental values "Responsible" ($p < .05$) and "Capable" ($p < .05$) higher than the combined median. Significantly more EL than AC addicts, however, ranked the instrumental values "Cheerful" ($p < .05$) and "Imaginative" ($p < .05$), and the terminal value "A world of beauty" ($p < .05$) above the combined medians.

The AC addicts seem to differ from the EL addicts in terms of a greater concern with task-oriented values ("Responsible" and "Capable") needed to pass successfully through treatment. Thus to remain in and complete treatment is possibly seen as behaving in a responsible, capable,

Table 2
Combined Medians, Chi-Square Values, and Levels of Significant Differences Between the AC Group (n = 89) and EL (n = 28) and NSAC (n = 49) Groups

Groups[a]	Combined median	Chi-square	Significance level
AC-EL			
AC Higher-EL Lower			
Responsible (I)	5.00	4.87	.05
Capable (I)	8.56	4.47	.05
AC Lower-EL Higher			
Cheerful (I)	11.58	4.97	.05
Imaginative (I)	12 56	4.92	.05
Beauty (T)	13.35	4.05	.05
AC-NSAC			
AC Higher-NSAC Lower			
Wisdom (T)	4.70	7.01	.01
AC Lower-NSAC Higher			
Obedient (I)	14.83	7.25	.01

[a] (I), Instrumental value; (T), terminal value.

competent manner. EL addicts, however, seem to value competency less and appear more to value personal inner states ("Cheerful" and "Imaginative") which are not dependent on external social judgment and do not require sustained task-orientation. The EL addicts also seem to be somewhat more aesthetically oriented, e.g., "A world of beauty." This pattern, contrasted with the AC group's apparent valuing of treatment as a good thing, aids in understanding why one group (EL addicts) leaves abortively (half even before their acceptability is determined) and the other group continues. This suggests further a possible difference in EL and AC addicts' perception of "the life" on the street and what the balance of its rewards and costs may be.

AC–NSAC Comparison. Significantly more AC than NSAC addicts ranked only the terminal value "Wisdom" ($p < .01$) higher than the combined median of the two groups. Significantly more NSAC addicts ranked the instrumental value "Obedient" ($p < .01$) higher than the combined median. Otherwise, the AC and NSAC groups hardly seem to differ in their value structures. Again, the AC group appears to be relatively concerned with "Wisdom" as an important end state of existence.

Being significantly less concerned with "Wisdom" while more concerned with "Obedient" suggests that the NSAC group, unlike the AC group, might be more oriented toward making superficial adjustments during the treatment—"going along with the program." That is, they present a picture of docile, dependent acceptance of treatment requirements rather than some more inner or self-determined purpose which seems more characteristic of the ACs. These values are consistent with distinguishing persons who, under treatment, make superficial adjustments but are unable to make changes which are deep enough or sustained enough to lead the staff to believe that they are suited for continued aftercare treatment.

Self- or Forced Elimination

EL–NSAC Comparison. A final question arises in the comparison of the two groups NSAC and EL, one of which is eliminated from treatment by hospital staff decision and one of which is self-eliminated (half even after being accepted for treatment). Table 3 shows that significantly more EL than NSAC addicts rank the instrumental value "Cheerful" ($p < .05$) higher than the combined median, while significantly more NSAC than EL addicts ranked the instrumental value "Capable" ($p < .025$) higher than the combined medians.

Apparently, EL addicts show more concern with the interpersonal-affective type value ("Cheerful") while NSAC addicts appear to be like AC addicts in their emphasis on the task and achievement-oriented value ("Capable"). The data suggest that an in-residence process may not be in harmony with the EL addicts' needs or desire for reasonably light-heared surroundings and a happy affective state and thus they go elsewhere; NSAC addicts, on the other hand, may not find the treatment process overly demanding to their less unconventional values and thus they make some attempt to remain in treatment.

Table 3
Combined Medians, Chi-Square Values, and Levels of Significant Differences Between the EL (n = 28) and NSAC (n = 49) Groups

Groups[a]	Combined median	Chi-square	Significance level
EL-NSAC			
EL Higher-NSAC Lower			
Cheerful (I)	10.60	3.93	.05
EL Lower-NSAC Higher			
Capable (I)	8.38	6.03	.025

[a] (I), Instrumental values; (T), terminal values.

CONCLUSION

The results show that a value analysis of a residential addict population is highly useful to understanding and predicting major preferences and priorities in an addict's life. The value analysis approach to the study of addicts is particularly helpful to understanding and predicting success in an addiction treatment program.

The results of the present study support the finding by Miller et al. (1973) that addicts are a heterogeneous group. To assume that all addicts share the same attributes and characteristics because they share the same categorical tag is naively simplistic. Not only do addicts differ as a function of race and sex, they also vary in terms of value patterns appropriate to selection into and continuation in the treatment program. In light of this heterogeneity, the need for several alternative methods of addiction treatment should be stressed. Hopefully, this and other studies of addicts' value systems will help to improve the "fit" of addicts to appropriate treatment alternatives.

If the four groups discussed in the present study are placed on a continuum running over time from institutional admittance, through treatment, and into aftercare, value patterns characteristic of the four groups become quite distinctive. Of special interest is a definite progression from a hedonistic carefree pattern to an apparently serious minded, task-oriented pattern of values and priorities. Thus NST addicts, who are terminated during the initial evaluation phase, hold values which seem most hedonically oriented ("Pleasure" and "Exciting life"). EL addicts, who as a group bridge the evaluation and treatment phases, and who at some time eliminate themselves from the program, also manifest concern with hedonic, carefree values though to a less extent than NST addicts. More characteristic of EL addicts is an emphasis on values stressing interpersonal interaction and pleasant affective states. NSAC addicts, who experience forced termination from the treatment phase before its completion, evidence a greater concern with task-oriented values than EL addicts and thus appear to a degree similar to AC addicts who complete the in-residence program. Finally, the AC group seems to be the most task- and achievement-oriented of the four groups. Especially characteristic of the AC group is a large concern with "Wisdom."

A major question that might be raised at this point is to what extent success in treatment is related to a particular value pattern found in some addicts. For example, the initial selection or rejection procedure can be construed as an attribution process whereby NST addicts are selected out and rejected on the basis of their characteristics which are felt to be inconsistent with successful therapeutic goals. The working assumption of this paper has been that the addict is responsible for his own good or bad outcome, so that if he has the appropriate value patterns, he will use these values to emit appropriate behaviors leading to success in the program. However, a common finding in other studies has been that the social correspondence between therapists and patients has an effect on the selection of patients for treatment. It is possible, therefore, that the addict's selection is also a function of "significant others" (therapists, aides, etc.) and *their* perceptions and characteristic attributions. To the extent that this is the case, an enhanced predictor of success would incorporate the relation of the addict's values to those of these significant others.

Further investigation would include, then, determining whether values of AC addicts correspond positively with therapists' values, whether selection of addicts for treatment is a function of similarity of value systems, and whether successful completion of treatment is determined by progressive change of values in the direction of similarity to therapists' values. Investigation into some of these areas has been initiated.

REFERENCES

ALLPORT, G. W., VERNON, P. E., and LINDZEY, G. *A Study of Values.* Boston: Houghton, Mifflin, 1960.

KLUCKHOHN, F. R., and STRODTBECK, F. L. *Variations in Value-Orientation.* Evanston, Illinois: Row, Peterson, 1961.

MILLER, J. S., SENSENIG, J., and REED, T. E. Risky and cautious values among narcotic addicts. *Intern. J. Addictions* 7(1): 1–7, 1972.

MILLER, J. S., SENSENIG, J., STOCKER, R. B., and CAMPBELL, R. Value patterns of drug addicts as a function of race and sex. *Intern. J. Addictions* 8(4): 589, 1973.

MORRIS, C. W. *Varieties of Human Values.* Chicago: Univ. of Chicago Press, 1956.

ROKEACH, M. *Beliefs, Attitudes, and Values.* San Francisco: Jossey-Bass, 1968a.

ROKEACH, M. A theory of organization and change in value-attitude systems. *J. Social Issues* 24: 13–133, 1968b.

ROKEACH, M. Value systems in religion. *Rev. Religious Res.* 11: 3–23, 1969.

ROKEACH, M. The measurement of values and value systems. In G. Abcarian (ed.) *Political Participation and Social-Psychological Processes.* Columbus, Ohio: Merril, 1970.

ROKEACH, M. The measurement of values and value systems. In G. Abcarian (ed.) *Social Psychology and Political Behavior.* Columbus, Ohio: Merril, 1971.

ROKEACH, M., and PARKER, S. Values as social indicators of poverty and race relations in America. *Ann. Amer. Acad. Political Social Sci.* March 1970.

ROKEACH, M. MILLER, M. G., and SNYDER, J. A., Jr. The value gap between police and policed. *J. Social Issues* 27: 155–171, 1971.

STONER, J. A. F. Risky and cautious shifts in group decisions: the influence of widely held values. *J. Exp. Social Psych.* 4: 442–458, 1968.

THOMAS, W. I., and ZNANIECKI, F. *The Polish Peasant in Europe and America.* Vol. 1. Boston: Badger, 1918.

The International Journal of the Addictions, 9(1), pp. 137–144, 1974

A Comprehensive Military Drug and Alcohol Program

Allen Frances, M.D.*

Fort Jackson, Columbia, South Carolina

INTRODUCTION

The Army has, since mid–1971, initiated Drug and Alcohol Programs at 34 United States installations, an effort which represents a singificant opportunity to study the efficacy of varied approaches to the addictions. This paper describes one such program, at Fort Jackson, Columbia, South Carolina, and addresses some of the theroretical and practical issues encountered during its evolution. (Statistical outcome and process studies are underway.) The catchment area includes 4,000 permanent party, 20,000 basic trainees who are transients being replaced every few months, 50,000 dependents and retirees, and 3,000 civilian employees.

The physical plant includes four adequate, if not elegant, adjoining buildings which once served as hospital wards. The staff includes 11 civilian counselors, 11 nursing service personnel (including three RN's), 10 enlisted military counselors and administrative people, an education coordinator, four regular and many part-time volunteers, several former patients designated "sponsors," and members of local Alcoholics Anonymous (AA) and Alanon chapters. Leadership is provided by a military

* Organizer and consultant to the program described. Present address: Albert Einstein Medical Center and Bronx State Hocpital, New York, New York.

officer who handles administration, a chaplain who oversees the in-patient service, and a psychiatrist who is general consultant. Most of these staff positions were filled by early 1972 and the program has experienced rapid, at times painful, growth in its brief existence.

COMPONENTS

The program's orientation and strength is in its effort to provide comprehensive, flexible, complementary, and unified services; the total being more productive than the sum of the individual components. Rehabilitation, community relations, and staff training will be discussed.

REHABILITATION

Depending upon his needs and preferences, the patient will participate in one or more of the programs described below. At present a total of more than 400 patients are involved in therapy, and a like number of their family members are seen regularly.

1. In-patient-partial hospitalization (25 beds): Provides the initial experience for those who cannot be seen as outpatients from the outset. Detoxification is accompanied by daily occupational, recreational, and group therapy. Active duty and retired men with jobs usually begin outside work within a week and are discharged within 2 weeks to continue in one or another of the outpatient therapies. "Down and out" retirees remain for several months, if necessary, with transitional steps including work therapy at designated jobs on post and positions in patient government.
2. A Halfway House for older alcoholics is in an adjoining building and provides a less supervised, self-governing experience for reliable graduates in need of such transition to the outside. They sponsor, counsel, and serve as role models for less advanced members.
3. A second, separate Halfway House serves active duty, usually young, "binge type," multiple drug abusers in a nonregressive, structured military environment. All patients work during the day and have rap sessions in the evening.
4. Day care consists of a program of occupational, recreational, work, and group therapy activities for women and is staffed with many volunteers.
5. Teenage drug abusers participate in daily after-school recreation and therapy. One technique effective in the groups is the playing of

recorded popular music to stimulate emotional reactions that can be discussed and promote cohesiveness. The parents are seen once weekly in therapy or discussion groups.

6. The outpatient division serves the majority of patients using various techniques. Many are seen by counselors in individual, family, and/or group therapy (including couple groups). Home visits are made when indicated. For some patients the major contact is with a nurse or patient sponsor. There is a weekly family social night to encourage "sober" fun and to congratulate successful members. A 24-hour "hot-line" and crisis intervention services are provided. There are nightly informal rap sessions for outpatient drug abusers, and twice weekly group therapy for abusers confined to the stockade.

7. Alcoholics Anonymous and Antabuse are adjuncts that are available and often critically helpful to alcoholics at all levels of the program. There is a local post AA chapter and several affiliated ones in town. The early rivalry between them and the growing army program is now becoming more of a mutual dependency. One continuing contention is over Antabuse, which is regarded with contempt by many AA members as a "crutch." The post also has Alanon and Alateen chapters.

8. The primary benefit of Antabuse is that it strengthens the patient's impulse control by reducing to one the number of times a day he must decide whether or not to drink. It is useful in attracting and holding people during the difficult early stages when drop outs are most likely. They come each morning to receive the medication, affording a friendly, communal contact with the nurse and other patients. Antabuse results in a dramatic, early abstinence which raises hope, reduces the need for inpatient care, and shortens the time away from work and family. Commanding officers, supervisors, and spouses are more likely to accept the patient back if they feel there is some guarantee of his abstinence. They may dispense the medicine daily to him.

9. There is a behavior modification program for obese "food addicts" and another is envisioned for cigarette abusers.

COMMUNITY RELATIONS

To have an impact on the military and surrounding community, the program must become related to it closely and, in our experience, must take the initiative in doing this. The attitude of the commanding general is obviously of great importance in promoting widespread acceptance. The program has individuals and education teams who speak regularly before all trainees, permanent party, and representatives of the VA, retired, and civilian personnel. They give high school assemblies, run discussions at the local colleges, and address civic organizations. Formal courses, varying in length from 4 to 32 hours, are provided for commanding officers, army drug specialists, parents, and other interested parties.

A consultation with family court leads to referral of teenagers; and anyone caught driving under the influence must participate in an evaluation and treatment, if indicated. Urine testing to screen and identify drug abusers is routinely performed on trainees, as a spot check for permanent party, and twice weekly for program staff and patients. There are frequent open houses and tours of the facilities for interested groups and individuals. A federal grant has been awarded and a committee established to determine ways of integrating the military with local civilian efforts.

Each patient is a liaison challenge requiring close cooperation between program and unit to coordinate rehabilitation and prevent manipulations, regression, and acting out. A kind of "extended family" therapy between the man and his unit supervisors is performed in conjoint sessions. Each unit provides a volunteer who is trained as a Drug Education Specialist to create education and counseling programs within his unit, and to refer patients when appropriate.

STAFF TRAINING

The nursing and administrative personnel have required supervision and direction rather than intensive training. The training efforts have been developed primarily for the counselors, a group of college graduates who had little or no prior experience as therapists. They vary widely in personality, background, defenses, depth of affective response, psychological aptitude, and value orientation. The goal has been to foster their personal maturity as well as to convey information, and to promote in them a sense of therapeutic identity, style, and confidence. Since the enthusiasm and skill with which an approach is applied may determine its effectiveness more than any objective superiority, the counselor is encouraged to choose those techniques that make sense to him and are most consonant with his character. Insofar as is possible, training is individualized.

Some counselors have developed a surprising understanding of psychodynamics, which they apply to deepen and intensify relationships with patients. Others are more comfortable with a here and now attitude, confrontational and/or supportive. Several are attracted to behavioral or transactional approaches and are supervised by a clinical psychologist in these. One, a former chaplain, has a fatherly, ministerial style with religious emphasis. Patient-therapist match-ups are often made by the psychiatrist, using educated guesses as to who and what will work best. If these are incorrect, patients can choose another therapist, unless this is felt to be an acting out that could be worked through. There are two teaching conferences each week, as well as supervision on individual and group therapy. There is a weekly staff group therapy that serves both a didactic and treatment function. As with other mental health workers, a fair number of the counselors enter therapy, which further deepens their skills. The training program may be educating them beyond their civil service job descriptions and pay, and we may lose several to graduate schools of social work.

The staff has a strong institutional transference to the program, which is in many ways helpful and only sometimes a problem. The program is often perceived as a powerful, protective umbrella under which they can achieve tasks they would otherwise shrink from undertaking. They become disappointed when the program fails, as it sometimes must, to meet their delegated omnipotent fantasies about it. Thus the staff alternates between periods of confidence and doubt. Since expectations may become self-fulfilling prophesies, leaders must interpret and support the staff through low periods. To succeed in this difficult work, a measure of grandiosity is probably necessary. It is difficult to separate the staff's transference to the program from its transference to its leaders. Allowing the staff to regard the leader as an omnipotent reservoir of good or evil is helpful only when his energy and delegated "magic" is needed to institute new programs and when they need a source of strength or someone to blame in especially trying situations. The transference elevation of the leader requires interpretation when individual staff members lose confidence in themselves or when group cohesion is compromised. It is obviously in this area of staff interaction that programs succeed or fail.

FORMULATIONS

The content of a program's theoretical formulations, conscious and implied, is probably less important to its success than are the enthusiasm they engender and the consistency and direction with which they are applied. The following works for us, but we claim no legitimacy or special originality for it.

To succeed with an addict, the program must find ways to meet his dependency and other needs to alleviate the painful affects that drive him to the addicting substance. His powerful self-absorption can be punctured only by providing a compelling alternative and by counteracting his inhibitions to relatedness. The program appeals simultaneously to different psychic structures: to id dependency (and perhaps angry and sexual impulses), to ego self-interest (family, job, health), and interacts in complex ways with superego pressures. Some patients require external controls and/or injunctions to curb regression (especially applicable to young drug users). Others lack, at least temporarily, the ego capacity to use guilt in promoting self-regulation. They have been overburdened by it already and respond positively to the absolution of guilt they feel upon starting the program. In the early stages the patient has a limited frustration tolerance which must be cultivated by gradually expecting him to assume more responsibility, including that he contribute to the progress of others.

The program attempts to minimize the frequent high drop-out rates experienced with addicts without limiting itself to highly motivated patients. The wide range of possible treatment alternatives is meant to satisfy various needs and tastes. Patients find it hard to drop out as a tenacious contact is maintained with them. Every patient starts treatment with at least some manipulative motives, conscious or unconscious. These must be challenged judiciously in such manner that he finds other reasons for continuing as he loses his manipulative ones. The level of conscious motivation reflects only dimly a complex and changing ambivalence toward change, which is amenable to therapeutic intervention. A program that tries can be successful with a fair percentage of people who seem poorly motivated at the outset. Some especially difficult patients, who had failed frequently before, have done remarkably better within a program they perceive as strong, constantly available, and unlikely to become intimidated by and reject them. Patients stay with a program they feel is helping, and this must be demonstrated to them quickly. Transferential, magical progress is valuable in itself and in restoring people to a level of functioning necessary to undertake other forms of change. Contrary to our preconceived notions, cessation of addictive behavior much more often reduced than increased depression, anxiety, and other acting out.

COMPARISON WITH CIVILIAN PROGRAMS

A military program has special opportunities and obstacles. In no other setting could there be such rapid provision of resources and such a clearly defined catchment population. The army constitutes an intense, global experience for its participants, providing structure, caring for needs, but also expecting acceptable behavior. The institutional transference to the program reflects feelings held for its parent, the army. The older career man often improves dramatically upon entering the barracks-like ambience of the rehabilitation center (especially does this typify retirees whose heavy drinking stems, in part, from an often poignant sense of loss of the army). Young trainees and Vietnam returnees are often more ambivalent and hostile to the army and its program. Unlike most civilian programs, we are a part of a tightly knit community which maintains close ties with the patient and affords an easy transition from program to community. For many clients, especially trainees, the goal is not to get them involved with the program per se, but rather to improve their relatedness with the army. This is necessary because they will be transferred to other installations within a short time and must learn to function in and have their needs met by the army as a whole. The most effective modalities for severe heroin dependency—methadone and long-term therapeutic communities—are both inapplicable in the army, and such patients usually require separation and referral. For those with less intense drug abuse, the rehabilitation is in providing a structured community involvement, peer pressure, and group experiences. This worked well with Vietnam heroin users (most of whom were more like pot smokers) and with those trainees who previously felt isolated and have found a home in the army.

Army alcoholics have an unusually good prognosis; they have usually performed well in the past, feel intense transference to the army and fear losing it, and have a tradition of discipline. The obstacles to success in this group are the widespread acceptability, and even encouragement, of drinking in the military, and frequent transfers which may separate them from family and the program.

One problem that army programs face is that with time they may be forced to conform to one model; the military depends upon regulated uniformity. This is unfortunate both because various army communities serve different functions and have differing needs which can best be met by locally devised solutions, and because each staff has a personality of its own and will be most effective working within a system that conforms with it.

CONCLUSION

The army has the capability of creating the first nationwide system of coordinated addiction programs. The military is in some ways a paradigm for community psychiatry, and ideas that work within it may also be effective in civilian communities. There is likely to be increased cooperation and cross fertilization between the army programs and local civilian agencies. Just as each program should be flexible and comprehensive, the total effort should allow for individualized responses to local needs. The paper describes a program that has evolved quickly and represents a promising global approach. Training and rehabilitation issues are discussed.

The International Journal of the Addictions, 9(1), pp. 145–150, 1974

Factors Related to Imprisonment in Female Heroin Addicts

A. E. Raynes, M.S., M.D.

C. Climent, M.S., M.D.

V. D. Patch, M.D.

F. Ervin, M.D.

City of Boston Department of Health and Hospitals
Boston, Massachusetts

Heroin addiction is a phenomenon which effects males approximately four times more frequently than females as measured by requests for treatment. Probably bacause of this, heroin addiction in females has received little attention in the literature. In 1966 Ellinwood et al. reported characteristics of 30 women in the USPHS narcotics hospital in Lexington. From clinical impressions it would appear that the natural history of addiction in women is similar to that in men, i.e., recurrent physical illnesses, arrests, incarcerations, overdoses, and high age specific mortality rates. Imprisonment is a major and not infrequent occurrence in an addict's life. However, not all addicts find their way into the prison system. While little is known about the female addict, even less is known about those factors which protect female addicts against incarceration. This study is an attempt to compare two populations of female addicts, one currently in prison and the other never having suffered imprisonment.

Variables related to imprisonment in female narcotic abusers can then be identified.

METHOD

The prison population consisted of 46 female narcotic addicts currently at the Correctional Institution for Women in Framingham, Massachusetts. These women had all been incarcerated for drug-related offenses.

Data concerning the hospital population was drawn from the Drug Detoxification Unit of Boston City Hospital. This is an in-patient and day care program serving a similar area to the Framingham prison. This group consisted of 49 consecutive voluntary female admissions who had had no previous imprisonments. Data was collected from the two groups by standardized questionnaires.

RESULTS

The mean age of the prisoners was 25.15 years, while that of the patients was 24.79 years. This difference was not significant (see Table 1). There were also no differences as regards the distribution of race and religion between the two groups. Twenty-two percent of the prisoners were married and living with their spouses prior to imprisonment, while 49% of the patients were living with their spouses. When the other categories are collapsed and compared with this variable, the difference is significant at the .02 level. Thirty-four (74%) of the prisoners had children, while only 26 (35%) of patients had children. However, among those who had children, the prisoners tended to have more.

The distribution of schooling and time in the longest job held showed little differences between the two groups.

Fifty-four percent of the prisoners had a history of having had previous psychiatric treatment, while only 27% of patients had had such treatment. This difference was significant at the .001 level.

Sixteen (35%) of the prisoner group had suffered paternal deaths and nine (20%) had suffered maternal deaths. These figures for the patients were eight (16%) and six (12%), respectively (see Table 2). There was little difference between the two groups as regard parental alcoholism and criminality (by arrests), but the prisoners had a higher prevalence of psychiatric illness among their mothers. Although these figures were small (13% for prisoners and 2% for patients), the difference is marked. Twenty-three (50%) of prisoners' parents were still living together, while 18 (37%)

Table 1

	Prisoners			Patients	
	No.	%		No.	%
N	46			49	
Mean age	25.15 years			24.79 years	
Race					
Black	20	44		20	41
White	25	54		29	59
Other	1	2		0	0
Religion					
Protestant	18	39		22	45
Catholic	25	54		22	45
Jewish	2	4		3	6
Other	1	2		2	4
Marital status					
Single	26	55		20	41
Married	10	22	($p < .02$)	24	49
Divorced	4	9		1	2
Separated	5	11		4	8
Widowed	1	2		0	0
Mean no. of children	2.0 ($N = 34$)			1.6 ($N = 26$)	
Mean no. years in school	10.3			8.5	
Longest job held					
Less than 6 months	18	40		16	33
6 months to 1 year	16	35		20	41
More than 1 year	12	25		13	26
Previous psychiatric treatment					
No	21	46		36	73
Yes	25	54	($p < .001$)	13	27

of the patients' parents were still together. This difference was not significant.

The first drug used most commonly for both groups was marijuana, with amphetamines being the second commonest drug of initiation. Neither of the two groups used heroin as their first drug of abuse. Overall, the pattern of initiation into drug abuse was similar for the two groups (see Table 3).

The prison group tended to have used marijuana at an earlier age; 16.8 years as opposed to 18.1 years among the patients. The use of amphetamines and hallucinogens, however, began earlier among the patient group. The mean age of onset of heroin use for prisoners was 18.9 years and 19.2 years for the patient group. This difference was not significant.

Table 2
Parental History

	Prisoners		Patients	
	No.	%	No.	%
Paternal				
Death				
Yes	16	35	8	16
No	30	65	41	84
Psychiatric treatment				
Yes	2	4	2	4
No	44	96	47	96
Alcoholism				
Yes	13	28	15	31
No	33	72	34	69
Arrested				
Yes	5	11	2	4
No	42	89	47	96
Maternal				
Death				
Yes	9	20	6	12
No	38	80	43	88
Psychiatric treatment				
Yes	6	13	1	2
No	40	87	48	98
Alcoholism				
Yes	5	11	5	10
No	42	89	44	90
Arrested				
Yes	1	2	0	0
No	46	98	49	100
Parental marital status				
Still together	23	50	18	37
Separated	24	50	31	63

No differences were found between the two groups as regards means of supporting their addiction. Only 13% of the imprisoned group and 14% of the hospital group were in legitimate employment. There were no differences between the two groups in the distribution of the types of illegal activity used to support their drug habits.

DISCUSSION

Ellinwood reported in 1966 that the major difference between male and female heroin addicts at the USPHS hospital at Lexington was in the

Table 3
Drug History

	Prisoners		Patients	
First drug taken	No.	%	No.	%
Marijuana	35	75	40	82
Amphetamine	8	17	4	8
Hallucinogen	1	2	1	2
Barbiturate	2	4	2	4
Opium derivative	0	0	0	0
Cocaine	1	2	2	4
Mean age (years) at 1st use	Mean age		Mean age	
Marijuana	16.8 ($N = 46$)		18.1 ($N = 43$)	
Amphetamine	18.2 ($N = 37$)		17.3 ($N = 30$)	
Hallucinogen	19.9 ($N = 31$)		17.8 ($N = 29$)	
Barbiturate	18.5 ($N = 39$)		19.4 ($N = 19$)	
Opium derivative	18.9 ($N = 44$)		19.2 ($N = 49$)	
Cocaine	19.0 ($N = 17$)		21.1 ($N = 27$)	
Means of supporting habit	No.	%	No.	%
Legitimate work	6	13	7	14
Stealing	8	17	9	18
Dealing	13	29	13	27
Prostitution	5	11	4	8
Dependent on male partner	14	30	16	33

absolute difference in numbers. The average age of his population was 30.9 years, 5 years older than this current population. The 1966 study, however, found that 40% of the women addicts were married. This may be accounted for by their greater mean age. In the current study, 22% of prisoners were married, but 49% of patients were married. Taking into account the younger mean age of the current study subjects, it would appear that being married protects against incarceration among heroin addicts. While 45% of the prisoners were or had been married, 74% had children. These figures for the patients were 59% and 51%. It therefore appears that there was a greater proportion of unmarried mothers among the prisoners.

As in the 1966 study, approximately 73% of the patients had no history of psychiatric illness. However, only 46% of the prisoners were free of such a history. Female heroin addicts who have a history of psychiatric treatment are more likely to find themselves in jail than those who do not have this kind of history. It is perhaps ironic that women who exhibit the greatest pathology end up in jail, while those who are not so afflicted are treated in hospitals.

As regards parental history, the prisoners suffered a higher prevalence of both maternal and paternal deaths. This may be associated with the greater proportion of previous psychiatric illness. There was also a higher proportion of psychiatric illness in the mothers of the prisoners. It is possible that the girls that are incarcerated have a further disadvantage in the inadequacy of the maternal identification figure.

Overall, there were few differences in the use of drugs between the two groups, other than the earlier use of marijuana among the prisoners. The age started and use of heroin as the initial drug was similar for the two groups.

In summary, the unmarried girl, who probably has children, who already has a previous history of psychiatric illness, and who has probably suffered more parental loss and more maternal psychiatric illness starts on marijuana earlier and ultimately finishes up in jail for her drug-related crimes. In short, the female addict who finishes up in jail usually starts with greater social and emotional disadvantages. Ultimately this may mean that she is relatively inept as a criminal or that she is at a disadvantage in providing adequate defense in court.

While prison systems do little more than isolate and further alienate people, it must be of great concern to the professional psychiatric community that in the midst of this present heroin epidemic it is the socially and emotionally disadvantaged women, having the greatest need, who receive the poorest treatment.

REFERENCE

ELLINWOOD, E. B., SMITH, W. G. and VAILLANT, G. E. Narcotic addiction in males and females: a comparison. *Intern. J. Addictions* 1: 2, 1966.

The International Journal of the Addictions, 9(1), pp. 151–159, 1974

Psychological Differentiation in Heroin Addicts

Dan Arnon, M. D.

Marc H. Kleinman, M.S.

Benjamin Kissin, M.D.

Division of Alcoholism and Drug Dependence
Department of Psychiatry
Downstate Medical Center, State University of New York
Brooklyn, New York

ABSTRACT

Thirty male and 31 female heroin addicts were tested for field dependence using the Portable Rod and Frame Test. Scores were compared to results obtained by Oltman of a normal population. The addicts as a group were found to be more field-dependent than normals. The female addicts, however, were significantly more field-dependent than male addicts who, conversely, appeared similar to normal males. Both addict samples were characterized by marked variability, suggesting that heroin addicts represent a strongly heterogeneous population and not a homogeneous one as suggested by earlier studies of the disorder.

Throughout the literature one notes a divergence of opinion as to the underlying personality structure leading to addiction. In the analytic literature, stress is placed on the commonality of the underlying dynamic processes and personality in all forms of addiction, be it to narcotics, alcohol, cigarettes, or food (Fenichel, 1954; Savitt, 1968). Other authors, however, have viewed addiction as a more complex problem in which economic, social, and psychological factors all have a role (Kolb, 1962; Chein, 1964; Berzins et al., 1971).

Witkin et al. (1959) and Karp (1963, 1965) have applied the easily quantifiable perceptual function of field dependence to investigations of personality in alcoholics. Considerable work has been done by Witkin and his co-workers (1954, 1962) in clarifying the relationships between this measure of cognitive style and other aspects of personality. Both field-dependent and field-independent cognitive style are associated with separate clusters of personality characteristics. Field-dependent individuals depend on their surrounding environment for structure and support. They have difficulty in dealing analytically with the world around them and characteristically react to it in a passive manner. They tend to have a poor sense of separate identity, a relatively primitive, undifferentiated body image, poor control over their impulses, and tend to use the more primitive defenses of denial and repression. Field independence, on the other hand, is associated with the ability to separate oneself from his environment and to deal with it in a more critical and analytic way. Field-independent persons are characterized by activity and independence in relation to the world around them, better impulse control, higher self-esteem, a more mature body image with a well-developed sense of separate identity and more differentiated defenses based on isolation and intellectualization.

Studies of field dependency in alcoholics by Witkin (1959) and Karp (1965) have repeatedly demonstrated that alcoholics of all types (males and females, out-patients and in-patients, members of Alcoholics Anonymous) are significantly more field-dependent than normal controls. Karp et al. (1970) reports that the mean performances of alcoholic groups tend to be 1 to 2 standard deviations above that of control groups in the direction of field dependence. He also notes that, in spite of the extreme field dependence of alcoholics as a group, female alcoholics are significantly more field-dependent than males. These results appear to corroborate clinical observations (Knight, 1937; Lisansky, 1960) describing alcoholics as a relatively homogeneous group characterized dynamically by intense conflict centering around powerful and unresolved dependent strivings. Field dependency has also been found in patients suffering from other clinical entities regarded as having similar dynamic roots including peptic ulcer, obesity, and asthma (Gordon, 1953; Karp, 1965; Fishbein, 1963).

If the hypotheses of a common personality organization and psychopathological process rooted in orality and dependence underlying all forms of addiction is correct, one would expect results in heroin addicts with respect to cognitive style to be similar to alcoholics in that heroin addicts would be a relatively homogeneous field-dependent group when compared to a normal population. If, on the other hand, our clinical impression that heroin addiction subsumes a wide variety of personality and psychopathology is correct, we would expect a greater range of scores with a large proportion of subjects appearing field-independent on testing. Hence, the present study was undertaken to test the relative validity of these two hypotheses.

METHOD

Subjects. Thirty male and 31 female heroin addicts were tested. All subjects were voluntary patients in a methadone maintenance clinic at Kings County Hospital Center, Brooklyn, New York. Male subjects comprised a random sample, while the female subjects comprised the total female population of the clinic, except for two patients whom we were unable to test.

Both male and female subjects had similar distributions of age, ethnic composition, and years of drug use. The average age of the males was 29, and 39.7% were Black, 16.9% were Puerto Rican, and 43.4% were White. The average age of the females was 27, and 46.0% were Black, 16.5% were Puerto Rican, and 37.5% were White. The male addicts had used drugs an average of 8.9 years prior to admission to the methadone program; the female addicts 5.9 years.

TESTS

Field dependence in these subjects was assessed by Oltman's portable modification of Witkin's Rod and Frame Test (Oltman, 1968). This is a simply administered instrument in which the subject's task is to align a rod to the vertical position when the frame in which the rod is placed is tilted at an angle of 28° either to the right or the left of the subject and in the absence of other visual cues.

Each subject was given eight trials. The subject's score was the sum of the deviations from the vertical measured in degrees for all eight trials. Scores were compared using *t* and *f* tests to data obtained by Oltman (1968) for normal subjects.

RESULTS

Examination of the results revealed that the total addict group, including male and female subjects, was significantly more field-dependent than Oltman's normal subjects ($p < .001$). The addicts' test score variance, however, was significantly higher than that of normal subjects ($p < .01$), suggesting the presence of a heterogeneous population (Table 1).

Table 1
Comparison of Means, Standard Deviations, t *and* f *Values for Normal and Addict Samples*

I.	Male normals	vs	Female normals
	$\bar{X} = 45.8$		$\bar{X} = 52.4$
	$s = 36.9$		$s = 41.0$
	$t = 1.07$ = not significant		
	$f = 1.23$ = not significant		
II.	Male addicts	vs	Male normals
	$\bar{X} = 63.8$		$\bar{X} = 45.8$
	$s = 62.03$		$s = 36.9$
	$t = 1.48$ = not significant		
	$f = 2.83 = p < .01$		
III.	Female addicts	vs	Female normals
	$\bar{X} = 129.4$		$\bar{X} = 52.4$
	$s = 71.7$		$s = 41.0$
	$t = 5.46 = p < .001$		
	$f = 3.17 = p < .01$		
IV.	Male addicts	vs	Female addicts
	$\bar{X} = 63.8$		$\bar{X} = 129.4$
	$s = 62.03$		$s = 71.7$
	$t = 3.73 = p < .001$		
	$f = 1.39$ = not significant		
V.	Total addicts	vs	Total normals
	$\bar{X} = 193.2$		$\bar{X} = 98.2$
	$s = 133.7$		$s = 77.9$
	$t = 5.22 = p < .001$		
	$f = 3.01 = p < .01$		

A comparison of male and female addicts revealed that female addicts were significantly more field-dependent than male addicts ($p < .001$). There was no difference in test score variance between male and female addicts (Table 1).

The male and female addicts were than compared separately to Oltman's male and female normals. Female addicts were found to be significantly more field-dependent than female normals ($p < .001$). No significant difference was found, on the other hand, between male addicts and normal males. Both male and female addicts had significantly higher test score variances than their normal counterparts ($p < .01$) (Table 1).

A comparison of the distributions of addicts and normal subjects' test scores revealed a bimodal distribution for addicts with peaks in the field-dependent and field-independent range. In contrast, the normative sample had a unimodal distribution, with its peak in the field-independent range (Fig. 1 and Table 2).

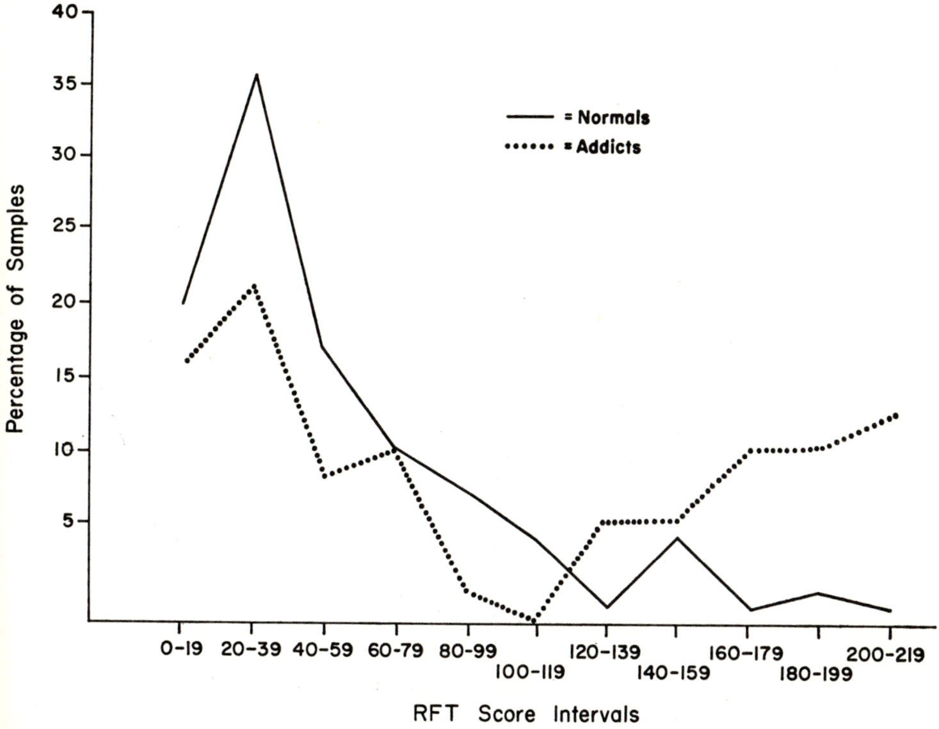

Fig. 1. Comparison of RFT scores for addict and normal populations.

Table 2

Frequency Distribution of Addict and Normal RFT Scores in Percentages

RFT score Intervals	Male addicts, %	Female addicts, %	Total normals, %
0–19	23	10	20
20–39	30	13	36
40–59	10	6	17
60–79	13	6	10
80–99	3	0	7
100–119	0	0	4
120–139	3	6	1
140–159	3	6	4
160–179	0	19	1
180–199	10	10	1
200–219	3	23	1
N	30	31	163

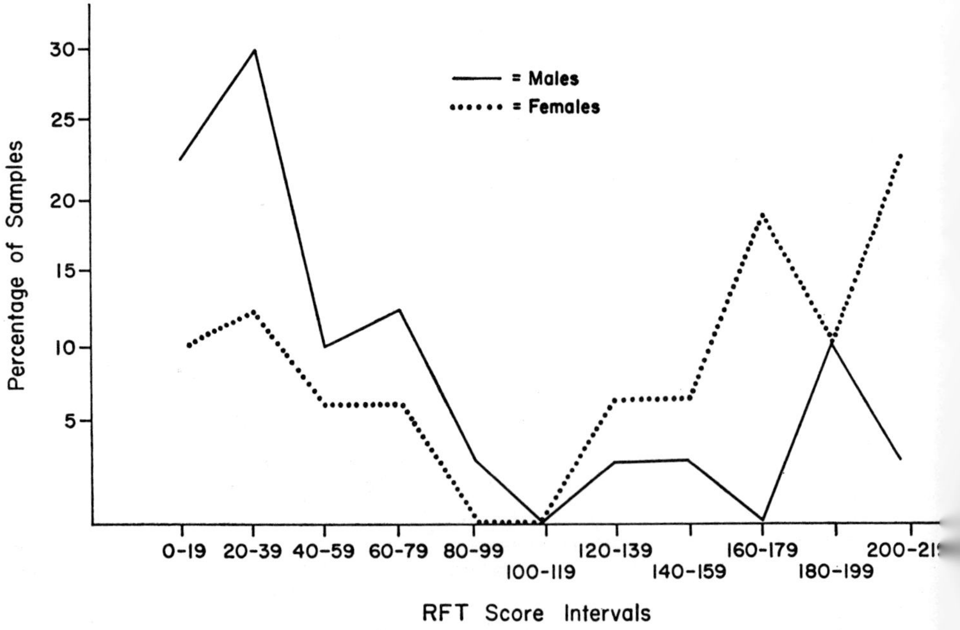

Fig. 2. Comparison of RFT scores for male and female addicts.

A comparison of the distributions of the male and female addict samples again revealed characteristic bimodal distributions for both groups. The distribution of male addicts, however, is marked by a large peak in the field-independent range of the distribution, with a smaller peak in the field-dependent range. A converse distribution appeared for the sample of female addicts (Fig. 2).

DISCUSSION

The present results suggest that a unitary concept of the addictive personality, while perhaps valid for most alcoholics, is not true for heroin addicts. The addicts studied showed greater variability in field dependence. The distribution of their test scores appeared bimodal, with subjects concentrated at the extremes of the spectrum. This is in marked contrast to alcoholics, among whom field-independent subjects are rare. This finding is also in contrast to the unimodal distribution of scores obtained by Oltman's normal subjects. The significance of the latter difference is not entirely clear since the normal subjects consisted of a relatively homogeneous group of white middle-class college students who had been exposed to very different environments and life experiences than those encountered by our addict subjects. It also should be noted that our sample of addicts may not be truly representative of the addict population as a whole, as it included only addicts who voluntarily requested treatment. Hence, in replicating this study, it would be useful to include addict subjects from other sources (civil commitments, jails, different treatment programs, etc.) and to use controls matched to the addict group in socioeconomic variables.

The results indicate that within the addict sample there is a marked difference in psychological differentiation between males and females, men being better differentiated than women. In this respect the female addicts were closer to alcoholics than male addicts. Thus it may well be that the psychoanalytic concepts of the addictive personality may hold for women but not for many men.

An explanation for these findings may lie in the possibility that, at least in the poorer socioeconomic areas of Brooklyn, significant environmental pressure for experimentation with heroin is exerted on many youngsters during adolescence, much like the pressure for experimentation with alcohol of former years. With alcohol, however, only those people with the personality characteristics described previously went on to serious addiction. In contrast, the rapid onset of physiological addiction with heroin dictates the continued use of the drug no matter what the underlying personality characteristics.

The findings suggest that men are more strongly subjected to the initial environmental pressure than are women, perhaps because drug use among male adolescents represents a lesser degree of social deviancy than among females of the same areas. Conversely, women may be more strongly drawn to heroin use as a means of resolving intra-psychic conflict rather than through strong adolescent peer-group pressure. Our clinical experience suggests that this conflict in women does appear to center around the need for environmental structure and for relationships of a dependent nature characteristic of those with poor psychological differentiation.

The wide variations in psychological differentiation in addicts with its concomitant differences in character structure and psychopathology lends further support to the need for a multimodality approach to the treatment of heroin addiction. It may be that addicts who are reasonably well differentiated and in whom the initial impetus toward drug use came through adolescent peer-group pressure may require little more than relief of physiological addiction and persistent drug craving to reorganize their lives in a more adaptive manner. The distribution of addict test scores as shown in Fig. 1 shows many subjects falling in the extremes of the spectrum where, as has been indicated, psychopathology is most likely to occur. It may be that poor treatment outcome is more prevalent among these latter patients than the former because of underlying psychopathology presently going undetected and untreated.

It is possible that much of the responsibility for failure in the treatment of addiction is due to a lack of appreciation of the great individual psychological differences between addicts who, in fact, comprise a quite heterogeneous population. These differences are, at present, little understood. Their clarification, however, is essential if a truly rational multimodality treatment approach is to be realized.

REFERENCES

BERZINS, J. I., ROSS, W. F., and MONROE, J. J. A multivariate study of the personality characteristics of hospitalized narcotic addicts on the M.M.P.I. *J. Clin. Psychol.* 27: 174–181, 1971.

CHEIN, I., et al. *The Road to H.* New York: Basic Books, 1964.

FENICHEL, O. *The Psychoanalytic Theory of Neurosis.* New York: Norton, 1954.

FISHBEIN, G. M. Perceptual modes and asthmatic symptoms: an application of Witkin's hypothesis. *J. Consult. Psychol.* 27: 54–58, 1963.

GORDON, B. An experimental study of dependence-independence in a social and laboratory setting. Unpublished doctoral dissertation. University of Southern California. Los Angeles, California, 1953.

KARP, S. A., KISSIN, B., and HUSTMYER, F. E., JR. Field dependence as a predictor of alcoholic therapy dropouts. *J. Nervous Mental Disease* 150: 77–83, 1970.

KARP, S. A., and KONSTADT, N. L. Alcoholism and psychological differentiation: long range effects of heavy drinking on field dependence. *J. Nervous Mental Disease* 140: 412–416, 1965.

KARP, S. A., and PARDES, H. Psychological differentiation (field dependence) in obese women. *Psychosom. Med.* 27: 238–244, 1965.

KARP, S. A., POSTER, D. C., and GOODMAN, A. Differentiation in alcoholic women. *J. Personality* 31: 386–393, 1963.

KARP, S. A., WITKIN, H. A., and GOODENOUGH, D. R. Alcoholism and psychological differentiation: effect of alcohol on field dependence. *J. Abnormal Psychol.* 70: 262–265, 1965a.

KARP, S. A., WITKIN, H. A., and GOODENOUGH, D. R. Alcoholism and psychological differentiation: effect of achievement of sobriety on field dependence. *Quart. J. Studies Alc.* 26: 580–585, 1965b.

KNIGHT, R. P. Psychodynamics of chronic alcoholism. *J. Nervous Mental Disease* 86: 538–548, 1937.

KOLB, L. *Drug Addiction, A Medical Problem.* Springfield, Illinois: Thomas, 1962.

LISANSKY, E. S. The etiology of alcoholism: the role of psychological predisposition. *Quart. J. Studies Alc.* 21: 314–343, 1960.

OLTMAN, P. K. A portable rod and frame apparatus. *Percept. Motor Skills* 26: 503-506, 1968.

SAVITT, R. A. The psychopathology of the addiction process. *J. Hillside Hosp.* 27: 277–286, 1968.

WITKIN, H. A., DYK, R. B., FATERSON, H. F., GOODENOUGH, D. R., and KARP, S. A. *Psychological Differentiation.* New York: Wiley, 1962.

WITKIN, H. A., KARP, S. A., and GOODENOUGH, D. R. Dependence in alcoholics. *Quart. J. Studies, Alc.* 20: 493–504, 1959.

WITKIN, H. A., LEWIS, H. B., HERTZMAN, M., MACHOVER, K., MEISSNER, P. B., and WAPNER, S. *Personality through Perception.* New York: Harper 1954.

The International Journal of the Addictions, 9(1), pp. 161–165, 1974

Reliability of Interview Data Concerning Current Heroin Use from Heroin Addicts on Methadone

Thomas J. Cox, Ph.D.

Bill Longwell, B.A.

Hope Center
Tucson, Arizona

ABSTRACT

In a methadone maintenance program with 110 heroin addicts, data concerning current heroin use from 175 interviews was correlated with the results of urinalysis for heroin. In 86% of the interviews, the patients truthfully reported the extent of their current heroin use to the interviewer.

INTRODUCTION

The question of the reliability of interview data from heroin addicts is becoming increasingly important as methadone clinics continue to proliferate across the country and more and more addicts are being interviewed (Jaffe, Zaks, and Washington, 1969; Gearing, 1969).

Ball (1967) sampled 59 addicts and compared responses during interviews with hospital records, arrests records, and urine tests as an attempt to find out the degree to which one can rely on patient responses. The responses to questions of current drug use were tabulated from a relatively small number of patients (25) who were also tested by urinalysis. The results of the interviews and the urinalysis agreed in 92% of the patients, with 71% of those using heroin admitting such use to the interviewer.

METHOD

Hope Center has a methadone maintenance clinic where approximetely 110 heroin addicts are being maintained as out-patients on methadone. Of these, 106 (24 females and 82 males) were included in the sample (Table 1). The number of interviews for each addict ranged from one to eight, with the total number of interviews being 175. The mean age for the sample was approximately 28. All patients had been in treatment for a minimum of 3 months.

The research design of the program requires an initial interview concerning current drug use, past history of incarceration, work history,

Table 1
Background Characteristics of the Sample (N = *106*)

	%	No.
Sex		
Male	77	82
Female	23	24
Ethnic group		
Chicano	51	55
Caucasion	32	34
Black	5	5
Indian	10	10
Other	2	2
	Median	**Range**
Age	27	18–64
Age of initial drug use	17	12–32
Number of drug arrests	3	1–28
Number of previous treatments	0	0– 7
Months on methadone maintenance	5	3–21
Highest grade of school completed	11	1–14
Years of heroin use	9	2–25

and other data. Every 3 months thereafter the patients are again interviewed. These subsequent interviews include a question about current (over the last 3 months) heroin use. The question is phrased so that the subject can choose an average frequency of use over the last 3 months. Possible responses are: Not at all, Less than once a month, Once a month, Once a week, Once a day, and More than once a day.

All interviews were done by the same person (Cox). The patients were told that any information given to the interviewer would not be used in any way to jeopardize their position in the program. A definite effort was made by the interviewer to put the patient at ease, and the interviewer made it a point to talk to all the patients in a casual way at different times when they came to the dispensary.

Under federal guidelines, all patients' urines are tested at least once a week. The results are recorded as percentage of heroin free urines for a 3-month period (12 urines) as follows: Less than 20% (<2.4), 21–30% (2.5–3.6), 31–40% (3.5–4.8), 41–50% (4.9–6.0), 51–60% (6.1–7.2), 61–70% (7.3–8.4), 71–80% (8.5–9.6), 81–90% (9.7–10.8), and 91–100% (10.9–12).

The day of the week the patients were required to give a urine sample was arrived at by randomly selecting numbered peas out of a bottle.

All urine samples were given under the surveillance of a counselor or nurse. No patients were aware ahead of time that they were to give a urine sample. If a patient claimed he was unable to void, or refused to void, then this was recorded as a positive. It is assumed that a patient who refuses to void, or claims he is unable to void, has used heroin and knows his urine results will be positive. The urines were analyzed by a thin-layer chromatographic procedure (Dole, Kim, and Eglitis, 1966).

RESULTS

The responses to the question of current heroin use for all interviews after the initial interview were compared with the actual percentages of positive urines obtained during the same period of time. The data were organized into high and low use as determined from the interview data, and high and low use as determined from the results of the random urinalysis. Fifty percent or less heroin-free urines was arbitrarily taken as high use, and greater than 50% heroin-free urines was taken as low use. Usage could vary from 0% heroin-free urines (all positive urines) to 100% free urines (no heroin use), and the midpoint (50% heroin free urines) was chosen to separate high and low usage. Interview responses to the

Table 2

Correlation of Amount of Heroin Use as Determined from Interview Data and Urinalysis Results

	Interview data	
	High use	Low use
High use (urinalysis results)	25	10
Low use (urinalysis results)	15	125

$\chi^2 = 55.141$, $df = 1$, $p < .001$
$C = .489$

frequency of heroin use were grouped as follows: high use, once a week or more frequent; low use, once a month or less frequent.

The data were grouped in a 2×2 contingency table to estimate the association between heroin use as reported and heroin use as determined from urinalysis (Siegals, 1956). A contingency coefficient (C) was calculated. A chi-square value was computed to test the significance of the association. The 5% significance level was used to indicate a statistical significance.

In 25 interviews the patients reported high heroin use (they claimed to have used heroin at least once a week), and the results of the urinalyses verified high use (Table 2).

In 125 interviews the patients reported low use (maximum use of once a month), and results of their urinalyses also fit into the low use category. Of the 25 patients whose responses regarding their current heroin use did not agree with the amount of heroin use determined from the urinalysis results, 10 reported less use than the urinalyses showed and 15 more use than shown in their urinalyses.

Thus, in 86% of the interviews, the patients admitted to the interviewer the extent of their current heroin use, low or high.

In those interviews where the results of urinalysis showed high use, 29% reported low use in their interviews. In 135 interviews, the urinalysis results were low use, while 11% reported high use in these interviews. Thus, in those interviews where urinalyses showed high heroin use, a larger percent (29 vs 11%) did not correctly report the extent of their heroin use to the interviewer when compared with those in the low use category.

Because of the research design of the program, in those interviews with 91–100% heroin-free urines it was not possible to determine the interviews in which there was no heroin use (100% heroin-free urines). But in 105 of the 175 interviews where the results of the urinalysis showed some heroin use (90% or less heroin-free urines), 70% admitted to the interviewer that they had used heroin.

The correlation, expressed by a contingency coefficient between heroin use as reported in the interviews and heroin use from urine results was $C = .489$. For a 2×2 contingency table the maximum value C can attain is .707. The chi-square value is 55.141, significant at the .001 probability level.

SUMMARY

In 175 interviews from 110 heroin addicts in a methadone maintenance program, the extent of heroin use from interview data and urinalysis results was correlated. In 86% of the interviews the patients admitted to the interviewer the extent of their heroin use, low or high. In the interviews where the patients had reported high heroin use, a larger percentage (29 vs 11%) did not correctly report the extent of their heroin use when compared with those reporting low use.

In 105 of the 175 interviews where the results of the urinalysis showed some heroin use, 70% admitted to the interviewer that they had used heroin.

These results indicate that the response of addicts to questions regarding frequency of drug use can be relied upon to a high degree. This is in itself an important consideration when one considers the cost of urine testing in government-sponsored programs.

REFERENCES

BALL, J. C. The reliability and validity of interview data obtained from 59 narcotic drug addicts. *Amer. J. Sociol.* 72(6): 650–654, May 1967.

DOLE, V. P., KIM, W. K., and EGLITIS, T. Detection of narcotic drugs, tranquilizers, amphetamines, and barbiturates in urine. *J. Amer. Med. Assoc.* 198: 115–118, 1966.

GEARING, R. F., Evaluation of methadone maintenance treatment for heroin addiction. A progress report read before the Epidemiology Section of the American Public Health Association, Philadelphia, 1969.

JAFFE, J. H., ZAKS, M. S., and WASHINGTON, E. N. Experience with the use of methadone in a multi-modality program for the treatment of narcotics users. *Intern. J. Addictions* 4: 481–490, 1969.

SIEGAL, S., *Nonparametric Statistics for the Behavioral Sciences.* New York: McGraw-Hill, 1956.

The International Journal of the Addictions, 9(1), pp. 167–170, 1974

Short-Term, Ambulatory Detoxification of Opiate Addicts Using Methadone

Harry Silsby*

Major, Medical Corps, United States Army

Forest S. Tennant, Jr.†

Major, Medical Corps, United States Army Reserve

ABSTRACT

Twenty-one young opiate addicts entered an ambulatory, low dose methadone detoxification program which lasted 7 days. Eight (38%) did not successfully complete detoxification. At the end of 6 months only two (9.5%) addicts were found to be free of opiate drugs. Although low dose methadone detoxification can easily be accomplished on a short-term ambulatory basis, the high relapse rate to opiate use indicates that this procedure should only be attempted with selected, motivated individuals.

* Regimental Surgeon, 2nd Armored Cavalry Regiment, U.S. Army, Europe.

† Formerly: Chief, Special Action Office for Drug Abuse, U.S. Army, Europe. Requests for reprints should be addressed to Dr. Tennant at the Department of Preventive Medicine and Social Medicine, UCLA School of Medicine, Los Angeles, California 90024.

INTRODUCTION

Due to increasing numbers of heroin addicts seeking treatment and the high cost of hospitalization, ambulatory detoxification of heroin addicts has emerged as a treatment modality of great interest. Recent reports of short-term ambulatory detoxification of heroin addicts indicate little success with this form of therapy (O'Malley, Anderson, and Lazare, 1972; Gay, Matzger, Bathurst, and Smith, 1971). O'Malley et al. (1972) offered ambulatory detoxification with methadone to 58 heroin addicts at the Massachusetts General Hospital in Boston but none even returned for their second visit to complete the withdrawal program (O'Malley et al., 1972). At the Haight-Ashbury Free Clinic in San Francisco, Gay and co-workers (1971) treated 435 young heroin addicts, using nonmethadone withdrawal techniques (Gay et al., 1971). Thirty-eight percent dropped out of the ambulatory detoxification program after only one clinic visit, and only 5.5% were abstinent from heroin usage for 1 month or more following detoxification. In an effort to determine if ambulatory detoxification can be accomplished by a physician in office practice, we attempted to detoxify 21 young, soldier addicts using methadone. Since the military provides an environment in which maximal control can be exerted over an individual's habits, this setting permits extremely close follow-up of patients and an excellent opportunity to elucidate defects in therapeutic procedures and determine outcomes of treatment.

METHODS

The subjects for this study were U.S. Army soldiers stationed in Nurnberg, West Germany. Ages ranged from 18 to 21 years. Subjects voluntarily presented for treatment between July and December 1971 and requested opiate detoxification. All initially indicated a desire to finish their army tour of duty. Opiate drugs, including crude opium, morphine, and heroin, are more readily available and cheaper in West Germany than in the United States (Tennant, 1972). No patient was rejected for treatment. Each was determined to be opiate dependent by a history of daily, multiple opiate injections; the physical presence of needle marks; and confirmatory history by a peer or superior officer.

Patients were given a routine physical examination and initially administered methadone up to 20 mg/day depending on severity of dependence. A low dose methadone regimen was selected to reduce the opiate users' compulsive drug-seeking behavior or "drug hunger" as hypothysized by Dole and Nyswander, as well as to alleviate symptoms of the opiate abstinence syndrome (Dole, Nyswander, and Kreek, 1966). Methadone was administered in decreasing doses for a period of 7 days. Each day the patient returned to the physician and was given medication. Following detoxification, patients were followed by mandatory appointments for group therapy and individual counseling at least once per week for at least 6 months or until the individual left the U.S. Army, Europe. At each follow-up visit the patient was questioned concerning opiate and other drug use, and a urine test for opiate drugs was collected. The individual's supervisors were contacted weekly to help document relapse to opiate use.

RESULTS

Eight (38%) subjects either dropped out of the detoxification program or failed to cooperate by using opiate drugs during detoxification. Thirteen (62%) subjects successfully completed ambulatory detoxification. All 13 detoxified patients experienced mild opiate withdrawal symptoms consisting primarily of nausea, vomiting, restlessness, sleeplessness, and rhinorrhea. Six months following ambulatory detoxification, two (9.5%) were found to be opiate-free. This was determined by patient history, urine testing, and confirmation with the individual's superior officers. Urine testing and/or personal interview revealed that all other subjects relapsed to at least occasional opiate use within 3 months following detoxification. Nine of the 21 (43%) subjects eventually required premature discharge from the U.S. Army due to treatment failure, recurrent narcotic abuse, and inability to perform military duties.

DISCUSSION

This study shows that low dose methadone withdrawal on an ambulatory basis is easily accomplished in individuals who voluntarily seek treatment. The high opiate relapse rate of the subjects, however, indicates that short-term, ambulatory detoxification is not usually associated with long-term abstinence. Studies of addicts detoxified in a hospital report variable results, but generally show more favorable detoxification and abstinence rates than do studies of addicts detoxified on an out-patient basis (Gudeman, Shader, and Hemenway, 1972; Vaillant, 1966; Richman, Perkins, Bihari, and Fishman, 1972). In this study, as in other outpatient studies, the only criteria to enter ambulatory detoxification was a request on the part of the addict (O'Malley et al., 1972; Gay et al., 1971). Addicts may seek ambulatory detoxification treatment to temporarily suppress abstinence symptoms or reduce the size of their opiate habit rather than from a desire for complete abstinence. The reported greater detoxification rates of addicts detoxified in a hospital may be related to limited access to opiate drugs in a hospital setting.

ACKNOWLEDGMENTS

The opinions contained herein are the private views of the authors and are not to be construed as official or as reflecting the views of the Department of the Army or the Department of Defense.

REFERENCES

GUDEMAN, J. E., SHADER, R. F., and HEMENWAY, T. S. Methadone withdrawal in the treatment of heroin addiction. *Diseases Nervous System* 33: 297–303, 1972.

GAY, G. R., MATZGER, A. D. BATHURST, W., and SMITH, D. E. Short-term heroin detoxification on an outpatient basis. *Intern. J. Addictions* 6(2): 241–264, 1971.

DOLE, U., NYSWANDER, M., and KREEK, M. Narcotic blockade. *Arch. Int. Med.* 118: 304–309, 1966.

O'MALLEY, J. E., ANDERSON, W. H., and LAZARE, A. Failure of outpatient treatment of drug abuse: I. heroin. *Amer. J. Psychiat.* 128: 865–868, 1972.

RICHMAN, A., PERKINS, M. E., BIHARI, B., and FISHMAN, J. J. Entry into methadone maintenance programs: a follow-up study of New York City heroin users detoxified in 1961–1963. *Amer. J. Public Health* 62: 1002–1007, 1972.

TENNANT, F. S., JR. Drug abuse in the U.S. Army, Europe. *J. Amer. Med. Assoc.* 221: 1146–1149, 1972.

VAILLANT, G. E. A twelve-year follow-up of New York narcotic addicts: the relation of treatment to outcome. *Amer. J. Psychiat.* 122: 727–737, 1966.

A Statement of Purpose

INSTITUTE FOR THE STUDY OF DRUG MISUSE, Inc.

The Institute for the Study of Drug Misuse, Inc. (formerly the Institute for the Study of Drug Addiction) was established in 1965 as an international organization to develop clear channels of communication and to encourage research in the field of drug abuse. To fulfill its goals, the Institute participates in research, professional training, and education. In addition, it serves as a consulting agency in the establishment of treatment programs in the United States and abroad. As professional, government, and lay concern increases in the field of drug abuse, the Institute has been called upon to serve as a resource agency for the dissemination of scientific materials through the press, television, radio, and other media.

In order to achieve its purposes, the Institute for the Study of Drug Misuse:

Sponsors the INTERNATIONAL JOURNAL OF THE ADDICTIONS, published by Marcel Dekker, Inc.

Sponsors national and international conferences and workshops in cooperation with universities, medical teaching centers, governmental agencies, and private industry.

Sponsors a lecture series "The Use and Misuse of Drugs and Alcohol," for professionals and interested lay people.

Sponsors international awards for significant research reports focusing upon various aspects of drug abuse.

The expanding programs of the Institute have been dictated by the present crisis in drug abuse. It is apparent that in the United States and in the world at large, certain social forces are at work which have magnified the scope of the problem. In order to insure that the Institute reaches the broadest group of interested individuals, it has become necessary to establish several categories of membership.

Membership in the Institute for the Study of Drug Misuse is tax exempt.

For membership information, write:

Institute for the Study of Drug Misuse, Inc.
111 Fifth Avenue
New York, N.Y. 10003

INFORMATION FOR AUTHORS SUBMITTING MANUSCRIPTS

Send a clear double-spaced typewritten original and two duplicate copies to the Editor, *International Journal of the Addictions*, Institute for the Study of Drug Misuse, Inc., 111 Fifth Avenue, New York, N.Y. 10003. DOUBLE-SPACE the entire manuscript; do not use single spacing anywhere.

Include authors' academic degrees and present affiliation. If applicable, cite auspices under which work being reported was done. Specify address to which requests for reprints should be sent.

Begin your TITLE with a word useful in indexing. Put news of your finding or a statement of the problem first. Major and minor headings may be used in the text; indicate major headings by typing in capitals. Provide a 100-word SUMMARY at the end.

Use METRIC UNITS of measure. If measurements were made in English units, give metric equivalents.

Cite all TABLES and FIGURES in the text. Tables should have titles, and figures should have brief legends. In tables, give each column a heading. Indicate units of measure in parentheses in the heading for each column. Do not use vertical rules. Do not use horizontal rules other than those in the heading and at the bottom. Submit PHOTOGRAPHS as glossy prints, untrimmed and unmounted; identify each with pencil lightly on the back and indicate top.

ARTWORK will not be returned unless specifically requested, and will be disposed of three months after publication.

REFERENCES in the text should be enclosed in parentheses and include the author's surname and the date of the item cited. Keep footnotes to a minimum.

The BIBLIOGRAPHY (double-spaced) should be given at the end of the article in alphabetical order. Journal references should include authors, title, name of journal abbreviated according to *Chemical Abstracts List of Periodicals,* inclusive page numbers, and date. Book references should include authors, title, place of publication, publisher, and date.

THE INTERNATIONAL JOURNAL OF THE ADDICTIONS

Published by Marcel Dekker, Inc., New York
Sponsored by The Institute for the Study of Drug Misuse, Inc., New York

THE INTERNATIONAL JOURNAL OF THE ADDICTIONS

Volume 9 Number 1 1974

CONTENTS

British Opiate Users: I. People Approaching London Drug Treatment Centres: Herbert H. Blumberg, S. Daryl Cohen, B. Elizabeth Dronfield, Elizabeth A. Mordecai, J. Colin Roberts, and David Hawks 1

Effects of the Vietnam Experience on Subsequent Drug Use Among Servicemen: Michael Rohrbaugh, Gerald Eads, and Samuel Press 25

Rehabilitation of Drug and Alcohol Abusers in the U.S. Army: Harvey L. Ruben 41

Values, Expectations, and Drug Use Among High School Students in a Rural Community: Roderick S. Carman 57

Drug Abuse Training and Education: The Physician: Stanley Einstein 81

Psychological Effects, Personality and Behavioral Changes Attributed to Marihuana Use: Gary Fisher and Allan Steckler 101

Value Structure as a Predictor of Type of Discharge Among Residential Addicts: Jerome S. Miller, John Sensenig, and Jonathan S. Raymond 127

A Comprehensive Military Drug and Alcohol Program: Allen Frances 137

Factors Related to Imprisonment in Female Heroin Addicts: A. E. Raynes, C. Climent, V. D. Patch, and F. Ervin 145

Psychological Differentiation in Heroin Addicts: Dan Arnon, Marc H. Kleinman, and Benjamin Kissin 151

Reliability of Interview Data Concerning Current Heroin Use from Heroin Addicts on Methadone: Thomas J. Cox and Bill Longwell 161

Short-Term, Ambulatory Detoxification of Opiate Addicts Using Methadone: Harry Silsby and Forest S. Tennant, Jr. 167

MARCEL DEKKER, INC., New York

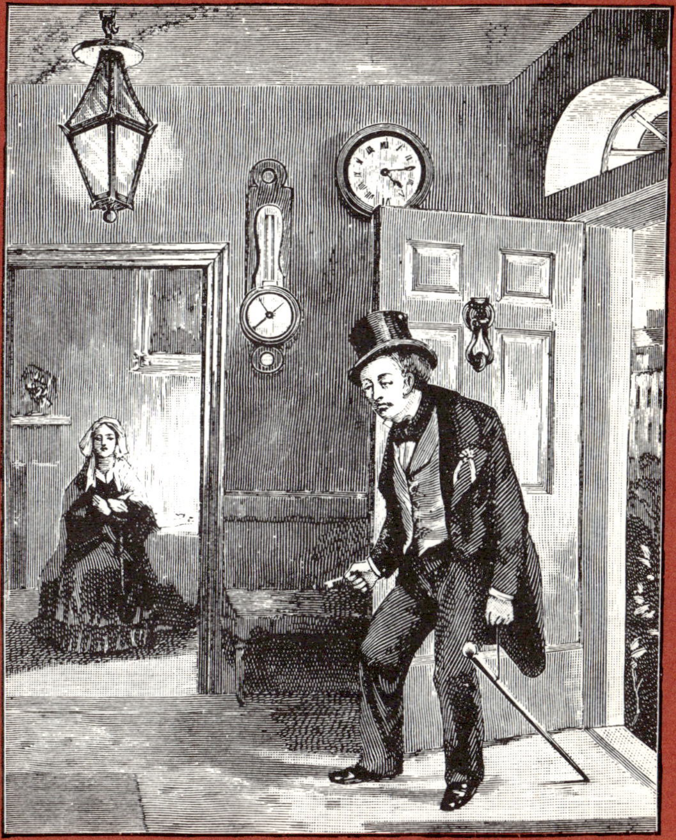

THE INTERNATIONAL JOURNAL OF THE Addictions

Volume 9 Number 2 1974

THE INTERNATIONAL JOURNAL OF THE ADDICTIONS

The International Journal of the Addictions, April 1974

Published six times annually—February, April, June, August, October, December—by Marcel Dekker Inc., 270 Madison Avenue, New York, N. Y. 10016. The subscription rate for Volume 9 (1974) containing 6 issues is $40.00 (prepaid). Postage outside the United States is $5.10 per volume for all subscriptions. The special discounted rate for individual professionals and students is $20.00. Back volume prices will be sent on request. Please *mail payment with order* to the following address: Marcel Dekker Journals, P. O. Box 11305, Church Street Station, New York, New York 10249.

Second-class postage paid at New York, N. Y., and at additional mailing offices.

The International Journal of the Addictions, 9(2), 171–183, 1974

Chemical Mutagenesis and Drugs of Abuse in Man—A Current View of the Problem

Arthur Falek, Ph.D.

Human and Behavior Genetics Research Laboratory
Georgia Mental Health Institute
Department of Psychiatry
Emory University
Atlanta, Georgia

From 1958 through 1962 evidence accumulated that the drug thalidomide, when taken by pregnant women between the 34th and 50th day after the first day of the last menstrual period, resulted in ear and limb deformities to the fetus. The drug, given by prescription throughout Europe, acted in such specific fashion that the observed types of malformations could be correlated with the time of drug ingestion (Lenz, 1971). The teratogenic action of this presumably mild tranquilizer on the fetus not only alarmed the general population but most forcefully alerted the medical community to the possible harmful potential of other chemical agents on man. Concern was voiced in many quarters about the need to evaluate other drugs and chemicals with regard to their possible interference with fertility, production of malformations in the offspring, or carcinogenesis in the individual himself. Just a few years later, in 1967, the phenomenon of chemical mutagenesis as it extended to the chromosome level was dramatically brought to the attention of an already alerted public. In that year chromosome aberrations were reported from *in vivo* and *in vitro* cultures of human leukocyte chromosomes in which the drug under evaluation was lysergic acid diethylamide (Cohen, Marinello, and Back, 1967; Irwin and Egozcue, 1967).

In fact, evidence that chemicals could induce mutations and chromosome damage was known to the geneticists prior to 1967. In studies conducted during World War II and finally permitted publication in 1947, Auerbach and Robson (1947) reported on the induction of mutations by mustard gas, and in that year Darlington and Kohler (1947) presented evidence that mustard gas produced chromosome aberrations similar to those found with ionizing radiations. Studies demonstrating genetic damage as a result of ionizing radiations had been reported almost a generation earlier by J. H. Muller (1927). These early findings were conducted in the fruitfly *Drosophila* and in the plant *Tradescanthia*. Human chromosome damage by chemical agents had been reported in the early 1960s (Cohen, Shaw, and Craig, 1963). Information on human chromosome damage is rather recent in origin because techniques were not available until 1956 (Tjio and Levan, 1956) to carefully examine chromosomes from human tissues, and relatively rapid procedures using peripheral blood leukocytes from human subjects were first described in 1960 (Moorhead et al., 1960).

Cytogenetic studies which reveal evidence of chromosome damage are one method of monitoring the potential harmful effects of new drugs and chemicals. This paper reports on some of the procedures considered to be of value in investigating mutagenic, teratogenic, carcinogenic and chromosome damaging abilities of various drugs and chemicals in man. What are their strengths and limitations, and to what extent have these procedures been employed in the investigation of drugs of abuse?

Many different classes of compounds in man's environment have been shown to break chromosomes. Biological, physical, and chemical agents which cause chromosome damage have been named as clastogens by Shaw, and she recently listed approximately 200 chemical agents which are suspected of being clastogens or mutagens (Shaw, 1970). Chemical agents which are clastogenic may also, of course, be mutagenic, teratogenic, or carcinogenic. The majority of the 200 chemical agents reported by Shaw were investigated using an *in vitro* procedure. This test method is based on the addition of a chemical agent to cultured human leukocytes or fibroblasts for varying times and in specified concentrations. A comparison of chromosome damage in the treated cultures with that found in the untreated control cultures indicates the *in vitro* clastogenic potential of the drug or chemical under investigation. *In vitro* studies are useful as a screening mechanism to determine toxic levels of the agent at various concentrations, and to obtain information regarding a dose-response relationship between chromosome damage in comparison with drug concentration and length of time of exposure.

In vivo cytogenetic studies are conducted in a similar manner except the cultures are established with lymphocytes obtained from individuals treated with the drug or chemical in question. The most useful investigations, of course, are those in which the cytogeneticist has no knowledge of whether or not he is evaluating patient or control cells for chromosome damage. Furthermore, the lymphocyte cultures should be established for both 48 and 72 hours in order that the chromosome aberrations can be evaluated after the first division in culture and compared with chromosome aberrations obtained during the second or third division in culture. This will indicate whether the chromosome anomalies were present in the cells during their residence in the body or are a reflection of their response to the trauma of tissue culture.

Chromosome aberrations are of two kinds, stable and unstable. The unstable chromosome aberrations include breaks, dicentrics, exchange figures, ring chromosomes, and acentric fragments (Figs. 1 and 2). These anomalies are the ones most readily detected in tissue cultures. They are unstable since they will be unable to go through mitotic or meiotic cell divisions. Such chromosome aberrations will most often result in the death of the cell in question.

Stable chromosome rearrangements include deletions, duplications, insertions, inversions (which are either paracentric and result in a change in gene order or pericentric and result in a change in gene order and a shift in centromere position), as well as translocations of chromosome material between two nonhomologous chromosomes, and aberrant centromere division which results in the duplication of one chromosome arm and the formation of an isochromosome. The stable chromosome rearrangements can successfully proceed through mitosis. Unless they cause an alteration in chromosome number or a marked change in configuration, they are difficult to recognize. The unstable rearrangements, however, are the ones which also indicate the occurrence of stable chromosome alterations.

In addition to chromosome studies, there are other methods of approach to chemical mutagens. Vogel and Rohrborn (1970) recommend the dominant lethal and the host mediated assay systems as two procedures for which results in mammals other than man can be extrapolated most readily to man.

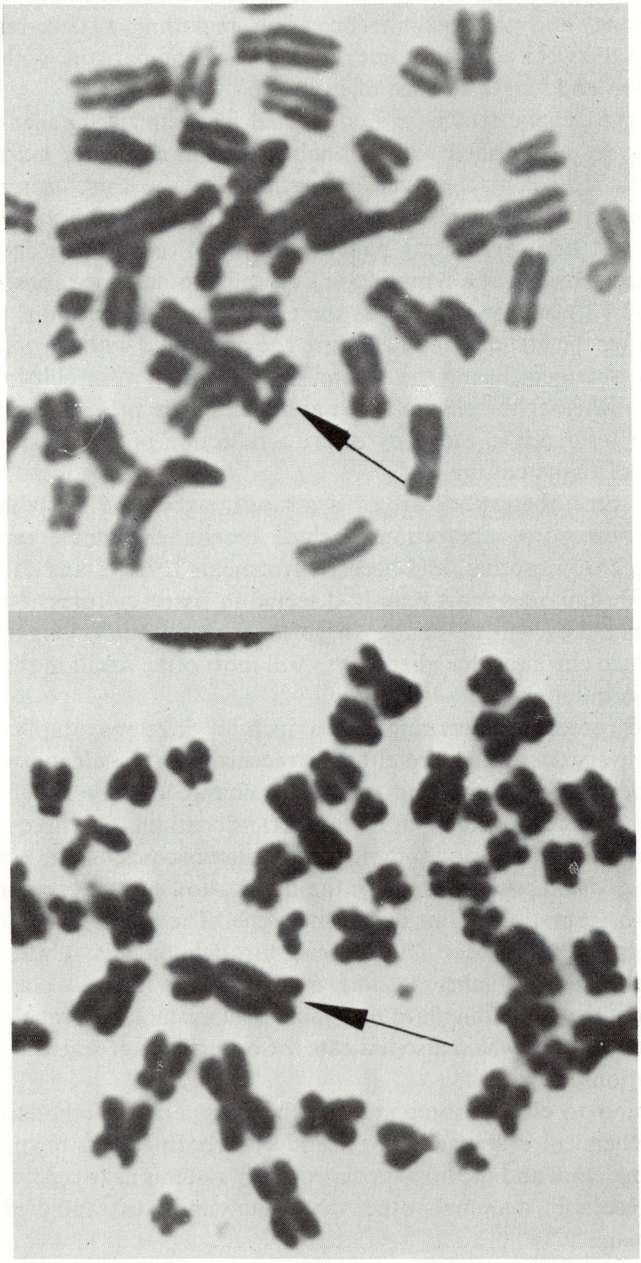

Fig. 1. Chromosome aberrations. Left: Dicentric chromosome. Right: Exchange figure.

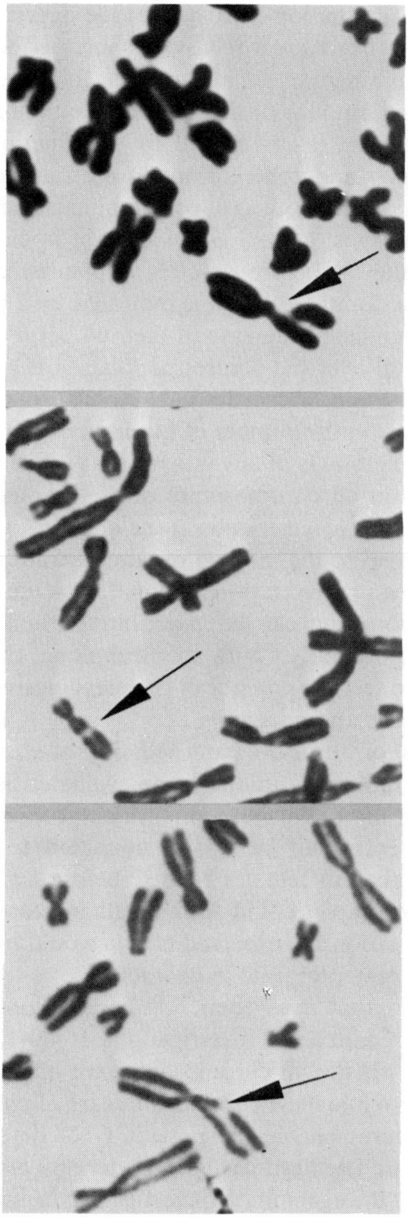

Fig. 2. Chromosome aberrations. Left: Single chromatid gap. Center: Double chromatid gap. Right: Single chromatid break.

The dominant lethal method evaluates germ cell response to chemicals and drugs through an examination of early cleavage stages. Rodents are the animals of choice since they have a relatively short period of pregnancy. The procedure in the dominant lethal method is as follows: male or female mice are given a defined amount of drug at specific time intervals before mating. The time of mating is ascertained by examination for a vaginal plug, and both the study and control females are sacrificed at approximately 15 days' gestation. In both groups of animals the fertilized eggs, the living and dead embryos, as well as evidence of implantation sites of embryos which died shortly before or after implantation, are counted. The determination of a dominant lethal is indicated by a preimplantation loss of eggs, while a significant increase in the number of dead implantations in the experimental over the control population is good evidence of an induced lethal mutation. According to Rohrborn (1970), the best method of comparison is in the number of live implants in the control and test populations. This method is of advantage as (1) it facilitates the analysis of mutation events in all chromosomes of the mammalian germ line within a reasonable length of time, and (2) the chemical treatment in this procedure can be adapted to the method of administration used for man. The chemical or drug can be given to the animal by acute, subacute, or in long-term administration, and can be given intraperitoneally, intramuscularly, intravenously, or orally. With this technique, therefore, experiments can be devised to test the potency of the presumptive mutagen at all stages of spermatogenesis and oogenesis.

The disadvantages of the dominant lethal procedure are that the number of observable point mutations to be evaluated is generally very small and, in addition, the point mutations which produce early lethality in mice or other rodents may be totally unrelated to those in man. Rohrborn also notes that in females treated before conception, endometrium lesions, for example, could lead to an increased rate of dead implants. In such a situation the observed effects would not be mutagenic but, in fact, would be preteratogenic in character.

It is also suggested that cytogenetic studies be conducted in these animals along with dominant lethal investigations. It must be remembered, however, that in mice all the 40 chromosomes are acrocentric and very similar to one another. While these chromosomes are of uniform character, recent banding procedures enable the possibility of detecting structural chromosome alterations. The need has been to develop a system such that it is possible to evaluate the agent under investigation in animals other than man after it is (1) concentrated in the serum, (2) distributed to the body tissues, or (3) detoxified by the liver and excreted in the urine. Some of these requirements have been met by the following host mediated assay system.

This system, established for evaluating potential mutagenic agents in man, is based, according to Legator (1970), on the universal nature of the genetic code. While he notes that there are numerous compounds that are not mutagenic in microorganisms but become active mutagens in animals and vice versa, it is his opinion that there is no basis for assuming that the action of a mutagen would be markedly different in bacteria from that in man. The host mediated assay system was, therefore, developed to determine the ability of laboratory animals to either potentiate or detoxify the mutagenic ability of the compounds in question. In this procedure a mammal such as a mouse is innoculated with an indicator microorganism for which a mutation frequency can be measured during treatment with a potential mutagenic agent. The potential mutagen and the indicator microorganism are always administered differently. After a sufficient length of time, microorganisms are withdrawn from the animal and the kind and frequency of mutagens of the microorganism are determined. Comparison of the mutagenic activity of the agent when given directly to the microorganism as compared with results obtained from the host mediated assay system is indicative of the ability of the host to either detoxify the compound or, as a result of the metabolic activities in the test animal, to form mutagenic compounds in mutant microorganisms. This procedure, now used by Legator and his colleagues at the Food and Drug Administration, employs among indicator organisms the histidine auxotroph *Salmonella* as well as the forward mutation system in *Neurospora*. The animal host of choice in this system is that of the mouse, and Legator reports that hamsters, rats, and guinea pigs have also been used with success. A large series of mutants are available for evaluation with the indicator organisms used in this technique. While this indirect test does not take into account DNA repair mechanisms in the host, differences in the metabolism of the rodent, host, and man or variation in response to an agent by a complicated organism such as man in comparison to that of a microorganism, it was pointed out by Vogel and Rohrborn (1970) that until more practical *in vivo* systems are established to investigate point mutations, the host mediated assay system should be used for routine evaluations.

Long-range planning also envisages the examination of the germ cells in meiosis. Studies are under way in our laboratory, as well as others (Steinberger, Ficher, and Steinberger, 1970; Ellingson and Yao, 1970; Schleiermacher, 1970), to establish mammalian spermatogenesis in culture.

Despite all of these sophisticated procedures, at the present time scientists have no reliable method for the early detection of a genetic catastrophe which may be introduced into the environment by new chemicals and drugs presented for evaluation. As pointed out by Shaw (1970), our methods at present only permit indirect experimental genetic studies which would not detect a rapid increase in damage to the human gene pool which was not anticipated. In a recent paper, Auerbach (1971) also pointed out the dilemma caused by current test procedures and the problems created in the attempt to extrapolate plant, bacterial, and other animal test data to man. According to Auerbach, the difficulties engendered in this type of testing are threefold: (1) specificity of response, (2) correlation between types of damage and, (3) dose-effect relationships. With regard to specificity of response, it is well known that chemicals have a wide range of different genetic effects based on differences between species, strains, sex, and individuals. As pointed out, even in the same individual, different cells and cells in different stages of the cell cycle may vary in response. For example, urethane has been found to act via a metabolite in both rabbits and mice, but only in mice did it induce tumors. If these related mammalian species showed such striking differences in response to a chemical mutagen, it would be hazardous to extrapolate between distantly related species such as mouse and man.

Auerbach, furthermore, noted that there was difficulty in the correlation of stable and unstable chromosome damage. She emphasized that chromosome breakage not followed by reunion would only result in a dominant lethal and early abortion and that there were no procedures to evaluate whether such animals could also produce more stable mutants which would survive and reproduce. Finally, sufficient knowledge was not available to determine whether it was possible to extrapolate from a system which resulted in a genetic effect at a high dose of a potential mutagen to a possible effect at a lower dose. Possibly, physiologically acceptable doses would be well below the threshhold for genetic effects. It was her belief that relevant data in this area might be obtained from determination of the dose-effect curves for weak mutagens.

This suggestion has also been proposed by Crow (1971) who indicated that the most frequent class of mutants produced in the human population by environmental mutagens consisted of those with mild effects. From *Drosophila* data he suggested that the spontaneous mutation rate produced by mildly deliterious mutants was about 15 times as high as the rate for lethal mutations which was estimated at approximately 0.014 per gamete. The average effect of such homozygous mutants according to Crow would reduce the probability of survival to adulthood by 2 to 3%. Furthermore, he observed that such mutants were not completely recessive, and also had an effect on the heterozygote. While in the heterozygote these mildly deliterious mutants did not produce significant genetic disorders, they could remain in the population for many generations. If they affected the physical, physiological, and mental ability of individuals, to ignore them would be to ignore the submerged part of the iceberg.

Drugs of abuse, on the other hand, are located on the most visible portion of the iceberg. What evidence is there that drugs of abuse such as LSD, heroin, or marijuana result in genetic damage to the individual or his offspring? With regard to LSD, an extensive review of studies by Dishotsky and his colleagues (1971) revealed contradictory results. These contradictory findings were observed even in studies employing similar test systems. Analysis of the *in vitro* leukocyte studies with LSD indicated no consistent dose-response relationship, and there was evidence by some that the reported chromosome damage was well within the range of that induced by physiological concentrations of a proprietary drug such as aspirin (Kato and Jarvik, 1969). *In vivo* cytogenetic studies on 310 LSD users indicated a significant increase of chromosome damage among illicit LSD users as compared with subjects on pure LSD. A portion of the LSD abusers also reported using other drugs. Teratogenic effects in rodents indicated a wide variation in individual, strain, and species response to LSD. The effect was found to be highly specific to a time early in gestation, and no effect was found when exposure occurred late in pregnancy. It has been suggested that a similar critical period exists for man. While this has not been confirmed, there is some evidence of early abortions in pregnant women ingesting illicit LSD. There are no data available on congenital malformations in human offspring exposed before birth to pure LSD, although there are several cases in which women on illicit LSD produced children with an increased frequency of chromosomal aberrations. In addition, there are six reports in the literature of malformed infants born to women who used LSD prior to or during pregnancy. In our own studies we have recently found that one infant with trisomy Down's syndrome and chromosome damage was born to parents who abused drugs. In fact, the mother had hepatitis at the time of delivery. In both mother and child, however, the unstable chromosome damage was transitory. Furthermore, this one case does not imply that the risk of Down's syndrome is increased in the offspring of drug abusers. While several cases of leukemia and persons with a Ph_1-like chromosome have been reported, there is little data at present to substantiate that LSD is a carcinogen. The evidence, as summarized by Dishotsky and his colleagues

(1971), suggests that LSD is a weak mutagen which results in an elevated rate of spontaneous abortions in pregnant women exposed to the illicit drug.

On the other hand, would this chemical be considered a safe drug according to current methods of evaluation? It is unfortunate that there are no reports based on the host mediated assay system about the potential mutagenic aspects of LSD. An experimental design recently suggested by Robson (1970) is as follows: If a drug's teratogenicity is open to challenge, a measure of value would be the ratio of the dose toxic to 50% of the mothers (LD_{50}) over the concentration which produces teratogenic effects in the fetus. It was determined by Robson that a ratio of 10 or better would reject the main human teratogens. Based on this information, the reports by Auerbach and Rugowski (1967) in mice and Alexander and his colleagues (1967) in rats with pure LSD have teratogenic ratios well over the mark required for the rejection of this compound. From their results, standard FDA procedures should require that LSD in the pure as well as in the illicit state be rejected. If, on the other hand, we selectively reject the FDA conclusions on selective drugs, what procedures will be available to replace them? Without a consistent drug testing policy, all of us will be exposed to constant danger. The need is to improve procedures and make them relevant, not to remove them. To determine the mutagenic and teratogenic aspects of a drug, what is needed in addition to information on its metabolism and elimination is the passage of these drugs and their metabolites into the embryo.

From the FDA point of view, heroin presents a more simplified problem. The ease of addiction and mental clouding as well as the physical and somatic effects due to the heroin habit are sufficient to have designated this opiate as a drug of abuse. Evidence is available that heroin has stronger effects and reaches peak degrees relatively earlier than does morphine (Smith and Beecher, 1962; Smith, Senke, and Beecher, 1962). These studies also indicate that at 1/3 the dose of morphine, heroin produces greater impairment of mental acuity and physical inactivity. From the standpoint of the production of undesirable side effects, therefore, heroin is medically of less value than morphine. There is also considerable evidence to demonstrate that the addictive effects of heroin can be transmitted in pregnancy to the fetus. The teratogenic effect of heroin and morphine has been described in a dominant lethal study of hamsters by Geber (1972). At very high levels of these drugs there is a marked increase in malformations in the offspring, while at physiologic concentrations there is no evidence of malformations or a decrease in fertility. Unfortunately, there are no other dominant lethal studies to compare with this one, and there is no study reported on the host mediated assay system for the evaluation of the potential mutagenic effect of either heroin or morphine. The only chromosome study of morphine is an *in vitro* one examining the effects of this drug in human lymphocytes at $3\times$, $1\times$, $1/3\times$, $1/6\times$ and $1/12\times$ the physiological level (Falek et al., 1972). The data from these *in vitro* investigations revealed no increased frequency of chromosome breakage even at the highest concentrations of this drug. Data from *in vivo* studies with heroin and morphine are based on studies of an illicit drug population (Falek et al., 1972). Individuals in this population also abused a multiple number of other drugs. There is evidence from that study of an increased frequency of unstable chromosome damage in 72 hour cultures. Since no such increase in clastogenic activity was noted in the 48 hour cultures, these findings suggested that this unstable damage might be indicative of chromosome fragility of cells in culture from some individuals abusing multiple drugs.

Until a few years ago there was very little material available for the study of marijuana. Since that time the federal government has established a farm in Mississippi and a research program to evaluate the biologic, psychologic, and sociologic aspects of marijuana use. The intoxicant ingredients in marijuana are the tetrahydrocannabinols. The information thus far is very limited, but it is expected that in the near future there will be data to clarify questions with regard to tolerance, withdrawal symptoms, physical dependence, and behavioral changes. It would seem that in common with many other drugs it may be that the subjective effects are in large measure related to the expectation of the user. The dominant lethal test by Geber and Schramm (1969) indicated that at high doses of marijuana there was an induction of congenital malformations in the fetal hamster and rabbit. Dominant lethal studies by other investigators have not as yet been reported nor has any study utilizing the host mediated assay system. No *in vitro* or *in vivo* chromosome studies with marijuana have been presented.

It appears, therefore, that much work has to be done in evaluating drugs of abuse with regard to their mutagenic, teratogenic, and carcinogenic effects. It is highly desirable that such data be obtained, particularly with marijuana since it is used so extensively in the population which includes a high proportion of persons in their reproductive period of life.

REFERENCES

ALEXANDER, G.J., MILES, B.E., GOLD, G.M., and ALEXANDER, R.B. LSD: injection early in pregnancy produces abnormalities in offspring. *Science* 157: 459, 1967.

AUERBACH, C. The dilemma of testing: is the medium of the test the message of our conclusions. *Environmental Mutagen Soc. Newsletter* 4: 16, 1971.

AUERBACH, C., and ROBSON, J.N. The production of mutations by chemical substances. *Proc. Roy. Soc. Edinburgh* B62: 271, 1947.

AUERBACH, R., and RUGOWSKI, J.A. Lysergic acid diethylamide: effect on embryos. *Science* 157: 1325, 1967.

COHEN, M.M., MARINELLO, M., and BACK, N. Chromosomal damage to human leukocytes induced by lysergic acid diethylamide. *Science* 155: 1417, 1967.

COHEN, M.M., SHAW, M.W., and CRAIG, A.P. The effects of streptonigrin on cultured human leukocytes. *Proc. Nat. Acad. Sci. U.S.* 50: 16, 1963.

CROW, J.F. The meaning of mutagenicity for society. *Environmental Mutagen Soc. Newsletter* 4: 16, 1971.

DARLINGTON, C.D., and KOHLER, P.C. The chemical breakage of chromosomes. *Heredity* (London) 1: 187, 1947.

DISHOTSKY, N.I., LOUGHMAN, W.D., MOGAR, R.B., and LIPSCOMB, W.R. LSD and genetic damage. *Science* 172: 431, 1971.

ELLINGSON, D.J., and YAO, K.T.S. Growth and observation of Chinese hamster seminiferous epithelium in vitro. *J. Cell Sci.* 6: 195, 1970.

FALEK, A., JORDAN, R.B., KING, B.J., ARNOLD, P.J., and SKELTON, D.W. Human chromosomes and opiates. *Arch. Gen. Psychiat.* 27: 511, 1972.

GEBER, W.F. Personal communication.

GEBER, W.F., and SCHRAMM, L.C. Marijuana extract: induction of congenital malformations in the fetal hamster and rabbit. *Toxicol. Appl. Pharmacol.* 14: 276, 1969.

IRWIN, S., and EGOZCUE, J. Chromosomal abnormalities in leukocytes from LSD-25 users. *Science* 157: 313, 1967.

KATO, T., and JARVIK, L.S. LSD-25 and genetic damage. *Diseases Nervous System* 30: 42, 1969.

LEGATOR, M.S. The host mediated assay system, a practical procedure for evaluating potential mutagenic agents. In F. Vogel and G. Rohrborn (eds.) *Chemical Mutagenesis in Mammals and Man.* New York: Springer, 1970, Chap. 15.

LENZ, W. How can the teratogenic action of a factor be established in man? *South. Med. J.* 64 (Suppl. 1): 41, 1971.

MOORHEAD, P.S., NORWELL, P.C., MELLMAN, W.J., BATTIPS, D.M., and HUNGERFORD, D.A. Chromosome preparation of leukocytes cultured from human peripheral blood. *Exp. Cell Res.* 20: 613, 1960.

MULLER, H.J. Artificial transmutation of a gene. *Science* 66: 84, 1927.

ROBSON, J.M. Testing drugs for their teratogenicity and their effects on fertility. *Brit. Med. Bull.* 26: 212, 1970.

ROHRBORN, G. The dominant lethals: method and cytogenetic examination of early cleavage stages. In F.Vogel and G. Rohrborn (eds.) *Chemical Mutagenesis in Mammals and Man.* New York: Springer, 1970, Chap. 4.

SCHLEIERMACHER, E. Histological and cytogenetic investigation methods on mammalian spermatogenesis. In F. Vogel and G. Rohrborn (eds.) *Chemical Mutagenesis in Mammals and Man.* New York: Springer, 1970, Chap. 7.

SHAW, M.W. Human chromosome damage by chemical agents. *Ann. Rev. Med.* 21: 409, 1970.

SMITH, G.M., and BEECHER, H.K. Subjective effects of heroin and morphine in normal subjects and placebo in normal subjects. *J. Pharm. Exp. Therap.* 136: 47, 1962.

SMITH, G.M. SENKE, C.W., and BEECHER, H.K. Objective evidence of mental effects of heroin and morphine. *J. Pharm. Exp. Therap.* 136: 54, 1962.

STEINBERGER, A., FICHER, M., and STEINBERGER, E. Studies of spermatogenesis and steroid metabolism in cultures of human testicular tissue. In E. Rosemberg and C.A. Paulsen (eds.) *The Human Testis.* New York: Plenum, 1970.

TJIO, J., and LEVAN, A. The chromosome number in man. *Hereditas* 42: 1, 1956.

VOGEL, F., and ROHRBORN, G. Concluding remarks. In F. Vogel and G. Rohrborn (eds.) *Chemical Mutagenesis in Mammals and Man.* New York: Springer, 1970, Chap. 29.

The International Journal of the Addictions, 9(2), 185–204, 1974

Multidrug Use: Supplementary Perspectives

Paul C. Whitehead

Department of Sociology
University of Western Ontario
and Lake Erie Region
Addiction Research Foundation
London, Ontario, Canada

The phenomenon of multiple drug use has been examined for a number of different types of groups ranging from "normals" (Blum et al., 1969) to psychiatric patients (Frosch, 1969; Rockwell, 1969; Rickels and Brand, 1969) to opiate users (Lucas et al., 1972). Most attention has been devoted to marihuana smokers (Goode, 1969; Whitehead et al., 1972; Grupp, 1971). Each of these studies has found high rates of multiple drug use among the populations in question. That is, each study suggests that users of any one drug are more likely to use other drugs than those who do not use that drug. However, the validity of this conclusion has yet to be tested for a variety of other types of drugs, e.g., alcohol, tobacco, and speed. Previous studies suggest that there may be some etiological significance that is attached to the use of a drug in terms of increasing the probability of using other drugs. However, this needs to be further examined in terms of other substances, and this is the purpose of this paper.

METHOD

Sampling. The survey involved 1,606 students from Grades 7, 9, 11, and 12, representing the Metropolitan Halifax (Nova Scotia) school attendance area. A 25% random sample of classes in each of the four grades mentioned above was chosen (63 classes from 26 schools) and the students in each of these classes completed a questionnaire concerning their use of drugs (cf., Whitehead, 1970a). Other research findings (Whitehead and Smart, 1972) allow us to attach considerable credibility to self-reported drug use.

Subjects. Fifty-one percent of the students were male and 49% were female. Their ages were as follows: 11–13 years, 24.0%; 14–16 years, 40.6%; 17–19 years, 33.7%; and 20 and over, 1.7%. Ninety-two percent of their mothers and fathers were born in North America and English was the only language spoken in 96% of their homes. Half of the students came from homes where the religious preference was Catholic and 44% from Protestant homes. Only 1.5% of the students were Jewish. Eight-nine percent of the students lived with both their parents. Almost 12% of the fathers did not work. The occupational categories within which the others fell were the following: professional or managerial, 24.7%; proprietor, 5.3%; clerical or sales, 17.1%; skilled or technical, 19.2%; and semiskilled, 22.1%. (Analysis and discussion of the relationship between the use of drugs and the following variables are available elsewhere: religious affiliation [Whitehead, 1970b), academic performance (Whitehead, 1971), and broken homes (Whitehead and Laforest, 1971).]

RESULTS

Of the 1,606 students in the survey, 704 did not acknowledge having used any of the following 10 drugs during the 6 months prior to the survey: tobacco, alcohol, solvents, LSD, tranquilizers, stimulants, marihuana, barbiturates, other hallucinogens (e.g., STP), or opiates. Hence, the current paper is based on the 902 students who acknowledged having used at least one of these drugs.

Table 1 indicates the number and percentage of students reporting the use of the 10 drugs examined in the Halifax study. The 6.6% of the sample that reported use of marihuana will not be commented on further here as their multiple drug use was the subject of a previous paper (Whitehead et al., 1972).

Table 1
Rates of Drug Use Among Halifax Students, 1969 (N = *902*)

Drug	*N*	%
Tobacco	764	84.7
Alcohol	643	71.3
Solvents	137	15.2
LSD	82	9.1
Tranquilizers	79	8.8
Stimulants	77	8.5
Marihuana	106	6.6
Barbiturates	44	4.9
Other hallucinogens	41	4.6
Opiates	27	3.0

Tobacco. Tobacco was used by 85% of the students. There were no significant differences between the users and nonusers of tobacco in their use of alcohol, tranquilizers, marihuana, stimulants, solvents, or other hallucinogens. While none of the nonsmokers of tobacco had ever used opiates, 3.5% of the smokers had. Over two times as many tobacco smokers as nonsmokers had used LSD, and eight times as many had used barbiturates. These three differences are significant at the 0.05 level (Table 2; Fig. 1).

Table 2
Comparison of Rates of Drug Use Between Users and Nonusers of Tobacco (N = *902*)

	A Users ($N = 764$)		B Nonusers ($N = 138$)			
Drug	*N*	%	*N*	%	Ratio A/B	Chi-square
Stimulants	70	9.2	7	5.1	1.8	2.0
Opiates	27	3.5	0	0.0	—	3.9*
Tranquilizers	66	8.6	13	9.4	0.9	0.0
Alcohol	542	70.9	101	73.2	1.0	0.2
LSD	76	9.9	6	4.3	2.3	3.8*
Marihuana	176	23.0	34	24.6	0.9	0.1
Other hallucinogens	39	5.1	2	1.4	3.6	2.8
Solvents	120	15.7	17	12.3	1.3	0.8
Barbiturates	43	5.6	1	0.7	8.0	5.0*

*$p < .05$.

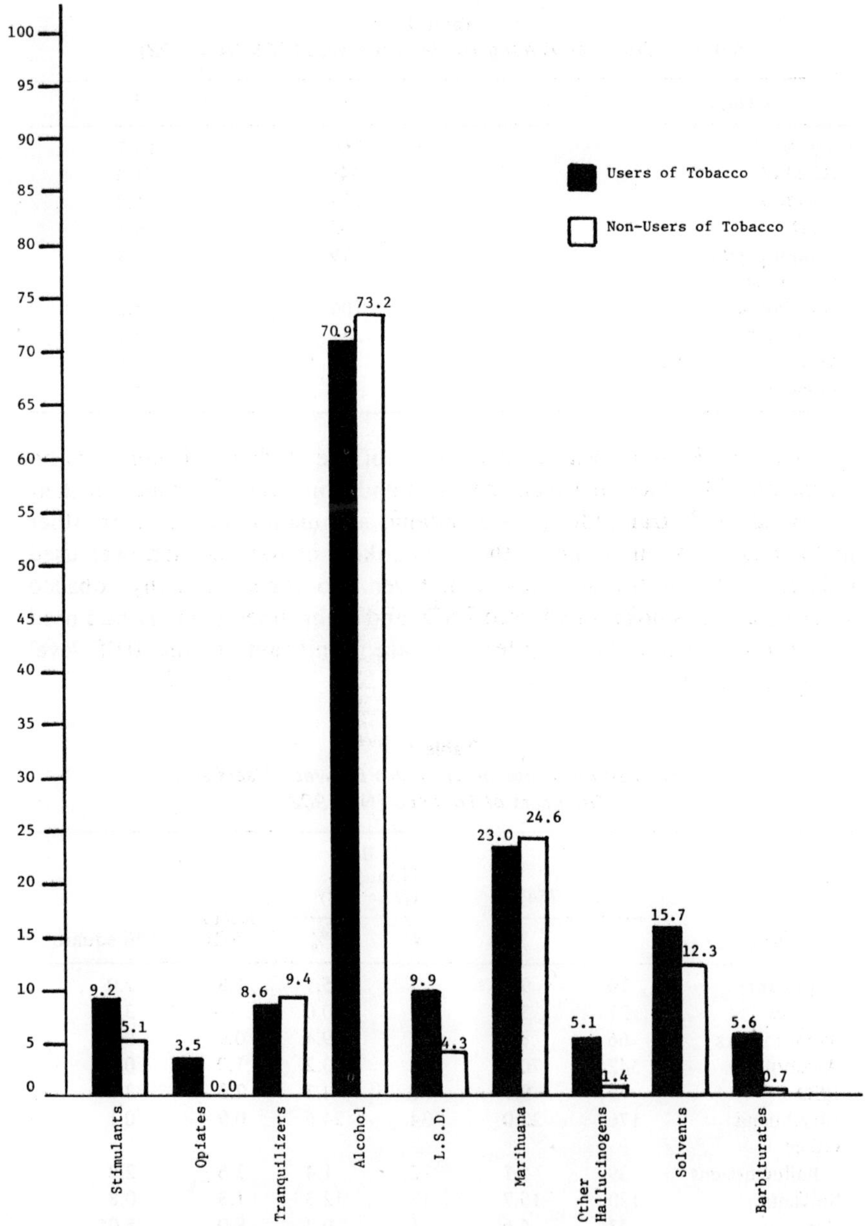

Fig. 1. Graphic comparison of rates of drug use between users and nonusers of tobacco.

Table 3
Comparison of Rates of Drug Use Between Users and Nonusers of Alcohol (N = *902*)

Drug	A Users ($N = 643$)		B Nonusers ($N = 259$)		Ratio A/B	Chi-square
	N	%	*N*	%		
Stimulants	67	10.4	10	3.9	2.7	9.3**
Opiates	27	4.2	0	0.0	—	9.8**
Tobacco	542	84.3	221	85.3	1.0	0.2
Tranquilizers	67	10.4	12	4.6	2.3	7.0**
LSD	76	11.8	6	2.3	5.1	19.0**
Marihuana	184	28.6	26	10.0	2.9	34.6**
Other hallucinogens	38	5.9	3	1.2	4.9	8.5**
Solvents	114	17.7	23	8.9	2.0	10.5**
Barbiturates	41	6.4	3	1.2	5.3	9.7**

$^{**}p < .01$.

Alcohol. Alcohol users comprise 71.3% of the students surveyed. Of these, 84.3% had used tobacco. A comparable 85.3% of the nonusers had used tobacco. Two to three times as many alcohol users as nonusers had also used stimulants, tranquilizers, solvents, and marihuana. Almost five times as many users had used other hallucinogens and over five times as many had ever used LSD and barbiturates. These differences, except for the negligible one on tobacco use, are significiant at the 0.01 level (Table 3; Fig. 2).

Solvents. Fifteen percent of the high school students had used solvents (Table 4; Fig. 3). Among these users, the use of opiates was almost 14 times as frequent as it was among nonusers of solvents. Thirteen times as many solvent users as nonusers had used barbiturates; almost eight times as many had used stimulants or other hallucinogens; five and one half times as many users had also used LSD, while almost five times as many had ever used tranquilizers, over three times as many had used marihuana, and 1.2 times as many had used alcohol. These differences are all significant at the 0.01 level. There is no significant difference in the proportion of solvent users and nonusers who had also used tobacco.

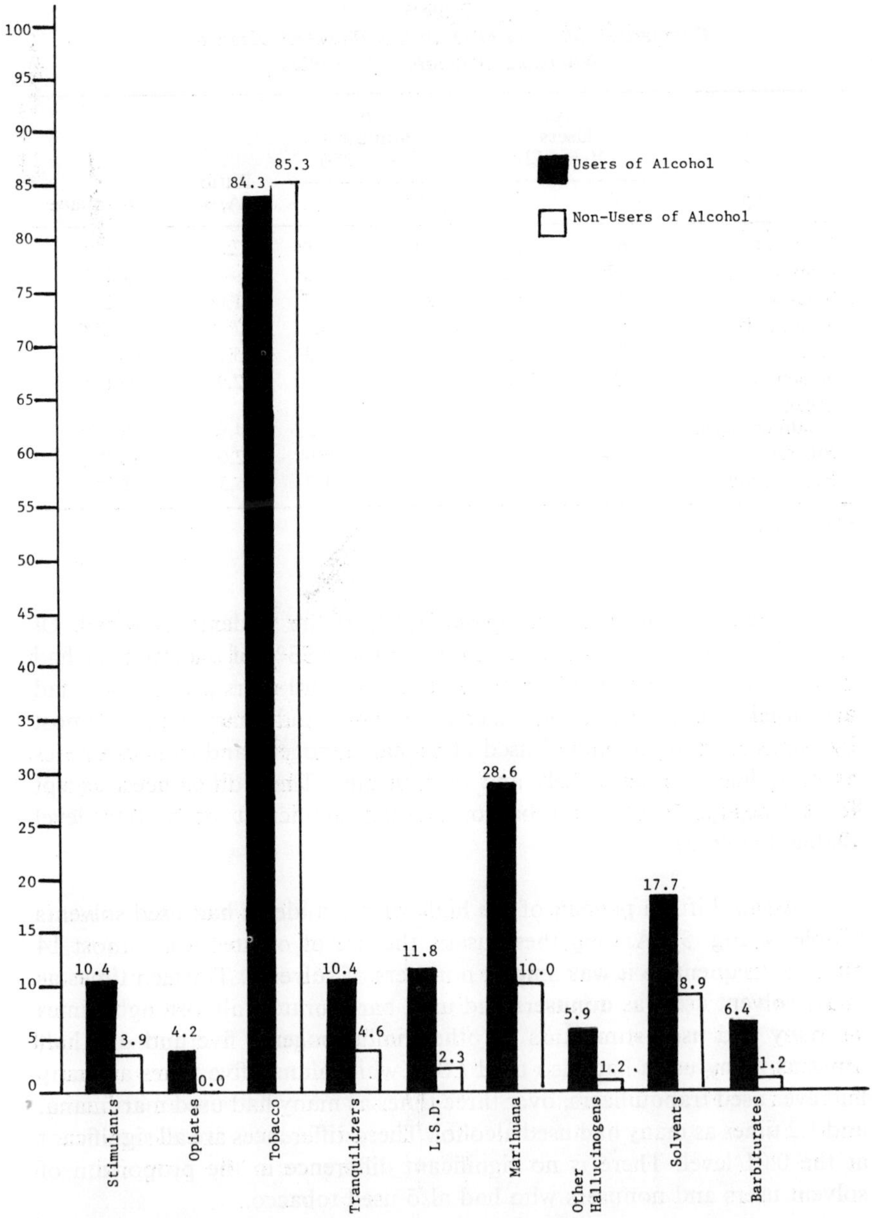

Fig. 2. Graphic comparison of rates of drug use between users and nonusers of alcohol.

Table 4
Comparison of Rates of Drug Use Between Users and Nonusers of Solvents (N = 902)

Drug	A Users (N = 137)		B Nonusers (N = 765)		Ratio A/B	Chi-square
	N	%	N	%		
Stimulants	45	32.8	32	4.2	7.8	118.6**
Opiates	19	13.9	8	1.0	13.9	61.4**
Tobacco	120	87.6	644	84.2	1.0	0.8
Tranquilizers	36	26.3	43	5.6	4.7	59.5**
Alcohol	114	83.2	529	69.2	1.2	10.5**
LSD	41	29.9	41	5.4	5.5	81.9**
Marihuana	80	58.4	130	17.0	3.4	109.2**
Other hallucinogens	24	17.5	17	2.2	7.9	59.2**
Barbiturates	31	22.6	13	1.7	13.3	105.2**

**$p < .01$.

Table 5
Comparison of Rates of Drug Use Between Users and Nonusers of LSD (N = 902)

Drug	A Users (N = 82)		B Nonusers (N = 820)		Ratio A/B	Chi-square
	N	%	N	%		
Stimulants	43	52.4	34	4.1	12.8	216.5**
Opiates	20	24.4	7	0.9	27.1	134.2**
Tobacco	76	92.7	688	83.9	1.1	3.8**
Tranquilizers	21	25.6	58	7.1	3.6	29.8**
Alcohol	76	92.7	567	69.1	1.3	19.0**
Marihuana	78	95.1	132	16.1	5.9	256.2**
Other hallucinogens	26	31.7	15	1.8	17.6	146.6**
Solvents	41	50.0	96	11.7	4.3	81.9**
Barbiturates	30	36.6	14	1.7	21.5	188.0**

**$p < .01$.

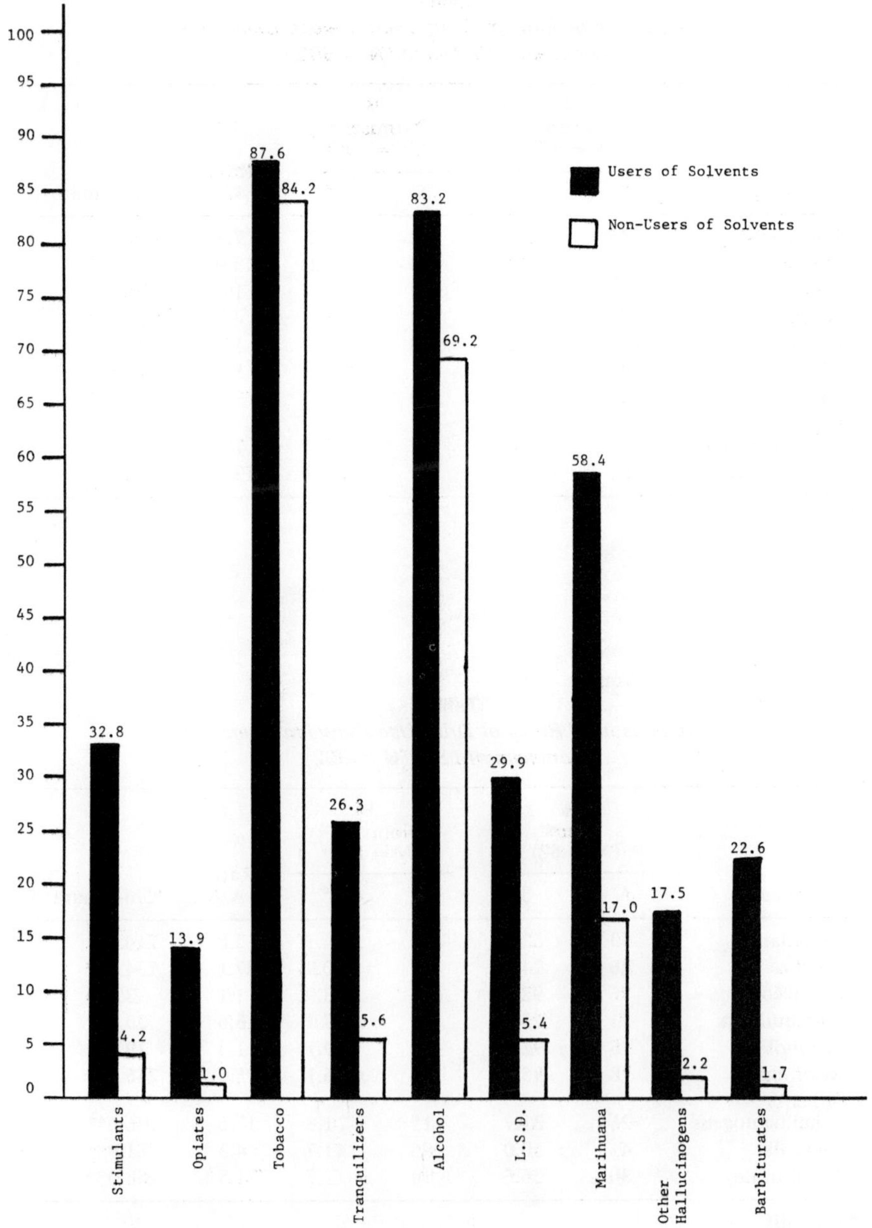

Fig. 3. Graphic comparison of rates of drug use between users and nonusers of solvents.

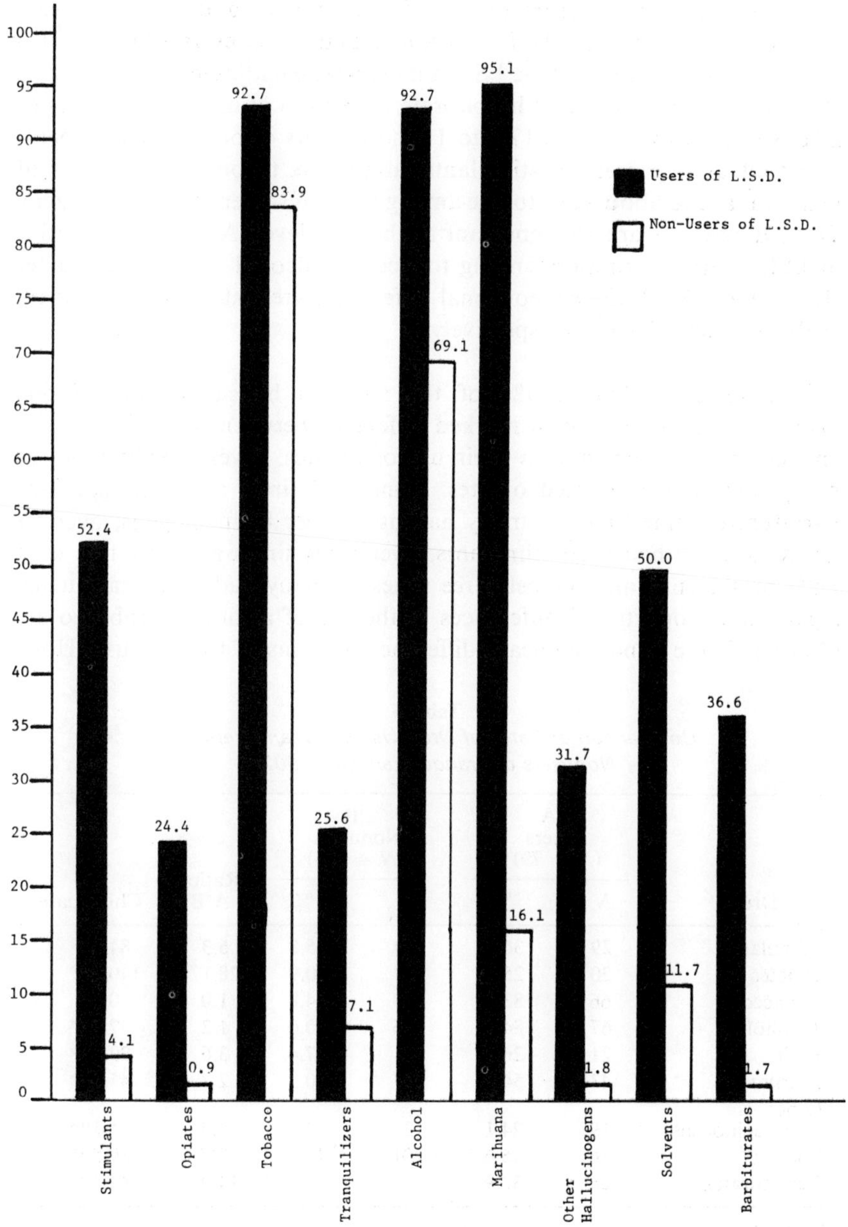

Fig. 4. Graphic comparison of rates of drug use between users and nonusers of LSD.

LSD. When LSD users (9.1% of the sample) and nonusers were examined (Table 5; Fig. 4), it was found that those users who had also used opiates outnumbered the LSD nonusers who had used opiates 27 to 1. Of those who had also used barbiturates, the ratio of users to nonusers of LSD was 21.5 to 1. It was 17.6 to 1 among users of other hallucinogens, 12.8 to 1 among users of stimulants, almost six to one among users of marihuana, and about four to one among users of solvents or tranquilizers. These differences are all significant at the 0.01 level. Although the ratios of LSD users to nonusers among tobacco or alcohol users were smaller (1.1: 1 and 1.3: 1), the proportional differences are statistically significant at the .05 and .01 levels, respectively.

Tranquilizers. Almost 9% of the students had used tranquilizers (Table 6; Fig. 5). The most marked difference between tranquilizer users and nonusers occurred with their use of opiates. Twenty-eight times as many users had also used opiates. Almost 15 times as many had used barbiturates, nine times as many had used other hallucinogens, over six times as many had used stimulants, over three times as many had used LSD or solvents, and almost three times as many had used marihuana. Again, the proportional differences in the use of alcohol or tobacco are reduced. There is no significant difference in terms of tobacco use. How-

Table 6
Comparison of Rates of Drug Use Between Users and Nonusers of Tranquilizers (N = *902*)

Drug	A Users ($N = 79$)		B Nonusers ($N = 823$)		Ratio A/B	Chi-square
	N	%	*N*	%		
Stimulants	29	36.7	48	5.8	6.3	84.1**
Opiates	20	25.3	7	0.9	28.1	140.3**
Tobacco	66	83.5	698	84.8	1.0	0.0
Alcohol	67	84.8	576	70.0	1.2	7.0**
LSD	21	26.6	61	7.4	3.6	29.8**
Marihuana	43	54.4	167	20.3	2.7	45.1**
Other hallucinogens	19	24.1	22	2.7	8.9	71.1**
Solvents	36	45.6	101	12.3	3.7	59.5**
Barbiturates	26	32.9	18	2.2	14.9	140.1**

**$p < .01$.

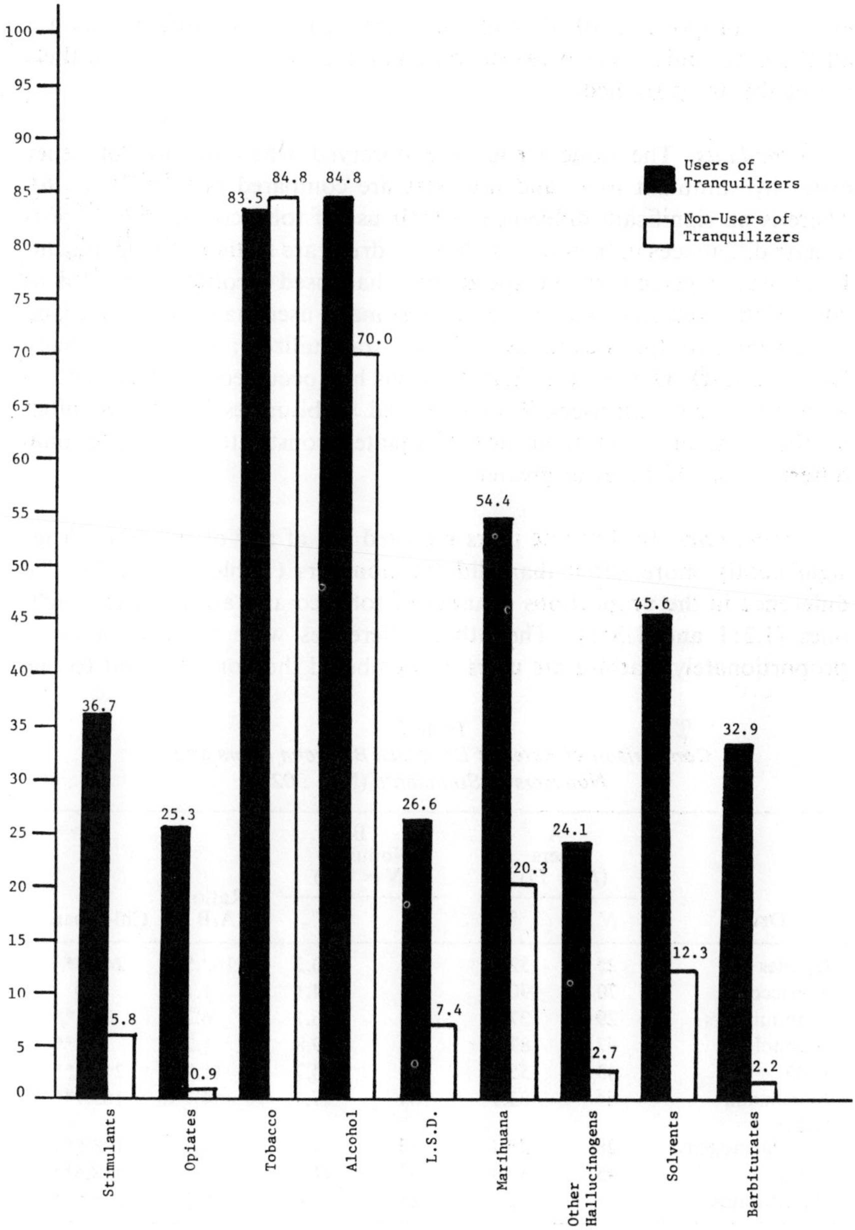

100
95
90
85
80
75
70
65
60
55
50
45
40
35
30
25
20
15
10
5
0
Users of Tranquilizers
Non-Users of Tranquilizers
36.7
5.8
25.3
0.9
83.5
84.8
84.8
70.0
26.6
7.4
54.4
20.3
24.1
2.7
45.6
12.3
32.9
2.2
Stimulants
Opiates
Tobacco
Alcohol
L.S.D.
Marihuana
Other Hallucinogens
Solvents
Barbiturates

ever, the proportions of alcohol users are significantly different, as are all the other differences between tranquilizer users and nonusers in their use of the drugs studied.

Stimulants. The same trends are observed when the use of other drugs by stimulant users and nonusers are compared (Table 7; Fig. 6). There is no significant difference in their use of tobacco, but the proportionate differences in their use of all other drugs are statistically significant. Eighty-seven percent of the speed users had used alcohol, compared to 70% of the nonusers. About five times as many users had used marihuana or solvents; six times as many had used tranquilizers; 12 times as many had used LSD. Use of other hallucinogens had occurred 23 times as often among the stimulant users. They had used barbiturates 25 times as often as the nonusers, and their use of opiates constitutes a proportional difference of 162 times or greater.

Barbiturates. Barbiturate users reported use of any of the other drugs significantly more often than did the nonusers (Table 8; Fig. 7). The difference in the proportions of users of tobacco and alcohol were slight ones (1.2:1 and 1.3:1). The other differences were more prominent: proportionately, barbiturate users outnumbered the nonusers four to one

Table 7
Comparison of Rates of Drug Use Between Users and Nonusers of Stimulants (N = *902*)

	A Users ($N = 77$)		B Nonusers ($N = 825$)			
Drug	N	%	N	%	Ratio A/B	Chi-square
Opiates	25	32.5	2	0.2	162.5	240.9*
Tobacco	70	90.9	694	84.1	1.1	2.0
Tranquilizers	29	37.7	50	6.1	6.2	84.1**
Alcohol	67	87.0	576	69.8	1.2	9.3**
LSD	43	55.8	39	4.7	11.9	216.5**
Marihuana	64	83.1	164	17.7	4.7	165.1**
Other hallucinogens	28	36.4	13	1.6	22.7	188.5**
Solvents	45	58.4	92	11.2	5.2	118.6**
Barbiturates	31	40.3	13	1.6	25.2	218.9**

*$p < .05$.
**$p < .01$.

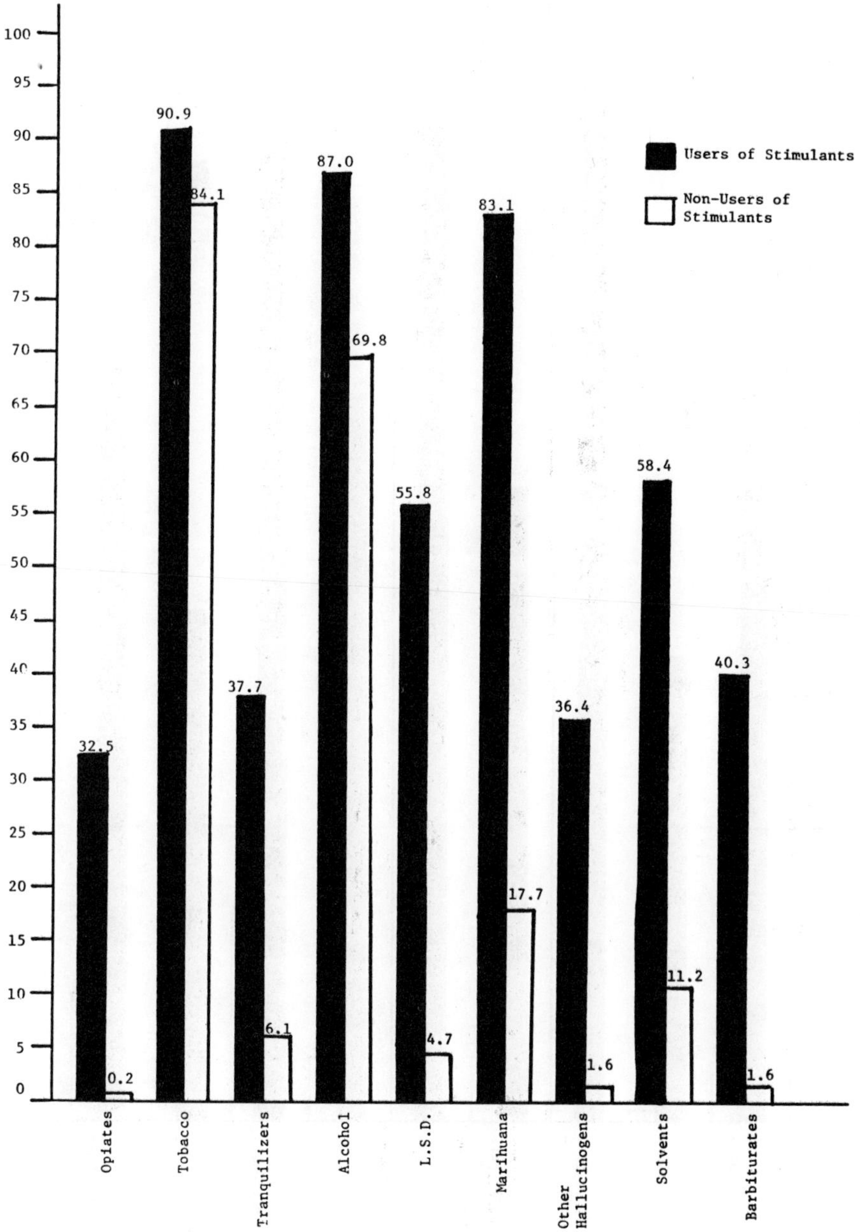

Fig. 6. Graphic comparison of rates of drug use between users and nonusers of stimulants.

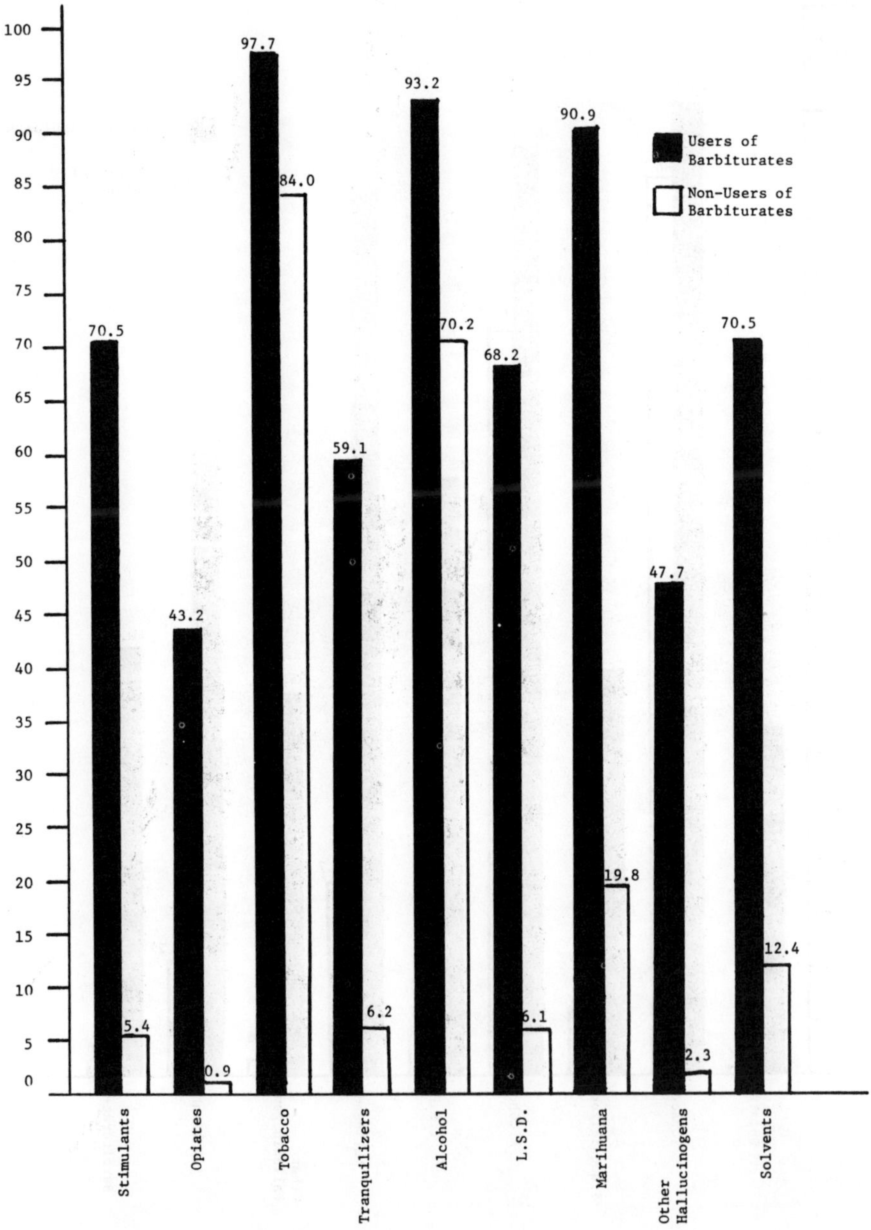

Fig. 7. Graphic comparison of rates of drug use between users and nonusers of barbiturates.

Table 8
Comparison of Rates of Drug Use Between Users and Nonusers of Barbiturates (N = *902*)

Drug	A Users (*N* = 44)		B Nonusers (*N* = 858)		Ratio A/B	Chi-square
	N	%	*N*	%		
Stimulants	31	70.5	46	5.4	13.1	218.9**
Opiates	19	43.2	8	0.9	48.0	242.9**
Tobacco	43	97.7	721	84.0	1.2	5.0*
Tranquilizers	26	59.1	53	6.2	9.5	140.1**
Alcohol	41	93.2	602	70.2	1.3	9.7**
LSD	30	68.2	52	6.1	11.2	188.0**
Marihuana	40	90.9	170	19.8	4.6	114.5**
Other hallucinogens	21	47.7	20	2.3	20.7	188.5**
Solvents	31	70.5	106	12.4	5.7	105.2**

*$p < .05$.
**$p < .01$.

Table 9
Comparison of Rates of Drug Use Between Users and Nonusers of Other Hallucinogens (N = *902*)

Drug	A Users (*N* = 41)		B Nonusers (*N* = 861)		Ratio A/B	Chi-square
	N	%	*N*	%		
Stimulants	28	68.3	49	5.7	12.0	188.5**
Opiates	20	48.8	7	0.8	61.0	293.8**
Tobacco	39	95.1	725	84.2	1.1	2.8
Tranquilizers	19	46.3	60	7.0	6.6	71.1**
Alcohol	38	92.7	605	70.3	1.3	8.5**
LSD	26	63.4	56	6.5	9.7	146.6**
Marihuana	39	95.1	171	19.9	4.8	119.9**
Solvents	24	58.5	113	13.1	4.8	59.2**
Barbiturates	21	51.2	23	2.7	19.0	188.5**

**$p < .01$.

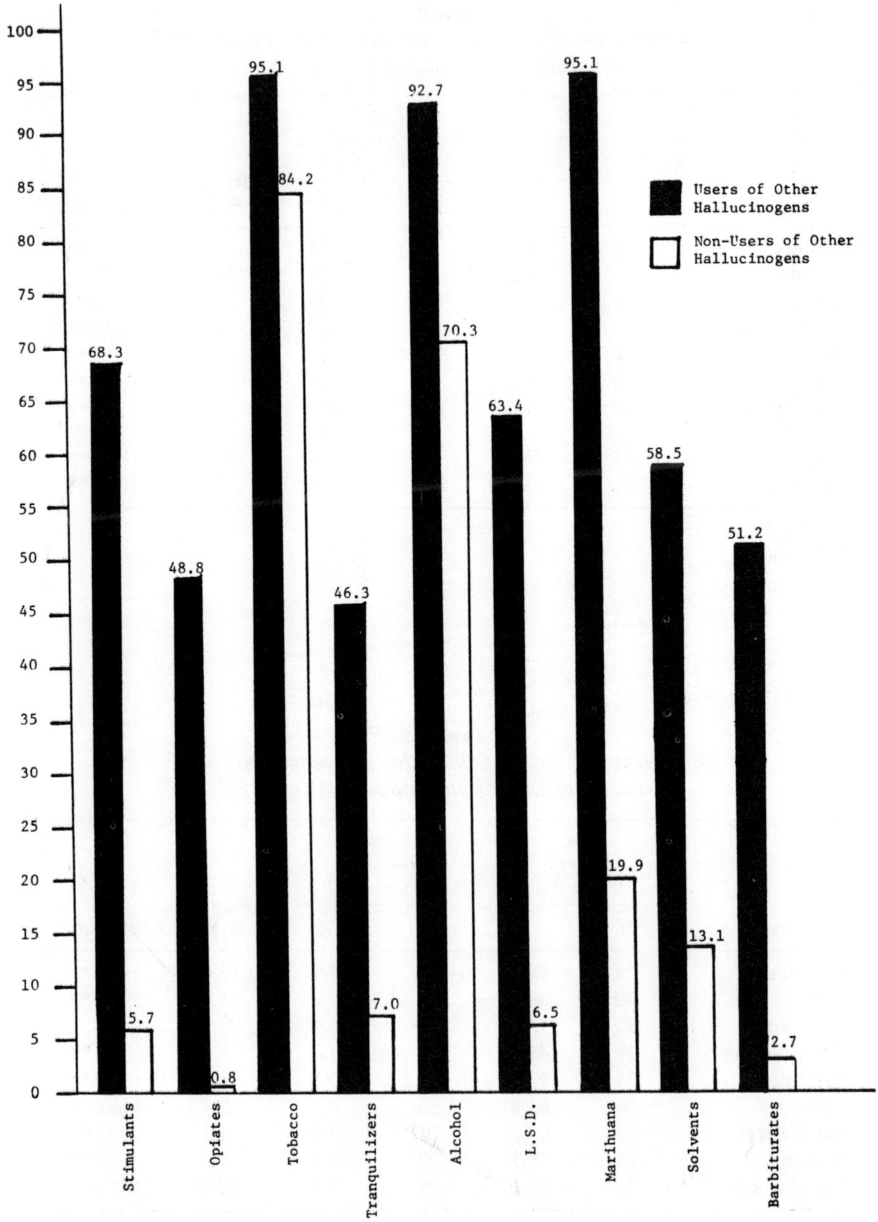

Fig. 8. Graphic comparison of rates of drug use between users and nonusers of other hallucinogens.

in their use of marihuana, almost six to one in the use of solvents, over nine to one in tranquilizer use, 11 to 1 in LSD use, 13 to 1 in use of stimulants, almost 21 to 1 in their use of other hallucinogens, and 48 to 1 in their use of opiates and other derivatives.

Other Hallucinogens. The use of other hallucinogens was reported by 4.6% of the sampled students (Table 9; Fig. 8). These students did not differ significantly from the nonusers in their use of tobacco, but the differences in their comparative uses of all the other drugs studied are statistically significant. Almost five times as many users as nonusers had used marihuana or solvents, 6.6 times as many had used tranquilizers, almost 10 times as many reported having used LSD, 12 times as many had used stimulants, 19 times as many used barbiturates, and 61 times as many reported opiate use.

Opiates. Only 27 of the Halifax students reported using opiates (3.0%). Their use of other drugs was significantly different from that of nonopiate users of these drugs. As Table 10 and Fig. 9 show, fully 100% of the users used tobacco and alcohol. About five times as many users of opiates had also used marihuana or solvents as nonusers; 10 to 15 times as many had used LSD, tranquilizers, and stimulants; over 24 times as many had used barbiturates; and 31 times as many had used other hallucinogens.

Table 10

Comparison of Rates of Drug Use Between Users and Nonusers of Opiates (N = *902*)

Drug	A Users ($N = 27$)		B Nonusers ($N = 875$)		Ratio A/B	Chi-square
	N	%	N	%		
Stimulants	25	92.6	52	5.9	15.7	240.9**
Tobacco	27	100.0	737	84.2	1.2	3.9*
Tranquilizers	20	74.1	59	6.7	11.1	140.3**
Alcohol	27	100.0	616	70.4	1.4	9.8**
LSD	20	74.1	62	7.1	10.4	134.2**
Marihuana	26	96.3	184	21.0	4.6	78.9**
Other hallucinogens	20	74.1	21	2.4	30.9	293.8**
Solvents	19	70.4	118	13.5	5.2	61.4**
Barbiturates	19	70.4	25	2.9	24.3	242.9**

*$p < .05$.
**$p < .01$.

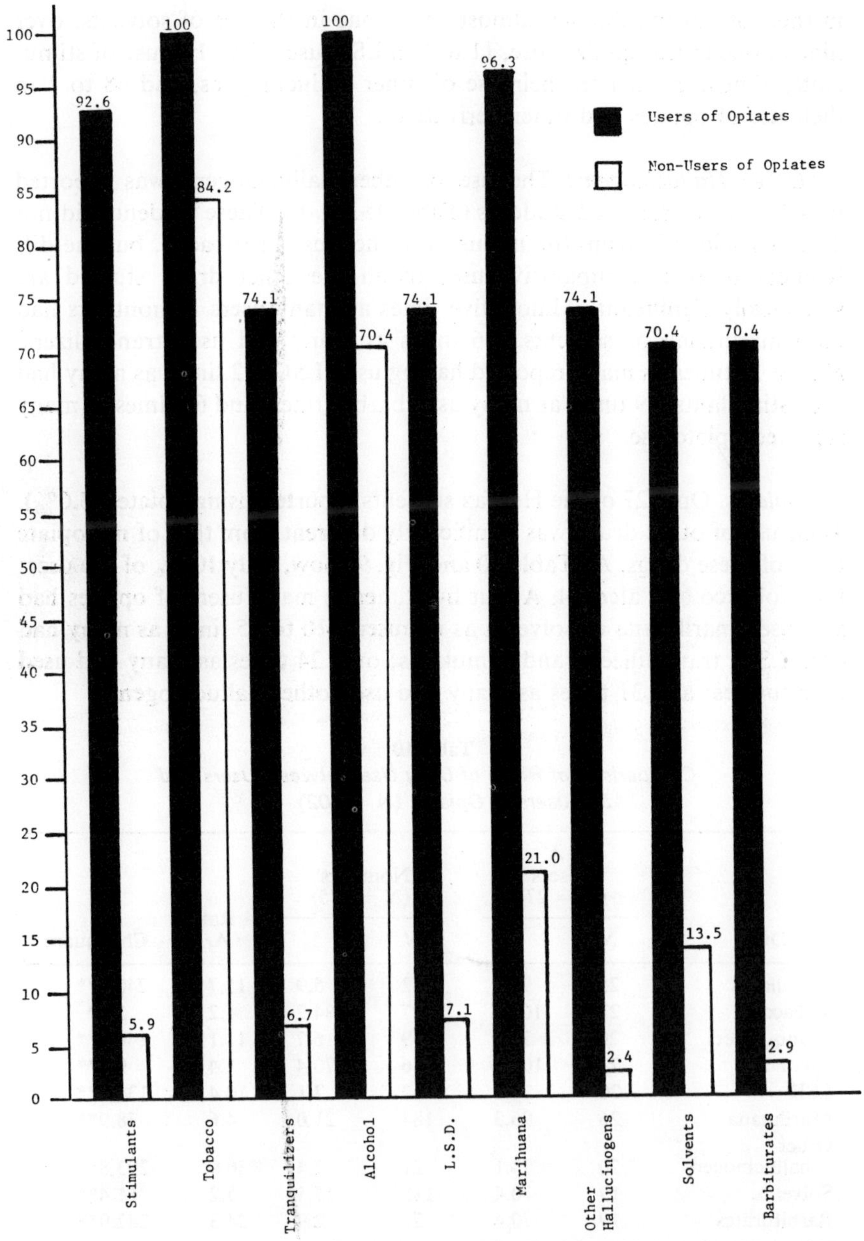

Fig. 9. Graphic comparison of rates of drug use between users and nonusers of opiates

DISCUSSION

The data presented above provide substantial support for the general proposition that users of most drugs are more likely to use almost any other drug than are nonusers. An examination of the trends within these data allows us to ascertain that not all drugs have the same etiological significance in terms of multidrug use. Specifically, there is a sizeable association between the use of such drugs as stimulants, opiates, marihuana, and LSD and multidrug use. This association is greater than that between alcohol use and multidrug use. And, the association is least in the case of tobacco smoking which appears to have little relationship to broader patterns of multiple drug use. Future research should be designed to ascertain the place of other drugs, such as aspirin, stomach remedies, and other over-the-counter preparations, within this framework of polydrug use.

The substance least often reported used was opiates. Users of drugs of this type tend to have used every other drug. At least 70% of the opiate users had used the other nine drugs, and all of them (100%) had used those drugs used most often by the student sample—tobacco and alcohol.

These results strongly support the notion that the use of a drug that was not formerly part of one's drug using repertoire tends to have a cumulative rather than a replacement effect relative to other drugs. Furthermore, there is a direct relationship between the use of drugs that fall outside the realm of generally acceptable social norms and the use of drugs that are generally more acceptable.

These findings complement those of previous research on the distribution of drug use that led to the conclusion that the use of drugs is a general phenomenon where a variety of communalities exist among the use of different drugs (cf., especially Smart and Whitehead, 1972; but also Smart et al., 1971). That is, the usage of drugs in our society does follow some discernible patterns which, rather than simply being characteristic of specific drugs, tend to cross-cut broader aspects of drug use.

This very much suggests that efforts designed to change some drug using practices must take into account the potential impact of such a change on other drug using practices. Furthermore, it leads to a partial appreciation of the forces against change that can result from the intimate relationship between some drug using practices and other, related, and sometimes firmly-established drug using practices.

REFERENCES

BLUM, R.H., BRAUNSTEIN, L., and STONE, A. Normal drug use: an exploratory study of patterns and correlates. In J.J. Cole and J.R. Wittenborn (eds.) *Drug Abuse: Social and Psychopharmacological Aspects*. Springfield, Illinois: Thomas, 1969, pp. 59–92.

FROSCH, W.A. Patterns of response to self administration of LSD. In J.J. Cole and J.R. Wittenborn (eds.) *Drug Abuse: Social and Psychopharmacological Aspects*. Springfield, Illinois: Thomas, 1969, pp. 27–38.

GOODE, E. Multiple drug use among marijuana smokers. *Social Problems* 17: 48–64, 1969.

GRUPP, S.E. Multiple drug use in a sample of experienced marihuana smokers. *Intern. J. Addictions* 7(3): 481–491, 1971.

LUCAS, W.C., GRUPP, S.E., and SCHMITT, R.L. Single and multiple drug opiate users: addicts or nonaddicts? *HSMHA Health Reports* 87(2): 185–192, 1972.

RICKELS, K., and BRAND, M.E. Incidence of nonnarcotic drug addictions at a large city hospital. In J.J. Cole and J. R. Wittenborn (eds.) *Drug Abuse: Social and Psychopharmacological Aspects*. Springfield, Illinois: Thomas, 1969, pp. 49–58.

ROCKWELL, D. Amphetamine use and abuse in psychiatric patients. In J.J. Cole and J. R. Wittenborn (eds.) *Drug Abuse: Social and Psychopharmacological Aspects*. Springfield, Illinois: Thomas, 1969, pp. 39–48.

SMART, R.G., and WHITEHEAD, P.C. The consumption patterns of illicit drugs and their implications for prevention of abuse. *Bull. Narcotics* 24(1): 39–47, 1972.

SMART, R.G., WHITEHEAD, P.C., and LAFOREST, L. The prevention of drug abuse by young people: an argument based on the distribution of drug use. *Bull. Narcotics* 23(2): 11–15, 1971.

WHITEHEAD, P.C. The incidence of drug use among Halifax adolescents. *Brit. J. Addiction* 65: 159–165, 1970a.

WHITEHEAD, P.C. Religious affiliation and the use of drugs among adolescent students. *J. Sci. Study Religion* 9(Summer): 152–154, 1970b.

WHITEHEAD, P.C. Head or brain: drug use and academic performance. In J.E. Gallagher and R.S. Lambert (eds.) *Social Process and Institution: The Canadian Case*. Toronto: Holt, Rinehart, Winston, 1971, pp. 364–370.

WHITEHEAD, P.C., and LAFOREST, L. Observations relatives aux foyers desunis et l'usage deviants des drogues. *Toxicomanies* 4(April-June): 199–203, 1971.

WHITEHEAD, P.C., and SMART, R.G. Validity and reliability of self-reported drug use. *Can. J. Criminology Corrections* 14(January): 83–89, 1972.

WHITEHEAD, P.C., SMART, R.G., and LAFOREST, L. Multiple drug use among marijuana smokers in Eastern Canada. *Intern. J. Addictions* 7: 179–190, 1972.

The International Journal of the Addictions, 9(2), 205–220, 1974

British Opiate Users: II. Differences between Those Given an Opiate Script and Those Not Given One

Herbert H. Blumberg, Ph.D.

S. Daryl Cohen, M.B., B.Ch.

B. Elizabeth Dronfield, B.A., Dip. Crim.

Elizabeth A. Mordecai, B.A.

J. Colin Roberts, B.A., Dip. Soc. Admin.

David Hawks, Ph.D.

Addiction Research Unit
Institute of Psychiatry
University of London
London, England

A previous paper (Blumberg et al., 1974) described British opiate users who had approached the drug treatment centers ("clinics") in Greater London for the first time during 1971. One of our intentions was to examine how the present population differs from that described by

Stimson and Ogborne (1970), which required that we obtain a sampling frame comparable to that used in earlier studies, where only those opiate users who were in regular contact with the clinics were included. This meant separating our data into two groups: one including respondents who were ultimately given an opiate script (the "Script Group") and the other from those who were not (the "No-Script Group").

Most research to date has been centered on samples equivalent to the Script Group—i.e., it has investigated those opiate users who are known to researching bodies by virtue of their receiving medical treatment or being in prison (Beckett and Lodge, 1971; Bewley, 1965a, 1965b; Chapple, 1966; Chapple and Gray, 1968; Crawley, 1971; Gardner and Connell, 1970, 1971; George and Glatt, 1967; Hewetson, 1967; Hewetson and Ollendorf, 1964; James, 1969, 1971; Mahon, 1971; d'Orban, 1970; Willis, 1969, 1971; Wright and Turner, 1971).

In the course of our work it became clear that there were important differences within our own sample between the two groups—i.e., between the 113 respondents who were started off on a regular opiate script (as at least one component of their treatment) and the 61 who were not given one. As a result, this paper is devoted to these differences and to a description of this latter, largely unresearched group. Historical changes in the British opiate-using population remain the subject of a future paper.

Empirically, in our data, it turns out that being issued a regular opiate script by a clinic is very closely associated with a person's urine having been analyzed as opiate-positive. Some possible reasons for failures to produce opiate-positive urine are considered at the end of this paper. It should be noted that the majority of the No-Script Group do claim to be using opiates.

METHOD

As with the first paper in the present series, identical analyses have, in general, been carried out separately on "odd numbered" and "even numbered" respondents. The *even* group were used to attempt to replicate the findings arising from the *odd* group. Most of the findings reported in this paper have been thus replicated. But for a few of the analyses, the odd and even groups were combined at the outset in order to have a sample of adequate size. All of the findings reported in this paper (unless described as trends or tendencies) were statistically significant at least at the 5% level in *both* groups (or in the single combined group for those few analyses that were carried out only once). The odd and even groups were each further divided into "Script" and "No-Script" Groups (see Table 1).

Table 1
Frequency Subdivisions of the Sample

Condition	Odd	Even	Total
Script Group	62	51	113
No-Script Group	34	27	61
(Script decision not yet made)	16	20	36
Total	112	98	210

A respondent is counted as being in the No-Script Group if he/she did not receive from the clinic one or more prescriptions (to cover at least about 8 days) for heroin and/or methadone. And, conversely, the Script Group consists of people who were at least started off on a regular opiate script but excludes those *only* given drugs other than opiates such as tranquilizers), and also excludes those not given any drugs. For 36 respondents (17% of the sample) the script decision was unknown or had not been made at the time of the main data analyses for the present paper—these cases are excluded from comparisons between the Script and No-Script Groups.

As mentioned above, nearly all of the people in the Script Group had produced an opiate-positive urine specimen (as part of their assessment at clinic), while most of the people in the No-Script Group did not produce one at the time. (There were several exceptions, in both directions, to this rule—just under 10% of the sample—but they were too few to permit analysis.) These facts must be carefully borne in mind when assessing the implications of the differences between the Script and No-Script Groups. Thus whenever a difference is reported between the two groups, one must be careful not to infer that the difference was a contributing *cause* of the script decision. Indeed, it would seem to be the case that *much* of the decision-making process, which determines whether or not a respondent is given a regular opiate script or not, is associated with his/her ability or failure to produce a specimen of opiate-positive urine; and for the most part other factors seem to play less part in this decision process—though once the decision to give a regular script has been made, they may, of course, influence other components of the treatment, including the size of the script given.

It must also be borne in mind that though for the most part the No-Script Group failed to produce an opiate-positive urine at the time of clinical assessment, this does *not*, of course, exclude the possibility that such respondents had been using opiates in the recent past and that they might be desirous of obtaining a legal supply of them.

In summary, reported differences between the Script and No-Script Groups should, for the time being, be regarded as descriptive rather than allowing inferential analysis.

Although very few people who wanted opiates and were able to produce opiate-positive urines at clinics are turned away without a script, this must be seen in the following perspective: approximately half of the scripts given at the commencement of treatment or maintenance were for amounts of about 30 mg or less of opiate (median = 33 mg). This figure may be contrasted with the median amounts *claimed to be used* by the respondents in this same Script Group, which was of the order of 50 mg. Because the minority who claimed to be using relatively large amounts of heroin were not given very large scripts, the discrepancy between means is greater than that between medians: mean script was for 40 mg (7 mg heroin plus 33 mg methadone—these are means, and very few respondents received *both* heroin and methadone) while mean claimed opiate use was 111 mg.

In all of the analyses which follow in this paper, where a difference is reported between the Script and the No-Script Groups, supplementary analyses are also reported whenever the difference seems possibly to be an artifact of other variables. (As part of the data analysis relevant to this point, correlation matrices were produced, and factor analyses were carried out separately for the odd and even subsamples for all variables that differentiated between Script and No-Script Groups).

In addition, all of the results reported in the first paper of this series apply about equally to both the Script and No-Script Groups except where differences are specified in the present paper in the results and discussion sections (which follow).

PROCEDURAL VARIABLES

The ratio of respondents given opiate scripts to those not given them differed from clinic to clinic and from doctor to doctor but—contrary to the opinions of some respondents and clinic staff—the differences were not significant (but given the small numbers of people representing each clinic, large differences would have been required to generate statistical significance). In our tabulations the respondents, doctors, and clinics have been assigned numbers and thus rendered effectively anonymous for purposes of data storage and analysis.

Our interviews were more likely to take place *after* the script decision in the case of the Script Group than in the case of the No-Script Group—possibly (1) because the script decision might have taken longer in the cases of those ultimately not given an opiate script, (2) in some few cases the interviewer might have felt that it was safer to delay those interviews where it was known that a respondent would be getting an opiate script and could be easily contacted at clinic, and (3) although the nonresponse rate in the present study was under 10%, a disproportionately large amount of this nonresponse probably represents interviews within the No-Script Group which "would" have taken place after the script decision.

PERSONAL BACKGROUND

Family and Demographic Variables

Sex. Apart from people for whom no script decision had been made at the time these figures were compiled, there were 134 male respondents, of whom 61% are in the Script Group; and 36 female respondents, 75% of whom are in the Script Group (the difference between the proportions is not quite statistically significant).

In this connection it is not the case that women per se are more likely to be given an opiate script than men, but rather that *anyone* who is "going with" someone who fixes is more likely to be in the Script Group, and as women are more likely than men to be going with someone who fixes (according to our findings), they are therefore only circumstantially more likely to be given an opiate script.

As a further point, not only is it the case that at least until recent years the proportion of women among "addicted persons" known to the Home Office had been falling (Hawks, 1971), but also our figures suggest that the proportion of women in the overall British opiate-using population may be even smaller than might be inferred from the Home Office figures, inasmuch as more women are given an opiate script once they do approach a clinic and would therefore be expected to stay with the clinic and remain "on the books."

Age. A trend was observed in which older aged respondents were more likely to be in the Script Group than younger respondents.

Age was also positively correlated with age of first fix. But this was to be expected simply because older respondents had more of a chance to have their first fixes at a later age. However, "age of first fix" is not substantially related to whether a respondent is in the Script or the No-Script Group.

Those results dealing with birth place and family background, and reported in the first paper of this series, apply about equally to the Script and No-Script Groups.

The mean school-leaving age was 15.6 years for the Script Group and 15.3 for the No-Script Group—and although this small difference was statistically significant, it is very probably no more than an artifact arising from the Script Group tending to be older and therefore having had a slightly greater chance to continue full-time education to a later age.

Employment. People in the Script Group had worked an average of 31 weeks in the year preceding the interview and those in the No-Script Group an average of 22 weeks.

Personality and Attitude

Included in the interviews were a variety of attitude items which had been found to be related to key items in the data collected by Stimson and Ogborne (1970). Those items which yielded consistent significant differences between the Script and No-Script Groups are listed in Table 2. The last four items (in Table 2) yielded successive positive intercorrelations.

These attitude items paint a picture of the No-Script Group as tending to take a negative and passive view of things (compared with the Script Group). Is it possible that some of those in the No-Script Group who wanted an opiate script might have "forgotten" to fix in time for their urine tests?

Although the No-Script Group tended (more than the Script Group) to be interviewed before the script decision was made, we cannot rule out the possibility that in some cases this "negative passive view" might be a response to the script decision itself.

Table 2
Attitude Items Differentiating between the Script and the No-Script Groups[a]

1. Heroin/Physeptone makes me better able to concentrate (Script Group)
2. Most people who fix regularly are unable to face up to difficulties (No-Script Group)
3. Heroin/Physeptone makes me less aware of my feelings (No-Script Group)
4. Most people who fix regularly would be happy doing nothing for the rest of their lives (No-Script Group)
5. Most people who fix regularly find the world almost too bewildering (No-Script Group)
6. I find the world almost too bewildering (No-Script Group)
7. I suffer from feelings of inferiority (No-Script Group)

[a]The Group whose members were more likely to endorse a particular item is indicated (in parentheses) after the item.

Social Agencies, Friends, and Residence

As regards contacts with social agencies, the only difference between the Script and the No-Script Groups was that the latter had reported fewer contacts with the Ministry of Social Security. This is not in keeping with their having worked for fewer weeks in the preceding year, unless the No-Script Group found that it was too much trouble to have to "sign on" regularly at a particular time, day, and place, or unless they were more likely to have money from other sources.

The Script Group also reported being acquainted with more people who had fixed than did the No-Script Group (a rough index of involvement with other opiate users). This at least indicates that the clinics are especially likely to be serving those who are more central in the social network of opiate users.

While the largest number of respondents in both the Script and No-Script Groups were living with their families (place occupied longest in the 12 months prior to interview), the remainder of the Script Group tended to be especially likely to live with a cohabitee, while the No-Script Group tended more to live only with other nonrelatives—perhaps suggesting that they are relatively distant from other people.

Illegal Activities

Of those with no drug convictions in the past year, 63% were in the Script Group while only 46% of those with at least one such conviction were in this group.

DRUGS

Early Use

There were no differences between the Script and No-Script Groups on the variables relating to early drug experience.

Recent Use

Frequency of Use. Members of the No-Script Group claim to make *more* frequent use of amphetamines (both orally and intravenously), "sleepers" and tranquilizers (orally and intravenously), and psychedelics than did the Script Group—and *less* frequent use of methadone. (Some respondents might not have understood that these questions applied to the 4 weeks *prior* to coming to a clinic; the more frequent use of methadone by the Script Group may partly reflect the clinic prescriptions—so one should treat this finding with caution.)

The Script Group were also more likely than the No-Script Group to indicate that they were using more methadone at the time of the interview than at the time 12 months prior to the interview. Members of the No-Script Group were more likely *currently* to be fixing barbiturates than were members of the Script Group. Respondents were asked about their most recent fix, and even for this one fix the No-Script Group were more likely to have fixed barbiturates (1 out of 99 in the Script Group, 8 out of 43 in the No-Script Group).

Among respondents in the Script Group, 80% claimed to have been spending more than £10 per week on drugs (excluding tobacco and alcohol) while only 45% of those in the No-Script Group were spending over £10. One must bear in mind that these figures and amounts relate to the period just before the respondents came to a clinic, and for this reason may be higher (or lower, for lack of available supplies?) than they would have been otherwise. Indeed, many respondents cite the high cost of their drug use as one reason for their coming to a clinic.

Liking, Need, Obtainability, and Intent. A number of items yielded significant differences between the Script and No-Script Groups, and these differences are summarized in Table 3. Indeed, a number of these distinguishing items are significantly intercorrelated in such a way that it is meaningful to talk about *clusters* of items that distinguish the Script and No-Script Groups. The grouping of items into clusters was based on the entire list of variables that significantly and consistently distinguished between the Script and No-Script Groups, and was carried out in such a way that: for both the odd and even subsamples, all or most of the correlations *within* clusters are statistically significant, and (except as noted) none of the correlations *between* clusters are. All of the main clusters are, in fact, represented in the present section except for two which have already been discussed—those dealing with degree of employment and those dealing with sex differences. This is an appropriate place, then, to consider all of the other main clusters that distinguish the two groups.

In part because of the questions we chose to include in the surveys, the main clusters of items that separate the Script and the No-Script Groups correspond to the main drugs asked about. One cluster of five items has to do with *Chinese heroin*: those given an opiate *script* have, on average, a greater need, liking, and frequency of use of Chinese heroin. They also spend more on drugs and "go to the Dilly" more often (i.e., buy drugs near Piccadilly Circus; in pilot studies it was clear that for respond-

Table 3
Characteristics of Drug Use: Differences between the Script and No-Script Groups

Characteristics and drug[a]	Script	No-Script
Frequency, amphetamines[b]	1.2	1.8
methadone ampules	3.8	2.8
sleepers and tranquilizers[c]	1.4	1.8
psychedelics	1.1	1.6
Liking, heroin[d]	4.7	4.1
Need, amphetamines[b]	1.2	1.6
methadone ampules	2.9	2.3
opiates other than heroin and methadone	2.0	1.4
sleepers and tranquilizers	1.4	1.8
Obtainability, heroin[d]	4.1	3.6
methedrine ampules	1.3	1.8

[a]Frequency is measured on a scale ranging from 1 (not taken in the past four weeks) to 5 (taken daily). The liking scale ranges from 1 (dislike) to 5 (like a lot). The need scale ranges from 1 (no need) to 4 (strong need). The obtainability scale ranges from 1 (very difficult to obtain) to 5 (very easy). All entries are mean values for those respondents who have at least tried the drug in question.

[b]The means refer to oral amphetamines. Figures for injected amphetamines are similar, except that frequency is even greater for the No-Script Group (who also have significantly greater liking than the Script Group).

[c]Means refer to injected sleepers and tranquilizers, oral being used more frequently and disliked less by both groups.

[d]Means refer to English heroin, but the figures for Chinese heroin are similar except as follows. Chinese heroin was used more frequently—and was needed more—by the Script Group than by the No-Script Group, and both groups found it easier to obtain than English heroin.

ents in the present population, frequency of going to Piccadilly Circus is about the same as that of going to Gerrard Street, where Chinese heroin is most commonly sold—see Walker, 1972).

Another cluster of items has to do with *methadone* ampules. On average, for those in the *Script Group* there was: greater frequency of use, greater need, greater actual claimed use, greater use at the time of interview than at the point of time a year prior to interview, greater liklihood of getting a methadone script, and a greater likelihood for the doctor to indicate that the respondent asked for methadone. Moreover, respondents who were high on the cluster of methadone items were more likely to be still under treatment at the clinic 2 months later (than were the No-Script Group).

As a third cluster of items, those in the *No-Script Group* had a *greater* frequency of fixing *amphetamines* as well as having both more liking and a greater need for doing so. They were also more likely to be given a prescription for tranquilizers.

A fourth cluster of items concerns the fixing of *sleepers*. Those in the *No-Script Group* have a *greater* frequency of fixing sleepers and also of using psychedelics. Frequency of fixing sleepers is significantly correlated with need to fix sleepers, which in turn had significant positive correlations with need for oral amphetamines and average need for all drugs. (The foregoing correlations notwithstanding, claimed average drug need was higher for the Script Group than for the No-Script Group.)

Several other correlations are relevant to those items that are listed in Table 3, but as they were more to be expected, they do not merit further comment.

To complete the picture, there are yet more distinguishing features between the two groups—the most important of which are that those in the Script Group have had fewer court convictions (already mentioned) and fewer physical complications (to be discussed below).

Abstention

The Script and No-Script Groups do not differ with respect to past or intended future abstention(s).

Physical Complications

The results of a number of questions dealing with physical complications, in the preceding year and prior to that, are shown in Table 4. The definition of each complication was left up to the respondent. In most cases, except for hepatitis, claimed incidence was *greater* in the No-Script Group than in the Script Group, but because of the small frequencies, many of the differences were not statistically significant. Reported hospitalizations in the past year were more frequent in the No-Script Group, and there was a tendency for the No-Script Group to say that they had had more overdoses in the 12 months prior to interview (than did the Script Group). Both hospitalizations and overdoses in the year prior to interview were significantly related to the respondent's stated need to fix sleepers. Also, these and other physical-complication variables were, in some cases, significantly correlated with one another. For example, as one would expect, hospitalizations and overdoses were significantly correlated.

It may be that those who most resort to fixing sleepers are people who

Table 4
Frequencies[a] *of Physical Complications*

Complication	Past year No-Script	Past year Script	Prior No-Script	Prior Script
Septicaemia	10 (17%)	6 (5%)	8 (13%)	8 (8%)
Hepatitis	6 (10%)	21 (19%)	9 (15%)	29 (26%)
Abcesses	23 (39%)	22[b] (20%)	12 (20%)	30 (29%)
Overdose	25 (43%)	38 (34%)	28 (47%)	40 (36%)
Other injury or disease	17 (30%)	15[c] (14%)	31 (54%)	35[d] (32%)
Drug-related hospitalizations	25 (42%)	28[e] (25%)	21 (35%)	27 (24%)
Nondrug hospitalizations[f]	5 (9%)	8 (8%)	16 (27%)	53[g] (48%)

[a]Frequencies refer to the number of respondents who have had a particular complication at least once in the relevant time period. Percentages are based on the total number in the No-Script—or Script—Group for whom there was a clear positive or negative response. The following significance tests are based on differences in incidence between the Script and No-Script Groups.
[b]$\chi^2 = 6.12, p < 0.02$.
[c]$\chi^2 = 5.87, p < 0.02$.
[d]$\chi^2 = 7.77, p < 0.01$.
[e]$\chi^2 = 4.35, p < 0.02$.
[f]Excluding respondents who had any drug-related hospitalizations in the particular time period.
[g]$\chi^2 = 6.32, p < 0.02$.

on occasion cannot obtain opiates or cannot afford the price. Such people might be likely to come to a clinic when they need but cannot get opiates, would possibly produce opiate-negative urine, and might therefore find themselves in the No-Script Group. (In other words, for some opiate users the chances of opiate-negative urine might be *greater* at the time of coming to clinic than at other times.)

CONTACT WITH CLINIC

A series of questions were asked separately of the respondent and the doctor about the initial consultations up until the time the doctor conveyed to the respondent a final decision about his/her preparedness, or otherwise, to prescribe opiates or other drugs.

Respondents in the Script Group were more likely to have their overall doctor/patient relationship rated by both the respondent and the doctor as a good one compared with those in the No-Script Group.

While most respondents in both groups said there was no "pressure" from family, GP, or friends to come to a clinic, there was a significantly higher proportion of respondents in the No-Script, as compared with the Script Group, who did in fact say that there had been pressure from their GP's.

It seems essential to discuss, however speculatively, the possible reasons why the No-Script Group produced opiate-negative urine at the clinic. A sizeable minority of the group did not claim to be using opiates currently and came to the clinic for some other purpose (e.g., wanting sedatives or amphetamines or supportive treatment); in these cases the reason for opiate-negative urine is self-evident. For the remainder of the No-Script Group, seven possible reasons—which are not to be taken as mutually exclusive—come to mind: (1) *Nonconstant use*—opiates may have been used currently but not recently enough to appear in urine; (2) *false negatives*—imperfections in the test procedure itself, such as opiates being masked or diluted (cf. Montalvo et al., 1972); (3) *good intentions*—some respondents may have thought that to appear at a clinic "drug-free" would recommend their case for being given a gradually diminished opiate prescription; (4) *ambivalence*—some might not want to be recognized as "drug dependent," and might thus have avoided opiate use in the period immediately before coming to clinic; (5) *unobtainability*—subjects may have come to clinic *because* they needed opiates and (perhaps temporarily) lacked a source of supply or could not afford to obtain them—in support of this, one notes that the No-Script group were more likely to have been fixing barbiturates at the times of their appointments; (6) *bad deals*—although there is no documentation that this has occurred in Britain, a person may have unknowingly purchased a supply of "Chinese heroin" consisting solely of impurities, and the resulting side effects or opiate withdrawal symptoms could have *led* to his coming to clinic. In each of these six situations a person may be a regular user of opiates and still not produce an opiate-positive urine at clinic. As a seventh reason, one cannot rule out the possibility that (7) some subjects were trying to "con" the clinics into prescribing drugs which could then be sold illicitly; however, one might reasonably think that the majority of such people would know to fix opiates before coming to clinic. Although urine analysis may be an unreliable index of a person's regular use of opiates, it is probably preferable to any more subjective assessment in decisions involving the issuing of scripts.

CONCLUSIONS

The salient characteristics of the No-Script Group, relative to the Script Group, are summarized in Table 5.

Most studies of opiate users have concentrated on those in receipt of a prescription from one of the drug treatment centers. The particular contribution of the present study is that it provides information on that little-studied group of people who, while notified by the clinics, are not prescribed opiates by the clinics and who, in some cases, because of the dissatisfaction they express with the clinic system, are unlikely to stay in contact with clinics. While the present study does not allow us to discern whether this subgroup will, at some time in the future, receive opiate prescriptions, at least some of the implications of their present refusal can be surmised. One of the ways that the No-Script Group was differentiated from the Script Group was in terms of their use of barbiturates; it appeared that the No-Script Group's lack of access to opiates (or less recourse to opiates) was associated with a higher incidence of physical complications in the past and can presumably be expected to result in more complications in the immediate future. The No-Script Group were also more often unemployed and engaged more in illegal activities. It might be argued, although the data available do not unequivocally demonstrate this, that the fact that the No-Script Group do not receive a prescription for opiates may be partly a result of—and partly cause of furthering—their illegal activities, their unemployment, and also their injection of barbiturates.

Table 5
Relative Reported Characteristics of the No-Script Group as Compared with the Script Group (partial list)

Item	Characteristic
Sex	Tend to be male
Age	Tend to be younger
Employment	Worked fewer weeks in preceding year
Attitude	"Negative passive"
Friends	Fewer acquaintances who had fixed
Court convictions	More with drug conviction(s) in preceding year
Drug use	Greater frequency for amphetamines-oral, amphetamines-fixed, sleepers-oral, sleepers-fixed, psychedelics; less frequent use of methadone and Chinese heroin
Complications	More abcesses and hospitalizations; trends toward more septicaemia and overdoses, less hepatitis

The decision to prescribe opiates was closely associated with the results of urinary analysis. Despite the fact that the majority of those who did not receive a script claimed to have used opiates in the recent past, most did not have a positive urine. While in some cases attendance at a clinic may have been motivated by the desire to receive opiates which might then be sold, in others the user may have felt that refraining from using opiates immediately before attending the clinic would have recommended his case—whereas in fact it served to deny him a prescription for opiates. In other cases the person giving a negative specimen may have approached the clinic precisely because he was unable to obtain opiates; the fact of his not having used opiates in the immediate past need not, however, attest to his not having used them at all.

As yet we are unable to say whether the decision not to prescribe opiates is more often associated with long-term abstinence than is the receipt of a prescription. In the meantime one can only wonder whether the decision not to prescribe in all cases where a negative urine is found is functional. It may be, of course, that the alternative of prescribing opiates to some individuals who have no opiates in their urine is an even less desirable alternative. Clearly, more research is needed regarding the identification of opiate use among those who would under present circumstances be refused an opiate script.

Whatever the implications of not prescribing opiates for the No-Script Group may be, comfort can be taken from the fact that those given a prescription are the people who tended to have more often used powdered heroin in the recent past and to be more integrated into a heroin-using scene. To the extent that their receiving a script results in their using less powdered heroin, the policy of prescribing followed by the clinics would appear to have beneficial consequences.

SUMMARY

The interview data from some of the people approaching London drug clinics during the 1-year period beginning mid-November 1970 were used to compare two groups of subjects: those who were given a regular opiate script (113 people) and those who were not (61 people who, for the most part, did not produce an opiate-positive urine at the time). People who were given such a script were likely to have been using more illicit heroin or methadone (than were people not given an opiate script), and the script given was usually a small quantity of methadone. Significantly higher rates of unemployment, illegal activities, and physical complications were demonstrated in the group who were *not* given a regular opiate script; further differences between the Script Group and the No-Script Group are also described.

ACKNOWLEDGMENTS

We express our gratitude to the Medical Research Council and the Department of Health and Social Security for their joint funding of this completely independent research. We are extremely grateful to the clinic consultants and staffs, the respondents, the University College Computer Centre Staff, and the office staff.

REFERENCES

BECKETT, H.D., and LODGE, K.J. Aspects of social relationships in heroin addicts admitted for treatment. *Bull. Narcotics* 23(4): 29–36, 1971.

BEWLEY, T. Heroin addiction in the United Kingdom (1954–1964). *Brit. Med. J.* 5473: 1284–1286, 1965a(2).

BEWLEY, T. Heroin and cocaine addiction. *Lancet* 7389: 808–810, 1965b(1).

BLUMBERG, H.H., COHEN, S.D., DRONFIELD, B.E., MORDECAI, E.A., ROBERTS, J.C., and HAWKS, D. British opiate users: I. People approaching London treatment centres. *Intern. J. Addictions* 9: 1–23, 1974.

CHAPPLE, P.A.L. Some clinical and biochemical problems of British narcotic users. *Excerpta Medica International Congress, Washington, D.C.*, March 1966, Series 129, 258–262.

CHAPPLE, P.A.L., and GRAY, G. One year's work at a centre for the treatment of addicted patients. *Lancet* 7548: 908–911, 1968(1).

CRAWLEY, J.A. A case-note study of 134 out-patient drug addicts over a 17-month period. *Brit. J. Addiction* 66: 209–218, 1971.

GARDNER, R., and CONNELL, P.H. One year's experience in a drug-dependence clinic. *Lancet* 7670: 455–458, 1970(2).

GARDNER, R., and CONNELL, P.H. Opioid users attending a special drug dependence clinic 1968–69. *Bull. Narcotics* 23(4): 9–15, 1971.

GEORGE, H.R., and GLATT, M.M. A brief survey of a drug dependency unit in a psychiatric hospital. *Brit. J. Addiction* 62: 147–153, 1967.

HAWKS, D.V. The dimensions of drug dependence in the United Kingdom. *Intern. J. Addictions* 6: 135–160, 1971.

HEWETSON, J. Treatment of heroin and cocaine dependence in general practice. *Nursing Times* 516–518, 1967.

HEWETSON, J., and OLLENDORF, R. Preliminary survey of 100 London heroin and cocaine addicts. *Brit. J. Addiction* 60: 109–114, 1964.

JAMES, I.P. Delinquency and heroin addiction in Britain. *Brit. J. Criminology* 9: 108–124, 1969.

JAMES, I.P. The changing pattern of narcotic addiction in Britain—1959 to 1969. *Intern. J. Addictions* 6: 119–134, 1971.

MAHON, T.A. An exploratory study of hospitalized narcotic addicts in Great Britain. *Acta Psychiat. Scand.* Supplementum 227, 1971.

MONTALVO, J.G., SCRIGNAR, C.B., ALDERETTE, E., HARPER, E., and EYER, D. Flushing, pale-colored urines, and false negatives—urinalysis of narcotic addicts. *Intern. J. Addictions* 7: 355–364, 1972.

d'ORBAN, P.T. Heroin dependence and delinquency in women—a study of heroin addicts in Holloway Prison. *Brit. J. Addiction* 65: 67–78, 1970.

STIMSON, G V , and OGBORNE, A.C. A survey of a representative sample of addicts prescribed heroin at London clinics. *Bull. Narcotics* 22(4): 13–22, 1970.

WALKER, M.J. *The London street addict*. London: Institute of Community studies, 1972 (unpublished manuscript).

WILLIS, J.H. Drug dependence: some demographic and psychiatric aspects in United Kingdom and United States subjects. *Brit. J. Addiction* 64: 135–146, 1969.

WILLIS, J. Delinquency and drug dependence in the UK and USA. *Brit. J. Addiction* 66: 235–248, 1971.

WRIGHT, D.J., and TURNER, A.G. An analysis of the effects of drug abuse as seen and treated in a casualty department. *Brit. J. Addiction* 66: 77–80, 1971.

The International Journal of the Addictions, 9(2), 221–227, 1974

The Relationship between Age and/or Negative Experiences and Success on a Methadone Maintenance Program

Thomas Henchy, Ph.D.

Byron Eckerson, M.A.

Jesse L. Paez, A.C.S.W.

Santa Barbara County Mental Health Services
Santa Barbara, California

PROBLEM

It is clear that funding agencies require that addicts fulfill certain criteria before they are allowed to enter a methadone maintenance program. What is not so clear is whether or not their assumptions lead to the most beneficial result. For example, the requirements are typically that an addict has to have been addicted a certain number of years, has to have been in treatment a specified number of times for the addiction, and has to have been in jail a certain number of times. While this may assure that someone is indeed a chronic addict before he is put on a potentially lifelong alternate dependence, it does not necessarily guarantee therapeutic success. Thus we decided to investigate whether it is the younger or older addict who benefits most from a methadone maintenance program and also whether addicts who have been subjected to a greater or lesser number of negative reinforcements (e.g., incarceration) are most likely to benefit from a methadone maintenance program.

The latter variables are of interest since it can be argued that addicts with more negative reinforcements, i.e., with more doors shut to them, and/or older addicts are more likely to benefit from methadone maintenance because it is their last resort. However, an equally compelling argument can be made for a younger addict faced with, most likely, fewer negative reinforcements and fewer closed doors than his fellow older addict. This type of client may see methadone maintenance as his chance to avail himself of a greater number of opportunities. In the present study, age and number of negative reinforcements as two main independent variables are separated as much as possible to determine which is the better predictor of successful methadone maintenance and/or eventual freedom from heroin use.

The answer to these questions can have far-reaching impact in terms of policy concerning the criteria for putting a person on methadone maintenance. That is, with limited resources it would be best to put those people on the program who have the characteristics which have been demonstrated to be good predictors of success. For example, in an inpatient methadone program in St. Louis (Knowles, Lahiri, and Anderson, 1971), it was found that persons over 25 were more likely to complete the program (70%) than those under 25 (30%) (n = 103). Gearing (1971), in an evaluation of New York's programs, reported that men have a higher probability than women of remaining on a program from month to month, but that younger addicts (20–29) had a higher probability than older addicts, and that whites and other nonblacks had a slightly higher probability than blacks of remaining on the program.

Williams and Johnston (1972), in comparing a group of drop-outs with those remaining, found the average age of the drop-outs to be 27.5 (n = 185), while the average age of those remaining was 39.7 (n = 115). Moreover, in comparing the number of years addicted prior to their present treatment, they found that the drop-out group showed an average addiction of 5.5 years, compared with 12.5 for those remaining on the program. Williams and Johnston (1972) also found that the number of previous treatment experiences was greater for those who remained on the program than for those who had dropped out (2.6 and 1.4, respectively). In addition, 80% of those remaining on the program and only 40% of the drop-outs had spent time in jail between onset of the addiction and first seeking treatment. Also, months spent in jail per year addicted were higher for those remaining than for the drop-outs (3.8 vs 2.1). Both groups showed approximately the same average number of convictions prior to addiction, and both groups were judged similar with respect to education and employment histories. In short, those remaining on the program showed a history of more negative experiences than those who dropped out. Whether this is to be explained mainly by their higher average age (i.e., simple exposure) or by some tendency to chronic failure and dependence (thus also explaining their longer tenure in the methadone program), the results seem to indicate that the probability of staying on the program increases with age and/or negative experiences.

The present study was conducted in the Santa Barbara County methadone program which has two sites, one in North County and one in South County. Both facilities are located adjacent to a hospital which has some facilities for detoxification. Additional services provided at both clinics are out-patient drug-abuse counseling and nonnarcotic out-patient medication in a "kick clinic." The subjects in the present study all started on the program when it opened in December 1970.

METHOD

Information concerning experiences prior to entering the program was taken from the intake interview given all clients.* This intake interview had been used extensively in the Contra Costa County methadone programs. There were 133 clients, 29 of whom had left the program at the time of the study. It is from this data that we derive our independent variables of age and negative experiences. Our dependent variable is whether or not the client is still on the program. Background characteristics of the sample are presented in Table 1.

An initial question is whether or not age and negative experiences are correlated. Rationally, it would be expected that they would be, in which

*On the reliability and validity of this kind of information, see Stephens (1972). It should be pointed out that although the Santa Barbara County methadone program is billed as a research program (for reasons of funding and administration), addicts might see it differently. That is, addicts might feel there is more at stake in their answers than in any ordinary research project which has little personal consequence for the participants. However, according to Stephens (1972), addicts do not distort their responses, in contradistinction to what has been commonly assumed.

Table 1
Background Characteristics of the Sample[a]

Age	29 (mean), 26.5 (median), 19–55 (range)
Sex	84% male, 16% female
Ethnic group	53% Chicano, 41% White, 6% other
Marital status	33% never married; 41% married/common law; 23% once married, now single; 3% unknown
Education, in years	14% 1–8; 47% 9–11; 23% 12; 15% 13–16; 1% unknown
Work history	60% worked in past; 26% working now; 3% never worked; 11% no information

[a]Only certain aspects of the input interview were deemed necessary for this study. Thus some demographic data have not yet been analyzed.

case we would be talking about one variable. However, when correlation coefficients were computed between age and the various negative experiences, age was significantly correlated ($p < 0.001$) only with age at first arrest and with the number of terms served for drug-related offenses. Thus we can conclude that age and the other negative experiences operate some-

Table 2
Program Status by Negative Experiences (medians and ranges)

	Remaining		Left		Total	
Number of previous convictions	2.0	0–18	1.4	0–12	1.9	0–18
Number of times hospitalized	1.7	0–10	1.9	0–12	1.7	0–12
Age at first arrest[a]	16.0	8–45	15.7	5–33	16.0	5–45
Terms served for drug-related offenses	1.5	0–8	0	0–6	1.1	0–8
Terms served for nondrug-related offenses	0	0–6	0	0–6	0	0–6
Times picked up, not charged, drug-related offenses	0.8	0–6	0	0–6	0.7	0–6
Times picked up, not charged, nondrug-related offenses	0.6	0–7	0	0–6	0	0–7
Months since picked up, any charge	7.6	1–72	8.1	1–84	7.8	1–84
Medical complications	26% yes		8% yes		22% yes	
Action pending	85% none		71% none		82% none	
	$n = 104$		$n = 29$		$n = 133$	

[a]Not all subjects reported arrests; figures for those reporting arrests only.

what independently. (Negative experiences measured are listed in Table 2 for those remaining on the program and for those who have left.)

RESULTS

Our measure of success is whether the client is still on or has left the program (21% of those who left the program are in jail):*

1. In terms of age, the older the client the more likely he will remain in the program ($p < 0.10$). The largest group of drop-outs are in the age range 21–25; above the age of 31, clients tend to remain in the program.
2. In terms of ethnic group, Chicanos are more likely than whites to stay in the program.
3. In terms of medical complications (half of which are definitely drug usage related, e.g., hepatitis and overdose), those who have had medical complications are more likely to stay in the program ($p < 0.10$).
4. With respect to terms served for nondrug offenses, those who have served greater than six terms stay in the program ($p < 0.02$). Those who drop out of the program tend to have not served a term or have served a low number of terms.
5. In terms of action pending, those who have court action pending (half of whom are on parole) tend to stay in the program significantly more than those with no action pending against them ($p < 0.01$).

CONCLUSIONS

It can safely be concluded that those clients who are older and/or have had more negative experiences as a consequence of their heroin addiction are more likely to remain in a methadone maintenance program. Some negative experiences, among others, that are related to a client's tenure in the program are as follows:

1. Being on parole or having other action pending.
2. Never having worked more than a year at one job.
3. Being a minority group,† e.g., Chicanos.

*For problems involved in using various measures of "success" in methadone maintenance programs, see Maddux and Bowden (1972). Also Perkins and Richman (1972).
†The reasoning here is that being a member of a minority group increases the likelihood of having a greater number of negative experiences than being a member of the dominant Anglo culture.

4. Having had medical complications as a result of their addiction.
5. Having served a large number of terms for non-drug offenses.

Thus our research findings are that those people who have had more doors shut to them, i.e., have had their options reduced, are more likely to remain on a methadone maintenance program.

In terms of policy implications, the use of entrance requirements (e.g., being older, having been in jail) seems justified in terms of the present data.

Therefore our research leads us to the conclusion that methadone maintenance is more likely to be successful for older addicts with more negative experiences.* Clearly, we are equating success with staying on the program. This follows from the fact that those who leave often wind up in jail, and that methadone maintenance was adopted as a therapeutic strategy because very little else helped. Also, a corollary implicit in our findings is that other treatment modalities, such as "kick clinics" and detoxification centers, requiring more involvement and staff time, would appear to be better geared to the younger and/or less negatively experienced addict. However, further research is being conducted to determine if staying on the program results in more successful social functioning than leaving.

ACKNOWLEDGMENT

The authors gratefully acknowledge the tireless assistance of Evelyn Ludington in all phases of this study.

REFERENCES

GEARING, F.R. Evaluation of methadone maintenance program. In S. Einstein (ed.) *Methadone Maintenance*. New York: Dekker, 1971, pp. 171–206.

KNOWLES, R., LAHIRI, S., and ANDERSON, G. Methadone maintenance in St. Louis. In S. Einstein (ed.) *Methadone Maintenance*. New York: Dekker, 1971, pp. 61–70.

LEVINE, D.G., LEVIN, D.B., SLOAN, I.H., and CHAPPEL, J.N. Personality correlates of success in a methadone maintenance program. *Amer. J. Psychiat.* 129(4): 116–120, 1972.

MADDUX, J.F., and BOWDEN, C.L. Critique of success with methadone maintenance. *Amer. J. Psychiat.* 129(4): 100–106, 1972.

PERKINS, M.E., and RICHMAN, A. Prevalence of participation in methadone programs. *Amer. J. Psychiat.* 129(4): 107–110, 1972.

*For a study relating success in a methadone maintenance program to *personality* factors, see Levine et al. (1972).

STEPHENS, R. The truthfulness of addict respondents in research projects. *Intern. J.* Addictions 7(3): 549–558, 1972.

WILLIAMS, H.R., and JOHNSTON, W.E. Factors related to treatment retention in a methadone maintenance program. In *Proceedings, Fourth National Conference on Methadone Treatment.* New York: National Association for the Prevention of Addiction to Narcotics, 1972, pp. 439–442.

The International Journal of the Addictions, 9(2), 229–239, 1974

Evolution of a Treatment Approach for Young Heroin Addicts. Comparison of Three Treatment Modalities

Raymond A. Lloyd, M.D.

Richard N. Katon, M.D.

Robert L. DuPont, M.D.

Narcotics Treatment Administration
Washington, D.C.

A program for treating young heroin addicts was developed during the spring of 1970 with an initial thrust toward out-patient abstinence. In mid-1970 a 65-bed detoxification facility and a 25-bed residential therapeutic community were opened. There was a unique commitment to treat all those who sought help without regard to age or associated illnesses. Ex-addicts comprised most of the initial staff.

In mid-1970 a youth medical staff was developed and short-term methadone detoxification was introduced. Youthful addicts were placed on small doses of methadone (10–30 mg) and detoxified as rapidly as possible (10–30 days) on an out-patient basis. This approach was supported by counseling plus vocational and educational services to the limit of the small staff. Abstinence therapy was made available to those who chose that form of treatment.

By December 1970 the first research evaluation of the youth program demonstrated remarkably high drop-out and arrest rates. (Clients Functioning in the Youth Division Program: May 15, 1970 through November 15, 1970. Division of Research and Development, Narcotics Treatment Administration, Washington, D.C.) For example, the arrest rate at 6 months for the adult program was 19% whereas it was 42% for the youth program. The drop-out rate was 45% for the adult program and 82% for the youth program. In comparing data obtained from both programs, there was a striking similarity in the performance of the youth program which initially used little methadone and the adult abstinence program. Patients who were receiving counseling without methadone frequently failed to achieve abstinence and made the major contribution to the drop-out rate.

During these first months we found that there were few heroin addicts under the age of 15 and that most young patients were 17 to 20. At that time the consensus of opinion around the country was that addicts under 18 years should not be treated with methadone. In reviewing our experience with abstinence in this population, it seemed that the accepted approach might not be in the best interest of many patients.

The initial experience with methadone detoxification in addicts under 18 had shown that they generally needed lower dosages—usually in the range of 10 to 30 mg daily. Our experience suggested that schedules lasting for longer periods of time enabled us to help the patients more successfully change their life style.

In January 1971 the youth program was restructured, concentrating primarily on out-patient methadone detoxification but using the therapeutic community and in-patient beds in appropriate cases. Youth who repeatedly failed at short-term in-patient and out-patient detoxification were placed on prolonged detoxification schedules lasting for 6 months at doses up to 45 mg a day. If this approach at detoxification failed, the patient was offered the opportunity to go on a temporary low-dose maintenance schedule generally under 60 mg. It was hoped that methadone maintenance would last from 3 to 18 months, thus allowing for more extensive psychosocial changes prior to another attempt at detoxification to abstinence.

METHODS

Two hundred and one patients were placed on short- or long-term detoxification and low-dose maintenance schedules based on the duration of addiction, detoxification failures, a careful clinical history, and physical signs. Those patients initially on short-term detoxification (STD) who failed to curb their use of heroin were transferred to long-term detoxification schedules (LTD). Patients who failed at detoxification, up to the highest dosage schedule, were placed on low-dose temporary maintenance. Assignments to specific dose schedules were clinical decisions and not made by research design. The counselor–patient ratio was 1 : 30.

The short-term detoxification schedule started with 10 to 30 mg daily as a single dose. This dosage was decreased by 5 mg at 3 to 7 day intervals—the longest detoxification period being 6 weeks.

The long-term detoxification schedules lasted for 6 months with initial dosages of 20 to 35 mg. Patients then received 5 mg increases weekly for 4 weeks, bringing them to dosages of from 40 to 55 mg. This dosage was maintained for 8 weeks. At this point the dosage was reduced to 0 mg over a 12-week period by decrements of 5 mg every 7 to 17 days.

The low-dose maintenance schedules started at the level of the patient's last dose. Five milligram increases were given at 3 to 7 day intervals up to a final dose of 40 to 70 mg. Most patients received 40 to 60 mg daily.

All patients requesting help were treated based on the clinical picture, and those leaving the program did so voluntarily. Signed parental consent was obtained for all patients 18 years and under.

Urines were taken routinely twice a week on scheduled days under a staff member's observation and then tested for the presence of methadone, heroin and other opiates, cocaine, and quinine. Any evidence of quinine, whether alone or in combination with other drugs, was interpreted as evidence of heroin use. Prescribed methadone in the urine was considered negative.

Arrest records were searched from adult and juvenile correctional institutions of the District of Columbia. Included were all persons arrested on felony charges and all persons arrested for nontraffic misdemeanors. However, arrests outside of the District of Columbia would be known only to the extent that they preceded arrests recorded by D.C. correctional units.

RESULTS

Two hundred and one patients who entered the NTA youth program between August and October 1970 were studied retrospectively. The study period ended in March 1971. Sixty-four patients were initially on STD, 79 were initially on LTD, and 58 were on LDM at the beginning of the study and at the intake period. Patients on LDM had failed to achieve abstinence on STD and/or LTD prior to the study period. The average ages in the groups were 18.19, 18.32, and 17.98 years, respectively. Ninety-two percent of the patients were Black, and 84% were male (Table 1).

Eighty-four percent of the patients were voluntary admissions and 16% were referred through the criminal justice system (Table 2). The average length of time enrolled in the program after the start of the study period was 3.2 months, 6.85 months for those still enrolled at the end of the study, and 1.9 months for those who left the program. The average length of time enrolled in the program by treatment categories was STD 2.9 months, LTD 6.6 months, and LDM 7.3 months (Table 3).

Follow-up Status of Patients by Treatment Categories

At the end of the study period, 27 patients (42%) from the STD group were active compared to 16 (20%) on LTD and 31 (53%) on LDM.

Table 1
Age, Race, and Sex Distribution

	STD	LTD	LDM	Total
Average age (years)	18.19	18.32	17.98	18.18
Age range	14–20	16–20	16–21.5	14–21.5
Race: Black	55 (86%)	74 (94%)	55 (95%)	184 (92%)
White	9 (14%)	5 (6%)	3 (5%)	17 (8%)
Sex: Male	59 (92%)	60 (78%)	49 (84%)	168 (84%)
Female	5 (8%)	17 (22%)	9 (16%)	31 (16%)

Table 2
Type of Admission

	STD	LTD[a]	LDM	Total
Voluntary	59 (92%)	60 (78%)	49 (84%)	168 (84%)
Criminal justice system	5 (8%)	17 (22%)	9 (16%)	31 (16%)

[a]Information not available for two patients.

Table 3
Duration in Program

	STD	LTD	LDM
Average duration of active patients according to initial treatment category	9.3	6.6	7.3
Actual average duration in treatment category	2.9	6.6	7.3
All Patients			
Average length of time enrolled			3.2 months
Average length of time for inactive patients			1.9 months
Average length of time for active patients			6.85 months

Seventy-four patients (36%) of the entire study group were still active (Table 4).

Tables 5, 6, and 7 show the disposition of the patients according to treatment modality. Of the 64 patients initially on STD, three (4.7%) achieved abstinence and remained abstinent up to the last contact (Table 8). All were inactive, having dropped out of the program or transferred to other treatment categories. Seven patients (10.4%) who started on

Table 4
Retention in NTA Programs

	STD	LTD	LDM	Total
Active	27 (42%)	16 (20%)	31 (53%)	74 (36%)
Inactive	37 (58%)	63 (80%)	27 (47%)	127 (64%)
Total	64 (100%)	79 (100%)	58 (100%)	201 (100%)

Table 5
Disposition of STD Patients[a]

Patients[b]	Active	Inactive
D-A	—	3 (4.7%)
D-A-M	1 (1.4%)	—
D-D	—	16 (25%)
D-D¹	20 (30%)	—
D-M	6 (9%)	—

[a]Volume drops without completing schedule 18 (28%).
[b]D = STD; A = abstinence; M = LDM; D¹ = LTD.

Table 6
Disposition of LTD Patients[a]

Patients[b]	Active	Inactive
D^1-A	2 (2.5%)	2 (2.5%)
D^1-A-M	—	4 (5%)
D^1-A-D	—	18 (22.8%)
D^1-M	8 (10%)	—
D^1-D^1	6 (7.6%)	—

[a]Volume drops without completing schedule 39 (49.2%).
[b]D^1 = LTD; A = abstinence; M = LDM; D = STD.

Table 7
Disposition of LDM Patients[a]

Patients[b]	Active	Inactive
M	26 (44.8%)	—
M-D	5 (8.6%)	7 (12%)
M-D-A	—	3 (5.1%)

[a]Volume drops without completing schedule 17 (29.2%).
[b]M = LDM; D = STD; A = abstinence.

Table 8

	STD	LTD	LDM
Completed schedule, attained abstinence with four clean urines	3 (4.7%)	2 (2.5%)	2 (3.2%)
Completed schedule, attained abstinence without four clean urines	1 (1.4%)	1 (1.2%)	1 (1.5%)
Patients achieving abstinence, active or inactive	4 (6.1%)	26 (32.8%)	3 (5.1%)

STD were on LDM, and 20 patients (30%) were on LTD 6 months later. Eighteen patients (28%) had dropped out without completing the initial attempt at detoxification, and 16 (25%) dropped out during the second attempt.

Of the 79 patients initially on LTD (Table 6), four (5%) achieved abstinence and two (2.5%) remained active at the end of the study period. Twelve patients had been placed on LDM and eight (10%) remained active. Twenty-four patients (30.4%) were transferred to higher dosage schedules and six (7.6%) remained active. Thirty-nine patients (49.2%) dropped out without completing the first attempt at detoxification.

There were 58 patients on LDM (Table 7) and 31 (53%) remained active in the program 6 months later. Twelve patients (20.6%) had transferred to a LTD schedule and five (8.6%) remained active in the program. Three patients placed on STD achieved abstinence and were inactive. Seventeen patients (29.2%) dropped out of the program while still on the LDM schedule.

Illicit Drug Usage

The results of patient urinalyses were evaluated during the 4-week period prior to the end of the study. Surveillance was maintained on 73 (99%) of the 74 patients at the end of the study period. A total of 587 urinalyses were performed, an average of 7.69 for STD patients, 8.13 for LTD patients, and 8.29 for LDM patients (Table 9).

Of the patients initially in STD, 19 (73%) of 27 active patients had 50% or more urines clean (none of these patients were abstinent or on STD at the end of the study period. Sixteen patients (100%) of the active

Table 9
Urine Surveillance During Last 4 Weeks of Study Period

	STD	LTD	LDM
Number of urines	200	130	257
Average number of urines per active patient	7.69	8.13	8.29
Clean urines	130 (65%)	111 (85%)	218 (85%)
Dirty urines	70 (35%)	19 (15%)	39 (15%)
Number and percent with 50% or more clean urines	19 (73%)	16 (100%)	31 (100%)
Number and percent with less than 50% clean urines	7 (27%)	0 (0%)	0 (0%)

Table 10
Percent Positive Urines Among Active Patients by Treatment Modality

	STD[a]	LTD	LDM
0	4 (15%)	4 (25%)	11 (35%)
1–25	10 (37%)	8 (50%)	11 (35%)
26–50	5 (18.5%)	4 (25%)	9 (29%)
51–75	6 (22.2%)	—	—
76–99	—	—	—
100	1 (4%)	0 (0%)	0 (0%)

[a]No active clients were still on this regime. Information not available for one patient.

patients from LDM had 50% or more negative urines. Among active patients (Table 10), four (15%) in STD, four (25%) in LTD, and 11 (35%) in LDM had all tests negative. One patient (4%) from the STD group and none from the LTD and LDM groups had all positive urines. There were no patients from the LTD or LDM groups with more than 50% positive urines.

Employment Status

Table 11 shows the available information on employment. There were no data available for 18 active patients. Thirty-five (63%) of the 55 patients for whom this information was available were in training or full- or part-time jobs. Fourteen patients were full-time students and six were unemployed.

Arrest Data

Fifty-six of 107 patients (52.3%) in this study interviewed at intake regarding previous arrests reported having been arrested at least once prior to their entering the program. Fifty-four (50%) of this group had been arrested at least once during the preceding 3-year period. The average number of arrests per month was 1.9 the first year, 3.6 the second, and 5.8 the third year (Table 12). During the follow-up period, 27 (21.5%) of these clients were arrested 33 times, an average of 5.5 arrests per month. Fourteen patients (13%) were arrested while in the program, and 12 (12%) were arrested after voluntarily leaving the program. One-hundred percent of the patients on maintenance, 78% of the LTD patients, and 72.6% of the patients on STD were not arrested during the study period either while in the program or after leaving it (Table 13).

Table 11
Employment Status of Active Patients

	STD	LTD	LDM	Total
Full-time job	6 (27%)	0	5	11 (20%)
Full-time job training	3 (14%)	1	5	9 (16%)
Full-time student	7 (32%)	5	2	14 (25%)
Part-time job	5 (23%)	2	4	11 (20%)
Part-time training or student	1 (4%)	1	2	4 (7%)
Unemployed	0 (0%)	6	0	6 (11%)
Total	22 (100%)	15	18	55[a] (99%[b])

[a]Less than number of active patients since employment status was not available for 18 patients.
[b]Less than 100% due to rounding.

Table 12
Arrest Rates

	No. of arrests	Average no. of arrests per month
First year	23	1.9
Second year	43	3.6
Third year	70	5.8
Six month follow-up	33	5.5

Table 13
Treatment Categories in Relation to Incidence of Arrests

	STD	LTD	Maintenance
Arrested while in program	6 (18.7%)	8 (12.8%)	0 (0%)
Arrested after leaving program	6 (18.7%)	7 (10.0%)	0 (0%)
Not arrested	20 (72.6%)	41 (78.0%)	19 (100%)

DISCUSSION

The shift to out-patient methadone detoxification and a changing philosophy about using methadone for longer periods in youth led to a measurable improvement in the performance of the program. An NTA Research Study (Clients Functioning in the Youth Division Program: December 1971. Bureau of Research and Development, Narcotics Treatment Administration, Washington, D.C.) showed increased retention, increased employment, decreased use of illegal drugs, and decreased arrests among youth in the program. Fifty percent of the patients interviewed had been arrested at least once during the previous 3 years, with an average of 5.8 arrests per month during the third year. During a 6-month follow-up period, 21% of these patients were arrested. Thirty-five percent of the patients active after 6 months reported at intake that they were in training or in school or had jobs, whereas 51% of the active patients at the end of the study period were so employed.

At the end of the study period, 36% of the 201 patients remained active. Ten patients (5%) had achieved abstinence and remained so up to the last contact. On the LTD program, 26 (32.8%) of the patients achieved abstinence whereas only four (6.1%) of the patients on STD and three (5.1%) on LDM achieved this goal. LTD was 5.4 times more effective at achieving abstinence; however, abstinence was not maintained by most patients (Table 8). There were 10.4% of patients in the STD group and 15% of the LTD patients transferred to LDM. Seventeen patients (29.2%) from the LDM group dropped out of the program while still on treatment and without attempting detoxification. Although 35% of the patients on LDM had all negative urines, 65% had occasional positive tests.

There were 37.4% of STD patients arrested while in the program or after having dropped out whereas 22% of LTD patients and 0% of LDM patients were arrested. Twenty-seven (21.5%) patients from the whole group were arrested during the study, an average of 5.5 arrests per month. Since the arrest rates of this group had increased dramatically during the preceding 3 years (1.9, 3.6, and 5.8 arrests per month, respectively), the slight decrease in average number of arrests per month during the study period would appear to be significant. Fifty percent of the patients had been arrested prior to the study, whereas 75% had no arrests while in treatment.

Although there was 42% retention among patients on STD, no patients were retained in their original modality. Retention in the program is probably the most important factor if we are to influence the addicts' life style. It is therefore essential that we employ modalities that promote such retention. STD patients remained in the program for an average of 2.9 months.

In order to achieve any substantial overall retention rate, many techniques must be used because of the diversity in individual needs when one patient is compared to another and even for the same patient at different points in time. Note that if STD had been the only available modality, the retention rate at 6 months would have been 0%.

These results are far from satisfactory and they have prompted further changes in our approach to treating youth. New youth clinics will be smaller, each treating about 200 out-patients with a staff of 24 full-time and two part-time employees. More emphasis will be placed on the follow-up of drop-outs, encouraging them to return to the program.

The youth staff developed for this program had received no special training for their unique assignment other than an initial orientation to the treatment plan, concentrating on the properties and use of methadone in detoxification and maintenance treatment. Many of the staff were former addicts and, therefore, while they may have been lacking in an academic knowledge of addiction and treatment, they had a great deal to offer in the way of street expertise. The entire staff was generally enthusiastic about this assignment because of the opportunity it gave them to work with the youthful drug abuser and help these individuals not enter a life style from which it becomes increasingly difficult to withdraw. Future plans for staff include increased training in the academic areas of addiction and counseling, as well as increased attention to identifying the special needs of youth and meeting these needs with additional services.

The community within which this program resides raised no great difficulties for the adequate functioning of the program. Indeed, a number of parents of the patients were actively involved in volunteer activities and participated in family-oriented therapy sessions. Future plans include increased attention to this potential source of support for any program geared to youth. Continued active community involvement would serve to encourage the participation of the patient population in program activities, which would in turn reinforce the need for a commitment of support by the community.

Our experience points to the fact that physicians' hesitation over the use of methadone in youth may be detrimental to many patients. Of course, more study is needed in this area, but early results suggest that methadone on a prolonged detoxification basis and methadone maintenance as part of a comprehensive program will add to the success of youth undergoing treatment for heroin addiction. It may be unpleasant for some critics to recognize this reality, but it is even more unpleasant to realize that heroin overdose is the leading cause of death in most cities in the population aged 15 to 35 years. (Report of the Laboratory for Addictive Drugs, Office of the Chief Medical Examiner of New York. Michael M. Baden, M.D., Director, Laboratory for Addictive Drugs. Presented at the International Conference on Poison Control, June 3, 1969 in New York City.)

Finally, the response to treatment is variable and complicated. Treating youthful addicts represents an exercise in clinical medicine that does not lend itself readily to research protocols. Treating an unselected population of people in the environment in which they initially became addicted and to which they return each day is very difficult. We must reassess our definitions of success and failure since it may be that any reduction in illegal drug use or increase in prosocial functioning is very significant. The data that we have presented must be evaluated in this light.

ACKNOWLEDGMENTS

To Deborah Miller and Sally Glendinning for their assistance in compiling these data.

The International Journal of the Addictions, 9(2), 241–253, 1974

The College Opiate User

Betty Crowther, Ph.D.

Southern Illinois University
Edwardsville, Illinois

ABSTRACT

Interviews were conducted with 43 known opiate users who had attended college. An analysis of the information obtained suggested that these student users were more similar to their college peers than the street addict studied in hospitalized samples. They were multiple drug users who reported experimentation with many different types of drugs including a large number of hallucinogens. Most came from middle-class families with no apparent history of deviance. Unlike the street addict, these users did not have a delinquent history prior to their drug use. Nearly all of the subjects interviewed expressed plans of finishing college. One variable, the use of heroin, did appear to differentiate two groups of users. The heroin users tended to start their drug careers at an earlier age, they had used a wider assortment of different drugs, and they tended to come from slightly lower socioeconomic backgrounds than did the nonheroin users.

There is no doubt that drugs have invaded the college scene over the past 10 years. Newspaper accounts of raids, busts, and dramatic misfortunes illustrate the public's concern for this problem. On many campuses college officials have developed clinics or drug abuse programs to aid the user in understanding his behavior. Estimates of marijuana use among college students often suggest that over 50% of the population have at least experimented with the drug. Survey researchers also consistently find that a relatively large proportion of the students have used other drugs such as LSD, speed, or downers. Most studies, however, suggest that opiates, and heroin in particular, have typically been avoided by these college drug users. Despite an apparent low rate of use, rumors aided by sensational accounts in the mass media have focused a good deal of attention on this problem. As Goode points out, "If a half-dozen students out of a college population of 10,000 use heroin more than a dozen times, a great stir is created, and an epidemic is claimed for that campus" (1969).

Most questionnaire surveys of drug use among students find a very low percentage of users claiming even experimental use of heroin. The University of Michigan study in 1969 (Frances and Patch, 1969) is one of the few surveys finding a relatively large percent (16.9%) of the students reporting opiate use. Other studies usually find less than 5% opiate users among normal student populations (Barter, Mizner, and Werme, 1970; Morrison, 1969; Goldstein et al., 1970; Blum, 1969). Even Yablonsky (1968), in his study of approximately 700 hippies, found only 2.8% reporting heroin use. These survey results confirm the notion that opiates, while present on the college campus, are not a common drug used by the student population.

Goode (1969) argues that heavy marijuana use will increase the individual's likelihood of using other drugs, if and only if they are approved of by the using subculture. He maintains that marijuana use may lead to opiate use in working class urban areas but not college campuses where such use is frowned upon. Blumer (1969) suggests that heroin addicts are viewed by the majority of drug-using adolescents as persons who have "lost their cool" and who are "weakminded." Thus one reason why heroin is not used on the college campus revolves about the generalized negative connotation students attach to the drug.

A second argument, however, is perhaps just as strong. According to Goode (1969, p. 62), "among college students . . . there is very little probability that the one [marijuana] will lead to the other [heroin], simply because the chances of meeting those involved with heroin are extremely limited." He goes on to say that middle-class college users are generally supplied with their drugs by a middle-class college dealer. Such a dealer is unlikely to handle heroin or even have contact with professional criminals. Similar statements are found in Blumer's discussion of attitudes toward addiction. According to him, "the majority of youthful drug users have no association with heroin users and no access to heroin. Without such association and access, youthful drug users cannot enter the arena of drug use" (Blumer, 1969, p. 85).

Thus it would appear that the college opiate user is a different type of individual than the average college user. Not only has he violated a college norm against the use of heroin or other opiates, but he has sought out or somehow made contact with a source of supply. The present study was designed to examine some of the characteristics of such persons.

The data for this study was obtained in the fall of 1971 and spring of 1972 through interviews with known opiate users in a Midwest metropolitan area. Due to the difficulty in obtaining subjects, there was no attempt to draw a probability sample of users. Subjects were found by sending out a request for volunteers among the drug-using population. The criteria for inclusion in the sample was twofold: the individual must presently be or have been a college student, and he must have used an illicit opiate at least once. Although nearly all the treatment programs in the metropolitan area were contacted, the majority of subjects were obtained through the informal communication structure existing among drug users. Dealers were the most valuable contacts, as they would often set up an interview with subjects. Interviewers were specifically instructed to omit names from the completed interview schedules. Thus even the principal investigator often could not identify individual subjects. In a few cases students cooperated by obtaining interviews themselves and submitting the data. Although these techniques made quality control impossible, it was felt that the information could not be obtained in any other manner.

Interviews were obtained with 33 males and 10 females meeting the criteria. Several questions concerning their scholastic records were asked to check whether or not their career as a student was valid. Of the entire sample, 63% were presently enrolled as students in a university. A similar percent reported that the majority of their friends were still in college even if they were not presently enrolled. When asked about their academic performance, only two persons reported a grade point average of under a "C." Thus it would appear that the majority of these persons are pursuing a serious college career. Further, on the basis of their own self reports, they seem to be succeeding relatively well in college and have adapted to the college environment.

Despite these responses from the subjects, their academic careers have not been smooth. A large percent (68%) had dropped out of school at least once. When asked the reason for this behavior, the majority stated that leaving school had nothing to do with their drug use. Nevertheless, the consistency of this response suggests a basic dissatisfaction with the educational system.

Twenty-four out of the 43 persons interviewed had used heroin. Since the use of heroin seemed to be the major differentiating characteristic between the two types of users found in the study, it has been used as a control variable.

BACKGROUND VARIABLES

Nearly all the subjects in this study were between the ages of 19 and 25. The actual age range, however, was from 19 to 42 with a median of 21.5. There is essentially no difference between the average age for heroin and nonheroin users although both of the older respondents had used heroin. The medians for these groups are 22 and 21.5.

The majority of the subjects (90%) lived with both of their parents for the first 16 years of their life. None of the nonheroin users and 17% of the heroin users reported some type of family disturbance (parental divorce, separation, death, etc.) during this time. Half of the subjects report one or two siblings in the home. Interestingly, 20% of the nonheroin users report four or more siblings as compared with 35% of the heroin users. When asked about father's education, 35% of the entire sample reported that their father had a high school education. This category is the median for both heroin and nonheroin users. However, a closer examination shows that 16% of the nonheroin users and 43% of the heroin users stated that their father had less than a high school education, and 16% of the nonheroin users and 5% of the heroin users stated that their fathers had more than a college education. These differences suggest that the nonheroin user tends to come from a better educated, higher socioeconomic status family than the heroin user. Both, however, tend to come from middle-class families, a vast difference from the addict population studied in the hospital.

One of the common findings in studies of heroin users is their lack of marital stability. Although the age factor contaminates the present study, similar results are suggested here. The majority of the sample (72%) were single and had never been married. Although the figures are too small to be significant, it is interesting that four persons reported a common-law arrangement of less than a month, while none reported a common-law arrangement of 6 months or more. Thirteen people responded that they had been married and, of these, four had been divorced.

Subjects were asked to state both their own religion and the religion of their parents. As might be expected from a Midwest community, 56% had been reared in the Protestant faith and 41% in the Catholic faith. At present, however, 55% of the entire sample state that they have no religious preference. A breakdown of the heroin and nonheroin users shows that 63% of the heroin users report no religious preference, as compared with 44% of the nonheroin users.

DRUG USE

In general, the heroin users tend to use a greater variety of different drugs than do the nonheroin users. Subjects were given a list of drugs prepared by a pharmacologist at the Lexington, Kentucky narcotic hospital and asked to check those that they had used. All of the heroin users stated that they had used at least three different opiate drugs and seven of this group reported use of 10 or more different opiates. The majority of the nonheroin users had used only one or two of the opiates listed. Thus it would appear that many of the nonheroin users have simply experimented once or twice with an opiate drug but never became regular users. These persons tend to confine their use to drugs other than opiates. In contrast, seven of the heroin users reported daily heroin use.

Although the differences are not as obvious, the heroin user also tends to have used a larger number of different types of barbiturates than the nonheroin user. All of the nonheroin users who responded to the question had used less than seven different barbiturates. In comparison, 74% of the heroin users had used seven or more of these drugs. Similarly, 11% of the nonheroin users and 38% of the heroin users report the use of more than five different stimulant drugs. Although there were no persons in the total sample who did not report amphetamine use, three stated that they had never used a hallucinogen. The majority of nonheroin users had used three or four different hallucinogens, with only 21% reporting more than five different drugs. The heroin users again reported a wider use of these drugs, with 63% reporting the use of five or more different hallucinogens. Only one person in the sample, a heroin user, reported no use of alcohol or marijuana. Thus the picture that emerges is one of a multiple drug user who has tried a wide variety of different drugs. The heroin user appears to be more deeply submerged in this drug culture and reports more experimentation with different types of drugs than does the nonheroin user.

The high rate of use of psychedelic drugs among this sample definitely

DRUG LIST

I. The "O" series (Narcotic Analgesics)

091 Bultar
001 Codeine
002 Cough syrups containing narcotics
059 Cyclazocine
051 Darvon/Propoxyphene/Dextropropoxyphene
052 Demerol/Meperidine
031 Dicodid/Hycodan/Dihydrocodeinone
032 Dilaudid
033 Dionin/Ethylmorphine
053 Dolophine/Methadone
093 Dorial
054 Dromoran/Racemorphan
044 Heroin
003 Laudanum
055 Leritine/Analeridine
056 Levodromoran/Levorphanol
034 Metopon/Methyldihydromorphinone
004 Morphine
035 Nalline/Nalorphine
057 Nisentil/Alphaprodine
036 Numorphan/Oxymorphone
005 Opium
006 Pantopon/Omnopon
037 Paracodin/Dihydrocodeine
007 Paregoric
038 Percodan/Oxycodone
058 Talwin/Pentazocine
008 Thebaine

II. The "1" series (Sedative Hypnotic Relaxants) excluding alcohol

110 Alurate/Aprobarbital
118 Amobarbital
111 Amytal/Blue Heaven/Blue Angels
150 Aqualude/Sopor/Methaqualone
192 Aravon
112 Barbital/Veronal
142 Bromides
131 Carbrital
132 Carbromal
133 Chloral Hydrate
113 Desbutal
134 Doriden/Glutethamide/Cibas
135 Equanil/Miltown/Meprobamate
193 Hartolid
136 Librium/Cholorodiazepoxide
114 Luminal/Phenobarbital/Idiot Pills/Pink Lady
115 Nembutal/Pentobarbital/Yellow Jackets/Nimbie
137 Noludar
138 Paraldehyde
139 Placidyl
116 Seconal/Secobarbital/Redbirds/Red Devils
151 Soma/Carisoprodol
152 Taractan
153 Tranpoise/Trepidome/Lenetran/Methenoxylone
117 Tuinal/Christmas Tree Lights
140 Valium/Diazepam

III. The "3" series (Stimulants)

310 Benzedrine/Amphetamine/Bennies
317 Caffeine (as a drug - not coffee, etc.)
302 Coca leaves
301 Cocaine or derivatives
311 Desoxyn/Desoxyephedrine
312 Dexedrine
313 Ephedrine
393 Etanol
314 Methedrine/Methamphetamine/Speed
315 Preludin/Phenmetrazine
316 Ritalin

IV. The "5" series (Psychotogens)

503 DET
504 DMT
505 DOM-STP
501 LSD
502 Mescaline
590 Petrovil
500 Peyote
506 Psilocybin/Psilocin
530 Belladonna alkaloids, unspecified
531 Scapolamine
532 Atropine

V. Other

101 Alcohol
600 Marijuana
201 Campazine/Procholorperazine
202 Mellaril/Thioridazine
203 Sparine/Promazine
204 Stelazine
205 Thorazine/Chlorpromazine
231 Harmonyl
291 Margotine
232 Reserpine/Serpasil
402 Elavil
430 Marplan
431 Nardil
432 Parnate
492 Petrovil
401 Tofranil
433 Catron/Pheniprazine
434 Marsilid/Iproniazid
435 Niamid/Nialamid

VI. Combination Drugs

045 Speedballs (Heroin + Cocaine)
046 Bambinos/Bambitos (Heroin + Amphetamines)
039 Footballs (Dilaudid + Cocaine)

sets them apart from the typical heroin addict. As reported by Cheek et al. (1969), hallucinogens are rarely used by the street addict. This drug tends to be used primarily by adolescents and college students. Another phenomenon rarely found among the street addicts is the use of a wide variety of different drugs (Crowther, 1972). The typical patient at the Fort Worth hospital had not used hallucinogens or tranquilizers and had used fewer than two different amphetamines or barbiturates. Over one-fourth of this group had only used one narcotic. Thus these college users tend to be more similar to those described by Blum in his study of high school and college drug users. The fact that they have experimented with a tremendously wide variety of drugs suggests that they are seeking different sensory experiences rather than the effects of a single drug. It is even possible that the use of different drugs has become a goal in itself, substituting for the physical effects of the drugs themselves.

All but one of the subjects interviewed reported the use of marijuana. Sixty-eight percent of the heroin users began their first marijuana use in high school, while 58% of the nonheroin users began in college. This difference in age may be due to the fact that heroin users report that marijuana was available to them at a younger age than nonheroin users. Forty-seven percent of the total sample reported that the drug had been offered to them before the first time they actually used it. Twelve percent of the nonheroin users and 58% of the heroin users said that it had been offered to them while still in high school.

The majority of the subjects (53%) stated that they had been given marijuana for their first experience by a close friend. Only 20% reported obtaining it from a dealer. These findings are consistent with previous research on initial contact with the drugs. If anything, 20% is a relatively high figure. Subjects were asked whether they got "high" the first time they tried marijuana. As previous reports have shown, many individuals do not obtain the subjective effects of the drug on their first experience. Interestingly, 74% of the heroin users and 47% of the nonheroin users said they did get "high." This finding again suggests a halo effect surrounding anything to do with drugs.

Eighty-six percent of the sample stated that they presently use marijuana. Some (33%) estimated that they used it more than they did before their first narcotic use, while 44% stated that they used it less. There is an interesting difference between heroin and nonheroin users in response to this question. Only 29% of the heroin users report less use today, as compared with 67% of the nonheroin users. Of those reporting present use, 71% of the heroin users stated that they used marijuana daily, as compared with 19% of the nonheroin users. This should not, however, be interpreted to mean that nonheroin users are not regular marijuana users. Of this group, 69% report use several times a week.

When asked what was the first narcotic ever used, 32% of the total sample replied opium. Since this is a relatively unusual drug, further questioning revealed that most of these individuals first obtained opium while in the armed forces. Thirty-nine percent of the heroin users started on heroin, and the only other significant category mentioned was that of cough syrups containing narcotics which were used by 16%. The majority (78%) took their first narcotic either orally or by smoking. Five of the 18 heroin users answering this question reported "IV" as their first route. Only one of the heroin users and four of the nonheroin users gave a medical reason for their beginning use.

Forty-three percent of the subjects stated that narcotics had been offered to them at least once before their initial use. When they did decide to first try the drug, the majority (70%) stated that they were with several males or a mixed sex group. As mentioned before, a large number of these people (33%) were living in the military at the time when they began their opiate use. Forty-three percent, however, were still living with their parents.

The majority of the subjects (73%) stated that there was nothing that they disliked about their first narcotic. There is no difference between the heroin and nonheroin user on this variable. Although only 21 persons answered the question of how long it was before they tried any narcotic again, 48% of these stated that their second narcotic was used within a single week. Furthermore, the majority who did try a narcotic again stated that it was the same drug that they had used initially (81%).

When asked what narcotic they primarily use now, 91% of the heroin users stated that they use heroin. Interestingly, however, when asked what drug they preferred, only 23% of the heroin users reported heroin. The others stated that they preferred either opium, morphine, or a nonopiate. Fifty percent of the nonheroin users who answered that question stated that they preferred a nonopiate.

As might be expected, the nonheroin users reported that smoking or oral ingestion are the primary means of ingesting the opiates they do use. In contrast, 85% of the heroin users mainline the drug. Although none of the nonheroin users think that they are addicted to the opiate presently used, eight of the 14 heroin users said that they were addicted. These findings are consistent with the fact that seven of the heroin users report daily use and two others use every weekend.

Most of these subjects did not begin their drug careers with an opiate. Fifty-eight percent of the nonheroin users and 74% of the heroin users report the use of other illicit drugs before their first narcotic use. When asked to describe the order of using several different drugs, the two most common patterns were "alcohol—marijuana—other narcotics—heroin—other drugs" and "alcohol—marijuana—other drugs—heroin—other narcotics." Unfortunately this question was slightly confusing and only 11 respondents, all of whom were heroin users, answered the question.

ANTISOCIAL BEHAVIOR

The majority of this sample (70%) stated that they had never been arrested. Of those that had, 11 out of 13 were picked up on a drug charge. Unlike the street addicts, these persons had not been in trouble with the law at a young age. Only one reported an arrest at the age of 13, and six were over 20. Sixty-seven percent stated that they had been arrested after both their first marijuana use and their first narcotic use. Only six of these persons had been in jail or reform school for 2 weeks or more. These figures should be compared with similar histories of street addicts. The author, in a study of patients at the Fort Worth hospital, found that 69% of the addicts had been arrested before their first narcotic use (Crowther, 1972). Fifty-five percent of her sample had been arrested before the age of 16. Similarly Chambers et al. (1970) found that nearly 80% of his Mexican-American sample had been arrested as juveniles. These figures suggest that a history of antisocial behavior and consequent arrests is the norm for the typical street addict but untrue for the college addict.

As noted previously, a relatively large proportion of these subjects reported that their initial opiate use had occurred while they were in the armed forces. Seventeen (40%) of the sample had served in the armed forces. All but two of this number had spent 19 or more months in the service. The majority of these subjects (88%) received an honorable discharge. These findings again illustrate the difference between the college and street addict. The majority of street addicts do not spend any time in the armed services (O'Donnell, 1968; Crowther, 1972). Of those who do, a large proportion receive a discharge that is other than honorable. O'Donnell, noting the consistency with which addicts report trouble in the service, has suggested that army records on this group are an excellent predictor of occupational success.

Fifteen of the 16 respondents who answered the question, "Did you use narcotics in the service?" answered in the affirmative. Thirty-three percent said they had used overseas, 40% said in the states, and 27% said in both places. These figures suggest that the present armed services are contributing to the drug problem in the United states.

As might be expected by the age of these respondents, only 50% report ever having held a full-time job. Forty-two percent, however, state they have held this job for 2 years or more, with six persons reporting a steady job for 4 or more years. These data reflect the difference between the college and the street addict. Bates (1968) found that most of the Negro addicts in his sample had never effectively entered the labor market. He argues that the primary orientation of the street addict is to antisocial behavior rather than to behavior such as work that is acceptable in American society. The relatively steady employment patterns of the college sample examined here does not suggest this pervasive antisocial orientation. Simply the fact of going to college is in itself a responsible action in our culture.

DISCUSSION

One finding that emerged consistently in this study was the difference between the heroin and nonheroin college user. The nonheroin user tended to come from a higher social class, he is less likely to reject the religious teachings of his parents, he is more likely to be successful in school, and he tends to have a less varied drug history. The heroin user, on the other hand, is a multiple drug user often having experimented with nearly all drugs listed. He tends to come from a larger family and has had a more erratic work and arrest history. His initial contact with drugs was at a younger age, and he reported a greater liking for them than his nonheroin counterpart. His enthusiasm for drugs is so great that it tends to be suspicious. It is hypothesized here that the use of drugs rather than the effects of the drugs has become a motivating force for this type of user. He seems to have sought out illicit drugs at a young age and pursued a drug career experimenting with nearly every type of drug available.

In general, the college opiate user appears to be more similar to the average college student "head" than the street addict. He not only tends to come from a middle-class background, but seems to have internalized the middle-class norm of achieving a college degree. He is a multiple drug user who has experimented with a wide variety of different types of drugs. Unlike the street addict who usually uses other drugs only to supplement the effects of heroin, the college user seems to try different drugs for their individual effects. Nearly all these users have experimented with psychedelic drugs as well as amphetamines and barbiturates.

Obviously, this study with a sample size of 43 can only be considered as exploratory in nature. Although the evidence seems to suggest that most college students do not experiment with opiates, a larger controlled study of all college drug users should be made. In this way it would be possible to confirm many of the findings suggested in this study. Further study should focus on that person who does deviate from the college population by using heroin.

The very fact that the individual in this study has attended college makes him different than the typical street addict who has no marketable job skills and little chance for successful rehabilitation. Such students can perhaps best be compared with professionals who become addicts. The professional has, in addition to marketable skills, a whole middle-class value system capable of producing alternate life styles unrelated to opiate use. Presumably it is this ability that accounts for the low recidivism rate among this group. The college addict similarly should be able to respond well to treatment directed toward substituting a different pattern of existence for the present drug related one. Existing treatment programs, however, are usually not designed for the middle-class clientele. If elimination of opiate use is the goal, treatment must focus on the reasons why the individual chose to use opiates. The research presented here suggests that boredom or a simple need to experiment appears to be at least one motivating factor in the decision to use drugs. Perhaps the need to experiment with any and all drugs is symptomatic of other difficulties encountered in the maturing process. If so, treatment for this group should attempt to substitute other more socially accepted activities for present drug-related ones.

Another finding of this study having practical significance is the fact that most of the heroin users started their drug career at a young age. Perhaps it would be possible to detect potential problems before they arise. This is not to say that all marijuana users will graduate to heroin use, but simply that a syndrome of need might be detectable long before heroin use. Obviously further study is needed to examine this possibility.

ACKNOWLEDGMENTS

I would like to thank Arthur Scholbe for his assistance in interviewing subjects in this study. I would also like to express my appreciation to the other students whose help made this study possible.

REFERENCES

BARTER, J.T., MIZNER, G.L., and WERME, P.H. *Patterns of Drug Use Among College Students: An Epidemiological and Demographic Survey of Student Attitudes and Practices*. Department of Psychiatry, University of Colorado Medical School, 1970.

BATES, W.M. Occupational characteristics of Negro addicts. *Intern. J. Addictions* 3: 345–350, 1968.

BLUM, R., and associates. *Students and Drugs*. San Francisco: Jossey-Bass, 1969.

BLUMER, H. Attitudes toward addiction. In E. Goode (ed.) *Marijuana*. Chicago: Aldine, 1969, pp. 85–88.

CHAMBERS, C.D., CUSKEY, W.R., and MOFFETT, A.D. Mexican-American opiate addicts. In J.C. Ball and C.D. Chambers (eds.) *The Epidemiology of Opiate Addiction in the United States*. Springfield, Illinois: Thomas, 1970, pp. 202–221.

CHEEK, F.E., NEWELL, S., and SARETT, M. The down-head behind an up-head—The heroin addict takes LSD. *Intern. J. Addictions* 4: 101–119, 1969.

CROWTHER, B. Patterns of drug use among Mexican-Americans. *Intern. J. Addictions* 7: 1972.

CROWTHER, B., The student opiate user. In W. Bates and B. Crowther (eds.) *The Typology of Drug Addiction*. Schenkman, 1974.

FRANCIS, J.B., and PATCH, D.J. *Student Attitudes Toward Drug Programs at the University of Michigan*. Study conducted under the auspices of the University Committee on Drug Education, September 1969.

GOLDSTEIN, J.W., et al. *The Social Psychology of Student Drug Usage: Report on Phase One*. A Report of the Carnegie-Mellon University Drug Research Project, June 1970.

GOODE, E. Multiple drug use among marijuana smokers. *Social Problems* 17(Summer): 48–63, 1969.

MORRISON, R.L. *Preliminary Report on the Incidence of the Use of Drugs at Sacramento State College*. May 15, 1969.

O'DONNELL, J.A. Social factors and follow-up studies in opioid addiction. *Assoc. Res. Nervous Mental Disease* 46: 333–346, 1968.

YABLONSKY, L. *The Hippie Trip*. New York: Pegasus, 1968.

The International Journal of the Addictions, 9(2), 255–266, 1974

Personality Characteristics of Heroin Addicts in a Methadone Treatment Program: An Exploratory Study

Arthur G. Cryns, Ph.D.

School of Social Policy and Community Services
State University of New York at Buffalo
Buffalo, New York

INTRODUCTION

Although in recent years the scientific literature on drug addiction has expanded spectacularly, systematic empirical research on the personality attributes of drug addicts seems to have lagged behind noticeably. To date, there exists only a limited number of data-based studies in this particular field of investigation. Moreover, most of the published research gives evidence of having been predominantly clinical in orientation, and thus of having been onesidedly geared to the discovery of pathological symptomatology in the addict. Beginning with the pioneering studies of Kolb (1925), Pescor (1939), and Felix (1944), the drug addict has invariably been described as psychopathic or neurotic with either defective impulse control or anxiety states and depression as his most frequently observed core symptoms (Gilbert and Lombardi, 1967; Hekimian and Gershon,

1968; Hill et al., 1960, 1962, 1968). However, there are other studies which seem to de-emphasize both psychopathic conditions and neuroticism as relevant clinical correlates of addiction (Gerard and Kornetsky, 1955; Monroe, Ross, and Berzins, 1971). Only the most recent past studies have been conducted with the focus on the *normal* psychological as well as the *psychiatric* attributes of the addict (Bewley, 1967; Cockett, 1971; Halstead and Neal, 1968; Kleckner, 1968).

This investigation probes the psychodynamics of the drug-addicted individual utilizing normal rather than clinical measures of inquiry. The specific questions it attempts to answer may be phrased as follows: Does the heroin addict submitting to methadone treatment differ significantly from similar addicts seeking no such treatment? Does methadone treatment, as such, effect changes in addict self-assessment over time? Do such subject variables as race and sex relate with any degree of consistency to obtained personality measures? Does psychotherapy or counseling provided in conjunction with methadone treatment significantly affect addict self-perception?

The study was not guided by any one, or any set of, formal hypotheses. It is to be conceived largely as an exploratory endeavor in a field that so far has yielded only limited empirical information.

METHOD

The Sample

The subjects of this study were $N = 70$ heroin addicts participating in a methadone maintenance program at a large metropolitan hospital in Buffalo, New York. They constitute an *unstratified random* sample of a $N = 255$ addict population being treated on an out-patient basis. Abstinence from heroin and commitment to rehabilitation were strictly enforced prerequisites for inclusion and continuance in the treatment program. Fifty-one of the subjects were male and 19 were females; 40 were black and 30 were white; 23 of the subjects were in methadone treatment for 3 months or less, 12 between 3 and 12 months, and 35 for 1 year or longer. Subjects ranged in age from 19 to 51 years, the median age being 28.4 years. Length of preexistent addiction to drugs ranged from 1 to 25 years, 2.8 years being the average. Almost all subjects had submitted to methadone treatment voluntarily; only three were court referrals for mandatory rehabilitation.

This study also reports psychological test scores on a small control group of $N = 11$ heroin addicts *not* on a methadone maintenance regime. The latter subjects were recruited from a small community drug counseling

Table 1
Background Characteristics of Sample Subjects in Methadone Treatment Group and Nonmethadone Control Group

Subject characteristics	Samples: Methadone treatment ($N = 70$)	Samples: Nonmethadone control ($N = 11$)
Sex: Male/female	51/19	7/4
Race: Black/White	40/30	6/5
Age (years): Median (range)	28.4 (19–51)	25.6 (18–40)
Marital status: Single/ married/divorced-separated	30/23/17	6/3/2
Length of Addiction: Median (range)	3.8 (1–25)	1.9 (1–19)
Rehabilitation treatment:[a]		
0–3 months	23	0
3–12 months	12	11
12 months and over	35	0

[a]Rehabilitative treatment = methadone treatment for methadone group and less than 6 months of informal group psychotherapy for control group.

clinic where they voluntarily participated in group psychotherapy sessions. It was composed of seven males and four females; six were black and five were white; its median age was 25.6 years and the average length of drug addiction was less than 2 years. Unlike the previous group, abstinence from illegal drugs or explicit commitment to rehabilitation were no prerequisites for participation in the therapeutic endeavor. The group therapy sessions were described as informal group discussions or "rap-sessions" led by a rehabilitated heroin addict.

Table 1 gives a summary account of the subject characteristics of both samples.

The Measuring Instrument

The measuring device utilized in this study was the Shostrom Personal Orientation Inventory (POI) (1965, 1966). It is an instrument for the measurement of positive mental health rather than of clinical defect; it is based mainly on Maslow's model of the self-actualizing person. The POI consists of 150 two-choice comparative value statements reflecting both values and behaviors seen to be important in normal human development. In responding to the test the subject is asked to select the one statement in each pair that is most true of himself. The instrument yields a total of 14 subscale scores: (1) *time incompetence* (TI)—degree to which person lives in past or future; (2) *time competence* (TC)—degree to which subject lives in the present; (3) *other-directedness* (O)—dependency upon others; (4) *inner-directedness* (I)—degree of personal autonomy, of self-support; (5) *self-actualizing value* (SAV)—tendency to prefer values generally held by mature persons; (6) *existentiality* (EX)—degree to which person is able to react flexibly to situations; (7) *feeling reactivity* (FR)—sensitivity to one's own needs and feelings; (8) *spontaneity* (S)—freedom to be oneself, to react spontaneously; (9) *self-regard* (SR)—feelings of self-worth, of self-affirmation; (10) *self-acceptance* (SA)—acceptance of self despite weaknesses or defects; (11) *nature of man* (NC)—degree to which subject views human nature positively or negatively; (12) *synergy* (SY)—ability to transcend dichotomies, to act synergistically; (13) *acceptance of aggression* (A)—acceptance of one's own natural aggressiveness; (14) *capacity for intimate contact* (C)—ability to relate intimately to others, emotional responsiveness to others.

The nonthreatening nature of the items and the interpretation of the scales in terms of perceived levels of self-development rather than of clinical symptomatology were prime considerations for selection of the instrument.

The literature reports test–retest reliability scores for the POI subscales ranging from 0.55 to 0.85, suggesting that the instrument's stability is comparable to that of most other objective personality measures (Knapp, 1971). As for the test's validity, Shostrom reports data to indicate that it discriminates significantly between clinically nominated normal and self-actualized groups and nonself-actualized groups as well as between other criterion groups of different levels of mental health; its correlations with other personality measures such as the MMPI were found to be consistent, in the expected direction and significant (Shostrom, 1966, pp. 25–32).

Analysis of Data

Two separate analyses were performed on the data obtained in this study. First, a comparison was made of the personality profiles of the methadone and nonmethadone addict groups. To that end, a simple randomized two-group design was used and the data subjected to multivariate and univariate, one-way analyses of variance. Second, the scores obtained from the methadone sample were analyzed in the context of a $2 \times 2 \times 3$ factorial design, with *sex* (male-female), *race* (black-white), and *duration of methadone treatment* (0–3 months; 4–12 months; 1 year and longer) as the independent variables. The 14 subscales scores were subjected to a three-way, fixed effects, multivariate analysis of variance as prescribed by Bock (1963) and Finn (1968).

The multivariate method of data analysis is based upon the psychometric assumption that the multiple dependent variable measures, yielded by each subject in a study, are not independent, and thus are to be treated simultaneously, as a set. Under the Bock-Finn linear program of multivariate data analysis, an exact partition of dispersion (variance and covariance) is obtained for a given ordering of effects in the ANOVA-model for both equal and unequal *N*-cases. In addition to multivariate *F* ratios, the program yields supplementary univariate *F*'s for all individual design factors and their interactions.

RESULTS

Methadone-Control Group Comparison

The mean POI subscale scores and the corresponding *F* ratios obtained by the methadone treatment group and the control group of nonmethadone treated addicts are given in Table 2; a graphical presentation of essentially the same data is presented in Fig. 1.

These data suggest that the methadone treatment group functions at a higher level of self-actualization and self-perceived maturity than

Table 2
Mean POI Scores and F *Ratios of Methadone Treatment Group and Nonmethadone Treated Addict Group*

POI Scales	Methadone group ($N = 70$)	Nonmethadone control group ($N = 11$)	F (univariate)
TI	8.06	6.91	1.21
TC	14.26	12.64	2.02
O	44.91	55.45	19.47**
I	78.09	74.45	0.85
SAV	18.27	16.64	1.62
EX	19.10	16.00	4.50*
FR	15.16	14.00	1.35
S	11.29	10.54	1.10
SR	12.61	7.54	3.74*
SA	15.44	10.36	3.84*
NC	11.23	9.91	0.32
SY	5.70	5.73	0.00
A	15.90	12.91	3.89*
C	19.00	16.09	2.42
	Multivariate $F = 4.97$**		

*Significant at $p < .05$.
**Significant at $p < .01$.

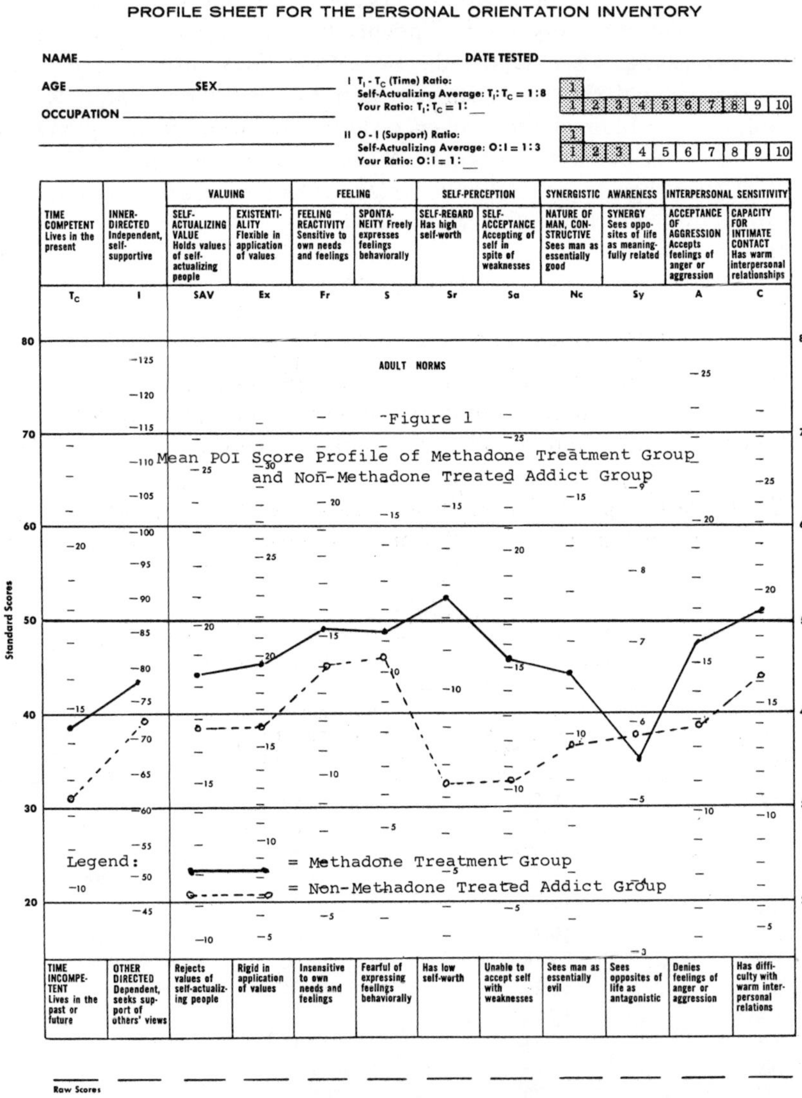

Fig. 1. Mean POI score profile of methadone treatment group and nonmethadone treated addict group. Reproduced with the permission of the Educational Testing Service, San Diego, California.

does the addict control group. It manifests a distinctly more elevated test profile than does the latter. The multivariate test of significance, considering the overall performance by both groups on *all* of the POI subscales, yields a F ratio of 4.97, the latter value denoting a statistically significant difference between the two groups ($p < .001$, $df = 14$ and 66). The univariate analysis of the 14 subscale scores, considered separately, registers significant differences between the two groups on five of those subscales. In comparison to the control group, the methadone sample scores significantly lower on *other-directedness*, but higher on *existentiality*, *self-regard*, *self-acceptance*, and *acceptance of natural aggressiveness*, respectively. Although the absolute magnitude of the test scores, actually achieved, is rather low (generally below T score values of 50), it would appear that the methadone treatment group manifests a generically higher level of maturational attainment than the addict control group: its lower level of other-directedness, but, more importantly, its greater tendency to behavioral flexibility, positive self-appreciation and self-regard, including tolerance of one's own native aggressiveness, suggests the prevalence of a significantly more favorable self-concept among the subjects of the methadone treatment group than among members of the control group.

Personality Profile Methadone Patient

Table 3 contains the mean POI subscale scores and the corresponding F ratios of the methadone treatment group differentiated by sex, race, and duration of methadone treatment.

The multivariate test of the three-way (sex × race × treatment) interaction as well as of all two-way (sex × race; sex × treatment; race × treatment) interactions between the independent variables, excluding main effects, failed to reach significance at $p < 0.05$. The parallel, but not independent, univariate F statistics for the 14 dependent variable measures, considered separately, also failed to reach significance, substantiating the lack of interaction *at any level* between the three design factors. As for main effects, the data in Table 3 indicate that neither sex or race nor duration of treatment registered sufficiently differential results to yield multivariate significance at $p < 0.05$. The corresponding univariate analyses, comparing all dependent variable scores separately, revealed that women methadone patients are significantly more sensitive emotionally than men patients (*FR-scale*) and that Black subjects may be significantly less flexible behaviorally than are their White counterparts (*EX-scale*). However, the latter results may be spurious in that the occur-

Table 3

Mean POI Scores and F Ratios of Methadone Patients Differentiated by Sex, Race, and Duration of Methadone Treatment

Shostrom POI scales	Methadone patients										
	Sex			Race			Duration of methadone treatment				
	Male ($N = 51$)	Female ($N = 19$)	F (univariate)	Black ($N = 40$)	White ($N = 30$)	F (univariate)	0–3 ($N = 33$) (1)	4–11 ($N = 12$) (2)	12 ($N = 35$) (3)	F (univariate) (1–2)	F (univariate) (2–3)
TI	7.90	8.47	0.42	8.10	8.00	0.006	8.39	8.50	7.69	0.32	0.65
TC	14.29	14.16	0.02	13.97	14.63	0.57	14.25	14.25	14.29	0.003	0.001
O	45.51	43.32	1.17	45.10	44.67	0.11	45.43	45.50	44.37	0.21	0.11
I	78.16	77.89	0.01	76.97	79.57	0.74	79.13	80.50	76.57	0.24	0.87
SAV	17.84	19.42	2.17	18.65	17.77	0.66	18.35	17.75	18.40	0.001	0.12
EX	19.06	19.21	0.01	18.00	20.27	5.40*	18.57	20.08	19.11	0.44	0.39
FR	14.71	16.37	4.33*	15.22	15.07	0.004	15.48	16.08	14.63	0.27	2.78
S	11.12	11.74	1.10	11.25	11.33	0.06	11.13	11.67	11.26	0.22	0.44
SR	13.22	11.00	0.91	11.65	13.90	1.02	11.96	10.75	13.69	0.16	1.23
SA	15.80	14.47	0.32	14.32	16.93	1.52	14.96	15.00	15.91	0.09	0.13
NC	11.57	10.32	0.36	10.42	12.30	0.93	10.30	10.25	12.17	0.44	0.63
SY	5.47	6.32	3.46	5.87	5.46	0.71	5.91	6.25	5.37	0.41	3.02
A	15.53	16.89	1.05	15.80	16.03	0.08	15.48	16.67	15.91	0.30	0.31
C	19.16	18.58	0.12	18.15	20.13	1.73	19.13	18.25	19.17	0.02	0.22
	Manova $F = 0.87$			Manova $F = 0.76$			Manova $F =$ (1–2) 0.57; Manova $F =$ (2–3) 1.77				

rence of two significant differences out of a total of 42 univariate comparisons is possible on the basis of statistical chance alone.

The findings, enumerated here, seem to suggest that no real differences in personality profile were found between male and female or between black and white addicts and, more importantly, that duration of methadone treatment does not result in significant modifications of addict self-perception: addicts who have been in methadone treatment for longer than 1 year do not assess themselves fundamentally differently than those with less rehabilitative exposure and experience.

Methadone Treatment and Psychotherapy or Counseling

Table 4 contains the mean POI-subscale scores and the corresponding *F* ratios of the methadone treatment group differentiated by psychotherapeutic or counseling service received. Approximately half of the sample subjects ($N = 36$) were on methadone maintenance only, but the remainder ($N = 34$) received some form of counseling in conjunction with their methadone treatment. The latter group included subjects who participated

Table 4
Mean POI Scores of Methadone Patients Differentiated by Psychotherapy or Counseling Received

Shostrom POI scales	Psychotherapy or Counseling: Yes	Psychotherapy or Counseling: No	*F* (univariate)
TI	7.36	8.79	3.62*
TC	15.28	13.18	6.78**
O	45.26	44.58	0.15
I	80.25	75.29	2.34
SAV	18.58	17.94	0.45
EX	19.69	18.47	1.20
FR	15.58	14.70	1.46
S	11.78	10.76	3.96*
SR	14.22	10.91	3.86†
SA	16.50	14.32	1.16
NC	12.39	10.00	1.74
SY	5.55	5.85	0.50
A	16.50	15.26	1.14
C	20.05	17.88	2.24
	Multivariate $F = 1.64$, $p < 0.09$.		

*Significant at $p < .05$.
**Significant at $p < .01$.
†$p < .06$.

in *group therapy* sessions at two-weekly intervals as well as a small number of subjects who had weekly *individual* counseling sessions.

The above data suggest that addicts who had been given some form of psychotherapeutic service obtained higher self-actualization scores than did the addict group who did not receive such service. However, the multivariate F ratio (1.64) indicates that the overall difference on all subscales combined is not significant ($p < .09$, 14 and 55 degrees of freedom). Univariately, three of the 14 subscales registered significant differences between the two groups of methadone patients: TI, TC, and S scales; a fourth subscale (SR) yielded a univariate F ratio of 3.86 with a p value that approaches significance ($p < .06$). These results suggest that the addict who did receive some form of counseling in addition to being the beneficiary of methadone maintenance is apt to have a significantly different personal time-perspective (TI, TC) and to manifest a significantly higher level of socioemotional spontaneity (S) and of self-worth (SR) than his noncounseled counterpart.

DISCUSSION

The preceding data appear to indicate (1) that the larger and most consistent differences in addict self-perception are those between addicts in methadone treatment and addicts receiving no such treatment, and (2) that methadone treatment per se does not effect significant changes in addict self-assessment over time. Only methadone maintenance in combination with psychotherapy or counseling seems to have the additive capacity of doing so.

The higher maturational level of the methadone treatment group, observed in this study, may best be interpreted in the light of its voluntary commitment to rehabilitation: addicts who freely submit to a drug rehabilitation program with such intrinsic constraints as continued abstinence from illegal drugs and with the espoused goal of making its patients ultimately drug-free must be necessarily more resourceful and self-esteeming than addicts who, at best, are willing to participate in group "raps," but without accepting further constraining or rehabilitative conditions. Thus the former group's commitment to drug rehabilitation, as evidenced by their participation in a methadone treatment program, may be seen as a function of its higher level of actual maturity. The contention that methadone maintenance is appealing to, and a viable option for, *all* illicit drug users seems not to be supported by the results of this study: a minimum level of preexistent maturational strength on the part of the addict may be an important self-selective variable among methadone maintenance patients.

The fact that methadone treatment does *not* alter addict self-assessment suggests that methadone maintenance, *in and by itself*, has no ego-enhancing impact upon its recipient: whatever benefits accrue to the patient, they do not seem to visibly alter his self-perception. Thus actual commitment to this form of drug rehabilitation or maintenance of the addictive condition through *legal* means and the consequent emancipation of the addict from illicit drugs and from the personal, social, judicial, and economic victimizations entailed in the latter does not seem to have the salutary psychological effect one would expect. The observation that the only consistent difference, noted within the methadone treatment group, was between those who had received some counseling and those who had not, indicates that only methadone maintenance in combination with psychotherapy or counseling has the cumulative capacity of effecting significant and positive changes in addict self-perception. The policy implication of this finding appears to be clear: effective treatment of the heroin addict requires that he be given the dual rehabilitative experience of being treated for both his addictive condition and for whatever personality problems he may carry with him into the treatment program.

Finally, it should be noted that the results obtained in this study were derived from rather small-sized samples. Consequently, they must be judged to be suggestive at best. Further and more extensive research will be required to establish the general validity of these findings.

SUMMARY

The present study was designed to assess some of the personality attributes of heroin addicts in a methadone maintenance program. The Shostrom Personal Orientation Inventory (POI) was administered to a randomly selected sample of 70 such addicts and to a control group of 11 nontreated heroin addicts. Multivariate and univariate comparisons of the two groups did indicate that the methadone group scored significantly higher in terms of level of maturational attainment and of self-actualization than did the control group. As for within-group differences in the methadone sample, no sex or race differences in personality scores were observed. It was also found that duration of methadone treatment is not significantly related to any change in addict self-perception over time. The only consistent difference noted was between methadone-treated addicts who did receive some form of psychotherapeutic counseling and those who did not. The former group was found to be significantly more expressive socioemotionally and self-esteeming than the latter. The study concludes with a discussion of the implications of the findings.

ACKNOWLEDGMENTS

The author wishes to express his indebtedness to Mrs. Judith Moscov, a graduate student, for her cooperation in the data-collecting phase of this study.

REFERENCES

BEWLEY, T.H. Some social, psychological, and environmental factors associated with drug dependence. *Health Educ. J.* 26: 60–66, 1967.

BOCK, R.D. Programming univariate and multivariate analysis of variance. *Technometrics* 5: 95–117, 1963.

COCKETT, R. *Drug abuse and personality in young offenders*. New York: Appleton, Century, Crofts, 1971.

FELIX, R.H. An appraisal of the personality types of the addict. *Amer. J. Psychiat.* 100: 462, 1944.

FINN, J. *Multivariance—Univariate and multivariate analysis of variance, covariance, and regression: A Fortran IV program*. Buffalo, New York: State University of New York at Buffalo, 1968.

GERARD, D.L., and KORNETSKY, C. Adolescent opiate addiction: Study of control and addict subjects. *Psychiat. Quart.* 29: 457–486, 1955.

GILBERT, J.G., and LOMBARDI, D.M. Personality characteristics of young male narcotic addicts. *J. Consult. Psychol.* 31: 536–538, 1967.

HALSTEAD, H., and NEAL, C.D. Intelligence and personality in drug addicts: A pilot study. *Brit. J. Addictions* 63: 237–240, 1968.

HEKIMIAN, L.J., and GERSHON, S. Characteristics of drug abusers admitted to a psychiatric hospital. *J. Amer. Med. Assoc.* 205: 125–130, 1968.

HILL, H.E., HAERTZEN, C.A., and DAVIS, H. An MMPI factor analytic study of alcoholics, narcotic addicts and criminals. *Quart. J. Studies Alc.* 23: 411–431, 1962.

HILL, H.E., HAERTZEN, C.A., and GLASER, R. Personality characteristics of narcotic addicts as indicated by the MMPI. *J. Gen. Psychol.* 62: 127–139, 1960.

HILL, H.E., HAERTZEN, C.A., and YAMAHIRO, R.S. The addict physician: An MMPI study of the interaction of personality characteristics and availability of narcotics. In *Association Research in Nervous and Mental Disease. The Addictive States*, Vol. 46. Baltimore: Williams and Wilkins, 1968.

KLECKNER, J.H. Personality differences between psychedelic drug users and non-users. *Psychology* 5: 66–71, 1968.

KNAPP, R.P. *The Measurement of Self-Actualization and Its Theoretical Implications.* San Diego, California: Educational and Industrial Testing Service, 1971.

KOLB, L. Types and characteristics of drug addicts. *Mental Hygiene London* 9: 300–313, 1925.

MONROE, J.J., ROSS, W.F., and BERZINS, J.I. The decline of the addict as "psychopath": Implications for community care. *Intern. J. Addictions* 6: 601–608, 1971.

PESCOR, M.J. The Kolb classification of drug addicts. *Public Health Rep. Suppl.* 155: 1–10, Washington, D.C.: Government Printing Office, 1939.

SHOSTROM, E.L. A test for the measurement of self actualization. *Educ. Psychol. Measur.* 24: 207–218, 1965.

SHOSTROM, E.L. *EITS Manual for the Personal Orientation Inventory.* San Diego, California: Educational and Industrial Testing Service, 1966.

The International Journal of the Addictions, 9(2), 267–287, 1974

Personality Traits and Attitudes and Their Relationship to Student Drug Using Behavior*

Joseph Powell Stokes, Ph.D.†

Department of Psychology
University of Illinois at Chicago Circle
Chicago, Illinois

Few issues in contemporary American life arouse more anxiety, fear, and irrationality than "student drug abuse." Opponents of drug use consider it self-indulgent and degenerate, a sign of psychological and moral weakness of American youth. The users and proponents of drug use, on the other hand, view psychedelic compounds as "mind expanders" which make life more meaningful and more enjoyable. There is little evidence to support either of these extreme views. What little evidence there is indicates one thing: the use of psychotropic drugs on college campuses is considerable. Whether this drug use per se creates a problem or whether the problem is created by the reactions of people to the drug use is a moot point. It has been said that the real problem is not the drug problem but

*This paper is based on a thesis submitted in partial fulfillment of the requirements for the degree of Doctor of Philosophy in Psychology in the Graduate College of the University of Illinois.

†Requests of reprints or information should be addressed to the author at Katharine Wright Psychiatric Clinic, 923 W. Wellington, Chicago, Illinois 60657.

the drug problem problem; that is, the real problem comes from the over-reaction of parents, administrators, and other community members to the drug use of students and the lack of communication and understanding which results from this reaction. Research designed to investigate the drug problem and the motivation of drug users can lead to a better understanding of the phenomenon and to more and better informed communication about this behavior.

Levy (1972) reviewed 22 published surveys of undergraduate and graduate student drug use. The oldest survey reviewed appeared in 1965, indicating that concern over student drug use is of rather recent origin. The many surveys which have been reported are not comparable because of differences in populations sampled, sampling techniques, response rates, etc., but in general they indicate that about 20 to 25% of undergraduate students have tried marijuana at least once and about 5 to 7% have some experience with other hallucinogens. Levy's own survey, which appears to be as good as any and better than most on methodological grounds, reveals much higher percentages. This might indicate that drug use among college students is increasing rapidly. Levy's 1971 survey found that 44.5% of the undergraduates at the University of Illinois at Chicago Circle and 54.6% at the University of Illinois at Urbana-Champaign have tried marijuana. In a survey conducted 3 years earlier at the Chicago Circle campus, Greenwald and Leutgert (1971) found that 24% of the undergraduates had some experience with hallucinogens (including marijuana). Levy's statistics for psychedelics such as LSD and mescaline (13.1% at Chicago and 16% at Urbana) are also among the highest ever reported.

In view of the tremendous amount of drug use on campus and in view of public concern over the growing use of illegal drugs, it is surprising to note the dearth of research on personality characteristics associated with drug use. Recently, however, some studies have investigated the differences in personality characteristics of students who use drugs not prescribed by physicians and those who do not partake of such drugs. Using the Cattell 16 PF personality inventory, Kleckner (1968) found that psychedelic drug users differed from nonsuers in that the former were brighter, more aloof, more anxious, more paranoid, more dominant, and had less ego and superego strength. Bottrill (1969) found that subjects who volunteered to take LSD scored higher on the hypochondriasis and paranoia scales of the MMPI than subjects who were not willing to take the LSD.

McGlothlin, Cohen, and McGlothlin (1967) recruited subjects for an experiment without telling the volunteers what the study would be. Of the 122 male graduate students qualifying as subjects (not prepsychotic, not in therapy), 25 refused to be in the experiment and 11 remained but were fearful when told that the experiment would involve taking LSD. The authors report that students who were against taking LSD were more extroverted, more organized, more conventional, and factual. Those in favor of taking LSD were more capable of regressive experience, more introverted, more spontaneous, more psychopathic, more bizarre, and more excitable.

Hogan, Mankin, Conway, and Fox (1970) administered the California Personality Inventory to students with varying degrees of experience with marijuana and found that users were more socially poised, open to experience, concerned with the feelings of others, impulsive, and rebellious. This description is based on the fact that users scored significantly higher than nonusers on the following scales: Capacity for Status, Social Presence, Flexibility, and Empathy. Nonusers scored higher than users on Responsibility, Socialization, Communality, and Achievement via Conformance.

Using the MMPI, McAree, Steffenhagan, and Zheutlin (1969) compared multiple drug users with marijuana only users and nondrug-using controls. The marijuana only group differed from the controls only on the Mf scale, but the multiple drug use group had significantly higher scores than the controls on Hy, Pd, Mf, Sc, Ma, and Si. Smart and Jones (1970) compared LSD users and nondrug-using controls and found that the former had higher scores on Hy, Pd, Mf, Sc, and Ma. These studies found that users of hallucinogens generally peak on the Pd and Ma scales of the MMPI and have profiles typical of character disorders rather than neurotic or psychotic personalities.

A massive study of student drug use by Richard Blum and associates (1969) included extensive psychological testing for a subsample of about 100 students specially chosen for their attitudes toward politics, religion, and drugs. A high rate of nonresponding (about 20%) makes it diffucult to draw any conclusions from this work, especially since, as Blum points out, most nonresponding was from the heaviest drug users. The Allport-Vernon Scale of Values revealed that illicit drug users (mostly marijuana and hallucinogens) place less emphasis on political and religious values and more emphasis on aesthetic values than nonusers. Nonusers were found to be more dogmatic on the Rokeach Dogmatism Scale. Users scored much higher than nonusers on the As Regressive Experience Scale, a measure of regressive-mystical experiences which is correlated with the ability to be hypnotized. Two subscales of the Myers-Briggs Type Indicator, a test derived from Jungian theory, successfully distinguish drug users from nonusers. On the sensing-vs-intuition subscale, drug users cluster toward the intuition end of the scale. On the judgment-vs-perception subscale, which measures liking for structure compared with spontaneity, significant differences are found with drug users showing a liking for spontaneity. The California Personality Inventory was administered to the subjects, but in this case nonresponding is a major problem since 33% of the drug users failed to complete the instrument. The only significant difference found nonusers scoring higher on Socialization. There were trends for nonusers to be more dominant, to score higher on Achievement via Conformance, and to score lower on Social Presence. These results are consistent with the findings of Hogan, Mankin, Conway, and Fox (1970) reported above, although the latter study found many more differences. This study was perhaps more sensitive than Blum's since it used more subjects and four, rather than two, levels of drug use.

Such research comparing personality characterisitcs of drug users and nonusers is interesting but is unlikely to lead to any real understanding of student drug use. Existing personality inventories are likely not adequate for investigating personality traits and attitudes that are predictive of drug use because drug use may be associated with attitudes or personality variables which cut across or correlate with several of the traditional categories or traits. Further, if one or a few constructs are related to drug use, it is likely that the constructs measured by existing personality inventories are not the ones most closely related to drug use. This study attempts to define constructs which are particularly relevant to drug use and to develop and validate an instrument to measure these personality traits and attitudes (hereafter factors). These constructs are based on popular concepts of the drug user and common sense explanations rather than analysis of traditional personality theory. The factors believed to be relevant to and predictive of drug use are as follows:

1. Hedonistic pleasure seeking. The author believes that too little attention has been paid to pleasure as a motive for drug use. This factor measures the degree to which a person is oriented toward pleasure and sensuality in general. People who score high on this hedonism scale would be people who have largely rejected the Puritan Ethic and who are highly oriented toward gratification of their desires. High scorers on this factor would be likely to use drugs.

2. Dissatisfaction with and a desire to change oneself. A popular conception (or misconception) about the student drug user is that he is unhappy with himself and turns to drugs to try to gain some insights into his own personality. The individual hopes drugs will provide him with a

better understanding of himself and will foster insight and creative growth. It is hypothesized that individuals who score high on this factor will likely be drug users. Blum and his associates (1969) obtained evidence to support this idea. They asked students if they had ever taken anything "to find out more about yourself" and found that students answering "yes" have had more experience in every drug class than those saying "no." The differences were particularly striking for marijuana (80% vs 12%) and for hallucinogens (34% vs 2%).

3. General tendency to use drugs. This factor measures the individual's general propensity to take drugs or to "pop pills." Presumably persons scoring high on this factor would be likely to use all kinds of drugs. Low scorers would avoid any drugs and would use very little medication of any kind. Blum and associates (1969, p. 97) found "a consistent trend for users of all drugs, whether social, medical, or illicit, to have had more experience with other psychoactive agents whether strong or mild." This finding supports the idea that there is a general tendency to use or not use drugs. Contradicting this idea that those who use one drug tend to use others also, some studies have found a negative relationship between use of alcohol and psychedelic drug use. Zinberg and Weil (1970) report that as marijuana use becomes regular for their subjects, alcohol use declines proportionally. Smart and Jones (1970), in comparing LSD users and nonusers, asked about alcohol use and found that twice as many nonusers of LSD as users drank alcohol as frequently as three times a week. Levy (1972), on the other hand, found a weak positive correlation among alcohol and marijuana use. Robbins, Robbins, Frosch, and Stern (1970) surveyed two colleges and found that in one alcohol consumption decreased as marijuana use increased while in the other no relationship was found. What little evidence there is, then, is not consistent. It may be that marijuana use substitutes for alcohol since, for some users at least, these drugs serve a similar social function. If this is the case, then marijuana and alcohol use would be negatively correlated for a particular individual across time but positively related across individuals at a given time period. In other words, one who has used alcohol or marijuana will tend to have used the other also, but not necessarily at the same time period in his life.

4. Fear of personal reaction to drugs. This factor taps how afraid one is of what will happen to him if he takes psychedelic drugs. It is predicted that the degree of this kind of fear is important in determining drug use habits. Individuals who score high on this factor will probably not use psychedelic drugs. Low scores are indicative of secure and self-controlled

individuals who feel invulnerable to adverse reactions from psychedelic drugs.

5. Respect for the illegality of psychedelic drug use. This factor purports to measure concern about the illegality of psychedelic drug use. High scorers on this factor will probably avoid psychedelic drugs at least in part because they are illegal. Low scorers would not be so concerned with the legality of the situation either because of lack of fear of getting caught or through active defiance of the law.

CONSTRUCTION AND VALIDATION OF THE INSTRUMENT

Statements were written or borrowed from existing instruments to represent each of the five hypothesized factors. A questionnaire was constructed by randomly ordering the 41 statements which define the five factors and asking subjects to respond to them with the following seven-point scale: disagree strongly, disagree mostly, disagree slightly, neutral—neither agree nor disagree, agree slightly, agree mostly, agree strongly. The questionnaire was administered to 738 subjects who volunteered for the experiment in order to fulfill a requirement for their introductory psychology course. These 738 subjects also responded to a questionnaire which asked about drug use habits.

One question about drug use was included to select out subjects who were answering dishonestly or carelessly. Subjects were asked about their use of "adrenochromes such as adrenolutin, carbazone or wagon wheels." Since it is not possible for a subject to have used this drug, subjects reporting any use of adrenochromes were eliminated from the study. Only one subject was eliminated for reporting that he used adrenochromes. This is encouraging in that it indicates that the reporting of drug use was honest.

To validate the factor structure, a principal components factor analysis with oblique rotation was chosen to factor analyze the 41 items. An oblique solution is appropriate since there is no reason to assume that the hypothesized factors will be uncorrelated with each other. Four of the five hypothesized factors appeared as predicted with dramatic clarity, but the hedonistic pleasure seeking factor did not appear. Instead, what originally had been considered one factor appears to have two interpretable components: one a philosophical kind of hedonism; the other a physical, sensual hedonism. The philosophical hedonism involves a rejection of the Protestant Ethic and an emphasis on independent thought and action at the expense of conventional expectations. The physical, sensual hedonism is more explicitly concerned with sensual, sexual pleasure.

As a check for concurrent validity for the factor dissatisfaction with and a desire to change oneself, a subset of 229 subjects was administered a self-description inventory devised by Dymond (1953) as a measure of self-concept. The instrument contains items which reflect good adjustment and items which indicate maladjustment. Subjects were asked to indicate for each item on the inventory whether the item is descriptive of themselves. This procedure yields a self-concept score for each subject as one point is scored for each well-adjusted item the subjects says is like himself and for each maladjusted item the subject says is not like himself. It was predicted that this score would correlate negatively with the factor being validated. The same subjects also responded to this instrument a second time under instructions to indicate for each item whether or not it is descriptive of how they would like to be. In other words, the subjects were asked to describe themselves as they would like to be. The number of items to which the subject responded differently under the two sets of instructions is a measure of self-concept–ideal self-concept discrepancy, with higher scores indicating greater discrepancy. As a further check on the validity of this factor, the same 229 subjects took the self-regard and the self-acceptance subscales of the Personality Orientation Inventory and the self-acceptance subscale of the California Personality Inventory.

Validation of a general tendency to use drugs was accomplished by seeing how well this factor predicts use of coffee and tea, tobacco, alcohol and nonprescription pain killers, stimulants, tranquilizers, and sedatives. All subjects responded to a questionnaire on drug use habits which included checks on frequency of use of these drugs as a validity check for this factor.

The factor respect for the illegality of psychedelic drug use purports to measure how concerned one is about the illegality of using psychedelic drugs. This factor was validated by asking 225 subjects to rank order reasons for not using drugs according to importance. Subjects who score high on the factor respect for the illegality of psychedelic drug use should rank the illegality of using marijuana as a more important reason than subjects who score low on this factor.

In every case these validation attempts yielded encouraging and statistically significant results. The factors appeared as predicted with the exception that the hedonistic pleasure seeking factor has two components: one physical or sensual, the other philosophical. Readers interested in

Table 1

The Six Factors and the Items which Load Most Heavily on Them

Factor I: Fear of personal reaction to drugs

I would be afraid of losing personal control under drugs.

I am afraid that drugs might cause me to say or do things I would later regret.

Even though a drug might not be physically habit-forming, I would be afraid of becoming dependent on it psychologically.

I would be suspicious of anyone who urged me to take a drug without a prescription.

I am afraid that psychedelic drugs might cause permanent changes in my personality.

I would be afraid for my younger brother or sister to try psychedelic drugs.

The use of psychedelic drugs often leads to serious mental health disorders.

I would take a drug which I did not need just to enjoy its pleasurable effects. (Loads negatively.)

I would be worried if I had to take a drug whose effects I knew little about.

Even if science proved that psychedelic drugs were in no way harmful, I would not use them until they were legal.

I get very afraid if I don't know what is happening to me.

I would never take any drug which requires a prescription except under the supervision of a doctor.

I would probably take psychedelic drugs if they were legal. (Loads negatively.)

Factor II: Dissatisfaction with and a desire to change oneself

Sometimes I think I am all mixed-up inside.

I wish I could get some help to achieve the "real" me.

I cannot seem to make up my mind as to what I really believe.

There are a lot of things about me I would like to change.

I would like to go through psychotherapy to find out more about myself.

I feel that I would be a much better person if I could gain more understanding of myself.

I sometimes wish I were someone else.

I sometimes question my motives for doing things.

Factor III: Respect for the illegality of psychedelic drug use

I am in favor of a very strict enforcement of all laws, no matter what the consequences.

It is never all right to break the law even if no one is hurt by it.

A person should be punished for breaking a law even if he thinks it is unreasonable.

Disobedience to any government is never justified.

Factor IV: Sensual hedonism

I would enjoy participating in an orgy with lots of food, drink, and sex.

I would enjoy going to a nude body painting party with my friends of both sexes.

I like to become sexually excited.

I would enjoy bathing in a tub filled with warm whipped cream.

I often sleep nude.

(*continued*)

Table 1 *(continued)*

Factor V: Philosophical hedonism
- I like to do what I please even if people I respect might consider it unconventional.
- I am more interested in being happy and enjoying myself than in being economically successful.
- I like to become sexually excited.
- I like to be able to come and go as I want to.
- People should spend more of their leisure time just enjoying themselves instead of trying to do something constructive.

Factor VI: General tendency to use drugs
- Sometimes I feel I have to take something to make me relax.
- If there were a drug which would make me feel less anxious, I would take it.
- Sometimes I feel I have to take something to stimulate me.
- I would take a drug which I did not need just to enjoy its pleasurable effects.
- When I do not feel good, I usually take something to make me feel better, even if it is only an aspirin.
- I would probably take psychedelic drugs if they were legal.
- I would never take any drug which requires a prescription except under the supervision of a doctor. (Loads negatively.)

obtaining a more detailed account of the validation efforts and their results are invited to write the author.

The six factors and the items which load most heavily on each one are presented in Table 1. Each subject was given a factor score for each factor. Each subject's response to each of the 41 items was converted to a standard score and multiplied by the factor score coefficient for that item for that factor. The sum of the weighted responses to each item, then, is the factor score.

THE FACTORS AND DRUG USE

The factors developed in this study were chosen because they had face validity in relation to drug using behavior. Tables 2 to 7 present data which depict the relationships of the six factors and drug use for the sample in this study. Chi-square statistics and Spearman Rank Order Correlations are presented. Response categories for the drug use questions have been collapsed where necessary to avoid unacceptably low expected values for cells in the contingency tables.

As can be seen from Table 2, Factor I (fear of personal reaction to drugs) is strongly and negatively related to use of tobacco, alcohol, marijuana, hallucinogens, and the prescription drugs (amphetamines, barbiturates, and tranquilizers). There are weaker relationships with nonprescrip-

Table 2
Relationship of Factor I (Fear of Personal Reaction to Drugs) and Drug Use

Drug	χ^2	*df*	*p*	*R*	*N*	*p*
Coffee and tea	11.91	20	n.s.	−.0458	735	n.s.
Tobacco	64.71	20	<.001	−.2614	737	<.001
Nonprescription pain killers	14.83	15	n.s.	−.0291	736	n.s.
Nonprescription sedatives	15.46	5	<.01	−.0833	736	<.05
Nonprescription tranquilizers	3.20	5	n.s.	.0031	737	n.s.
Nonprescription stimulants	15.72	5	<.01	−.1220	737	<.001
Alcohol	76.87	20	<.001	−.2868	737	<.001
Marijuana	339.13	25	<.001	−.5869	737	<.001
Hallucinogens	332.70	15	<.001	−.5529	737	<.001
Amphetamines	159.17	5	<.001	−.3947	736	<.001
Barbiturates	65.83	5	<.001	−.2553	737	<.001
Tranquilizers	39.61	5	<.001	−.1821	737	<.001

tion sedatives and stimulants, and no relationships with nonprescription pain killers, tranquilizers, and coffee and tea. It appears that fear is an important factor in determining drug using behavior, particularly for drugs about which very little is known (marijuana and hallucinogens) and for drugs whose adverse effects have been well publicized by the media (marijuana, hallucinogens, tobacco, alcohol and, to a lesser extent, amphetamines and barbiturates). It is interesting that fear of personal reaction seems to be influential in determining usage patterns for nonprescription stimulants (caffeine compounds) but not for coffee and tea. These latter drugs are so widely used and accepted that drinking coffee is viewed very differently from taking a caffeine pill. It is likely that smoking tobacco enjoyed this "nondrug" status until publicity about its adverse effects became widespread.

Factor II (dissatisfaction with and a desire to change oneself) is related to drug use but the relationships are the weakest of any of the factors (see Table 3). In every case, however, as one scores higher on Factor II, the probability of his using any of the drugs increases, even though the relationship is in no case a strong one. It would seem that the hypothesis that student drug users have turned to drugs to try to change themselves and to achieve a new or altered being is not strongly supported. This is not to say, of course, that a particular person would not experiment with

Table 3
Relationship of Factor II (Dissatisfaction with and a Desire to Change Oneself) and Drug Use

Drug	χ^2	*df*	*p*	*R*	*N*	*p*
Coffee and tea	32.48	20	<.05	.0935	735	<.01
Tobacco	21.69	20	n.s.	.0520	737	n.s.
Nonprescription pain killers	25.64	15	<.05	.1546	736	<.001
Nonprescription sedatives	12.87	5	<.05	.1067	736	<.01
Nonprescription tranquilizers	19.36	5	<.01	.1552	737	<.001
Nonprescription stimulants	2.86	5	n.s.	.644	737	<.05
Alcohol	42.90	20	<.01	.0723	737	<.05
Marijuana	37.21	25	n.s.	.1274	737	<.001
Hallucinogens	20.05	15	n.s.	.1177	737	<.001
Amphetamines	13.91	5	<.05	.1053	736	<.01
Barbiturates	13.47	5	<.05	.0861	737	<.05
Tranquilizers	10.82	5	n.s.	.0915	737	<.01

or abuse drugs in response to being unhappy or dissatisfied with himself. In general, however, this does not seem to be a major reason to account for student drug use.

Factor III (respect for the illegality of psychedelic drug use) is strongly related to marijuana and hallucinogen use, such that those with the strongest respect for the legality of the situation are less likely to be users (see Table 4). This factor also relates to use of the prescription drugs, a fact which is easily understood when one realizes that most students using these drugs are obtaining and using them illegally. It would seem that this factor would be irrelevant to use of legal drugs. This is true in the case of the nonprescription pain killers, sedatives, tranquilizers, and stimulants, and of coffee and tea, but high scorers on Factor III are not likely to use tobacco and alcohol. It could be that a general conservative, rigid personality pattern is being reflected. It seems likely that a family that emphasizes respect for the law to its children might tend to be a family that would discourage use of tobacco and alcohol. Such a family would likely produce children who would have great respect for the illegality of psychedelic drug use and who would not likely use alcohol or tobacco.

The sensual hedonism factor (Factor IV) follows the pattern of Factor III in that it is related to use of tobacco, alcohol, marijuana, hallucinogens, and the prescription drugs but not to coffee and tea and the nonprescription

Table 4
Relationship of Factor III (Respect for Illegality of Psychedelic Drug Use) and Drug Use

Drug	χ^2	*df*	*p*	*R*	*N*	*p*
Coffee and tea	23.09	20	n.s.	−.0642	735	<.05
Tobacco	54.96	20	<.001	−.1846	737	<.001
Nonprescription pain killers	19.63	15	n.s.	.0083	736	n.s.
Nonprescription sedatives	7.18	5	n.s.	−.0434	736	n.s.
Nonprescription tranquilizers	4.11	5	n.s.	−.0601	737	n.s.
Nonprescription stimulants	7.79	5	n.s.	−.0730	737	<.05
Alcohol	37.26	20	<.05	−.1417	737	<.001
Marijuana	178.90	25	<.001	−.4645	737	<.001
Hallucinogens	154.47	15	<.001	−.4114	737	<.001
Amphetamines	96.30	5	<.001	−.3435	736	<.001
Barbiturates	42.76	5	<.001	−.2236	737	<.001
Tranquilizers	23.56	5	<.001	−.1478	737	<.001

Table 5
Relationship of Factor IV (Sensual Hedonism) and Drug Use

Drug	χ^2	*df*	*p*	*R*	*N*	*p*
Coffee and tea	22.02	20	n.s.	.0498	735	n.s.
Tobacco	32.31	20	<.05	.1249	737	<.001
Nonprescription pain killers	16.01	15	n.s.	−.0238	736	n.s.
Nonprescription sedatives	5.58	5	n.s.	−.0030	736	n.s.
Nonprescription tranquilizers	4.60	5	n.s.	−.0725	737	<.05
Nonprescription stimulants	8.22	5	n.s.	.0787	737	<.05
Alcohol	110.28	20	<.001	.3270	737	<.001
Marijuana	171.93	25	<.001	.4317	737	<.001
Hallucinogens	89.25	15	<.001	.3133	737	<.001
Amphetamines	34.86	5	<.001	.1966	736	<.001
Barbiturates	12.33	5	<.05	.1180	737	<.001
Tranquilizers	16.21	5	<.01	.1124	737	<.001

Table 6
Relationship of Factor V (Philosophical Hedonism) and Drug Use

Drug	χ^2	*df*	*p*	*R*	*N*	*p*
Coffee and tea	19.94	20	n.s.	.0495	735	n.s.
Tobacco	31.42	20	<.05	.1631	737	<.001
Nonprescription pain killers	26.64	15	<.05	.0555	736	n.s.
Nonprescription sedatives	4.00	5	n.s.	.0177	736	n.s.
Nonprescription tranquilizers	6.36	5	n.s.	−.0079	737	n.s.
Nonprescription stimulants	4.80	5	n.s.	.0704	737	<.05
Alcohol	49.43	20	<.001	.1932	737	<.001
Marijuana	105.23	25	<.001	.3381	737	<.001
Hallucinogens	60.43	15	<.001	.2499	737	<.001
Amphetamines	25.90	5	<.001	.1574	736	<.001
Barbiturates	3.37	5	n.s.	.0625	737	<.05
Tranquilizers	5.83	5	n.s.	.0787	737	<.05

drugs (see Table 5). Of course, any of the drugs in this survey can be taken to attain a pleasurable state or alleviate an unpleasant one, but alcohol, marijuana, and hallucinogens are used exclusively for this purpose. It is not surprising, therefore, that these three drugs relate most strongly to the sensual hedonism factor.

Table 6 shows that for Factor V (philosophical hedonism) use of marijuana, hallucinogens, and alcohol once again are most closely related to factor scores. Of the prescription drugs, however, only amphetamine use is highly related to scores on Factor V.

Factor VI is a very good predictor of use of nonprescription, legal drugs. Only in the case of coffee and tea is the relationship boarderline. If one considers only the subjects who report drinking more than 12 cups of coffee of tea per week, 58% of these subjects scored above the median on Factor VI. If one considers only the heavy coffee and tea drinkers (more than 25 cups per week), the figure is 73%. For tobacco smokers, 63% of those who smoke at all and 68% of those who smoke more than a pack a day are above the median for Factor VI. For users of nonprescription pain killers, the corresponding figures are 70% (considering subjects who use these pain killers twice a month or more) and 88% (considering only those who use pain killers twice a week or more). The percentages of users of nonprescription sedatives, tranquilizers, and stimulants who are above the median on Factor VI are 84, 81, and 73%, respectively. Of the subjects

Table 7
Relationship of Factor VI (General Tendency to Use Drugs) and Drug Use

Drug	χ^2	*df*	*p*	*R*	*N*	*p*
Coffee and tea	34.63	20	<.05	.1270	735	<.001
Tobacco	83.85	20	<.001	.2854	737	<.001
Nonprescription pain killers	120.74	15	<.001	.3539	736	<.001
Nonprescription sedatives	30.29	5	<.001	.2085	736	<.001
Nonprescription tranquilizers	52.57	5	<.001	.2216	737	<.001
Nonprescription stimulants	64.75	5	<.001	.2722	737	<.001
Alcohol	118.06	20	<.001	.3555	737	<.001
Marijuana	193.71	25	<.001	.4654	737	<.001
Hallucinogens	178.45	15	<.001	.4441	737	<.001
Amphetamines	120.05	5	<.001	.3505	736	<.001
Barbiturates	66.03	5	<.001	.2526	737	<.001
Tranquilizers	55.49	5	<.001	.2602	737	<.001

who use alcohol once a week or more, 65% are above the median on Factor VI, while the figure is 74% for those who drink three times a week or more. These figures support the idea that there is an overall drug using personality trait or attitude and that Factor VI measures it. Table 7 confirms that this factor is also highly related to the use of illegal and prescription drugs.

Factor Scores for Selected Groups of Subjects

A second way to explore the relationships of the factors and drug use is to select subjects with a particular drug use pattern and examine their scores on the factors. For example, one could look at the nonusers of marijuana and compare their mean factor scores with the mean scores of the sample as a whole. The comparisons were made by treating the sample in this study as a population and comparing the mean of this population and the mean of a particular sample with the *Z* statistic. The standard error depends on the standard deviation of the population for the factor in question and on the size of the sample being compared to the population. Table 8 presents the *Z* scores obtained by comparing the means for the six factors of several groups of drug users and nonusers with the population means.

The principled nonusers of marijuana (subjects who have not and will not use marijuana) are extremely high on fear of personal reaction to drugs

Table 8

Z Scores Comparing Means of Subsamples with the Whole Sample Mean

Subject sample	N	Factor I $\bar{x} = 0.008$ SD = 0.897		Factor II $\bar{x} = 0.002$ SD = 0.650		Factor III $\bar{x} = 0.010$ SD = 0.853		Factor IV $\bar{x} = -0.002$ SD = 0.860		Factor V $\bar{x} = 0.009$ SD = 0.755		Factor VI $\bar{x} = 0.017$ SD = 0.852	
Entire sample	737	$\bar{x}$	Z	$\bar{x}$	Z	$\bar{x}$	Z	$\bar{x}$	Z	$\bar{x}$	Z	$\bar{x}$	Z
Principles nonusers of marijuana	317	0.508	9.921	−0.103	−2.877	0.414	8.434	−0.406	−8.364	−0.294	−6.722	−0.386	−8.413
Nonprincipled nonusers of marijuana	91	0.125	1.245	0.184	2.673	−0.074	−0.940	0.231	2.583	0.152	2.035	0.107	1.008
Former marijuana users who have quit	52	−0.030	−0.306	−0.043	−0.499	0.016	0.051	0.053	0.462	0.134	1.362	−0.016	−0.280
Users of marijuana who smoke more when alone	25	−0.812	−4.581	−0.168	−1.308	−0.411	−2.462	0.265	1.552	−0.048	−0.258	0.548	3.124
Heavy users of marijuana (several times/ week)	33	−1.293	−8.237	0.297	2.611	−0.920	−6.284	0.791	5.287	0.264	2.084	1.115	7.419
Principled nonusers of hallucinogens	564	0.296	7.619	−0.039	−1.496	0.194	5.125	−0.146	−3.978	−0.105	−3.019	−0.200	−6.045
Nonprincipled nonusers of hallucinogens	71	−0.657	−6.274	0.121	1.543	−0.376	−3.822	0.352	3.471	0.245	2.835	0.597	5.743
Heavy users of hallucinogens (five times +)	24	−1.657	−9.098	0.118	0.872	−0.968	−5.621	0.798	4.545	0.451	2.987	1.047	5.920
Alcohol nonusers	104	0.374	4.159	−0.192	−3.046	0.233	2.667	−0.505	−5.967	−0.364	−4.797	−0.467	−5.796
Heavy users of alcohol (three times/week or more)	61	−0.578	−5.096	0.051	0.589	−0.291	−2.761	0.484	4.418	0.137	1.510	0.552	4.908

and respect for the illegality of psychedelic drug use. They are very low on sensual and philosophical hedonism and on general tendency to use drugs. They are also significantly lower than the sample as a whole on dissatisfaction with and a desire to change oneself, but the mean difference is lower than for the other factors. As has been seen before, Factor II (dissatisfaction with and a desire to change oneself) is less powerfully related to drug use than the other factors. The nonprincipled nonusers (those who have never used marijuana but might in the future) tend to score in the opposite direction from principled nonusers on all factors except fear of personal reaction to drugs. On this factor the nonprincipled nonusers are not different from the sample as a whole. For the factors dealing with dissatisfaction with self and sensual and philosophical hedonism (Factors II, IV, and V), the nonprincipled nonusers are significantly different from the total sample in the opposite direction from the principled nonusers. The pattern of the factor scores for the nonprincipled nonusers looks much like the pattern for the heavy users, although the scores are less extreme. It seems that the nonprincipled nonusers will likely be users in the near future. Heavy users of marijuana have extreme scores on each factor, and in each case their score is in the opposite direction from the principled nonusers. The heavy user of marijuana has very low fear of personal reaction to drugs and very little respect for the illegality of psychedelic drug use. He is extremely high on the sensual hedonism and general tendency to use drugs factors and significantly higher than the sample as a whole on philosophical hedonism and dissatisfaction with and a desire to change oneself.

Those subjects who report that they have used marijuana but will probably never use it again do not differ from the sample as a whole on any of the factors. Important information as to the composition of this subsample was not obtained. This group is probably composed of at least two types: (1) people who at one time used a lot of drugs but no longer do, and (2) people who tried marijuana once or twice but never really used it with any frequency. Lack of information about these subjects makes speculation about the data they produced difficult.

A small group of marijuana smokers report smoking more by themselves than with others. This group of subjects is low on fear of personal reactions to drugs and respect for the illegality of psychedelic drug use. They are high on the general tendency to use drugs and not significantly different from the sample as a whole on the other factors. In short, their factor scores look like the scores of drug users but show no peculiarities.

The pattern for users and nonusers of hallucinogens is much like that for marijuana. The principled nonusers of hallucinogens are significantly higher than the whole sample on fear of personal reaction to drugs and respect for the illegality of psychedelic drug use. They are significantly lower on sensual and philosophical hedonism and on the general tendency to use drugs. All these factors are significantly different from the whole sample in the opposite direction for both heavy users of hallucinogens and for nonprincipled nonusers of hallucinogens. Again the nonprincipled nonusers have profiles which look like those of the heavy users but are less extreme. Neither the principled or nonprincipled nonusers nor the heavy users differ from the whole sample on Factor II (dissatisfaction with and a desire to change oneself).

Nonusers of alcohol are significantly different from the sample as a whole on all six factors, in each case in the direction which is characteristic of low drug use. The heavy users of alcohol are significantly low on fear of personal reaction to drugs and respect for the illegality of psychedelic drug use. This group is significantly higher than the sample as a whole on sensual hedonism and the general tendency to use drugs but not different from the whole sample on dissatisfaction with and a desire to change and philosophical hedonism.

Self-Concept, Self-Acceptance, and Anxiety Scores for Selected Groups of Subjects

The mean scores for the selected groups of drug users mentioned in the previous section on the measures of self-concept, self-acceptance, and anxiety were examined and compared with the mean scores for the whole sample. None of the subsample group means differed significantly from the whole sample mean on any of these measures, except that heavy alcohol and heavy hallucinogen users have lower mean ideal self-concept scores than the sample as a whole ($Z = -4.790$ for heavy alcohol users and $Z = -2.666$ for heavy hallucinogen users). The self-concept scores for these groups are almost identical to those for the whole sample. These two groups of heavy drug users have ideal self-concepts which are somewhat less well adjusted according to traditional definitions of adjustment than the ideal self-concepts of the sample as a whole.

Predicting Drug Use from Factor Scores

Instead of looking at the relationships of each individual factor with each drug, it might be interesting to try to predict drug use from all the factors simultaneously. A regression analysis was performed for each drug, using the scores for the six factors as predictors and each drug sur-

Table 9
Predicting Drug Use from Factor Scores

Drug	Multiple R of six factors with drug use	F for predictable component from regression	df	p
Coffee and tea	.160	3.155	6,721	$<.001$
Tobacco	.349	16.716	6,721	$<.001$
Nonprescription pain killers	.410	24.340	6,721	$<.001$
Nonprescription sedatives	.254	8.263	6,721	$<.001$
Nonprescription tranquilizers	.291	11.125	6,721	$<.001$
Nonprescription stimulants	.309	15.294	6,721	$<.001$
Alcohol	.451	36.949	6,721	$<.001$
Marijuana	.726	134.173	6,721	$<.001$
Hallucinogens	.669	97.414	6,721	$<.001$
Amphetamines	.476	35.175	6,721	$<.001$
Barbiturates	.318	13.485	6,721	$<.001$
Tranquilizers	.311	12.840	6,721	$<.001$

veyed as a criterion variable. The results shown in Table 9 include the multiple correlation of the six factor scores with drug use as well as a test of significance for the component of drug use predictable from the factors. In all cases the results are significant, but the size of the predictable component varies from quite small in the case of coffee and tea to rather substantial for marijuana and hallucinogens.

The Beta weights for the factor scores which best predict marijuana use are shown in Table 10. This weighted combination of factor scores yields a prediction score for marijuana use for each subject. A crude median split on this predictor correctly classifies 76.2% of the subjects as to whether they have or have not used marijuana. The miss rate (subjects who have smoked marijuana but who score below the median on the predictor variable) is just over 9%, but over 95% of the "misses" are subjects who once used marijuana but do not now use it or who have used it less than

Table 10
Beta Weights for Predicting Marijuana Use from Factors

Factor	I	II	III	IV	V	VI
Beta weights	−.34369	−.02753	−.18447	.15867	.08787	.29138

10 times or who use it no more than once or twice a month. Of the 72 subjects who report using marijuana once a week or more, only three scored below the median for the predictor variable.

The false alarm rate for prediction of marijuana use (subjects who score above the median on the predictor variable but have not used marijuana) is 14.7%. Of these "false alarms," 48% indicate that they might use marijuana in the future while 52% are principled nonusers. This is interesting since for the whole sample the ratio of principled nonusers of marijuana to nonprincipled nonusers is over three to one.

CONCLUSIONS

The relative magnitudes of the Beta weights for the six factors for predicting marijuana use confirms what the data have suggested previously: fear of personal reaction to drugs and the general tendency to use drugs are the most important factors for predicting drug use. The factors which predict drug use so powerfully could not be validated by concurrent testing because no measures exist which tap these concepts. Existing personality and attitude measures simply are not so sensitive to drug using behavior as an instrument designed with that specific behavior in mind.

The reasons given by subjects for not using marijuana confirm the idea that fear of personal reaction to drugs and the general tendency to use drugs are important factors in determining drug use. The most important reasons for not using marijuana were a general dislike for using any kind of drug or chemical agent and a fear that the drug would become a psychological crutch. These reasons parallel the two factors which are most powerfully related to drug use. Lack of access to marijuana or the illegal status of marijuana use were seldom given as important reasons for not using the drug.

A person's position on the factors which are most closely related to drug using behavior are probably determined largely by the attitudes of his family and peers toward drugs and drug use. A child reared in a home where drugs are casually and frequently dispensed is likely to have little fear of his personal reaction to drugs and will likely use all kinds of drugs frequently. Of course, it is possible that one could be made to fear his personal reaction to a particular drug, and the media have attempted to do that, particularly with respect to amphetamines and hallucinogens. Some attempts have been made to discourage use of marijuana by trying to increase one's fear of his personal reaction to the drug, but these attempts have been countered by official reports (such as by the President's

Commission) which fail to find any psychological or physiological damage resulting from marijuana use and by the personal reports of marijuana users who are often enthusiastically in favor of its use. It seems that the typical college student draws a distinction between marijuana-type drugs and other drugs which can be obtained and injested illegally. This distinction, which is probably a realistic and useful one, is reflected in the frequency with which various illegal drugs are used by students in this study.

It is encouraging to the author that the factor dissatisfaction with and a desire to change oneself is related very weakly to drug use. The typical student drug user is not turning to drugs out of despair or in order to try to alter himself. A particular person might turn to drugs in response to depression or personal dissatisfaction, but this does not appear to account for the bulk of student drug use. It would be interesting to select students who initially encountered illegal drug use in an attempt to change or run away from themselves or an unpleasant situation and follow their drug using careers. It seems likely that these students would be more likely to have "drug problems" than drug users whose initial use was motivated by curiousity and pleasure seeking. Studies designed to discover and study drug using situations which lead to dependency and other undesirable situations are needed, for it seems that extensive use of psychotropic drugs will continue to be characteristic of our society. It would seem that drug use, especially for marijuana-type drugs, will continue to increase. As more and more people use drugs and find their experience with drugs to be pleasant, fear of personal reaction to drugs will decrease and drug use will rise. That people will find their drug experiences to be pleasant is, of course, an assumption, but the rise of marijuana use in the past decade lends support to this assumption for this drug. Further, increased use of legal prescription and nonprescription drugs of the past decade are reflections of an increased general tendency to use drugs. The large sums of money which are being spent to promote nonprescription pain killers, sedatives, stimulants, and tranquilizers contribute to this increased drug using tendency. It would seem that drug use at all levels is here to stay, and a campaign aimed at eliminating social, nonmedicinal drug use is foolish and unrealistic. It is the responsibility of the behavioral sciences to try to understand this drug use and to try to define and to control the variables which differentiate drug use and drug problems.

A word of caution about the use of the instrument developed in this paper would seem to be in order. All the data reported in this paper which were used to develop and validate this instrument were collected anonymously and in groups large enough so that subjects could be sure that no one would know how they responded. Under these conditions the factors reported predict drug use rather well, but any attempt to use this instrument to predict drug use without guaranteeing anonymity to the respondents would be misguided. It is reasonable to assume that this instrument is fakable and that it will not be useful for predicting drug use when the respondents are identifiable.

REFERENCES

BLUM, R.H., and Associates. *Students and Drugs*. San Francisco: Jossey-Bass, 1969.

BOTTRILL, J.H. Personality change in LSD users. *J. Gen. Psychol.* 80: 157–161, 1969.

DYMOND, R.F. An adjustment score for Q sorts. *J. Consult. Psychol.* 17: 339–342, 1953.

GREENWALD, B.S., and LEUTGERT, M.J. A comparison of drug users and non-users on an urban commuter college campus. *Intern. J. Addictions* 6: 63–78, 1971.

HOGAN, R., MANKIN, D., CONWAY, J., and FOX, S. Personality correlates of undergraduate marijuana use. *J. Consult. Clin. Psychol.* 35: 58–63, 1970.

KLECKNER, J.H. An investigation into the personal characteristics and family background of psychedelic drug users. *Psychology*, 5: 66–71, 1968.

LEVY, L. *Drug Use on Campus*. Unpublished research report, 1972.

McAREE, C.P., STEFFENHAGAN, R.A., and ZHEUTLIN, L.S. Personality factors in college drug users. *Intern. J. Social Psychiat.* 5: 102–106, 1969.

McGLOTHLIN, W.H., COHEN, S., and McGLOTHLIN, M.S. Personality and attitude changes in volunteer subjects following repeated administration of LSD. Paper presented before the Fifth International Congress, Colligium Neuropsychopharmacologicum, March 1967.

ROBBINS, E.S., ROBBINS, L., FORSCH, W.A., and STERN, M. College student drug use. *Amer. J. Psychiat.* 126: 1743–1751, 1970.

SMART, R.G., and JONES, D. Illicit LSD users: Their personality characteristics and psychopathology. *J. Abnormal Psychol.* 75: 286–292, 1970.

ZINBERG, N.E., and WEIL, A.T. A comparison of marijuana users and non-users. *Nature*, 226: 119–123, 1970.

The International Journal of the Addictions, 9(2), 289–300, 1974

Patterns of Drug Abuse

Richard S. Campbell, Ph.D.

Jeffrey B. Freeland, M.A.

Clinical Research Center
Social Science Section
NIMH
Lexington, Kentucky

Abstract

A great deal of interest and debate has focused on the tendency of drug abusers to progress from one drug to another (e.g., the relationship between marijuana and heroin abuse). This paper presents methods and results from three types of analysis: (1) correlation between pairs of drugs, without regard for order of abuse; (2) measurement of the order in which pairs of drugs are abused; and (3) determination of what holistic patterns or sequences of drugs tend to be followed. Results indicate that patterns of abuse are not random, and that distinctions should be made between drugs on nonpharmacological grounds. The suggestion is made that the pattern of abuse may be useful in generating typologies of drug abusers.

INTRODUCTION

A great deal has been said and written in both the lay and professional press about progressive drug abuse, i.e., the tendency for abusers of one drug to have a history of the abuse of other drugs. Much of the recent debate about the legalization of marijuana, for example, has centered on the question of a progressive relationship between marijuana use and heroin addiction.

Earlier studies regarding sequences of drug abuse usually focused on particular pairs of drugs in isolation. Even the more comprehensive recent approaches have been limited to focusing on one drug and examining other drugs associated with it, rather than analyzing the holistic interrelationships between abused drugs (e.g., Weppner and Agar, 1971; Whitehead et al., 1972; Goode, 1969). In order to understand the significance and implications of multiple drug abuse sequences it is necessary to adopt a methodology that is not context limited, i.e., a way of analyzing all significant drugs of abuse and their interrelationships for all subjects in a sample. It is also useful if the method is easily replicable. Toward these ends, the major purposes of this research are threefold:

1. To present a reliable method of describing the sequential abuse of drugs in a more holistic context.
2. To determine whether sequences of drug abuse from significant patterns.
3. To point to applications of the methods described here to research problems in the field of drug abuse.

THE SAMPLE AND SOURCE DATA

The sample for this study consists of 3,583 narcotic addicts admitted to the NIMH Clinical Research Center, Lexington, Kentucky during the period from May 1969 through April 1971. Of these cases, 3,549 were selected for analysis, 34 being rejected for reasons of incomplete information or other errors. The mean age of respondents was 26.9 years, and the mean education 10.6 years. Seventy-two percent reported having had experience in "blue collar" occupations.

After withdrawal, each individual was interviewed using the Lexington Social Data Form, a schedule for collecting demographic, social, and drug-related information. The drug history section includes a list of 102 psychoactive drugs divided into 10 classes: narcotic analgesics, sedative-hypnotics, tranquilizers, antidepressants, stimulants, psychotogens, antihistamines, inhalants, marijuana, and alcohol.

Each subject is asked which drugs in each of the classes he has used and which ones he has seriously abused or been dependent upon. The

Table 1
Demographic and Social Characteristics of Sample (N = *3583*)

	White ($N = 1327$)		Minority ($N = 2256$)	
	M ($N = 1008$)	F ($N = 319$)	M ($N = 1861$)	F ($N = 395$)
Mean age at admission	26.2	26.0	27.4	27.2
Mean age at first arrest (for those arrested	17.3 ($N = 926$)	18.7 ($N = 257$)	17.0 ($N = 1728$)	18 5 ($N = 344$)
Mean age at first narcotics use	18.9 ($N = 985$)	19.4 ($N = 307$)	19.0 ($N = 1860$)	19.9 ($N = 394$)
Mean time served (no. months)	16.9 ($N = 1006$)	9.3 ($N = 319$)	26.0 ($N = 1853$)	17.1 ($N = 390$)
Mean no. years education	11.0	10.9	10.5	10.0
Occupation:				
Administrative, etc.	7.9%	3.7%	1.8%	0.8%
Clerical and skilled	41.7%	47.0%	28.7%	31.5%
Semiskilled and unskilled	47.9%	44.3%	67.6%	64.7%
Entertainers, etc.	2.5% ($N = 993$)	5.0% ($N = 300$)	1.9% ($N = 1814$)	3.0% ($N = 365$)
Percent married	67.1%	80.3%	73.7%	83.5%

subject is also asked his age at the time of first use and first abuse for each drug. These ages are rank ordered and stored with the social data collected at the same time. It should be noted that these data are relevant to the serial use and abuse of drugs, and do not provide information on the concurrent use or abuse of drugs.

For this study, primary interest is in those drugs which individuals have used regularly or habitually. Consequently, "abuse" was operationally defined as regular use, frequent use, use for sprees, or physical dependence. For purposes of reference, Table 1 presents the basic demographic and social characteristics of the sample.

PATTERNS OF ABUSE

There are three basic viewpoints which one can take in relation to patterns of drug abuse. First, there is the question of coappearance; i.e., the extent to which the abuse of pairs of drugs tends to occur together regardless of order or position. Thus narcotics and stimulants would be coappearing drugs in an individual case if they appeared together as narcotics followed by stimulants or as stimulants followed by narcotics. Coappearance simply reflects the degree of association of abused drugs.

Second is the question of directionality or progression; i.e., the propensity which certain drugs show to either precede or follow other drugs in an ordered sequence. Hypothetically, if narcotic abuse tended to precede the abuse of most other drug classes, narcotics would show a high directionality value as a precursor drug.

Third is the question of overall pattern. This is the most general view in which all significant drugs of abuse are considered holistically.

Each of these approaches is relevant to different kinds of research questions, and each requires a different method of determination.

Table 2 describes the number of individuals and percentages of the total sample which reported abuse of each drug class. Marijuana and alcohol are treated as separate drug classes because the abuse of these drugs and their relation to the abuse of other drugs has been of particular interest to many people.

Drug classes were used in the present study for purposes of simplicity. If, for certain purposes, specific drugs were of interest, the same methods could be used. It should be noted that since 98.5% of the sample are

Table 2
Number and Percentage of Subjects Abusing Each Class of Drugs (N = *3583*)

Drug class	Examples	Abbreviation	*N*	%
Narcotic, analgesics	Codeine, Demerol, Dilaudid, heroin	NARC	3494	98.5
Marijuana	Also hashish, THC	MARJ	1951	55.0
Stimulants	Benzedrine, cocaine, Dexedrine, methamphetamine	STIM	1571	44.3
Sedatives, hypnotics, relaxants	Barbiturates, Valium, Seconal	SED	655	18.5
Psychotogens	LSD, peyote, STP, psilocybin	PSYCH	431	12.1
Alcohol		ALCH	441	12.4
Tranquilizers	Compazine, Thorazine, reserpine	TRAN	244	6.9
Inhalants (organic solvents)	"Glue " sodium amytal	INHL	222	6.3
Antihistamines	Pyribenzamine, Tagathen, Atarax	AHST	86	2.4
Antidepressants	Elavil, Nardil, Marsilid, Niamid	ADEP	47	1.3

narcotic addicts, it is natural that narcotics are the most frequently reported drugs of abuse and hence show the highest degree of coappearance with other drugs. This finding would probably differ in studies with a smaller proportion of narcotic addicts in the sample.

Coappearance

While there are several ways of calculating coappearance, a good description of this kind of relationship is yielded by a simple row percentage cross-tabulation. Table 3 shows, for example, that of those people reporting abuse of narcotics, 54.9% also abused marijuana.

Table 3 indicates a wide range in the degree of coappearance (i.e., the percentage of subjects abusing drug X who also abused drug Y) between drug classes. Generally, it might seem that simple coappearance may be a function of the number of persons abusing each drug class independently; i.e., drugs which occur most often in the data show the highest coappearance values.

In order to account for the possibility that simple coappearance is an artifact of the chance relationships between the occurrence of abused drugs, a standardized indicator of coappearance was developed. This permits the detection of relationships between abused drugs which deviate from chance expectation.

The standardized coappearance measure indicating percentage departure from statistical independence is calculated by

$$C_{\mathrm{AB}} = \frac{O_{\mathrm{AB}} - E_{\mathrm{AB}}}{E_{\mathrm{AB}}}$$

where the expected coappearance frequency (E_{AB}) of two drug classes is calculated in the same manner as in a conventional chi-square test, and O_{AB} is the observed coappearance frequency. Instead of measuring statistical "significance," the measure is a restricted type of measure of association indicating the degree to which the relationship between two drugs departs from chance. (Because chi-square is a function of N and the sample is very large, significance is almost automatic and therefore meaningless.)

Table 4 shows a wide range in percentage departure from chance coappearance, varying from 300% greater than chance to 60% less than chance (negative numbers refer to coappearances less than chance). In itself, this finding strongly supports the notion that there are factors which significantly determine choices of drugs of abuse.

Inspection of the ranked coappearance values reveals some interesting

Table 3
Percentage Coappearance

	NARC	MARJ	STIM	SED	PSYCH	ALCL	TRAN	INHL	ADEP	AHST
NARC	—	54.9	44.0	18.0	11.9	12.3	6.7	6.2	1.3	2.4
MARJ	98.4	—	53.9	19.9	19.1	13.2	7.8	8.2	1.3	2.7
STIM	98.0	67.0	—	26.7	20.7	14.0	11.8	9.4	2.4	3.8
SED	96.0	59.2	64.1	—	22.7	19.8	19.7	10.1	5.2	4.0
PSYCH	96.3	86.3	75.4	34.6	—	16.9	18.6	18.8	4.4	3.5
ALCL	97.5	58.5	49.9	29.5	16.5	—	10.7	10.2	2.9	2.7
TRAN	96.7	62.7	76.2	52.9	32.8	19.3	—	11.9	17.2	8.6
INHL	98.6	72.1	66.2	29.7	36.5	20.3	13.1	—	1.8	1.8
ADEP	95.7	53.2	78.7	72.3	40.4	27.7	89.4	8.5	—	17.0
AHST	96.5	60.5	68.6	30.2	17.4	13.9	24.4	4.6	9.3	—

Table 4
Standardized Coappearance

>+10% Departure			+10% Departure			>−10% Departure		
	N	%		N	%		N	%
TRAN–ADEP	42	316.4	STIM–AHST	59	9.8	MARJ–AHST	52	−11.5
AHST–ADEP	8	161.4	INHL–NARC	219	9.3	NARC–AHST	83	−11.7
AHST–TRAN	21	68.8	STIM–TRAN	186	5.0	INHL–TRAN	29	−13.5
MARJ–NARC	1919	65.7	PSYCH–SED	149	2.7	ALCL–TRAN	47	−13.8
SED–ADEP	34	57.9	PSYCH–NARC	415	2.2	ADEP–STIM	37	−15.0
SED–TRAN	129	47.3	INHL–STIM	147	1.5	ALCL–PSYCH	73	−19.2
INHL–STIM	81	45.8	INHL–MARJ	160	0.9	MARJ–TRAN	153	−21.0
NARC–STIM	1539	45.5	ALCL–INHL	45	0.8	NARC–ADEP	45	−25.3
ALCL–NARC	430	31.9	ALCL–MARJ	258	0.1	PSYCH–AHST	15	−27.2
MARJ–STIM	1053	25.8	SED–AHST	26	−2.1	ALCL–AHST	12	−27 5
NARC–SED	629	20.2	ALCL–ADEP	13	−3.1	MARJ–ADEP	25	−47.5
PSYCH–TRAN	80	17.8	NARC–TRAN	236	−3.6	INHL–ADEP	4	−51.5
MARJ–PSYCH	372	15.9	MARJ–SED	388	−5.5	AHST–INHL	4	−60.7
PSYCH–ADEP	19	13.7	ALCL–STIM	220	−6.6			
NARC–HIST	83	11.7	INHL–SED	66	−7.8			
ALCL–SED	130	11.6						
STIM–SED	420	11.0						
STIM–PSYCH	325	10.8						

regularities. For example, the pairs of drugs which strongly tend to coappear more often than chance are those drugs which appear to have other characteristics in common. The three drug pairs with the highest coappearance, for example, are all "pills," i.e., medical drugs which are diverted to nonmedical use. Fourth highest is the pair marijuana–narcotics, which contains two illegal street drugs.

The drug pairs which appear far less often than chance are those which feature "pills" and street drugs together, or "pills" and "jailhouse drugs," such as inhalants and antidepressants, or antihistamines and inhalants. The data suggest that the combinations of drug classes a person uses over time is not a function of chance. Rather, it seems to be partly a function of nonpharmaceutical similarity, i.e., the degree of illegality of the drug classes.

Further, there were several patterns which contained the same drugs in different orders, such as the stimulant–narcotic and the narcotic–stimulant patterns. For example, the stimulant–narcotic pattern is more often a White pattern (62.6% White), while the opposite ordering (narcotic–stimulant), is more apt to be a minority pattern (69.2% minority or non-White).

Directionality

The question of progressive drug abuse is of interest to both laymen and professional researchers. In order to more fully explore this issue, a measure, G, was constructed to indicate the direction and strength of "progressive" tendencies in drug abuse:

$$G = \frac{N_{\mathrm{AB}} - N_{\mathrm{AB}}}{N_{\mathrm{AB}} + N_{\mathrm{AB}}}$$

where N_{AB} = the number of occurrences of drug A before drug B, and N_{AB} = the number of occurrences of drug B before drug A.

Table 5 presents the G values for all two-drug combinations. The table is ordered so that row entries generally represent the first drug and column entries represent the second or following drug. A negative value on a cell entry indicates a reversal of this order. For example, alcohol precedes inhalants 20% of the time when they occur in the same case, while antihistamines precede antidepressants (indicated by the negative sign) 25% of the time when they occur in the same pattern. Entries on the major diagonal (e.g., ALCL-ALCL, NARC-NARC, etc.) represent a generalized G value for that drug class, e.g., the tendency for abuse of that class to either precede or follow the abuse of other classes. This value (G_{A}) is cal-

Table 5
G *Values (excluding narcotic only cases)*[a]

	ALCL	INHL	MARJ	PSYCH	NARC	STIM	SED	TRAN	ADEP	AHST
ALCL	.443	.200	.070	.726	.595	.500	.477	.574	.692	.000
INHL		.460	.188	.531	.708	.510	.424	.793	.500	.000
MARJ			.717	.887	.849	.761	.624	.805	.680	.852
PSYCH				−.203	.325	.126	.087	.275	.368	.067
NARC					−.292	.173	.128	.568	.422	.783
STIM						−.260	.105	.495	−.568	.356
SED							−.193	.535	.529	.077
TRAN								−.509	.571	−.238
ADEP									−.067	−.250
AHST										.453

[a]Diagonal contains G_A values.

culated by

$$G_A = \frac{N_{A\#} - N_{\#A}}{N_{A\#} + N_{\#A}}$$

where $N_{A\#}$ = the number of times drug A precedes other drugs in a pattern, and $N_{\#A}$ = the number of times drug A follows other drugs in a pattern. (Cases involving only one drug of abuse are excluded from this computation.)

Of particular note here is the finding that, even with our sample of narcotic addicts, narcotics are not "terminal" drugs of abuse, but rather they commonly occur in midpositions in drug strings. Excluding those cases (23%) in which narcotics were the only drug of abuse, only in 40% of the cases were narcotics the last drug of abuse. The G_A value of − .292 indicates that narcotic abuse tends to follow the abuse of other drugs, but this is not as strong as the "following" tendency of .509 shown by tranquilizers. This further substantiates the idea that drug abuse must be conceived of within a holistic context, and illustrates the weakness of approaches which assume that a particular drug is the "end point" of an abuse career.

Further, examination of the directional relationships indicated in Table 5 shows that there is a variety of strong progressive relationships (e.g., MARJ-PSYC .88, MARJ-NARC .85, ALCL-NARC .60) which indicate that the pathways of progressive drug abuse are multiplex, probably involving variables other than the drugs themselves. As the next section on patterns will demonstrate, however, these pathways do not appear to be random. This leaves the question of explanation open in terms of discovering those variables which best account for the observed variations in patterns of abuse.

Patterns

For the 3,549 cases analyzed here, there were 567 distinct drug abuse temporal sequences or patterns. Of these distinct patterns, 19 account for over 70% of the cases. Since there are over 5,000 possible sequences just within the first four drug classes, it is remarkable that so few patterns actually appear.

The analysis was restricted to the first four drug classes out of a possible seven drug-class temporal sequence since the majority of subjects abused four or fewer drugs, hence simplifying the analysis (see Table 6).

The bulk of the remaining cases, i.e., those which differed from the most prevalent 19 patterns, appear to be minor variations in order or have an

Table 6
Number of Drug Classes Abused

Number of classes abused	*N*	%
1	835	23.5
2	1096	30.8
3	845	23.8
4	443	12.4
5	227	6.3
6+	85	2.3

additional drug added somewhere in the sequence. Rather than attempt to subsume these variants within the basic 19 patterns, our discussion here combines the variants under the category of residual patterns. Table 7 describes the basic patterns.

Table 7
Drug Abuse Patterns

Pattern	*N*	%
NARC	819	23.1
MARJ–NARC	586	16.5
MARJ–NARC–STIM	262	7.4
NARC–STIM	198	5.6
MARJ–STIM–NARC	125	3.5
STIM–NARC	79	2.2
ALCL–NARC	62	1.7
NARC–SED	49	1.4
MARJ–PSYCH–NARD	39	1.1
"Nonaddict"	34	1.0
ALCL–MARJ–NARC	29	0.8
MARJ–PSYCH–STIM–NARC	29	0.8
MARJ–ALCL–NARC	27	0.8
MARJ–STIM–PSYCH–NARC	26	0.7
SED–NARC	26	0.7
MARJ–SED–NARC	25	0.7
STIM–MARJ–NARC	23	0.6
NARC–MARJ–STIM	23	0.6
ALCL–NARC	22	0.6
Residual patterns	1066	30.0
Total	3549	99.8[a]

[a]Does not sum to 100.0 due to rounding.

The most prevalent pattern is that of narcotic abuse only. This one-drug sequence is, of course, the most direct progression to narcotic addiction. The marijuana–narcotic pattern is the second most prevalent pattern and one which has generated the most controversy. It should be stressed that the sample is almost entirely composed of narcotic addicts, so this relationship applies only to those who abused marijuana and who ultimately became narcotic addicts.

For 1,142 cases (32% of the cases), marijuana was the first drug in the basic 19 abuse sequences. Narcotics were the first or only drug class abused in 1,089 cases (30% of the total, even disregarding the residual patterns). This clearly indicates that narcotics are not universally the last drugs to be abused in some stepping-stone sequence of drug abuse. There is, however, a strong tendency for narcotics to be "following" drugs, as indicated by the G_A value in Table 5.

SUMMARY AND IMPLICATIONS

This paper has described aspects of drug abuse sequences for a sample of 3,549 narcotic addicts. These aspects include (1) the tendency for certain drugs to coappear in the drug histories of individuals, (2) the tendency for some drugs to precede others, and (3) the tendency for drug abuse sequences to fall into one of a small number of patterns.

These findings have suggested the need to gather data which can distinguish between concurrent abuse and serial abuse of two or more classes of drugs. Further, the findings have suggested that it may be worthwhile to separate legal from illegal drugs within drug classes. By gathering serial and concurrent abuse data from a sample containing nonnarcotic addicts and by making nonpharmacological distinctions between drugs, it should be possible to more clearly specify what types of individuals follow what types of drug abuse patterns.

This in turn may make it possible to match specific drug abuser types with the drug abuse theory which bests explains the pattern they follow. Similarly, this may suggest differing treatment modalities for differing kinds of drug abusers.

REFERENCES

GOODE, E. Multiple drug use among marijuana smokers. *Social Problems* 17: 48–64, 1969.

WEPPNER, R.S., and AGAR, M. Immediate precursors to heroin addiction. *J. Health Social Behavior* 12 (March): 10–18, 1971.

WHITEHEAD, P., SMART, R., and LAFOREST, L. Multiple drug use among Marihuana smokers in Eastern Canada. *Intern. J. Addictions* 7: 1972.

The International Journal of the Addictions, 9(2), 301–314, 1974

Patterns of Multiple Drug Abuse: 1969–1971

D. Dwayne Simpson, Ph.D.

S. B. Sells, Ph.D.

Institute of Behavioral Research
Texas Christian University
Fort Worth, Texas

Abstract

Information concerning types and frequencies of pretreatment drug abuse, obtained by interview from 11,380 patients included in the first two years (June 1969–June 1971) of the NIMH-TCU Drug Abuse Reporting Program, were examined with respect to patterns of usage. Twenty-eight patterns were defined, involving various combinations of drugs used and frequencies of use. The results indicated that the most frequent drug-abuse pattern in this patient sample, accounting for 28% of the entire sample, was the daily or weekly use of heroin with no other drugs. The daily or weekly use of heroin with cocaine, with marihuana, and with both cocaine and marihuana were also frequently observed patterns, and combined with the heroin-only pattern, they characterized the majority of all the patients. The most common patterns reported by the remainder of the patients were of poly-drug use, typically involving marihuana, amphetamines, and barbiturates, as well as heroin and cocaine.

An aspect of the drug abuse scene which is currently being viewed with widespread interest is that of multiple drug abuse. While usage patterns involving combinations of drugs are of great concern, relatively few studies have dealt factually or comprehensively with them, and thus little information has been available on their specific nature and prevalence. Even less appears to be known about how such patterns relate to other characteristics of those who abuse drugs.

Previously, investigators interested in the general area of drug-abuse patterns have focused attention on the frequency and motives involved in the use of individual drugs (Shick, Smith, and Meyers, 1970) and on the environmental and social climates in which drug abuse, particularly heroin, began (Ball, 1970; Sheppard, Gay, and Smith, 1971; Cohen, 1972). There have been studies involving specific drug combinations, such as heroin with marihuana (Ball, Chambers, and Ball, 1970) or heroin with barbiturates (Chambers and Moldestad, 1970), but such investigations provide no basis for comparisons across different patterns of drug abuse. A few studies (Perkins and Bloch, 1970; Collier, 1972; Fraser, 1972) have reported frequency tabulations for groups of drugs which were used concurrently by patients in treatment programs, but the drug combinations were loosely defined and incomplete with respect to frequency of use.

The data file compiled in the joint NIMH-TCU Drug Abuse Reporting Program (DARP) has filled an important gap in the field of drug abuse research by providing information relevant to the identification of patterns of multiple drug usage and a context in which the implications of such patterns may be examined. Their relationships with tenure in treatment, treatment outcomes, death rates, and other variables are important research questions which may lead to improvements in treatment effectiveness.

The present study was undertaken in the framework of the DARP-based research program on evaluation of drug-abuse treatment outcome, described below. One of its major objectives is to contribute to the program effort to provide a basis for classification of patients, in this case in terms of drug-abuse patterns at the point of admission to treatment. However, the results also have general importance in terms of examining and establishing the drug combinations which were observed most frequently in a large contemporary sample of drug abusers such as that represented by the DARP patient population. The association of the patient drug-usage patterns reported in the present study with demographic data (age, sex, and population group) and treatment information will be the focus of subsequent reports.

DESCRIPTION OF THE REPORTING AND RESEARCH PROGRAMS

The DARP is a system for monitoring patients entering drug-abuse treatment programs from admission to termination. It involves the maintenance of a computer file of Admission and Status Evaluation Reports on individual patients, submitted by participating treatment agencies throughout the United States which are supported by NIMH. The Admission Report is essentially a patient history, providing family background, social, educational, employment, drug and alcohol abuse, and criminality information on each patient, obtained at the time of admission. The Status Evaluation Report is a bimonthly report of patient status, up to the time of termination, providing information of treatment delivered and patient behavior with respect to residence, family relations, employment, drug abstinence and abuse, alcohol use and abuse, financial support, arrests, and time in jail during each 2-month report period. All reports are coded and entered in the computer file at TCU as received from each agency. Name, address, and all other identifying information have been excluded to protect the privacy of the patients who are identified only by agency case numbers. Individual patient files are maintained continuously, even in the event of readmission by the same agency after one or more terminations.

At the initiation of the DARP in June 1969, there were six participating agencies which provided treatment services primarily for narcotic (opiate) addicts. During 1971 the character of the program broadened due to the inclusion of new agencies which focused on a broader spectrum of drug abusers, including youthful nonopiate drug abusers, and the diversification of admissions to the older agencies. By the end of the second year of the program (May 1971), 23 agencies were participating and had reported a total of 11,380 patients admitted for treatment; 13 agencies were located in cities in the Northeastern region of the United States, two in the Southeast, four in the Midwest, three in the Southwest, and one in Puerto Rico. The types of treatment offered involved methadone maintenance (20 agencies), residential therapeutic communities (16 agencies), and outpatient drug-free programs (13 agencies). Seven agencies provided treatment programs including all three approaches, while four agencies offered only a single treatment approach (three MM and one TC). The remaining twelve agencies offered combinations of two types of treatment (six included MM and TC, four included MM and DF, and two included TC and DF).

The program of evaluative research, of which the present study is a part, was expanded in June 1972 with separate funding to carry out a series of investigations including a major evaluative study based on outcomes during treatment. In general the research will focus on the effects of various treatments for different types of patients and the identification of optimal matches between treatments and patients. In order to allow for a treatment and follow-up period of at least 1 year after admission, the research studies currently in progress are based primarily on the population of patients admitted to treatment during the first 2 years of the Reporting Program. These patients (3,131 from Year 1, and 8,249 from Year 2) serve as the basis for the present study. A description of the background characteristics of these patients is provided in Table 1.

Table 1

Description of the Patient Population (N = *11 380*)

	%
1. Age at admission	
<18	7.6
18–20	16.6
21–25	31.9
26–30	17.5
>30	26.4
2. Ethnic background	
Black	50.8
Puerto Rican	10.7
Mexican-American	7.0
Other White	30.0
Other	1.5
3. Sex	
Male	80.6
Female	19.4
4. Marital status	
Single	50.5
Married	27.9
Separated	14.0
Divorced	6.4
Widowed	1.2
5. Religious preference	
None	14.4
Protestant	38.0
Catholic	37.4
Other Christian	3.3
Hebrew	2.4
Muslim	2.1
Other non-christian	1.3
No information	1.1
6. Education (highest grade completed or attending)	
<7	3.4
7–9	21.7
10–12	65.4
13–14	6.3
>14	1.6
No information	1.6
7. Number of previous treatments for drug abuse	
None	49.6
1	21.5
2–3	17.3
4–5	4.9
>5	4.1
No information	2.7

FREQUENCY OF DRUG USE AND DEFINITION OF DRUG-ABUSE PATTERNS

The amount and types of illegal drug usage during the 2 months prior to admission to treatment were obtained by interviews with patients. The information reported in the Admission Record for each patient was coded in categories indicating daily use, weekly use, less than weekly use, or no use. These frequency categories were reported separately for eight drug classes: heroin, other opiates, barbiturates, cocaine, amphetamines, hallucinogens, marihuana, and "other drugs."

Table 2 presents the frequency of usage of each class of drugs for patients admitted during the first 2 years of the DARP; Year 1 (Report Periods 1–6) extended from June 1969 to June 1970, and Year 2 (Report Periods 7–12) extended from June 1970 to June 1971. The number of admissions in each year is shown at the top of the appropriate column, and the percentages of patients are reported for each drug class by frequency-of-usage alternatives. In summary, it is noted that over 72% of the admissions in both years reported daily use of heroin, while the frequency of usage of the remaining drugs was much lower.

On the basis of both logical and empirical analyses, a total of 28 drug-abuse patterns was defined as a first step toward providing a comprehensive description of drug use in the present patient population. These patterns reflect a wide range of drug habits but most of them include the abuse of opiates. The patterns are presented in Table 3. Pattern 1, which includes those cases with no reported drug use, is included for the purpose of completeness in the present description of the population (many of these patients were transferred from another treatment program and some were hospitalized or in jail during the 2 months prior to admission to treatment). Patterns 2 to 9 represent "single-drug specialists," or individuals who reported using only a single drug either daily or weekly. These categories are for heroin (H) only, other opiates (O Op) only, barbiturates (B) only, cocaine (C) only, amphetamines (A) only, hallucinogens (Ha) only, marihuana (M) only, and other drugs (O Dr) only.

Patterns 10 through 15 include categories for the joint use of heroin (daily or weekly) with either barbiturates (HB), cocaine (HC), amphetamines (HA), hallucinogens (HHa), marihuana (HM), or other drugs (HO Dr). Patterns 16 through 23 represent heroin users (daily or weekly) with two additional drugs used in combination. The first seven of these (16–22) reflect the most common specific combinations (HBC, HBA, HBM, HCA, HCM, HAM, and HHaM), while Pattern 23 (H + 2) includes all remain-

Table 2

Percentages of Patients Reporting Given Frequencies of Use for Eight Drug Classes During Year 1 and Year 2

Drug class	Frequency of use	Year 1 ($N = 3131$) %[a]	Year 2 ($N = 8249$) %[a]
Heroin	1. Daily	72.6	73.6
	2. Weekly	9.4	7.7
	3. <Weekly	2.2	2.5
	4. Not at all	15.2	15.4
Other opiates	1. Daily	2.7	3.7
	2. Weekly	3.8	4.9
	3. <Weekly	6.8	7.2
	4. Not at all	85.2	83.2
Barbiturates	1. Daily	4.5	4.6
	2. Weekly	8.6	9.0
	3. <Weekly	8.1	8.7
	4. Not at all	77.3	76.6
Cocaine	1. Daily	2.5	3.5
	2. Weekly	12.4	12.1
	3. <Weekly	17.6	16.6
	4. Not at all	66.1	66.8
Amphetamines	1. Daily	3.0	2.5
	2. Weekly	5.4	5.7
	3. <Weekly	5.6	5.8
	4. Not at all	84.4	85.0
Hallucinogens	1. Daily	0.6	0.6
	2. Weekly	4.2	3.8
	3. <Weekly	4.9	5.7
	4. Not at all	88.7	88.9
Marihuana	1. Daily	6.6	7.9
	2. Weekly	16.6	16.7
	3. <Weekly	16.4	15.1
	4. Not at all	58.8	59.2
Other drugs[b]	1. Daily	3.2	1.3
	2. Weekly	1.5	1.0
	3. <Weekly	1.0	0.7
	4. Not at all	92.7	95.7

[a]Percentages for each drug class do not add to 100 due to patient records with missing entries, which ranged from 0.6 to 1.6% across the classes.
[b]Primarily includes hashish and inhalants, such as glue and gasoline.

Table 3
Definition of 28 Drug-Abuse Patterns Based on Frequency of Use and Joint Use of Eight Drug Classes[a]

Pattern	Drug classes and frequency of use							
	H	O Op	B	C	A	Ha	M	O Dr
1. No use	4	4	4	4	4	4	4	4
2. H only	1, 2	4	4	4	4	4	4	4
3. O Op only	4	1, 2	4	4	4	4	4	4
4. B only	4	4	1, 2	4	4	4	4	4
5. C only	4	4	4	1, 2	4	4	4	4
6. A only	4	4	4	4	1, 2	4	4	4
7. Ha only	4	4	4	4	4	1 2	4	4
8. M only	4	4	4	4	4	4	1, 2	4
9. O Dr only	4	4	4	4	4	4	4	1, 2
10. HB	1, 2	4	1, 2, 3	4	4	4	4	4
11. HC	1, 2	4	4	1, 2, 3	4	4	4	4
12. HA	1, 2	4	4	4	1, 2, 3	4	4	4
13. HHa	1, 2	4	4	4	4	1, 2, 3	4	4
14. HM	1, 2	4	4	4	4	4	1, 2, 3	4
15. HO Dr	1, 2	4	4	4	4	4	4	1, 2, 3
16. HBC	1, 2	4	1, 2, 3	1, 2, 3	4	4	4	4
17. HBA	1, 2	4	1, 2, 3	4	1, 2, 3	4	4	4
18. HBM	1, 2	4	1, 2, 3	4	4	4	1, 2, 3	4
19. HCA	1, 2	4	4	1, 2, 3	1, 2, 3	4	4	4
20. HCM	1, 2	4	4	1, 2, 3	4	4	1, 2, 3	4
21. HAM	1, 2	4	4	4	1, 2, 3	4	1, 2, 3	4
22. HHaM	1, 2	4	4	4	4	1, 2, 3	1, 2, 3	4
23. H+2	1, 2	4	(any 2 must = 1, 2, or 3 ....)					
24. Op only	1, 2, 3	1, 2, 3	4	4	4	4	4	4
25. Op+	(either = 1, 2, 3)		(any 1 or 2 must = 1, 2, or 3..................)					
26. Poly	3, 4	3, 4	(any 3 or more must = 1, 2, or 3 ....)					
27. Poly and Op	(either = 1, 2)		(any 3 or more must = 1, 2, or 3 ....)					
28. All other								

[a]Drug classes include heroin (H), other opiates (O Op), barbiturates (B), cocaine (C), amphetamines (A), hallucinogens (Ha), marihuana (M), and other drugs (O Dr) and frequency-of-use categories include daily (1), weekly (2), less than weekly (3), and not used at all (4).

ing combinations of heroin with any two other drug classes, excluding other opiates. Combination opiate users (heroin with other opiates) who reported use of no additional drugs constitute Pattern 24 (Op Only), and Pattern 25 (Op+) includes opiate users who also use either one or two additional drugs.

Patterns 26 and 27 are for multiple or "poly-drug" users who reported using at least three of six drug classes (excluding heroin and other opiates). The poly-drug users who reported no use or less than weekly use of heroin and other opiates were placed in Pattern 26 (Poly), while those who reported more frequent use of opiates were placed in Pattern 27 (Poly and Op). Finally, those patients who remained unclassified after all of the hierarchical assignments to the preceding 27 categories were grouped in an "all other" category (Pattern 28).

The percentage of patients represented by each of the 28 patterns in Year 1, Year 2, and both years combined is shown in Table 4. It is noteworthy that the percentages for the 2 years are closely similar for all patterns. The pattern of H only (2) was by far the most frequent (over 28%) and the other seven most frequent patterns (ranging from 13.3 to 4.9% for Year 1 and Year 2 combined) were Poly and Op (27), HC (11), HM (14), Op+ (25), HCM (20), No use (1), and Poly (26). Together, these eight patterns accounted for approximately 85% of all patients.

Distributions of frequency of use of the different drug classes within 11 of the most common drug-usage patterns are presented in Table 5. Since the data were essentially the same for Year 1 and Year 2, they are combined in Table 5 and only those patterns representing more than 1% of the total population (see Table 4) are included, listed from the most frequent to the least frequent. For each pattern the frequency of use for the drug classes involved is shown in percentage form, and the number of patients in each pattern is entered in the right-hand column. A total of 12 patterns from Table 4 represented sufficiently large proportions of the population to be included in Table 5, but Pattern 1 (No use), not technically an abuse pattern, was omitted; the frequency of use for this category was "none" in all eight drug classes.

Of the 11 patterns included in Table 5, 10 involved frequent (daily or weekly) use of opiates, particularly heroin. In fact, the percentage of daily users of heroin in these 10 opiate-related patterns ranged from a minimum of 72% (Op+) to 96% (HC). The other drugs which were most often used concurrently with heroin, either singly or in combination, included barbiturates, cocaine, and marihuana. The percent of daily heroin users in each of the patterns in Table 5 that involve various combinations of

Table 4
Percentage of Patients in Each of 28 Drug-Abuse Patterns During Year 1 and Year 2

Pattern	Year 1 ($N = 3078$) %	Year 2 ($N = 8124$) %	Total ($N = 11{,}202$)[a] %
1. No use	6.7	7.0	6.9
2. H only	28.2	28.3	28.3
3. O Op only	0.4	0.7	0.6
4. B only	0.6	0.7	0.7
5. C only	0.0	0.1	0.1
6. A only	0.3	0.4	0.4
7. Ha only	0.0	0.1	0.1
8. M only	0.4	0.7	0.6
9. O Dr only	0.9	0.4	0.5
10. HB	2.3	2.5	2.4
11. HC	10.2	8.2	8.8
12. HA	0.5	1.0	0.8
13. HHa	0.0	0.0	0.0
14. HM	7.4	8.0	7.8
15. HO Dr	1.0	0.3	0.5
16. HBC	1.2	1.5	1.4
17. HBA	0.3	0.4	0.4
18. HBM	2.1	1.6	1.8
19. HCA	0.6	0.5	0.5
20. HCM	8.0	7.0	7.3
21. HAM	0.6	0.6	0.6
22. HHaM	0.5	0.5	0.5
23. H+2	0.8	0.7	0.8
24. Op only	1.4	1.3	1.3
25. Op+	6.6	8.3	7.8
26. Poly	5.6	4.7	4.9
27. Poly and Op	12.5	13.5	13.3
28. All other	0.9	1.0	1.0
Total	100.0	100.0	100.0

[a]*N* equals less than 11,380 since 178 patients were not assigned to patterns due to records with one or more missing drug entries.

Table 5

Frequency of Use for Drug Classes within Selected Drug-Abuse Patterns which Included over 1% of the Total Population in Year 1 and Year 2

Pattern	Frequency of use: 1 Daily, %	2 Weekly, %	3 <Weekly, %	4 None, %	No. patients (% of total)
1. H only (Pattern 2)					3168 (28.3)
a. Heroin	92	8	0	0	
2. Poly + Op (Pattern 27)					1486 (13.3)
a. Heroin	80	15	2	3	
b. Other opiates	8	16	21	55	
c. Barbiturates	12	34	34	20	
d. Cocaine	7	26	42	25	
e. Amphetamines	7	22	27	44	
f. Hallucinogens	2	14	27	57	
g. Marihuana	24	37	30	9	
h. Other drugs	3	4	3	90	
3. HC (Pattern 11)					983 (8.8)
a. Heroin	96	4	0	0	
b. Cocaine	13	39	48	0	
4. HM (Pattern 14)					876 (7.8)
a. Heroin	87	13	0	0	
b. Marihuana	12	41	47	0	
5. Op+ (Pattern 25)					876 (7.8)
a. Heroin	72	10	12	6	
b. Other opiates	18	27	44	11	
c. Barbiturates	8	10	9	73	
d. Cocaine	5	16	24	55	
e. Amphetamines	2	3	4	91	
f. Hallucinogens	0	1	3	96	
g. Marihuana	9	25	26	40	
h. Other drugs	1	1	1	97	
6. HCM (Pattern 20)					812 (7.3)
a. Heroin	93	7	0	0	
b. Cocaine	8	43	49	0	
c. Marihuana	11	41	48	0	
7. Poly (Pattern 26)					549 (4.9)
a. Heroin	0	0	24	76	
b. Other opiates	0	0	10	90	
c. Barbiturates	15	23	15	47	
d. Cocaine	1	4	13	82	
e. Amphetamines	21	29	11	39	
f. Hallucinogens	4	30	23	43	

(*continued*)

Table 5 *(continued)*

Pattern	Frequency of use 1 Daily, %	2 Weekly, %	3 <Weekly, %	4 None, %	No. patients (% of total)
g. Marihuana	26	37	21	16	
h. Other drugs	6	5	2	87	
8. HB (Pattern 10)					272 (2.4)
a. Heroin	90	10	0	0	
b. Barbiturates	23	41	36	0	
9. HBM (Pattern 18)					195 (1.8)
a. Heroin	86	14	0	0	
b. Barbiturates	14	39	47	0	
c. Marihuana	15	42	43	0	
10. HBC (Pattern 16)					161 (1.4)
a. Heroin	92	8	0	0	
b. Barbiturates	17	33	50	0	
c. Cocaine	9	37	54	0	
11. Op Only (Pattern 24)					148 (1.3)
a. Heroin	80	15	5	0	
b. Other opiates	36	28	36	0	
Total					9526 (85.1)

heroin with barbiturates, cocaine, and marihuana (HB, HC, HM, HBC, HBM, and HCM) ranged from 86 (HBM) to 96 (HC). The usage frequencies of barbiturates, cocaine, and marihuana for patients in these six patterns, on the other hand, indicated predominantly weekly or less than weekly use. Two other patterns involving frequent opiate use along with additional drugs (Op+ and Poly and Op) also showed that barbiturates, cocaine, and especially marihuana were abused more often than the remaining nonopiates. Finally, the only pattern in Table 5 which included no daily or weekly opiate users (Poly) revealed that the drugs abused most commonly by patients in that group were marihuana, amphetamines, and barbiturates.

Examination of agencies with respect to patient drug-abuse patterns revealed that in some cases there tended to be differences in the types of patterns admitted to different agencies. These differences appeared to exist between agencies within the same geographic regions as well as those in different regions. For instance, the number of patients reporting patterns involving frequent opiate abuse without additional drugs who were admitted to the different agencies ranged from 8 to 60%. Likewise, the frequencies of each of the patterns involving poly-use as well as heroin with either cocaine or marihuana (HC, HM, and HCM) fluctuated from approximately 0 to 15% or more of admissions for the different agencies. While the basis for such variations among agencies is not certain, factors such as the particular types of treatment offered by a program, background characteristics of the agency's clientele, and distribution channels for illegal drugs each appear to be important contributors.

DISCUSSION AND CONCLUSIONS

Data concerning the types and frequencies of pretreatment drug abuse obtained from the Admission Reports of 11,380 patients included in the first 2 years of the NIMH-TCU Drug Abuse Reporting Program provided a basis for this study of drug-abuse patterns. Based on the analysis of a comprehensive set of 28 patterns, it was revealed that the most prevalent pattern was the daily or weekly use of heroin with no other drugs; this pattern represented over 28% of the patients. The daily or weekly use of heroin with cocaine, with marihuana, and with both cocaine and marihuana were also frequently observed patterns, representing from 7.3 to 8.8% of the patients. These four patterns combined characterized slightly over 52% of the patients. Furthermore, a substantial number of patients (18%) revealed patterns of poly-use in which at least three nonopiate drugs were used and, of these, over two-thirds also used opiates either daily or weekly.

In considering the data examined in the present report, two important points must be emphasized. First, the data presented are based on interviews with patients concerning their drug usage during the 2 months prior to admission to treatment and, second, the data are based on drug abusers and addicts who have entered treatment for their drug problems. The first point involves the question of reliability and validity of the data since they were not based on objective observation, but rather on what the patients themselves related to the treatment agency personnel concerning drugs used. It is realized that such reports depend not only on the willingness of the patients to provide accurate information, but also on their ability to recall completely and accurately the details of their drug abuse. There is also the possibility that in procuring drugs "in the street," patients may have to some extent been uninformed (or misinformed) regarding the actual content of the drugs taken. Most of these potential problems are not accessible to independent checks of their magnitude, and the data have been accepted essentially at face value. It should be noted, however, that interview procedures have been standardized and that checks on the consistency of patient reports are routinely conducted as a part of the DARP file maintenance.

The second point has important implications which relate to the patient selection factors known to exist in the treatment program. First of all, there is the matter of self-selection whereby the patients have agreed to enter treatment for their drug problems. Furthermore, as noted previously, treatment agencies participating in the Reporting Program were oriented in the first 2 years primarily toward admitting opiate addicts, and abusers of other drugs were not generally admitted except when such use accompanied opiate abuse; this is illustrated by the prevalence of opiate-related drug-abuse patterns observed and the finding that over 80% of the total sample of patients reported either daily or weekly use of heroin.

It is apparent, therefore, that the selective factor of motivation on the part of individuals who entered treatment programs and the selective admission policies of the treatment agencies were both operative in determining the composition of the sample of patients included in the present study. The degree to which the present population sample is representative of 1969–1971 or current drug abusers and addicts in general is not specifically known and, hence, generalizations regarding the prevalence in the total population of the drug-abuse patterns developed from the present data must be qualified. As a result of the trend among treatment agencies toward broader-spectrum admission procedures concerning the types of drugs abused, it is expected that patients in later-year samples will constitute somewhat more representative samples of drug abusers than do those in the present study.

In addition to changes in the types of patients more recently being admitted to treatment by the agencies in the DARP, changes may also be anticipated from year to year with respect to the "in" drugs in conspicuous segments of the current drug culture. For instance, hallucinogens (or psychedelics) were given widespread publicity in the middle 1960s and they were later replaced in popularity by amphetamines or "speed." Since the June 1969 to June 1971 time interval represented in the present study, illegal methadone appears to have become a major problem. Information currently obtained in the DARP concerning drug abuse includes illegal methadone, and this may well be a potentially important candidate for future revision of the taxonomy of drug-abuse patterns as they are altered to incorporate trends in multiple drug use in the patient population. It is also anticipated that future pattern revisions or additions may involve finer breakdowns of the gross poly-user groups defined in the present report.

The comprehensive description given of trends in current drug-abuse patterns has provided important and heretofore unavailable information to drug research and rehabilitation personnel, but possibly of even more significance are the questions concerning associations of these patterns with other patient characteristics and treatment outcomes. Research is currently in progress to answer these and related questions based on data gathered in the NIMH-TCU Drug Abuse Reporting Program.

ACKNOWLEDGMENTS

Acknowledgment is made of the helpful criticism by Douglas J. McRae, Robert G. Demaree, George W. Joe, and Douglas K. Spiegel of the IBR Drug Abuse Treatment Evaluation Research Staff and the support in computer programming by Michael Abbamonte and Charles Kee, Jr. The research reported in this paper was completed as part of a program on evaluation of drug abuse treatment under contract with NIMH, Contracts No. HSM–42–69–6 and HSM–42–72–132.

REFERENCES

BALL, J.C. Two patterns of opiate addiction. In J.C. Ball and C.D. Chambers (eds.) *The Epidemiology of Opiate Addiction in the United States.* Springfield, Illinois: Thomas, 1970.

BALL, J.C., CHAMBERS, C.D., and BALL, M.J. The association of marihuana smoking with opiate addiction. In J.C. Ball and C.D. Chambers (eds.) *The Epidemiology of Opiate Addiction in the United States.* Springfield, Illinois: Thomas, 1970.

CHAMBERS, C.D., and Moldestad, M. The evolution of concurrent opiate and sedative addictions. In J.C. Ball and C.D. Chambers (eds.) *The Epidemiology of Opiate Addiction in the United States.* Springfield, Illinois: Thomas, 1970.

COHEN, S. Patterns of drug abuse—1970. In C.J.D. Zarafonetis (ed.) *Drug Abuse: Proceedings of the International Conference.* Philadelphia: Lea and Febiger, 1972.

COLLIER, W.V. *The 1971 Profile: Statistical Report on the Therapeutic Community Program of Daytop Village, Inc.* New York: Satellite Litho Corp., 1972.

FRASER, H.F. Patterns of abuse of narcotics: An historical view. In C.J.D. Zarafonetis (ed.) *Drug Abuse: Proceedings of the International Conference.* Philadelphia: Lea and Febiger, 1972.

PERKINS, M.E., and BLOCH, H.I. Survey of a maintenance program on methadone. *Amer. J. Psychiat.* 126: 1389, 1970.

SHEPPARD, C.W., GAY, G.R., and SMITH, D.E. The changing patterns of heroin addiction in the Haight-Ashbury subculture. *J. Psychedelic Drugs*, 3: 22–30, 1971.

SHICK, J.F.E., SMITH, D.E., and MEYERS, F.H. Patterns of drug use in the Haight-Ashbury neighborhood. *Clin. Toxicol.* 3: 19–56, 1970.

The International Journal of the Addictions, 9(2), 315–320, 1974

Heroin Addict Clients' Description of Their Families of Origin

Carolyn A. Eldred, Ph.D.

Barry S. Brown, Ph.D.

*Narcotics Treatment Administration,
Washington, D.C.*

Cynthia Mahabir

*Howard University
Washington, D.C.*

The roots of deviance are often sought in the family of origin, and the families of male heroin addicts have not escaped such attention. (See Seldin, 1972, for a review of this literature.) A composite picture derived from the previously reported findings summarized in Table 1 suggests that the addict's mother is typically the dominant and pathological parent, while the father is either weak or absent. Yet it is usually the mother who is seen in positive terms by the addict himself, and the father who is viewed negatively. Presumably in many cases the addict simply accepts his mother's negative view of his father. Some common consequences of this family situation have been reported: (1) the addict's mother may depreciate her son because she sees him as like her husband, and the addict may incorpo-

Table 1

Previous Findings Concerning the Families of Heroin Addicts

Study	Sources of data	Major relevant findings
Oltman and Friedman, 1967	69 addicts, 350 controls	Drug addicts more likely to have experienced parental loss through separation
Larner and Tefferteller, 1964	Clinical impressions	Addicts had either no relationship or a negative relationship with their fathers, thus lacking both a model of successful relations with women and a model of a breadwinner
Bess et al., 1972	17 former addicts and matched recidivists	Addicts able to renounce drugs typically grew up in intact families with fathers who provided suitable models for work roles
Chein et al., 1964	30 addicts, 29 controls	Father absent, emotionally distant, or hostile; relationships with mothers disturbed, hostile, or distant
Nyswander, 1956	Clinical impressions	Father seen by addict through mother's eyes and viewed as weak, ineffectual, and under mother's domination; mother is object of sympathy
Frazier, 1962	Clinical impressions	Fathers nonexistent, distant, or known only through hostile eyes of mother; anger toward father more easily expressed than hostility toward mother, which generally remains unconscious
Hirsch, 1961	Clinical impressions	Mothers narcissistic, seductive, and infantilizing, and use child to gratify their own needs; fathers weak and ineffectual and seen by addicts through mothers' eyes
Mason, 1958	Clinical impressions	Mothers possessive, controlling, infantilizing, ambivalent, narcissistic, and seductive; fathers in the background or physically absent
Mason, 1958	65 addicts	94% preferred their mother to their father
Vaillant, 1966	100 addicts	Although 20% had lost mothers prior to age 16, 72% were still living with mother after age 22, and 47% were living with a female blood relative at age 30
Weinrobe, 1968	45 adolescent addicts and their mothers	Mother depreciates husband and sees son as like him; sons' self-concepts reflect mothers' negative appraisals of them, but addicts' judgments do not reflect mothers' depreciation of husbands
Wolk and Diskind, 1961	Clinical impressions	Mothers infantilizing and inconsistent and may sabotage treatment of addict; fathers typically weak or absent; wives of addicts similar to mothers of addicts
Taylor et al., 1966	16 wives of addicts	Wives motivated to remain with weak men whom they can dominate and who make minimal adult heterosexual demands on them

rate his mother's negative appraisal into his self-concept; (2) the addict may experience unusual difficulty in achieving independence from his mother; (3) when he does, he may then select a similarly deviant woman for a mate; and (4) both wife and mother may unconsciously attempt to perpetuate the addict's drug use.

Half of the reports cited were based on clinical impressions, however, and only three utilized control groups. Thus some question remains as to whether the family of the heroin addict is actually different from other families or whether it is simply a convenient scapegoat. To learn more about this issue, heroin addict clients' perceptions of their families were compared with those of a similar group of nonaddicts. A secondary focus was on the conceptions of self which developed in these individuals out of their experiences with family and significant others.

METHOD

Subjects. The addict sample ($N = 20$) was drawn from one treatment center of the District of Columbia Narcotics Treatment Administration, a city government agency treating Washington's heroin addicts with counseling, urine surveillance, and/or methadone maintenance or detoxification.

The control group comprised 20 ambulatory patients at Freedmens Hospital in Washington, D. C., a teaching institution associated with Howard University. *S*s in this group were neither heroin addicts nor alcoholics.

The two groups were all male and all black and came from low socioeconomic backgrounds. The addict group had a mean age of 24.25 years, which was not significantly different from that of the control group, 24.80 years.

Procedure. Each *S* completed the Adjective Check List (ACL) (Gough and Heilbrun, 1965), a 300-item self-administered inventory, under three sets of instructions. He was asked to check the adjectives which (1) "best describe yourself," (2) "best describe your mother," and (3) "best describe your father."

RESULTS

Ten of the 24 ACL scales were selected as relevant to the present study. These included seven scales based on Murray's (1938) need-press system:

achievement (Ach), dominance (Dom), nurturance (Nur), aggression (Agg), succorance (Suc), abasement (Aba), and deference (Def); as well as the empirically developed scales for personal adjustment (Per Adj) and self-control (S-Cn) and a scale representing the number of favorable adjectives checked (Fav).

Differences between addict-clients and controls in their descriptions of their mothers, their fathers, and themselves were examined through profile analyses, carried out by means of three two-factor univariate analyses of variance. Here group membership constituted the first factor, and the 10 ACL scales comprised the 10 levels of the second factor; measures were repeated across this second factor.

Only the profiles of the fathers of the addict-clients and the fathers of the controls differed significantly from one another, as revealed by a significant interaction between group membership and ACL scale ($p = 0.017$). Differences between the two groups on the individual scales were examined by testing simple effects; the two levels of the group membership factor were thus compared at each level of the scale factor. This process revealed that the addict-clients described their fathers as significantly

Table 2

Description of Fathers by Addict Clients and Controls: Means and Standard Deviation on Five ACL Scales Expressed as Standard Scores

Scale	Fathers of addicts ($N = 18$)[a]	Fathers of controls ($N = 20$)	p
Favorable			
Mean	36.83	44.65	<0.01
(s.d.)	(12.39)	(10.02)	
Personal adjustment			
Mean	37.17	46.35	<0.01
(s.d.)	(10.50)	(6.73)	
Dominance			
Mean	49.94	56.10	<0.05
(s.d.)	(10.45)	(8.38)	
Nurturance			
Mean	38.22	48.35	<0.01
(s.d.)	(12.41)	(7.74)	
Succorance			
Mean	51.00	46.35	<0.05
(s.d.)	(8.03)	(7.56)	

[a]Two of the 20 *S*s were dropped from this analysis because they marked fewer than 20 of the 300 adjectives.

lower on the Fav, Per Adj, Dom, and Nur scales, and higher on the Suc scale than did the controls. Mean scores for the two groups on these scales appear in Table 2.

DISCUSSION

Gough and Heilbrun's (1965) interpretations of these scales suggest that, in general, the fathers of the addict-clients were described in less favorable terms by their sons than the fathers of the controls. They were viewed as less well-adjusted, less able to get along with others, less likely to assume a leadership role or to be influential in individual relationships, and less likely to extend material or emotional benefits to others, while simultaneously requiring more sympathy, affection, and emotional support from others than fathers in general.

These findings are consistent with reports in the literature which indicated that fathers of addicts were viewed in more negative terms by their sons, that they were liked less, and that they were seen as less effective and successful, particularly in meeting the requirements of the traditional male role, than fathers of controls. However, they contradict previous reports about the mothers, and they cast doubt on the assumption that mothers of addicts behave differently toward their children than other mothers. Also, the failure to find differences in the self-concepts of the addicts and the nonaddicts raises questions about the role of individual psychopathology in drug addiction.

Attempts to generalize from the findings must take into account the limitations of the study. First, of course, the samples utilized were not large. Second, the findings reflect conscious attitudes toward the parents, and it may be that differences between addicts and nonaddicts exist at lower levels of awareness. Indeed, Frazier (1962) postulates that the young addict's hostility toward his father serves to mask the fact that his real hostility is toward his mother. Nonetheless, if the mothers really were deviant, they should have been described in somewhat different terms than the controls, if only in an exaggeratedly positive way.

Another limitation relates to the population sampled. The results apply to a black, inner-city population, living in an environment where drugs are plentiful and drug use is prevalent. Family pathology may well play an even greater role in heroin addiction in a white, suburban population. Similarly, these findings apply only to male addicts. If such factors as the husband–wife power structure and identification with the like-sexed parent are important, then the family dynamics involved in female addiction may be very different. Further research will be required to clarify these issues.

ACKNOWLEDGMENTS

The authors are grateful for the assistance of Karen Pettigrew of the Biometry Branch, NIMH, and Hugh R. Baird of the Division of Computer Research and Technology, NIH, for their assistance with the data analysis.

REFERENCES

BESS, B., JANUS, A., and RIFKIN, A. Factors in successful narcotics renunciation. *Amer. J. Psychiat.* 128: 861–865, 1972.

CHEIN, I., GERARD, D.L., LEE, R.S., and ROSENFELD, E. *The Road to H.* New York: Basic Books, 1964.

FRAZIER, T.Treating young drug users: a casework approach. *Social Work* 7: 94–101, 1962.

GOUGH, H.G., and HEILBRUN, A.B. *The Adjective Check List Manual.* Palo Alto, California: Consulting Psychologists Press, 1965.

HIRSCH, R. Group therapy with parents of adolescent drug addicts. *Psychiat. Quart.* 35: 702–710, 1961.

LARNER, J., and TEFFERTELLER, R. *The Addict in the Street.* New York: Grove Press, 1964.

MASON, P. The mother of the addict. *Psychiat. Quart. Suppl.* 32: 189–198, 1958.

MURRAY, H. *Explorations in Personality.* New York: Oxford Univ. Press, 1938.

NYSWANDER, M. *The Drug Addict as a Patient.* New York: Grune, 1956.

OLTMAN, J.E., and FRIEDMAN, S. Parental deprivation in psychiatric conditions: III. In personality disorders and other conditions. *Diseases Nervous System* 28: 298–303, 1967.

SELDIN, N.E. The family of the addict: a review of the literature *Intern. J. Addictions* 7: 97–107, 1972.

TAYLOR, S.D., WILBUR, M., and OSNOS, R. The wives of drug addicts. *Amer. J. Psychiat.* 123: 585–591, 1966.

VAILLANT, G.E. Twelve-year follow up of New York narcotic addicts: 1. The relation of treatment to outcome. *Amer. J. Psychiat.* 122: 727–737, 1966.

WEINROBE, C.K. *The Male Adolescent Drug Addict and His Mother: Their Concepts of Themselves, Each Other, and the Addict's Father.* Unpublished doctoral dissertation, Columbia University, 1968.

WOLK, R.L., and DISKIND, M.H. Personality dynamics of mothers and wives of drug addicts. *Crime and Delinquency* 7: 148–152, 1961.

The International Journal of the Addictions, 9(2), 321–327, 1974

Marihuana Use by College Students: Three-Year Trends, 1970–1972

Douglas P. Ferraro, Ph.D.*

David K. Billings, B.A.

Department of Psychology
University of New Mexico
Albuquerque, New Mexico

One-year surveys of marihuana use at separate colleges have often been reported in the literature. While it is possible to infer long-term trends in college students' marihuana use from these studies (cf. HEW Congressional Report, 1972), such inferences are necessarily limited by several differences among the populations surveyed, not the least of which has been the geographical location of the survey college. In contrast, there exist only a very few recent surveys which have been repeated over consecutive years at the same college (e.g., Goldstein, 1970; McKenzie, 1970; Garfield, Boering, and Smith, 1971). By and large, these latter surveys have been conducted at either East or West Coast colleges. We now report the trends in marihuana use observed over a 3-year period at a large Southwestern state university.

*A copy of the questionnaire used may be obtained by writing the senior author at 176 Psychology Hall, University of New Mexico, Albuquerque, New Mexico 87106. Reprints are also available from him.

METHOD

Shortly after commencement of the Fall semester for the years 1970, 1971, and 1972, a 51-item, multiple-choice questionnaire was group administered to students attending introductory courses at the University of New Mexico. The questionnaire was divided into three parts. Part I consisted of 16 items regarding general background variables of the student. Part II consisted of 22 items on the illicit use of minor and major psychotropic drugs excluding marihuana. Part III contained 13 items on the use of marihuana.

The questionnaire was administered by the survey team during regularly scheduled classes on a voluntary basis. Students were instructed that the questionnaire was anonymous and that the survey was being carried out independently of the university administration or of local or federal law enforcement agencies. Practically 100% participation was obtained each year. The respective number of responders for the years 1970–1972 were 3,349, 3,123, and 3,173.

Only the data on background variables and marihuana use were analyzed for the present report. Since our primary objective was to study current trends in marihuana use rather than simply to describe absolute rates of drug use at the University of New Mexico, only those undergraduates under the age of 31 who responded consistently to all the relevant background variable and marihuana use questions were included in the final data sample. Consequently, the sizes of the samples for the years 1970–1972 were reduced to 3,076, 2,756, and 2,787, respectively.

RESULTS

Background Variables

Previous surveys of marihuana use by college students have fairly well established that the student marihuana user is a young, unmarried male from a middle- to upper-middle-class home who is somewhat active politically but who does not participate in formal religion. Accordingly, we chose to analyze the trends in four possible correlates of marihuana use: age, marital status, religious activity, and sex. Table 1 presents the percentage distributions that were obtained for these four variables from the student sample. A standard chi-square test of independence performed over the 3 survey years did not yield significance at the .05 level for the variables of age, marital status, or religious activity. Accordingly, the percentages presented for these variables in Table 1 are based on the total

Table 1
Percentage Distribution of Age, Marital Status, Religious Activity, and Sex for the Student Sample

Age	17	18	19	20	21	22	23	24	25–30
	7.5	30.9	22.2	13.4	8.8	4.9	3.5	2.6	6.2

Marital status	Single	Married	Widowed	Divorced
	86.3	12.0	0.2	1.5

Religious activity	Very active	Active	Barely active	Inactive	No religion
	4.7	19.2	25.5	21.0	29.6

Sex	Male	Female
1970	50.9	49.1
1971	47.4	52.6
1972	49.5	50.5

sample of 8,619 responders. A statistically significant difference was obtained in the ratio of males to females in the samples for the 3-year period ($\chi^2 = 7.30$, $df = 2$, $p < .05$). The yearly percentages given for sex of responder in Table 1 suggest that the samples contained higher percentages of females than males during the years 1971 and 1972.

All students were asked whether they were currently using marihuana. The answer to this question was correlated with the four background variables for each survey year. The correlations for religious activity and sex, but not for age and marital status, were statistically significant ($p < .001$) for each of the 3 survey years. Indeed, current marihuana users tended to be male and religiously inactive. More important, however, was the fact that there was no indication that these latter two variables were becoming less relevant over the 3-year period.

Trends in General Use of Marihuana

We attempted to obtain an estimate of the rate of increase in marihuana use by analyzing students' answers to five marihuana use questions across the 3-year survey. The questions asked were essentially: (1) Have you ever used marihuana; (2) Do you now use marihuana; (3) If given the opportunity in the future, would you ever use marihuana; (4) Have either of your parents ever used marihuana; and (5) Have any of your friends ever used marihuana?

Table 2
Percentage of "Yes" Responses and Percentage of Possible Change in Each of Five Questions Regarding Marihuana Use for the 3 Survey Years

	Percentage "yes"			Percentage change	
Question	1970	1971	1972	1970–1971	1971–1972
Have you ever?	55.6	63.9	68.0	18.7	11.4
Do you now?	37.2	44.6	46.5	11.8	2.9
Would you?	51.2	56.1	56.9	10.0	1.8
Have either of your parents?	4.9	7.0	8.6	2.2	1.7
Have any of your friends?	81.6	85.3	86.5	20.1	8.2

The left side of Table 2 presents the percentage of students answering "yes" to the marihuana use questions in each year of the survey. As expected, a standard chi-square test of independence indicated that the percentage increases shown for each question in Table 1 were significant ($p < .05$) across the 3 years. Approximately one-third of the students who had ever used marihuana were not current users. However, there was no trend in the tendency to discontinue use of marihuana over the 3-year period; the percentages of students who no longer used marihuana for the years 1970–1972 were, respectively, 33.1, 30.2, and 31.5. Furthermore, some of those students who had discontinued use of marihuana were apparently willing to use marihuana in the future if the opportunity arose. Of those students who had ever used marihuana, the percentages of those who disclaimed any intention of again using marihuana were 19.5, 19.2, and 22.4, respectively, for each survey year. With respect to those students who had never used marihuana, a sizeable proportion stated they would use marihuana if the opportunity provided itself but, again, there was no apparent trend in these percentages across the years 1970 (14.6%), 1971 (12.5%), and 1972 (13.2%).

The above data are clear in indicating that the use of marihuana by college students has been increasing and most likely will continue to increase. Nevertheless, there is strong suggestion in the data that the rate of increase in marihuana use may be diminishing. The right side of Table 2 presents the percentage of possible increase that actually occurred between successive years of the survey. This measure is a direct indicant of the rate of increase in marihuana use. As may be seen from Table 2, there was a marked reduction in the percentage change measure between 1971 and 1972 as compared to that between 1970 and 1971 for each marihuana use question.

Trends in First Use of Marihuana

That the first use of marihuana is occurring more and more often prior to the student's entrance into college is shown in Table 3. There was a significant increase ($\chi^2 = 83.9, df = 4, p < .05$) across the 3 survey years in the incidence of first marihuana use during both the junior high and senior high school grades. Whereas in 1970, 55.3% of marihuana users had experienced the drug prior to college, 70.7% had done so in 1972. More important, perhaps, is the observation that a larger proportion of precollege users of marihuana were drawn from the junior high school grades during each succeeding year of the survey.

Trends in Frequency of Marihuana Use

In order to avoid the confounding which would occur if students were surveyed in more than 1 year of the study, analyses of the trends in frequency of marihuana use were limited exclusively to those freshman students in each year's sample who had used marihuana at least once. The resulting sample sizes for the years 1970–1972 were 504, 484, and 541 freshman students.

The numbers of marihuana experiences for the freshman samples are presented in Table 4. A majority of the freshman marihuana users sur-

Table 3
Percentage of Marihuana Users Who First Used Marihuana in Junior High School, Senior High School, or Undergraduate College for Each Survey Year

Grade	1970	1971	1972
Junior high	4.4	8.6	11.1
Senior high	50.9	55.7	59.6
College	44.7	35.7	29.3

Table 4
Total Number of Maihuana Experiences for Those College Freshmen Who Had Ever Used Marihuana Given in Percentage for Each Survey Year

Number	1970	1971	1972
1	4.6	2.9	1.7
2–4	10.9	9.1	11.5
5–14	18.2	14.9	14.0
15–30	10.3	9.7	9.6
>30	56.0	63.4	63.2

veyed each year had extensive marihuana histories as is indicated by the fact that well over 50% of these students had used marihuana more than 30 times. Although there was a significant change in frequency of marihuana use for the 3 years ($\chi^2 = 15.2$, $df = 8$, $p < .05$), most of this change had taken place between 1970 and 1971 with little noticeable trend occurring between 1971 and 1972. The most notable observation for the 1970–1971 survey years was that of a sizeable increase in the percentage of students who had used marihuana more than 30 times.

The incidence of current marihuana use for the freshman samples did not differ significantly across the 3 survey years. For the 3 years combined, the breakdown of incidence of current marihuana use was as follows: less than once a month (19%); 1–4 times per month (30.2%); 1–3 times per week (25%); 4–6 times per week (12.5%), daily (13.3%).

SUMMARY

Between 1970 and 1972 the trend in marihuana use by college students at the University of New Mexico was clearly upward. Not only had an increasing number of these students ever used marihuana, but they had done so at an earlier age and more often in each succeeding year. At the same time, the rate with which marihuana use was growing appeared to be decelerating. That is, the rate of increase in marihuana use had diminished between 1971 and 1972 as compared to the preceding 2-year period. Whether this latter trend signals the onset of a changing interest in marihuana use among our college students or simply reflects the fact that the proportion of college students who have not yet experienced marihuana has been decreasing over the years cannot be definitely determined from the present work.

ACKNOWLEDGMENTS

Research supported, in part, by Drug Resources for University Groups and Department of Psychology, University of New Mexico. The authors thank Sandra O'Dell, Marsha Summers, and James Trost for their help in collecting the data.

REFERENCES

GARFIELD, E.F., BOERING, M.L., and SMITH, J.P. Marihuana use on a campus: spring 1969. *Intern. J. Addictions* 6: 487–491, 1971.

GOLDSTEIN J. *The Social Psychology of Student Drug Use.* Pittsburgh: Department of Psychology, Carnegie-Mellon University, 1970.

HEALTH, EDUCATION, AND WELFARE REPORT TO CONGRESS, *Marihuana and Health*. Washington, D.C. U.S. Government Printing Office, 1972.

McKENZIE, J.D. Trends in marihuana use among undergraduate students at the University of Maryland. College Park, Maryland: Counseling Center, University of Maryland, 1970.

The International Journal of the Addictions, 9(2), 329–335, 1974

Marijuana Use in Urban Secondary Schools: A Three-Year Comparison

Robert Bloom, Ph.D.

J. Ray Hays, Ph.D.

G. Michael Winburn, M.A.

Texas Research Institute of Mental Sciences
Houston, Texas

Abstract

In this study the use of marijuana by high school students ranking from the lower to the upper socioeconomic class and including Blacks, Mexican-Americans, and Anglos was compared over a 3-year period. Analyses of the data revealed that the Preston and Hays findings of the incidence of reported marijuana use were comparable, and the different instruments and methodologies used by each investigator yielded data that were similar in pattern and frequency. The major finding was that marijuana use varies according to the ethnic and socioeconomic group examined.

Within the past 3 years, two different researchers have investigated reported marijuana use among Houston's high school students (Preston, 1970; Hays, 1971, 1972). The intent of these three studies was to provide baseline data necessary to detect changes in the pattern of drug abuse. Since each study examined marijuana use in the same schools, an opportunity was presented for a longitudinal comparison of marijuana use.

Preston's (1970) study of 535 students specifically focused upon reported marijuana use among students in the tenth, eleventh, and twelfth grades. Preston purposely selected students within five different schools that represented a wide range of socioeconomic and cultural differences. Two of the schools were predominantly Black and were of relatively low socioeconomic status. A third school, chosen because it had a large number of Mexican-Americans, was ethnically heterogeneous and represented the low middle to middle range in socioeconomic status. The fourth school, composed predominantly of White students, comprised the low-middle or "working class" range, while the fifth school, also predominantly White, represented the upper-middle to lower-upper range of socioeconomic status.

Preston's (1970) respondents represented both sexes and were drawn from required classes. The respondents were given a structured interview based upon a questionnaire which was previously developed and pretested. The respondents anonymity was protected by not having them sign the questionnaire, by not having school personnel present during the interviews, and by having the interviews in large conference rooms in group-type situations.

The Hays (1971, 1972) studies of 5,908 and 5,819 students, respectively, were conceived as a wide-range investigation of drug abuse in Houston's school system. A 10% random sampling of the homerooms of each grade level from the seventh through the twelfth was attempted. However, due to absenteeism and students' exempting themselves from participation, a 6% sample was obtained which was approximately representative of the total secondary school population of students, including ethnic, religious, socioeconomic differences, and sex ratio. Both the Black and Mexican-American groups were slightly underrepresented in the sampling of the first study by Hays. The ethnic breakdown was as follows: 55% Anglo, 30% Black, 9% Mexican-American, and 5% others. The HEW Campus report for December 1, 1970 shows 33% Black, 55% White, 11% Mexican-American, and 5% others. This undersampling was not considered critical. There was no undersampling of ethnic groups in the second study by Hays. The Hays' studies included the schools surveyed by Preston. A total of 471 students in 1971 and 516 in 1972 were included in the five schools Preston surveyed.

The survey instrument was administered in the students' homeroom by nonschool personnel under anonymous conditions. The instrument was designed to show frequency of use of nine categories of substances during three time periods. The nine categories of substance were: marijuana, hallucinogens, opiates or cocaine, tobacco, alcohol, cough syrup, solvents, barbiturates, and stimulants. The three time periods were: ever used, used in the past six months, and used in the past seven days. In addition to drug use items, the questionnaire contained items devoted to demographic, attitudinal, and factual variables which were used to determine correlates of drug use.

The purpose of the present study is to compare reported marijuana use among Houston high school students in order to determine whether any shift in pattern of use among the socioeconomic classes has occurred and whether there has been a growth in reported use over the past 3 years. In order to examine such change, the Preston (1970) study was used as a base with which the Hays (1971, 1972) data could be compared. Since both Hays studies contained data from the five schools that Preston surveyed, a 3-year longitudinal comparison was possible.

RESULTS AND DISCUSSION

Table 1 contains a comparison of the Hays and Preston surveys of reported marijuana use by school. There were a total of 530 students surveyed in the Preston study, 471 in the first Hays study, and 516 in the second Hays study. A "yes" response indicates that a student reports he has used marijuana at least once and falls within the Hays "ever used" category. A "no" response indicates that a student denies ever using marijuana.

As a partial check on the comparability of the Preston and Hays data, Spearman rank order correlations were computed between all possible pairs of schools in the three surveys. Table 2 contains a summary of the correlations between rankings of schools by percentage of reported marijuana use across the 3 years the surveys covered. All correlations were significant at the 5% probability level. The possibility of repeated measurement of the same students is small due to the random sampling techniques employed and to the fact that homeroom and "required class" composition changed over the years.

As a further check on the comparability of the two types of survey

Table 1

Comparison of Hays and Preston Surveys of Reported Marijuana Use by School

		School									
		1 Black		2 Chicano		3 Black		4 Anglo-lower		5 Anglo-upper	
Marijuana use		*N*	%	*N*	%	*N*	%	*N*	%	*N*	%
Yes	Preston	17	13.8	17	23.3	5	5.0	28	24.8	58	48.3
	Hays, 1970	12	10.5	15	24.2	2	5.0	48	37.5	46	36.2
	Hays, 1971	19	13.4	35	36.5	8	19.0	51	44.0	63	52.5
No	Preston	106	86.2	56	76.7	96	95.0	85	75.2	62	51.7
	Hays, 1970	102	89.5	47	75.8	38	95.0	80	62.5	81	63.8
	Hays, 1971	123	86.6	61	63.5	34	81.0	65	56.0	57	47.5

Table 2
Correlation Between Ranking of Five Schools by Percent of Marijuana Use Across Three Studies

Study	Hays, 1971	Hays, 1972
Preston	.90*	.90*
Hays, 1971		.90*

*$p > .05$.

instruments employed, each set of data was subjected to a chi-square analysis in order to determine whether the pattern of reported marijuana use among schools remains constant between surveys. Expected frequencies were obtained for each school, and chi-square analyses were run. Table 3 contains the expected frequencies of reported marijuana use, the obtained frequencies, and a summary of the chi-square test. All tests were significant ($p < .001$). Inspection of the data reveal that in all cases Schools 1, 2, and 3 are underrepresented in terms of reported marijuana users and Schools 4 and 5 are overrepresented.

Table 3
Chi-Square Analysis Among Schools for Three Surveys

Survey		School 1	2	3	4	5	χ^2
Preston	Yes	17[a]	17	5	28	58	
		29[b]	17.2	23.8	26.7	28.3	
							66.8*
	No	106	56	96	85	62	
		94	55.8	77.2	86.3	91.7	
Hays, 1971	Yes	12	15	2	48	46	
		29.8	16.2	10.4	33.4	33.1	
							39.1*
	No	102	47	38	80	81	
		84.2	45.8	29.6	94.6	93.8	
Hays, 1972	Yes	19	35	8	51	63	
		48.4	32.7	14.3	39.6	40.9	
							54.7*
	No	123	61	34	65	57	
		93.6	63.3	27.7	76.4	79.1	

[a]Theoretical frequency.
[b]Obtained frequency.
*$p > .001$, $df = 4$.

As a final check on the comparability of the Preston and Hays studies, an overall chi-square was performed across all three studies upon the data generated by the "yes" responders. The results of the analysis were non-significant, revealing that the proportion of reported marijuana users in each school is independent of the method used in gathering the data. Thus it appears that Preston's and Hays' survey instruments and sampling techniques were comparable, and that each produces reliable information about reported marijuana use in secondary schools. The different instruments and methodologies used by each investigator yielded data which were similar in pattern and frequency. Thus each study is a cross validation of the other.

Since the Preston and Hays data are comparable, chi-square analyses were performed to determine whether reported marijuana use had changed over the 3-year period encompassed by the studies. The results of the analyses revealed that there was no change in reported marijuana use in Schools 1, 2, and 3 in the 3-year period studied. In School 4, the predominantly White school within the lower-middle range of socioeconomic status, there was a significant increase in reported marijuana use ($\chi^2 = 3.93$; $df = 1$; $p < .05$) between Preston and Hays (1970) and between Hays (1971) ($\chi^2 = 8.50$; $df = 1$; $p < .01$). However, there was no increase between the two Hays studies ($\chi^2 = 0.80$; $df = 1$; n.s.). In School 5, the White school representing the upper-middle to lower-upper range of socioeconomic status, the only significant increase was found to be between the Hays' studies of 1970 and 1971 ($\chi^2 = 5.99$, $df = 1$; $p < .02$).

The three studies demonstrated the probability of reported marijuana use among high school students was almost one in four. The investigators also found that the incidence of reported marijuana use varied according to ethnicity, with Anglos most likely to use marijuana, Blacks least likely, and Mexican-Americans between Anglos and Blacks. Concurrently, it was found that when obtained frequencies were compared to expected frequencies for the general population without regard to ethnicity, Black and Mexican-American students were underrepresented and Anglo students were overrepresented in user groups. This trend was consistent over the 3 years encompassed in the studies. In relation to the ethnicity data, it was found that the incidence of reported marijuana use was lower in the low to lower-middle range of socioeconomic status and higher in the middle to upper-class range.

Several trends are noted in the above study. It appears that the reported use of marijuana was fairly stable over the 3 years covered by the study. The only significant increases were found in schools serving the middle to upper-class students which were predominately composed of Anglos. There were no significant increases found in schools serving the Black or Mexican-American students. Further, the pattern of reported marijuana use was stable, that is, Black and Mexican-Americans representing the lower end of the socioeconomic scale were underrepresented as marijuana consumers and Anglo students were overrepresented. Each of these studies has indicated that socioeconomic factors are positively related to marijuana use. The increase among the White middle class can be attributed to increasing affluence among this group of students, increased availability of marijuana, and acceptance of its use among young people. Among the Black and Mexican-American communities there is less affluence, closer police surveillance, and less peer acceptance of marijuana use. These findings need to be substantiated for other substances of abuse and a comparison needs to be made among studies which have used a variety of techniques for investigating the incidence of use for other drugs.

The data in these studies appear to substantiate claims that increasing marijuana use is a problem of the White middle-class and not of the minorities. However, it must be noted that the use of marijuana by minority and lower socioeconomic groups has not declined, but only remained constant. Future research and treatment of marijuana users should take into account social and ethnic background as significant variables. The educational system, because of its general charge for drug education, should develop programs which take into account the differential rates of use of drugs among ethnic groups. Further, parental education should occur to alert parents to the fact that marijuana use is a particular problem among the middle socioeconomic class rather than among the lower socioeconomic class. The use of marijuana is pandemic but does vary with ethnic and socioeconomic groups.

REFERENCES

HAYS, J.R. The incidence of drug abuse among secondary school students in Houston. *St. Joseph Hosp. Med. Surg. J.* 6: 52–59, 1971.

HAYS, J.R. The incidence of drug abuse among secondary school students in Houston, 1971. *St. Joseph Hosp. Med. Surg. J.* 7: 146–152, 1972.

PRESTON, J.D., and FRY, P.A. Marijuana use among Houston high school students. *Social Sci. Quart.* 52: 170–178, 1970.

The International Journal of the Addictions, 9(2), 337–343, 1974

Addict Attitudes toward Methadone Maintenance: A Preliminary Report*

Patricia B. Sutker, Ph.D.

Albert N. Allain, M.S.

Medical University of South Carolina
and Veteran's Administration Hospital
Charleston, South Carolina

Charles E. Moan, Ph.D.

Tulane University School of Medicine
New Orleans, Louisiana

In the past several years it has become obvious that methadone maintenance is a popular, if not necessary, treatment approach to the problem of heroin addiction. Indeed, many addicts unable to function on a drug-abstinent basis are required, encouraged, or voluntarily request methadone maintenance as a relatively long-term situation. Proponents of this treatment modality point to a reduction in crimes committed, a significant decrease in heroin use, and a rise in steady employment among methadone

*Requests for reprints should be mailed to Psychology Service, Veterans Administration Hospital, 109 Bee Street, Charleston, South Carolina 29403.

clients as evidence of its success (Dole, Nyswander, and Warner, 1968; Dole, Robinson, Orraca, Towns, Searcy, and Caine, 1969; Dole, 1971). On the other hand, Brown and his colleagues (1972) sampled staff and client attitudes toward methadone maintenance using the Adjective Check List (Gough and Heilbrun, 1965) and noted that addict-clients may not share the enthusiasm for methadone exhibited by program administrators. Specifically, ratings of client psychological effectiveness and general maturity were found to vary as a function of drug use, whether methadone or heroin. Although methadone clients were described in more positive terms than addicts on heroin, highest and significantly more favorable personality descriptions were attributed to addicts who had become drug free.

Similarly, frequently voiced client complaints, focusing on a variety of psychological and physiological problems described as corollaries of methadone maintenance, are a source of conflict and dissension in many comprehensive drug treatment programs. In view of such client observations and a paucity of comment or interest in the general acceptability of methadone as a treatment alternative, albeit a frequent last choice among many addict-clients, this investigation was designed to explore further the current opinions regarding methadone maintenance with special focus on reported attitudes of addict-clients as a possible function of their experience with methadone.

METHOD

Subjects

A total of 207 heroin addicts was selected from two population sources: addicts applying to the Narcotic Addict Rehabilitation Act Program (NA RA) over a 2-year period ($n = 143$) and prisoners with a history of heroin addiction selected from a random sample of 154 inmates serving sentences for a variety of offenses in state and local correctional institutions within the State of Louisiana ($n = 64$). All *S*s were literate, completed the questionnaire on a voluntary basis, and reported a consistent history of heroin abuse. Prior use of methadone was not a prerequisite for inclusion in the total sample as even methadone-naive *S*s are theoretically sufficiently informed by "hearsay" evidence to have formed relevant opinions which would undoubtedly affect their future use of methadone as a treatment modality.

Materials and Procedure

A personal opinion questionnaire containing 21 true-false statements concerning methadone maintenance was developed on the basis of frequently voiced remarks regarding methadone recorded in interviews with 36 heroin addicts who had been maintained on daily dosages of methadone greater than 50 mg for a period of at least 6 months. Topics of conversation raised in more than 50% of the nondirective interviews were included in the questionnaire, which was designed primarily as a rudimentary screening device. The questionnaire was then presented to 207 *S*s who were assembled in small groups for administration of a battery of psychological tests. Prospective addict-clients for the NARA Program and prison addicts were cautioned that their responses would in no way be related to possible availability of methadone or interpreted as either criticism or praise for a particular program in the geographical area. *S*s completed the questionnaire by providing their name, pertinent information relative to their criminal convictions, and total time served in adult correctional institutions. For purposes of statistical analyses, addicts were divided into four groups on the basis of their previous experience with methadone on a recognized maintenance program: no methadone experience ($n = 91$), methadone for 1 to 6 months ($n = 66$), methadone for 7 to 12 months ($n = 26$), and methadone for more than 12 months ($n = 24$). Table 1 provides a detailed description of the four groups with statistical comparisons for such variables as age, education, and criminal convictions. As indicated, *S*s were characterized by similar educational and criminal backgrounds; however, older addicts reported more experience with methadone and heroin than younger addicts.

RESULTS AND DISCUSSION

Responses of the total 207 addicts as a group, regardless of experience with methadone, were favorable on approximately half of the opinion statements and unfavorable on remaining items. Application of the Kuder-Richardson Formula 20, a measure of homogeneity of test items, showed a high degree of intercorrelation among opinion statements ($r = 0.76$). Percentages of agreement and disagreement for each item are presented in Table 2, where it is evident that the majority of addicts regarded methadone as an agent which gives addict-clients a new outlook and a second chance in life. They described methadone programs as generally beneficial rather than a waste of time and money. There was also overwhelming agreement to support the experimentally demonstrated claims that methadone helps addict-clients maintain a steady job, reduce their involvement in criminal activities such as stealing, and remain free of incarceration.

On the other hand, opinions were less favorable on items regarding

Table 1
Subject Characteristic Data for Four Groups of Heroin Addicts Divided on the Basis of Experience with Methadone

	0 months ($n = 91$), $\bar{x}$	1–6 months ($n = 66$), $\bar{x}$	7–12 months ($n = 26$), $\bar{x}$	Over 12 months ($n = 24$), $\bar{x}$	F
Age	25.57	27.08	29.88	31.17	5.77*
Highest grade completed	9.43	9.22	9.73	9.33	0.11
Months addicted to heroin	51.27	60.05	94.38	91.78	4.35*
Months addicted to heroin prior to methadone use		50.72	84.65	54.78	2.44
Adult felony convictions	2.97	3.06	3.42	3.17	0.42
Total months incarcerated	23.73	25.60	32.38	29.96	0.14

*$p < .01$.

the effects of methadone on physical functioning. Methadone was reported to produce a longer lasting effect than heroin, although only slightly less than half of the *S*s were of the opinion that ever-increasing dosages were necessary to remain physically comfortable. There was also agreement that methadone impaired sexual functioning as does heroin, and almost half of the *S*s complained methadone interfered with sexual functioning more than heroin use. Similarly, at least 50% of the addicts reported that methadone involves more physical risks than heroin and stated their preference for heroin over methadone regardless of the situation. Other reservations were obvious in that 85% of the addicts agreed that kicking methadone "cold turkey" was worse than kicking a heroin habit, and over one-fourth stated that they feared methadone and its effects to the extent that they would maintain their heroin habit rather than take methadone. Similarly, addicts agreed that methadone is "just another addiction," though only a little more than half felt it was another way of not dealing with their problems. It is interesting to note that skepticism was relatively high regarding the role of methadone as a preventive agent with regard to illicit drugs, and a strikingly large number either responded in the negative direction or offered no opinion (39%) to the statement that doctors do not really know what they are doing with methadone.

In a comparison of addict responses as a function of experience with

Table 2
Addict Agreement and Disagreement in Percentages on the Methadone Opinion Questionnaire (N = 207)

Item	Agree	Disagree
1. I prefer heroin over methadone regardless of the situation.	55	45
2. I think that taking methadone involves more physical risks than heroin.	50	50
3. I think that methadone gives me a longer lasting load than heroin.	73	25[a]
4. I think that kicking methadone "cold turkey" is definitely worse than kicking a heroin habit.	86	13
5. I think that taking methadone every day definitely keeps addicts out of trouble.	79	21
6. Addicts steal considerably less taking methadone.	93	6
7. Methadone has helped many addicts maintain a steady job.	97	2
8. Methadone interferes with my sexual functioning.	63	32
9. Heroin interferes with my sexual functioning.	63	36
10. Methadone interferes with my sexual functioning more than heroin.	49	44
11. I think methadone is just another addiction.	72	27
12. Methadone is just another way of not dealing with my problems.	57	41
13. I think in general methadone programs are beneficial.	85	14
14. I actually fear methadone and its effects, and I will maintain my heroin habit rather than take methadone.	26	73
15. I think in general methadone programs are a waste of time and money.	8	92
16. A person really needs higher and higher doses of methadone to feel comfortable.	38	59
17. Methadone gives addicts a second chance in life.	84	16
18. Methadone keeps addicts from taking illicit drugs such as goof balls.	42	58
19. The methadone program gives addicts a new outlook on life.	77	22
20. Methadone is responsible for keeping many addicts out of prison.	93	7
21. Doctors don't really know what they are doing with methadone.	26	61

[a]Totals falling short of 100% reflect a certain percentage of "no responses" to the specific item.

methadone maintenance, opinions differed significantly from the overall sample on only a few items. Addicts having experience with methadone over time tended to agree with the statement that methadone interferes with their sexual functioning significantly more frequently than those who had never used methadone or had little experience with the drug ($\chi^2 = 16.13$, $df = 6$, $p < .05$). A similar trend was observed in response to the item stating that methadone interferes with sexual functioning more than heroin. Those having never used methadone endorsed this statement in only 31% of the cases, while the percentage rose to 70% for those who had used methadone for 1 year or more ($\chi^2 = 27.34$, $df = 6$, $p < 0.01$). Substantially fewer *S*s indicated that methadone keeps addicts from taking illicit drugs as their experience with methadone increased ($\chi^2 = 14.95$, $df = 6$, $p < .05$). Although not statistically significant, the percentage of *S*s who felt that methadone gives addicts a new outlook on life declined with increased methadone use.

In view of the rapid growth of methadone maintenance facilities and an ever-increasing emphasis on this treatment resource, it is interesting to note with Brown et al. (1972) that addict-clients have reservations regarding the use of methadone which have implications for planning more effective maintenance programs as well as individual rehabilitative strategies. In addition to their more general concern to be wholly free from any type of addiction, addicts become more preoccupied with problems in physical functioning as their experience with methadone increases over time. The constellation of physical concern includes a fear of kicking what they feel to be a more binding addiction and worry over inadequacies in sexual performance. Although convinced that methadone maintenance programs aid them in remaining free of criminal involvement and periods of incarceration, addicts admit that methadone in itself does not prevent them from obtaining and using illicit drugs. To what extent such opinions are influenced by staff attitudes is unknown; however, it is probably true that they are maintained in spite of staff reassurances and counterarguments. These preliminary results suggest that many addict-clients are dissatisfied with long-term methadone maintenance, though they find it significantly more beneficial than alternatives such as incarceration or continued heroin addiction. In addition, they highlight the need for increased efforts to find a heroin substitute with fewer physical corollaries, whether imagined or real, as well as careful attitude assessment, psychological preparation, and continued medical supervision for individual methadone clients.

ACKNOWLEDGMENTS

This research was supported in part by the National Institute of Mental Health, Health Services and Mental Health Administration, United States Department of Health, Education and Welfare, through Contract PH–43–68–1520 administered through the Department of Psychiatry and Neurology, Tulane University School of Medicine. Appreciation is expressed to Chester B. Scrignar and Gary H. Cohen, past and present directors of the NARA program which provided a source of unincarcerated heroin addicts.

REFERENCES

BROWN, B.S., BASS, U.F., GAUVEY, S.K., and KOZEL, N.J. Staff and client attitudes toward methadone maintenance. *Intern. J. Addictions* 7: 247–255, 1972.

DOLE, V.P. Methadone maintenance treatment for 25,000 heroin addicts. *J. Amer. Med. Assoc.* 215: 1131–1134, 1971.

DOLE, V.P. NYSWANDER, M.E., and WARNER, A. Successful treatment of 750 criminal addicts. *J. Amer. Med. Assoc.* 206: 2708–2711, 1968.

DOLE, V.P., ROBINSON, J.W., ORRACA, J., TOWNS, E., SEARCY, P., and CAINE, E. Methadone treatment of randomly selected criminal addicts. *New England J. Med.* 208: 1372–1375, 1969.

GOUGH, H.G., and HEILBRUN, A.B. *The Adjective Check List Manual.* Palo Alto, California: Consulting Psychologists Press, 1965.

The International Journal of the Addictions, 9(2), 345–350, 1974

Research Note

Epidemiological Studies of Female Prisoners. II: Biological, Psychological, and Social Correlates of Drug Addiction

Carlos E. Climent, M.D.

Universidad del Valle
School of Medicine
Cali, Colombia

Anthony Raynes, M.D.

Harvard University Medical School
Cambridge, Massachusetts

Ann Rollins, M.A.

Massachusetts General Hospital
Boston, Massachusetts

Robert Plutchik, Ph.D.

Albert Einstein College of Medicine
Boston, Massachusetts

*Reprints are available from the senior author.

INTRODUCTION

This paper is concerned with identifying some of the factors which are associated with heroin addiction among female criminals who are already in the prison system.

Types of variables studied include medical, psychiatric, and socio-demographic variables. The basic comparisons which are made are between female heroin addicts in the prison and those female prisoners who reported never using any kinds of illegal drugs.

One advantage of this method of approach is that it provides an approximate way of matching the women on degree of social deviancy. Differences which may then be found will reflect the influence of addiction rather than of incarceration per se.

METHOD

The study was carried out during May 1970 at the Framingham Institution for Women in Framingham, Massachusetts and was part of a larger study in which extensive information was obtained on about 96 prisoners (volunteers) out of a total population of 158 (Climent et al., 1973). The comparison was made between 42 women judged to be heroin addicts at the time of commitment and 24 women who did not use illegal drugs. Medical variables investigated included a medical neurological examination, dermatoglyphic analysis, and a standardized medical questionnaire. Psychiatric variables included psychiatric evaluation by a psychiatrist, the MMPI, and review of medical psychiatric records. Social variables included a standardized questionnaire and a review of criminal records.

The determination of whether or not a woman belonged to the heroin addiction group (H) or was a nondrug user (ND) was made through the agreement of the physician's evaluation and a self-assessment questionnaire. The presence of depressive elements was measured in three ways: (1) By the MMPI depression scale, (2) through clinical evaluation, and (3) according to a list of 13 objective symptoms considered indicative of depression. Childhood neuroticism was measured by a 20-item scale which collected information on pyromania, cruelty to animals, enuresis, thumb-sucking, and several other events. This instrument yields a quantitative score determined by the frequency of "yes" responses.

RESULTS

Sociodemographic Factors

As might be predicted, birth in an urban setting and continued urban dwelling are associated with heroin use. Table 1 shows that 21.7% of the ND user group were born in a big city (defined as having a population of more than 500,000) as compared to 34.1% of the heroin users; 30.4% of the ND group are urban dwellers in adulthood, while 51.2% of heroin addicts are urban dwellers.

Regarding age, the heroin group is somewhat younger, (29.5 vs 25.3 years), and using a *T* test for proportion, significantly more heroin users are under the age of 20 ($p < .05$). With respect to religious affiliation, the sample contains an almost equal number of Protestants and Catholics. Significantly more nondrug users are divorced than are heroin addicts, but there are no differences on any of the other marital statuses.

Table 1
Demographic Differences Between Female Prisoners Who Use Or Do Not Use Heroin

	Nondrug users (N = 24)		Heroin users (N = 42)	
Variables	%	No.	%	No.
Born in big city	21.7	5	34.1	14
Live in big city	30.4	7	51.2	21
Religion				
Protestant	56.5	13	40.5	17
Catholics	39.1	9	52.4	22
Jewish	0.0	0	4.8	2
None	4.3	1	2.4	1
Marital status				
Single	50.5	12	61.0	25
Married	12.5	3	19.5	8
Divorced	25.0*	6	7.3	3
Separated	8.3	2	9.8	4
Widowed	4.2	1	2.4	1
Age				
Under 20	16.7	4	40.5*	17
20–25	37.5	9	30.9	13
Over 25	45.9	11	28.6	12
Mean age	29.5		25.3	
Mean age of first conviction	20.7		20.7	

*Significant at the .05 level.

Descriptive and Psychological Aspects

Table 2 presents psychiatric information regarding the two groups under study.

The heroin users reported fewer "child guidance center contacts" but a substantially higher frequency of "adult psychiatric outpatient contacts." There were no differences between the two groups in the number of psychiatric hospitalizations.

Regarding the variable of "depression," no differences were found between the two groups on any of the measures used to evaluate depressive states. However, the heroin addicts reported more suicidal thoughts at a near significant level ($p < .10$) than did the nondrug users, and more suicide attempts (62% vs 46%). No differences between these two groups were found on MMPI scales.

Medical Parameters

Regarding EEG abnormalities, out of a total of 23 EEG's taken in the ND group, five were considered abnormal or borderline. In the heroin user group, out of 39 taken, seven were considered abnormal or borderline. None of these differences were significant. No significant differences were found on IQ (93 vs 88) or on frequency of birth problems, head trauma, seizures, neurological disorders, medical disorders in relatives, age of

Table 2
Psychological Differences Between Female Prisoners Who Use Or Do Not Use Heroin

	Nondrug users ($N = 24$)	Heroin users ($N = 42$)
Mean number of adult psychiatric out-patient contacts	1.0	3.8
Mean number of adult psychiatric hospitalizations	0.28	0.26
Mean number of child guidance center contacts	2.6	0.75
Mean number of symptoms indicating neuroticism in childhood	2.7	3.5
Number of subjects reporting suicidal thoughts	13	32*
Number of subjects reporting suicidal attempts	11	26

*$p = < .10$.

menarche, or menstrual patterns (duration, severity of flow, or extent of physical discomfort).

DISCUSSION

A number of medical and social history variables were studied in addition to the ones reported here. Few showed any significant differences between the H and ND groups. The major differences between the two groups seemed to be that the heroin addicts were somewhat younger, that they were less likely to be identified early as problem children in a child guidance clinic, that they had more psychiatric outpatient contacts as adults, and that they had more suicidal thoughts and suicide attempts than the nondrug users.

These findings suggest the hypothesis that heroin addiction is perceived by the addict as a painful, unpleasant state requiring psychiatric contact as an adult, and that the style of life associated with it which leads to prison incarceration increases the problem. The findings also suggest the possibility that the pattern of life leading to prison is different for the heroin addict than for the nonaddict prisoner. The fact that heroin addicts do not have early contact with child guidance clinics may imply that emotional problems for addicts occur later in life, and only as an adult does the addict and her family seek psychiatric help. The nonaddict prisoner is more likely to have a lifelong pattern of antisocial behavior. It is also likely that the types of crimes for which the two groups are incarcerated is also different.

As the addict enacts the life pattern created by addiction, she develops suicidal thoughts and tends to make suicidal attempts. As a practical implication, prison officials should consider that female prisoners who have a history of heroin addiction are more serious suicidal risks than are other prisoners. In addition, such prisoners are probably more likely to be accepting of psychiatric contacts and efforts at rehabilitation than the nonaddict prisoners.

Further research should look more closely into types of crimes associated with incarceration as well as the early life style characteristics of such prisoners.

ACKNOWLEDGMENTS

This research was supported by NDH grant No. Ro112119605 and LEAA Grant Ni 72–0230. We wish to thank Mrs. Betty Cole Smith, Dr. Ken Bishop, and all the staff at the Framingham Institution for Women for their cooperation and the inmates for their participation in the study.

REFERENCE

CLIMENT, C.E., ROLLINS, A., ERVIN, F., and PLUTCHIK, R. Epidemiological studies of female prisoners, I: Medical and psychiatric variables related to violent behavior. *Amer. J. Psychiat.* 130: 9, September 1973.

The International Journal of the Addictions, 9(2), 351–354, 1974

Research Note

Progression Time to Narcotic Use in a Southwestern Addict Population

Charles R. Lett, M.D.

C. Robert Ingram, Jr., Ph.D.

Methadone Clinic
Dallas County Mental Health and Mental Retardation Center
Dallas, Texas

The stepping-stone theory highlights the qualitative process of progressing from minor to major chemical abuse. The authors were interested in the time lapse in the progression from the first illicit drug to narcotics. Valid observations on the progression time should have both epidemiologic and therapeutic relevance. This study, therefore, investigated the time interval associated with this phenomena in a sample of narcotic users in Dallas, Texas.

All narcotic addicts presenting at the methadone clinic, Dallas County MH-MR Center, District VI, for evaluation and treatment from February 1970 to August 1972 were interviewed by a staff member. A questionnaire was completed by the staff member based on responses from the subject and included demographic, social, legal, psychological, and medical data. All 460 questionnaires received during the first 18 months of clinic operation were reviewed. Eight questionnaires were incomplete, 452 questionnaires were complete. For reasons unknown to the authors, very few

Mexican-American narcotic addicts ($N = 23$) presented at the methadone clinic. Because of this small sample size, they were excluded from the comparative analysis.

Responses to questions concerning sex, ethnicity, initial illegal drug used, age of first use of the illegal drug, and age of first use of heroin were obtained from the 429 remaining questionnaires. The difference between the age of first use of illegal drugs and first use of heroin was then calculated. This figure, along with the initial drug, were then subjected to statistical analysis.

The data of this study consisted of both the initial illicit drug used and the total number of years elapsed between first illicit drug usage and first experience with heroin. This data, categorized by sex and ethnic groups (Black and White), are presented in Table 1. Here will be found the total number of persons in each group who fall into each of the various "years elapsed" categories.

Data were initially analyzed using the Kruskal-Wallis analysis of variance for ranked data. The resultant value of "H" was greater than 40 ($p < .001$).

Table 1

Race–Sex Distribution of Progression Time

Progression time (in years) from first use of illicit drug to first use of heroin	Black male	White male	Black female	White female
Less than 1	32	32	25	20
1	23	26	22	5
2	16	5	8	5
3	22	5	8	4
4	13	9	6	3
5	13	8	6	2
6	8	2	3	1
7	15	2	2	2
8	6	3	2	0
9	6	1	1	0
10	2	1	1	0
11	5	0	0	0
12	11	1	3	0
13	5	0	0	1
14	1	0	11	1
15	2	0	0	0
16+	4	0	0	0
Median	3 years	1 year	2 years	1 year

Table 2
Mann-Whitney Comparisons

Groups compared	U	z
Black male vs White male	32,139	4+*
White male vs White female	4,676	4+*
Black female vs White female	4,030	4+*
Black female vs Black male	17,783	4+*

*$p < .001$.

In an attempt to shed light on the differences revealed in the above analysis, several two-group comparisons were made using the Mann-Whitney U test. The results summarized in Table 2 indicate that statistically reliable ($p < .001$) differences existed between the two groups in all four comparisons made. It is realized that these findings, along with those that follow, are based on a "post-hoc" view of the data; however, the major attempt of the present study is to describe differences found in an existing population of heroin addicts rather than to make inferences as a result of experimental manipulation.

A closer, more qualitative view of the data was then made in an attempt to investigate other areas of possible difference among the members of the population studies. These possible differences were subjected to analysis using the χ^2 technique.

One of the more obvious of these differences was found in the type of illegal drug used during one's first experience with illicit drugs. It appeared that a disproportionately larger number of Whites (both male and female) had their first drug experience with opiates while Blacks, for the most part, began their drug abusing history with either marihuana or barbiturates. For example, 16 Black males (9% of all Black males) and 10 Black females (10%) began their drug abuse with heroin while 14 White males (14%) and 6 White females (14%) used heroin in their first experience.

Another apparent difference that existed between the ethnic groups was in the time elapsed between the first experience with illegal drugs and first experience with heroin. Approximately 66% of the White subjects as opposed to less than 40% of the Black subjects began their narcotic use less than 2 years following their first illegal use of drugs. These differences, again, are statistically significant ($\chi^2 = 21.2$, $df = 3$, $p < .01$).

The major findings of the present study are that there were ethnic differences in progression time from first abuse of a drug to first abuse of heroin. Perhaps related to this finding were the supplemental results that the White drug abuser was more likely to begin his drug abuse history with the use of heroin and that significantly more Whites began using heroin within 2 years of their first experience with drugs.

It has been noted in past investigations that different classes of drugs attract persons of different psychopathological groups. Perhaps an explanation of the present data may be found at this level. In addition, there are some obvious suggestions for further research in the economic and social spheres. More important, however, are the implications related to the prevention of heroin addiction. In spite of the fact that persons do not usually present for therapy in a methadone clinic until addiction to heroin has become a fact, it is conceivable that preventive programs could be developed as natural outgrowths of these clinics. The present data could be of importance in these efforts.

SUMMARY

This study examined the time interval associated with the progression of first illegal drug use to narcotic use. Four hundred fifty-two questionnaires completed by narcotic addicts presenting at the Dallas County MH-MR Methadone Clinic were used to obtain data.

The results revealed differences in progression time for both sex and ethnic groups. The major ethnic groups in this sample were Black and White. The Chicano group was too small for valid analysis. Whites had a shorter progression time than Blacks. The Black male had a significantly longer progression time than the Black female, White female, or White male groups.

The lack of sufficient, relevant data in the literature precluded any valid comparative analysis with other narcotic samples.

The implications of this study should stimulate more exploration and investigations for validation and exploration of progression time to narcotic and should be useful in preventive efforts.

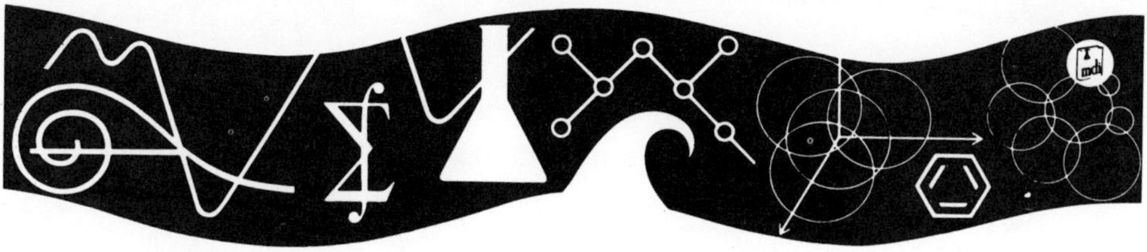

A Statement of Purpose

INSTITUTE FOR THE STUDY OF DRUG MISUSE, Inc.

The Institute for the Study of Drug Misuse, Inc. (formerly the Institute for the Study of Drug Addiction) was established in 1965 as an international organization to develop clear channels of communication and to encourage research in the field of drug abuse. To fulfill its goals, the Institute participates in research, professional training, and education. In addition, it serves as a consulting agency in the establishment of treatment programs in the United States and abroad. As professional, government, and lay concern increases in the field of drug abuse, the Institute has been called upon to serve as a resource agency for the dissemination of scientific materials through the press, television, radio, and other media.

In order to achieve its purposes, the Institute for the Study of Drug Misuse:

Sponsors the INTERNATIONAL JOURNAL OF THE ADDICTIONS, published by Marcel Dekker, Inc.

Sponsors national and international conferences and workshops in cooperation with universities, medical teaching centers, governmental agencies, and private industry.

Sponsors a lecture series "The Use and Misuse of Drugs and Alcohol," for professionals and interested lay people.

Sponsors international awards for significant research reports focusing upon various aspects of drug abuse.

The expanding programs of the Institute have been dictated by the present crisis in drug abuse. It is apparent that in the United States and in the world at large, certain social forces are at work which have magnified the scope of the problem. In order to insure that the Institute reaches the broadest group of interested individuals, it has become necessary to establish several categories of membership.

Membership in the Institute for the Study of Drug Misuse is tax exempt.

For membership information, write:

Institute for the Study of Drug Misuse, Inc.
111 Fifth Avenue
New York, N.Y. 10003

INFORMATION FOR AUTHORS SUBMITTING MANUSCRIPTS

Send a clear double-spaced typewritten original and two duplicate copies to the Editor, *International Journal of the Addictions*, Institute for the Study of Drug Misuse, Inc., 111 Fifth Avenue, New York, N.Y. 10003. DOUBLE-SPACE the entire manuscript; do not use single spacing anywhere.

Include authors' academic degrees and present affiliation. If applicable, cite auspices under which work being reported was done. Specify address to which requests for reprints should be sent.

Begin your TITLE with a word useful in indexing. Put news of your finding or a statement of the problem first. Major and minor headings may be used in the text; indicate major headings by typing in capitals. Provide a 100-word SUMMARY at the end.

Use METRIC UNITS of measure. If measurements were made in English units, give metric equivalents.

Cite all TABLES and FIGURES in the text. Tables should have titles, and figures should have brief legends. In tables, give each column a heading. Indicate units of measure in parentheses in the heading for each column. Do not use vertical rules. Do not use horizontal rules other than those in the heading and at the bottom. Submit PHOTOGRAPHS as glossy prints, untrimmed and unmounted; identify each with pencil lightly on the back and indicate top.

ARTWORK will not be returned unless specifically requested, and will be disposed of three months after publication.

REFERENCES in the text should be enclosed in parentheses and include the author's surname and the date of the item cited. Keep footnotes to a minimum.

The BIBLIOGRAPHY (double-spaced) should be given at the end of the article in alphabetical order. Journal references should include authors, title, name of journal abbreviated according to *Chemical Abstracts List of Periodicals,* inclusive page numbers, and date. Book references should include authors, title, place of publication, publisher, and date.

CLINICAL TOXICOLOGY

Volume 7 Number 2 1974

CONTENTS OF THIS ISSUE

CHARLES L. WINEK, EARLE R. DAVIS, W. D. COLLOM, AND S. P. SHANOR: Quinine Fatality—Case Report 129

P. H. JOUBERT AND J. A. OLIVIER: Fatal Suicidal Ingestion of Thioridazine 133

SYMPOSIUM ON COMPARATIVE TOXICOLOGY: THE RELATIONSHIP BETWEEN ANIMALS AND HUMANS

FREDERICK W. OEHME: Comparative Toxicology Is Where It's At 139

D. L. NELSON: Evaluation of the Safety of Agricultural Chemicals 141

W. E. RIDDER AND F. W. OEHME: Nitrates as an Environmental, Animal, and Human Hazard 145

PAUL M. NEWBERNE: The New World of Mycotoxins—Animal and Human Health 161

WALTER ED BREWER: Effects of Noise Pollution on Animal Behavior 179

Abstracts of Unpublished Papers Presented at the Symposium on Comparative Toxicology: The Relationship between Animals and Humans 191

RICHARD F. KEELER: Coniine, A Teratogenic Principle from Conium maculatum Producing Congenital Malformations in Calves 195

ABSTRACTS

The American Academy of Clinical Toxicology, San Diego, California; July-August 1973 207

NEWS ITEM 229

A complimentary copy will be sent on request

Contributions to This Journal Are Published Free of Charge

MARCEL DEKKER, INC., New York

THE INTERNATIONAL JOURNAL OF THE ADDICTIONS

Published by Marcel Dekker, Inc., New York
Sponsored by The Institute for the Study of Drug Misuse, Inc., New York

THE INTERNATIONAL JOURNAL OF THE ADDICTIONS

Volume 9 Number 2 1974

CONTENTS

Chemical Mutagenesis and Drugs of Abuse in Man—A Current View of the Problem: Arthur Falek ... 171

Multidrug Use: Supplementary Perspectives: Paul C. Whitehead ... 185

British Opiate Users: II. Differences between Those Given an Opiate Script and Those Not Given One: Herbert H. Blumberg, S. Daryl Cohen, B. Elizabeth Dronfield, Elizabeth A. Mordecai, J. Colin Roberts, and David Hawks ... 205

The Relationship between Age and/or Negative Experiences and Success on a Methadone Maintenance Program: Thomas Henchy, Byron Eckerson, and Jesse L. Paez ... 221

Evolution of a Treatment Approach for Young Heroin Addicts. Comparison of Three Treatment Modalities: Raymond A. Lloyd, Richard N. Katon, and Robert L. DuPont ... 229

The College Opiate User: Betty Crowther ... 241

Personality Characteristics of Heroin Addicts in a Methadone Treatment Program: An Exploratory Study: Arthur G. Cryns ... 255

Personality Traits and Attitudes and Their Relationship to Student Drug Using Behavior: Joseph Powell Stokes ... 267

Patterns of Drug Abuse: Richard S. Campbell and Jeffrey B. Freeland ... 289

Patterns of Multiple Drug Abuse: 1969–1971: D. Dwayne Simpson and S. B. Sells ... 301

Heroin Addict Clients' Descriptions of Their Families of Origin: Carolyn A. Eldred, Barry S. Brown, and Cynthia Mahabir ... 315

Marihuana Use by College Students: Three-Year Trends, 1970–1972: Douglas P. Ferraro and David K. Billings ... 321

Marijuana Use in Urban Secondary Schools: A Three-Year Comparison: Robert Bloom, J. Ray Hays, and G. Michael Winburn ... 329

Addict Attitudes toward Methadone Maintenance: A Preliminary Report: Patricia B. Sutker, Albert N. Allain, and Charles E. Moan ... 337

Research Notes

Epidemiological Studies of Female Prisoners. II: Biological, Psychological, and Social Correlates of Drug Addiction: Carlos E. Climent, Anthony Raynes, Ann Rollins, and Robert Plutchik ... 345

Progression Time to Narcotic Use in a Southwestern Addict Population: Charles R. Lett and C. Robert Ingram, Jr. ... 351

Cover illustration: "Sunrise oft proclaims its verdict and its woe."
From the Illustrated London News and Sketch, December 25, 1897.
Courtesy of the Picture Collection, The Branch Libraries, New York Public Library.

MARCEL DEKKER, INC., New York

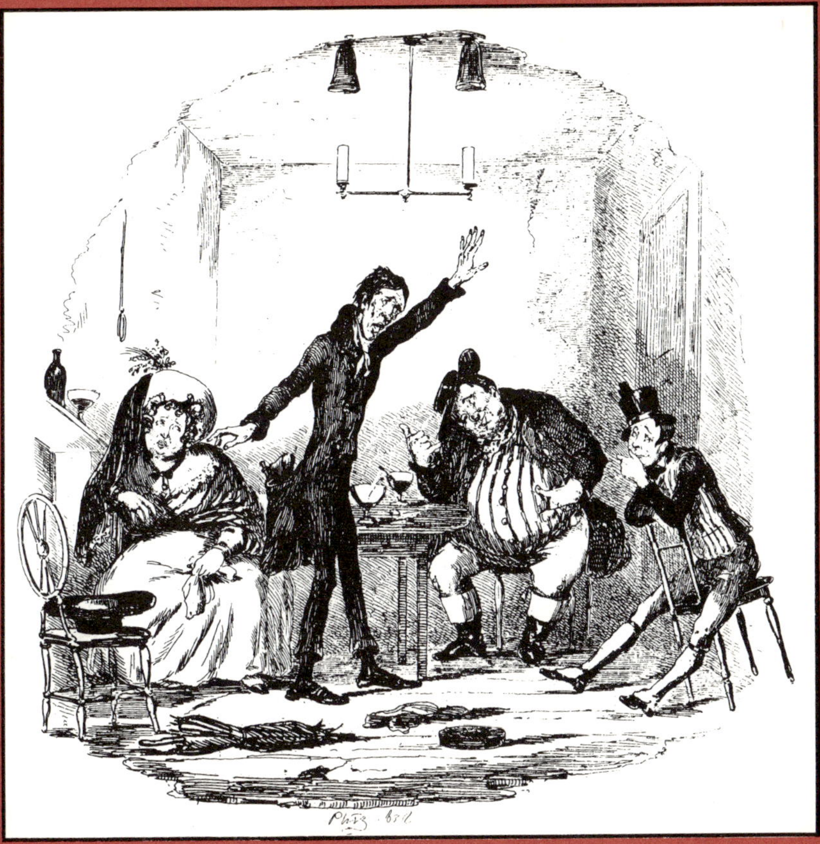

THE INTERNATIONAL JOURNAL OF THE Addictions

Volume 9 Number 3 1974

THE INTERNATIONAL JOURNAL OF THE ADDICTIONS

See inside back cover

The International Journal of the Addictions, June 1974

Published six times annually—February, April, June, August, October, December—by Marcel Dekker, Inc., 270 Madison Avenue, New York, N. Y. 10016. The subscription rate for Volume 9 (1974), containing 6 issues is $40.00 (prepaid). Postage outside the United States is $5.10 per volume for all subscriptions. The special discounted rate for individual professionals and students is $20.00. Back volume prices will be sent on request. Please *mail payment with order* to the following address: Marcel Dekker Journals, P. O. Box 11305, Church Street Station, New York, New York 10249.

Second-class postage paid at New York, N. Y., and at additional mailing offices.

Contributions to This Journal Are Published Free of Charge

The International Journal of the Addictions, 9(3), 355–363, 1974

Mortality in an Alcoholic Cohort

Raymond M. Costello, Ph.D.

Department of Psychiatry
The University of Texas Health Science Center at San Antonio
and Bexar County Mental Health and Mental Retardation Center
Alcohol Treatment Program
San Antonio, Texas

Sandra Lee Schneider, MT (ASCP) BB

Southwest Foundation for Research and Education
San Antonio, Texas

Numerous investigators have replicated the finding that members of alcoholic cohorts die at a rate far higher than expected on the basis of comparison with a general population. The finding has been found to be stable also when the appropriate age and sex corrections are applied to the general population data. If an issue yet exists in this regard, it involves only the precise measurement and not the form or general direction of the phenomenon. Tashiro and Lipscomb (1963), for example, reported an observed to expected ratio of about 2.5:1 for death from all causes, Schmidt and deLint (1972) reported a ratio of 2:1 for men and 3:1 for women, and Brenner (1967) reported a ratio of 7:1 for deaths from accidents of all types.

Yet at issue, however, is the role played by abuse of alcohol in the different modes of death and at different ages at death. Jellinek (1942) introduced the issue when he defined more precisely the phrase, "death from alcoholism" and when he exposed certain long-held beliefs as myths or methodological artifacts. More currently, Dahlgren (1951) has written that the social and mental consequences of alcohol abuse outweigh the physical damage consequences, as he found that excess mortality in alcoholic cohorts was accounted for primarily by the parameter of deaths by violent causes, drowning, accidents, and suicide. He also found that the chronological ages 40 to 55 were the primary years of excess mortality for his sample. Schmidt and deLint (1972) replicated the finding of excess mortality from violent causes, accidents, and suicides, but also reported that the largest share of excess deaths was attributed to heart disease, with other chronic physical disease states also overrepresented. They found excess mortality over an extended chronological age range from 22 to 60 years.

PROBLEM

This investigation sought to explicate certain aspects of the above issue. It sought to determine the case fatality rate in an alcoholic cohort, or the rate at which members of the alcoholic cohort died from all causes; to determine if the case fatality rate varied over time as the follow-up progressed; to determine alcoholic cohort cause-specific mortality rates, or the rate at which deaths in the sample were attributable to various causes; to determine if cause-specific mortality rates differed from like rates in the general population; to determine if age at death was related to specific causes; and to determine if cause of death varied over time as the follow-up progressed.

METHOD

The employed method of investigation was a retrospective, longitudinal cohort study (MacMahon and Pugh, 1970). The alcoholic cohort consisted of 400 clients of an alcoholic rehabilitation center, newly admitted to the center in 1963 ($N = 100$), 1964 ($N = 100$), 1967 ($N = 100$), and 1970 ($N = 100$). Only first admissions were included as the parameter "first admission to the center" was employed as an operational definition of first public identification of the individual as a chronic alcohol abuser. The local community, treatment resources and follow-up methodology have been previously reported (Costello, Bechtel, and Giffen, 1973). Circumstances of death and age at death were derived from the death certificate in each case and from autopsy reports when available. Deaths were recorded as of January 1 for each year following identification. Thus the 1963 sample was followed longitudinally for 9 years, the 1964 was followed for 8 years, the 1967 sample for 5 years, and the 1970 sample for 2 years.

RESULTS

Ninety-five cases, 28 from the 1963 group, 37 from the 1964 group, 20 from the 1967 group, and 10 from the 1970 group, were located as deceased. The overall case fatality rate was .0459, with 95 deaths tabulated for 2069 person-years of observation. The overall case fatality rate was only roughly compared to the local general population rate as this was not of primary interest in this investigation. Vital statistics of Bexar County deaths in 1970 indicated that 5,667 deaths occurred in a general county population of approximately 687,000. This would indicate a general uncorrected mortality rate of .0083 (this rate is representative also of the 5 years previous to 1970), a figure far less than the case fatality rate in the alcoholic sample. Although this is an uncorrected estimate, it is quite doubtful that a more accurate figure would contradict the conclusion that deaths in the alcoholic sample were far beyond expectations.

Table 1 displays the case fatality rate for each of the nine follow-up years successively, and for the cumulative person-years of observation. Mortality in excess of the overall case fatality rate was observed in follow-up years one, two, five, and six, and was less frequent in years three, four, seven, eight, and nine.

Table 1
Follow-up Intervals, Person-Years of Observation, and Case Fatality Rates, Successive and Cumulative[a]

I	PYI	NI	CFR/I	CPY	CN	CFR/CPY
1	400	21	.0525	400	21	.0525
2	379	19	.0501	779	40	.0518
3	270	11	.0407	1049	51	.0486
4	259	11	.0425	1308	62	.0474
5	248	12	.0483	1556	74	.0475
6	156	13	.0833	1712	87	.0508
7	143	4	.0279	1855	91	.0491
8	139	1	.0072	1994	92	.0461
9	75	3	.0400	2069	95	.0459

[a] I = interval; PYI = person-years per interval; NI = number of deaths per interval; CFR = case fatality rate; CPY = cumulative person-years; CN = cumulative number of deaths. Also, CFR/I = NI/PYI and CFR/CPY = CN/CPY.

Cause-specific mortality rates were: polycythemia vera (.0105), amytrophic lateral sclerosis (.0105), spinal meningitis (.0211), renal failure from various causes (.0316), pneumonia (.0316), cerebral lesions (.0632), carcinomas of all types (.0632), acute ethanol intoxication (.0737), cirrhosis (.0947), violent deaths (.2105), and cardiovascular disease of various types (.3895). Thirteen percent of the deaths were attributable to seven causes; none considered to play a significant role beyond expectations as determined by cause-specific rates in the general population. In fact, deaths attributable to carcinomas and cerebral lesions were underrepresented as Bexar County population rates for these causes for 1970 were 0.176 and 0.108, respectively. Seventeen percent of the deaths were attributable to two causes, both indicative of alcohol abuse (i.e., cirrhosis and acute intoxication). Only 2 % of the general population deaths in 1970 were attributable to these causes. The leading causes of death in the alcohol sample were cardiovascular diseases (39 %) and violent deaths (21 %), accounting for 60 % of all deaths. These two causes accounted for approximately 42 % of all deaths in Bexar County in 1970; 34 % attributable to cardiovascular diseases and 8 % to violent deaths.

Mean age at death for each cause of death was: polycythemia vera 81, SD = 0; amytrophic lateral sclerosis 56, SD = 0; spinal meningitis 40, SD = 0; renal failure 62.3, SD = 16.3; pneumonia 48.3, SD = 4.8; cerebral lesions 59.6, SD = 12.6; carcinomas 57.3, SD = 6.8; acute intoxication 44.6, SD = 6.1; cirrhosis 55.1, SD = 6.4; violent deaths 41.5, SD = 12; and cardiovascular disease 64.7, SD = 11.6. Overall mean age at death was 55.5 years. A one-way analysis of variance of ages, corrected for unequal numbers of observations per cell, was performed for each of the six leading causes of death to determine if age at death and cause of death were related. A statistically significant F of 11.05 ($p < .001$, $df = 5, 79$) was achieved. Violent deaths and deaths by acute alcohol intoxication occurred at younger ages, whereas deaths due to cardiovascular diseases, cirrhosis, carcinomas, and cerebral lesions occurred at older ages.

The criterion, proportion of deaths in interval minus proportion of deaths in total sample × 100, was calculated for each of the four leading causes of death to determine if cause of death was related to follow-up period. The greater the deviation from zero, the stronger was the association of cause with follow-up period. The follow-up intervals were collapsed to thirds for ease of visual display and of analysis of trends. Thus three follow-up periods were analyzed; 1–2–3, 4–5–6, and 7–8–9. Figure 1 displays the results of this analysis. Note that deaths due to cardiovascular diseases were strongly overrepresented in the follow-up period of years

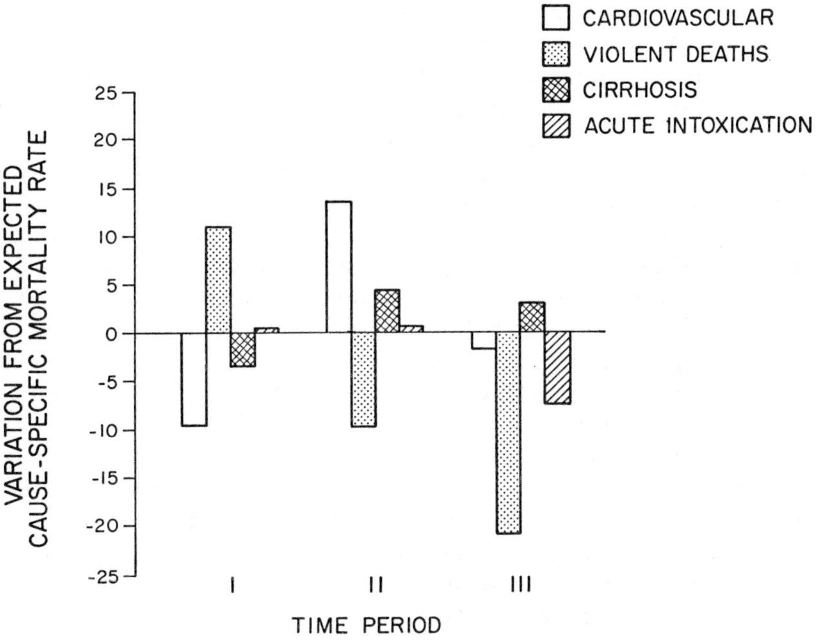

Fig. 1. Variation of cause-specific mortality over time.

4–5–6. Violent deaths were strongly overrepresented in the early follow-up period, years 1–2–3. Deaths due to cirrhosis occurred most frequently in the middle and late follow-up years. Deaths due to acute intoxication were observed in early and middle follow-up years, but did not occur in late follow-up years.

DISCUSSION

This investigation explored various facets of mortality in an alcoholic cohort. First, the observed case fatality rate (0.0459) and mean age at death (55.5 years) suggested that this group was selectively sampled from the general population.

Second, the case fatality rate varied over time, as did cause-specific mortality. The case fatality rate and violent mortality showed concomitant variation as these variables were observed to peak in the years soon after first identification of the cohort. It thus appeared that the early follow-up period was a time of crisis or violence for certain members of the cohort.

Risk of violent death appeared to be highest for those who were younger, most often between the ages of 29 and 53. Nine (45%) of the violent deaths involved automobiles. Six of these involved the victim as driver and three involved the victim as pedestrian. The victim-drivers died at ages 21, 29, 30, 30, 34, and 42, whereas the victim-pedestrians died at ages 47, 53, and 55. The victim-drivers posed both an acute individual and a social risk as they were young, mobile, and had an automobile at their disposal. The victim-pedestrians were older and could be stereotyped as chronic public inebriates. Carlson (1972) surveyed studies of the role of alcohol in automobile accidents and concluded both that alcohol was involved in many fatal crashes and that the inexperienced or young drinking driver was a very important contributor to alcohol-related crashes. Carlson reported that it was generally felt that reduction of alcohol-related automobile fatalities would be possible by influencing human factors (i.e., reduction of alcohol usage when driving) rather than by redesign of machine factors (i.e., occupant packaging systems). Payne and Selzer (1962) linked personality characteristics such as feelings of omnipotence, invulnerability, chronic rage, and depression with drinking drivers, and suggested that judicial court-enforced treatment might prove necessary to influence automobile alcoholic mortality.

Three violent deaths were ruled homocide at ages 30, 33, and 36. Three deaths were ruled suicide at ages 35 (gas asphyxiation), 59 (hanging), and 66 (stabbing). Five deaths were ruled accidental at ages 53 and 58 (burning), 38 and 38 (overdose), and 42 (drowning). The suicide mortality rate was formally .0316, but could have been as high as .0842 if the accidental deaths were also considered suicides. In either case, the rate was higher than the general population reference figure for 1970 of .0119. The high incidence of suicide in alcoholic cohorts has long been recognized. Mayfield and Montgomery (1972) have delineated two types, the abreactive and the depressed. The abreactives were described as displaying their suicide attempt after abrupt intoxication and in an interpersonal context of anger and hyperactivity. The depresseds were described as displaying their suicide attempt after prolonged heavy drinking while socially withdrawn, depressed, and hypoactive. Prophylaxis in either case is difficult as the abreactives are likely to be impulsive and situation specific, and the depresseds are not likely to be visible at the time of the event as they gradually become more isolated.

Third, the case fatality rate and cardiovascular mortality showed concomitant variation. These variables were observed to peak in the middle follow-up years and to occur in the older age ranges, most often between 53 and 75 years. Although death from chronic heart diseases was probably not greatly overrepresented in the alcoholic cohort, it did occur with some predictability so that specific prophylactic measures might be directed toward those people at greatest risk for this type of death. These individuals appeared to be chronic drinkers who avoided public identification until their fifth decade of life. Their life situation at time of identification appeared as less of an acute crisis and more as a chronic, gradual decline, most often observed to culminate 4 to 6 years after public recognition. Although neither Gillis (1969) nor Dahlgren (1951) found cardiovascular deaths overrepresented in their alcoholic cohorts, cardiovascular disease was the leading cause in either case. Schmidt and deLint (1972) found both that cardiovascular disease was the leading cause and that it accounted for the largest share of excess death in their cohort.

Fourth, the obviously alcohol abuse-related conditions of acute intoxication and liver cirrhosis accounted for a good share of the excess mortality. Deaths from acute intoxication, however, followed the pattern of violent deaths as they were observed in early and middle follow-up years and at young ages, but were not observed in late follow-up years. Conversely, deaths from cirrhosis were not observed in early follow-up years, but made their appearance only after progression of the chronic condition in later follow-up years and in older victims. Prophylaxis, in either form of death, obviously requires reduction of alcohol intake. In the case of chronic cirrhosis, Powell, Mortimer, and Harris (1971) have written that prognosis and survival varies according to the different manifestations and complications of the disease, but that the life span can be increased with abstinence and close supervision of medical complications. Early diagnosis and presenting symptoms not including massive bleeding from oesophageal varices are good prognostic factors.

Mortality data such as has been presented has ramifications for the design and delivery of alcoholism treatment services. First, indices of mortality are potential criteria upon which alcoholism treatment program effectiveness might be measured. Although excess mortality in alcoholic cohorts is consistently reported in studies which attend to this variable, a review, currently in preparation, of alcoholism treatment follow-up investigations revealed that only 21 of 58 or 36% of the studies reporting over a 1-year time span considered either case fatality rate or cause-specific mortality as an outcome dimension. Second, as Dahlgren (1951) suggested nearly two decades ago, different death scripts occur with regularity in alcoholic cohorts. The particular juncture at which an individual is first publicly recognized as behaving abnormally with respect to alcohol is extremely important for analysis and prescription of treatment stratagem. Dahlgren identified this juncture as evidence of an active "psychopathia" and expected that the risk of violent death, and by implication the risk of serious social consequences, was very high for 3 to 4 years following initial public recognition. If the period of active psychopathia is not resolved by early death, the probability of death by physical disability induced by chronic ingestion of alcohol, heavy cigarette smoking, poor diet, and other factors (Schmidt and deLint, 1972) is very high. The need for multiple treatment alternatives imbedded in a context of a coordinated network of social agencies must be underscored. Primary, secondary, and tertiary preventative efforts are variously appropriate for members of alcoholic cohorts of different ages or with different life styles of cohort entry. Community projects such as taxi-service for intoxicated citizens, highway sleep-off centers, suicide prevention centers, telephone crisis lines, and home-visiting family counseling teams are appropriate and necessary treatment efforts for the younger, less experienced drinker usually identified only after a social crisis such as an automobile crash or an abreactive suicide attempt. In these cases the abstinence criterion gives way to more flexible treatment goals, more adequately representative of the nature of the problem to be resolved. More traditional rehabilitative efforts might be more appropriate for the older, more experienced drinker. Here, abstinence as a goal of treatment might be required to halt the progressive march of internal organ disease.

SUMMARY

This investigation explored various aspects of the phenomenon of mortality in an alcoholic cohort. A retrospective, longitudinal cohort study of 400 new admissions to an alcohol rehabilitation center demonstrated: (1) a high case fatality rate (.0459) in the cohort with 95 deaths tabulated for 2,069 person-years of observation; (2) that the case fatality rate varied over time, peaking in years soon after first identification of the cohort (i.e., years 1 and 2) and in middle range follow-up years (i.e., years 5 and 6); (3) that cardiovascular diseases and violent causes accounted for the greatest numbers of deaths in the cohort; (4) that deaths from violent causes, acute intoxication, and cirrhosis were excessively over-represented; (5) that cause-specific mortality and age at death were significantly statistically associated, with deaths from violent causes and acute intoxication occurring at younger ages and deaths from cerebral lesions carcinomas, cirrhosis, and cardiovascular diseases occurring at older ages; (6) that cause-specific mortality and case fatality rate showed concomitant variation, with violent deaths peaking in early follow-up years and disappearing in late follow-up years; and cardiovascular deaths peaking in middle follow-up years.

ACKNOWLEDGMENTS

This investigation was supported by the Bexar County Mental Health and Mental Retardation Center, Alcoholism Treatment Program through its association with the university. The authors wish to thank the following for their contributions: R. M. Winningham, Jack Chance, Barbara Lewis, James Bechtel, and Dr. Reuben Santos.

REFERENCES

Annual Report of the Bexar County Medical Examiner's Office, 1970.

BRENNER, B. Alcoholism and fatal accidents. *Quart. J. Studies Alc.* 28: 517–528, 1967.

CARLSON, W.L. Alcohol useage of the nighttime driver. *J. Safety Res.* 4(1): 12–25, 1972.

COSTELLO, R.M., BECHTEL, J.E., and GIFFEN, M.B. A community's efforts to attack the problem of alcoholism: II. Base rate data for future program evaluation. *Intern. J. Addictions*, In press.

DAHLGREN, K.G. On death-rates and causes of death in alcohol addicts. *Acta Psychiat. Neurol. Scand.* 26: 297–311, 1951.

GILLIS, L.S. The mortality rate and causes of death of treated chronic alcoholics. *S. African Med. J.* 43: 230–232, 1969.

JELLINEK, E.M. "Death from alcoholism" in the United States in 1940: A statistical analysis. *Quart. J. Studies Alc.* 3: 465–494, 1942.

MacMAHON, B., and PUGH, T.F. *Epidemiology: Principles and Methods.* Boston: Little, Brown, 1970.

MAYFIELD, D.G. and MONTGOMERY, D. Alcoholism, alcohol intoxication and suicide attempts. *Arch. Gen. Psychiat.* 27: 349–353, 1972.

PAYNE, C.E., and SELZER, M.L. Traffic accidents, personality and alcoholism; a preliminary study. *J. Abdominal Surg.* 4: 21–26, 1962.

POWELL, L.W., MORTIMER, R., and HARRIS, O.D. Cirrhosis of the liver; a comparative study of the four major aetiological groups. *Med. J. Australia* 18: 941–950, 1971.

SCHMIDT, W., and deLINT, J. Causes of death of alcoholics. *Quart. J. Studies Alc.* 33 (1): 171–185, 1972.

TASHIRO, M., and LIPSCOMB, W.R. Mortality experience of alcoholics. *Quart. J. Studies Alc.* 24: 203–212, 1963.

The International Journal of the Addictions, 9(3), 365–372, 1974

International Issues in Drug Abuse*

David E. Raskin, M.D.

Department of Psychiatry
University of Chicago
Chicago, Illinois

HISTORY OF INTERNATIONAL INVOLVEMENT

The international movement to suppress drug abuse began as far back as the nineteenth century when, as a result of pressure from diplomats and missionaries, a treaty was passed which prohibited United States opium trade with China (Taylor, 1969).

Pre-World War I involvement was mainly concerned with the problems of drug traffic in the Far East. In the Hague Opium Convention of 1912 provisions were made to help China and other nations eliminate the drug problem. In post-World War I the United States made the discovery that drug traffic was not confined to the Far East. Ambivalence toward the League of Nations complicated international policy. The United States felt that the league's policies toward drugs reflected the interests of the opium growing countries. During this period the United States was developing a policy which consisted of the following: (1) Use of opium for other than medical or scientific means was considered a moral and

* At the time this article was written, Dr. Raskin was the NIMH Consultant to the State Department for Drug Abuse Control.

social evil. (2) The only legitimate transactions from production to consumption were those designed to meet medical and scientific means. (3) The basic solution to the drug abuse problem lay in limiting the production of raw materials to the quantities necessary to fill the world's legitimate requirements. During the 1930s the United States collaborated more closely with the league. The limitation of manufacturing of narcotic drugs was achieved but World War II interrupted attempts to extend controls to raw materials. The United States was able to lead the way during the periods described in the legislation of several multilateral treaties. Machinery had been devised to deal with manufacture and illicit traffic, which was supplemented by systems of national control in many countries.

Nevertheless, narcotics was still a pressing problem. And focus on demand, the provision of treatment and preventive services, had been given little consideration by the international community. Aspects of the history of the international drug abuse effort are described by a number of authors (Anslinger, 1953; Bemis, 1950; Claude, 1956; Eldridge, 1962; Schur, 1962).

THE UN AND DRUG ABUSE

In 1946 the Commission of Narcotic Drugs (CND) was established by the UN Economic and Social Council (ECOSOC). The commission is responsible for (1) supervising international treaties and carrying out functions previously vested in the League of Nations. These include preparation of reports on production, medical and scientific needs, and illicit traffic. (2) Advising ECOSOC on control of narcotic drugs and on any desirable changes in treaties, reports, and resolutions. (3) Performing other functions bestowed on the council by Article 624 of the UN Charter: "The Economic and Social Council may make or initiate studies and reports with respect to international economic, social, cultural, educational, health and related matters and may make recommendations with respect to the members of the United Nations, and to the specialized agencies concerned."

The commission is composed of the members of 24 governments, and observers from other governments, specialized agencies (WHO, UNESCO, etc.), the International Narcotics Control Board, etc. In its early years the CND focused its attention on implementation of narcotic treaties. In the mid-fifties it began to consider problems of defining narcotic drugs and keeping track of cocaine and cannabis. By the mid-sixties the CND was attending to a wide variety of nonlegal facets of the drug abuse problem: research, social, and economic facets of drug abuse; problems of psychotropic drugs; crop substitution; etc.

The Division of Narcotic Drugs is part of the UN Secretariat and is responsible to the Commission on Narcotic Drugs. The division runs a laboratory specializing in basic biochemical research and in addition maintains a library on basic research. The division publishes reports on the actions of international bodies, the implementation of treaties, statements on illicit traffic and abuse of drugs, etc. The division is also responsible for administering the UN Fund for Drug Abuse Control (described later).

Single Covention and the International Narcotics Control Board

The Single Convention on Narcotic Drugs was signed at New York on December 13, 1961: The convention (1) replaced prior treaties, (2) extended controls to plants (opium, coca leaves, and cannabis), and (3) simplified international control. The convention outlawed the nonmedical use of narcotic substances, and prohibited the production for nonmedical uses of opium, cannabis, and the coca leaf. Narcotic substances were limited to medical and scientific purposes, and to persons authorized to possess such substances. The convention incorporated the provisions of the Opium Protocol of 1953 which provided for the international control of all opium transactions to national opium monopolies. The countries permitted export privileges were Greece, India, Iran, Turkey, USSR, Bulgaria, and Yugoslavia. Opium production was only permitted by licensed farmers in areas and plots of land designated by the national monopoly (government agency).

Under the 1961 Convention, the main international organ for the implementation of that convention is the International Narcotics Control Board (INCB) (Steinig, 1971). Replacing its predecessors, the Permanent Central Opium Board and the Drug Supervisory Body created by the 1925 and 1931 Conventions, respectively, the International Narcotics Control Board inherited its responsibilities which were increased by new ones under the 1961 Convention. The new board, in order to exercise properly the functions of an independent judiciary organ of the international system of narcotics control and to meet its treaty obligations:

1. Administers the estimates system as well as the system of statistical control of all transactions concerning narcotic substances under the 1961 Convention.

2. Watches continuously the course of the international trade in narcotics with the view to preventing any country from becoming a center of illicit traffic.

3. Investigates matters relating to narcotic substances which may be brought to its attention under the provisions of the convention by a government or by United Nations or organs.

4. Seeks explanations in respect of apparent breaches of the treaties.

5. Brings the matter of treaty breaches before the Economic and Social Council of the United Nations.

6. Arranges for the publication of its reports; this confers upon the board the right of addressing itself to the public opinion of all countries; the convention stipulates expressly that "the Parties shall permit . . . unrestricted distribution" of the board's reports (Article 15).

7. Recommends in situations in which the aims of the 1961 Convention are being *seriously* endangered by *any* country, party or nonparty to the convention, that parties "stop the import of drugs, the export of drugs, or both, from or to the country or territory concerned, either for a designated period or until the Board shall be satisfied as to the situation in that country or territory" and to call upon a government "to adopt such remedial measures as shall seem . . . to be necessary for the execution of the provisions" of the 1961 Convention. The board, like any international body, is dependent upon the goodwill of nations to implement its functions.

In March 1972 the UN proposed several amendments to the Single Convention. It is proposed that the International Narcotics Control Board have the authority to limit opium cultivation and production in countries shown to be sources of illicit traffic. The INCB will have access to nongovernment information sources about illicit traffic, will conduct on-site examinations, and will notify the UN of any noncooperating nations. There will be greater ability to extradite and prosecute narcotics dealers. Recommendations will be made for technical and financial assistance to help nations carry out their treaty obligations. For the first time nations undertake an obligation to drug abuse prevention, education, treatment, rehabilitation, and social reintegration of drug abusers, as well as to law enforcement measures. The proposed amendments to the Single Convention are currently before the Congress.

The Psychotropic Convention represents an attempt to provide similar controls over central stimulants, depressants, and hallucinogenic drugs as that provided for in the Single Convention for narcotic drugs. Although the administration has pushed for ratification of this treaty, there have been protests raised by the medical and legal community. These have consisted of the following: Since the Single Convention has been ineffective in decreasing the amount of narcotic drug abuse, there is little reason to suspect that the Psychotropic Convention will be more successful; record keeping and inventory control will be expensive and inefficient; the decision process for adding new drugs to the schedules under the convention are not acceptable since (Kaplan, 1971; Koran, unpublished)

There is no provision for appeal of the commission's decision to international courts.

WHO does not have a veto in the decision-making process analogous to the secretary of HEW's veto under the American Comprehensive Drug Act 91–513.

Psychotropic is defined in such global terms as to include almost any substance.

A drug presently scheduled by the convention might be found to have important medical properties. If the United States ratified the convention, we would be required to ask the UN's permission before such a drug could be rescheduled. It is possible that we would not obtain the two-thirds majority necessary for positive action or the one-third necessary to veto those actions we disagree with. In addition, developing nations cannot carry out the terms of the convention.

The Psychotropic Convention would have major effects on research. The convention permits examination of research protocols, licensing of researchers, and keeping of detailed records, which must be open to inspection. There is no guarantee that record searches would be in the hands of health authorities. Clearly such steps would discourage research into these substances.

The convention indicates that prescriptions should accord with sound medical practices. This phrase is not interpreted, nor is it clear who shall provide the interpretation. A similar phrase in the Harrison Act was interpreted in a manner leading to the prosecution of doctors for dispensing narcotics.

The convention calls for the use of psychotropic drugs for limited medical and scientific purposes, but it is not clear as to who shall define limited medical and scientific purposes. Since the convention calls for the limiting of research to government-approved establishments, it is unclear whether or not this would eliminate private practitioners.

Although the administration has called for legislation which would maintain the role of the secretary of HEW, if the secretary recommends against controlling a substance which the UN Commission feels needs control, the United States will be obligated to provide minimal controls under the treaty.

At the request of Senator Hughes, the Senate Foreign Relations Committee has postponed action on the Psychotropic Convention. The draft has been referred to the Hughes Subcommittee on Alcoholism and Narcotics for futher hearings.

THE UN FUND FOR DRUG ABUSE CONTROL

The UN Fund was established in March 1971. In his aide-memoire the secretary-general indicates that drug abuse requires international measures. "Concerted and simultaneous action must be taken on the supply of drugs for purposes of abuse, on the demand for such purposes and on the illicit traffic which serves as a channel connecting production with demand. . . . The demand for drugs comes from large numbers of addicts and habitual abusers in many parts of the world, and it stimulates both production and the illicit traffic. To diminish demand, addicts and abusers must be treated and re-integrated as productive members of society. This treatment and reintegration cannot follow a wholly uniform pattern everywhere, but must be based on studies which take full account of social and economic conditions, cultural traditions, etc. in each country or region. Moreover, demand must also be reduced by preventive measures, which include education, particularly of young people, in the dangers of drug taking and addiction."

The fund was begun by a $10,000,000 United States contribution. Up to this point other governments have contributed $3,400,000. Suggested projects include (1) training seminars for law enforcement officials, (2) research into the effects of the chronic use of cannabis, (3) study of methadone maintenance programs, (4) development of medical campaigns, and (5) crop substitution projects. It is too early to evaluate the possible value of the UN Fund.

THE WORLD HEALTH ORGANIZATION

The WHO (Cameron, 1971) is one of the specialized agencies of the UN and thus has its own governing bodies and independent resources. Its relations with the UN are regulated by an agreement on reciprocal representation and common tasks. Since its inception WHO has been concerned with three interacting factors involved in drug dependence; (1) the properties and amounts of drugs taken, (2) characteristics of the drug user, and (3) sociocultural context of drug taking behavior. Both the Single Convention and Psychotropic Convention call upon WHO to make recommendations.

In September 1971 WHO sponsored its first interregional training course on "Problems of Alcoholism and Drug Dependence." Participants observed programs in three European countries and considered (1) drug taking behavior and societal response; (2) kinds of data necessary to evaluate drug problems and means of collecting such data; and (3) principles involved in treatment, rehabilitation, and evaluation. Another program is planned for 1972.

WHO convenes groups of experts to examine various questions concerning drug abuse and in addition provides limited fellowships and consultative services to governments. WHO is currently involved in developing a collaborative reporting system on drug abuse patterns throughout the world which would standardize international data collection.

Consideration is being given to developing research and training centers to train personnel, to stimulate research, and to participate in collaborative research projects.

Problems with the WHO programs are (1) a limited budget with only a small fund ultimately being used for drug abuse; (2) drug abuse and alcoholism are handled by separate agencies (alcoholism through mental health, drug abuse through pharmacology and toxicology); and (3) the relationship between the UN Division of Narcotic Drugs and the WHO has been competitive, with marked difficulties in working together. Hopefully this will change. The UN Fund has currently awarded WHO money for projects, but this is a relatively small amount of the total UN Fund resources.

UNESCO, through a grant from the UN Fund, will be holding meetings on the theme of "Education for the Prevention of Drug Abuse." Another theme will be the Evaluation of Mass Media Programs. The UN Secretariat is planning an interagency meeting to consider what the UN system should do in the social science field to assist the UN program. Naturally, in addition to the international agencies, a number of intergovernmental bodies such as the NATO group and the Council of Europe have meetings, proposals, etc. in regard to drug abuse. Bilateral programs continue to be developed. The United States is currently exploring possibilities for bilateral research with both Canada and Mexico. The international drug scene continues to be a fascinating area for psychiatrists interested in the interplay between health and politics.

REFERENCES

AIDE-MENOIRE, An Expanded United Nations Programme of Drug Abuse Control.

ANSLINGER, H., and TOMPKINS, W.F. *The Traffic in Narcotics.* New York: Funk and Wagnalls, 1953.

BEMIS, S.F. *A Diplomatic History of the United States.* 3rd ed., revised. New York: Holt, 1950.

CAMERON, D.C. *The Drug Dependence Programme of the World Health Organization*, 5th World Congress of Psychiatry, Mexico City, 29th November, 1971.

CLAUDE, I.L., JR. *Swords into Plowshares: The Problems and Progress of International Organization*, New York: Random House, 1956.

ELDRIDGE, W.B. *Narcotics and the Law: A Critique of the American Experiment in Narcotic Drug Control.* New York: American Bar Foundation, 1962.

KAPLAN, J. Vindication of John Bricker. *Nat. Rev.* December 17, 1971.

KORAN, L. Unpublished paper.

PRESS, DEPARTMENT OF STATE. Statement by Secretary of State William P. Rogers, March 27, 1972, No. 74.

SCHUR, E.M. *Narcotic Addiction in Britain and America: The Impact of Public Policy.* Bloomington, Indiana: Indiana Univ. Press, 1962.

SINGLE CONVENTION ON NARCOTIC DRUGS, 1961. Treaties and other International Acts, Series 6298, Department of State.

STEINIG, L. The International Aspects of Drug Control. Non-Medical Use of Dependence-Producing Drugs—Current Problems and Approaches. Council for International Organization of Medical Sciences, 1971.

TAYLOR, A. *American Diplomacy and Narcotic Drugs.* Durham, North Carolina: Duke Univ. Press, 1969.

UN CHARTER, Article 62, paragraph 1.

UNITED NATIONS ECONOMIC AND SOCIAL COUNCIL. United Nations Conference for the Adoption of a Protocol on Psychotropic Substances.

The International Journal of the Addictions, 9(3), 373–388, 1974

The Uses of an Epidemiology of Drug Use: The Canadian Scene

Reginald G. Smart

Addiction Research Foundation
Toronto, Ontario, Canada

Paul C. Whitehead

Department of Sociology
University of Western Ontario
and Addiction Research Foundation
London, Ontario, Canada

Epidemiology began as the science of epidemics originally investigating the source, spread, and control of communicable diseases (Rogers, 1965). This remains an important function in many parts of the world, but in North America more attention is given to epidemiological studies of noncommunicable diseases. A further novelty is the application of epidemiological methods to behavioral pathologies such as mental illness, drug abuse, and drug use in which physical illness is a minor element. Broadly speaking, epidemiology is "the study of all factors (and their interdependence) that affect the occurrence and course of health and disease in a population" (Rogers, 1965). It is this broader definition into which current studies of drug use fit since they only rarely bear upon disease or pathology. Such studies have been, at times, concerned with the *incidence* of drug use—the number of new users during some given period of time (usually 6 months or 1 year)—but mainly they have attempted to produced estimates of the *prevalence* of drug use—the proportion of some defined population (e.g., high school students in one city) that has used drugs at a given point in time (usually about the time the study was conducted). Generally speaking, less attention has been paid to broader aspects of factors that affect their occurrence. In many such studies the uses of epidemiology beyond the acturial have not been considered.

The best outline of the "uses" of epidemiology has probably been made by Morris (1964). The purpose of this paper is to outline how a large set of epidemiological studies of drug use relate to these "uses." This review is not intended to be an exhaustive survey of research in this area since such reports have been published previously (Smart and Fejer, 1971a; Berg, 1970). Also, this review concerns mainly the psychoactive and illicit drugs rather than alcohol and tobacco. The aim is more to illustrate how the uses of epidemiology outlined by Morris relate to current research in this area and what uses are underserved in current research on drug use.

The uses of epidemiology outlined by Morris (1964) are to:

1. Study the history of the health of populations, and of the rise and fall of diseases and changes in their character.
2. Diagnose the health of the community and the condition of the people.
3. Study the working of health services with a view to their improvement.
4. Estimate from the group experience the individual risks and chances, on average, of disease, accident, and defect.
5. Complete the clinical picture of chronic disease and describe its natural history.
6. Identify syndromes by describing the distribution, association, and dissociation of clinical phenomena in the population.
7. Search for causes of health and disease.

HISTORY OF DRUG USE

An important aim of epidemiological studies is to examine the history and development of health-related events, and make projections into the future. Relatively little interest has been taken in this aspect for drug use in Canada. The use of nonnarcotic drugs has only rarely been studied from a historical perspective. Campbell (1970) studied nonmedical drug use at Bishops University between 1965 and 1970, and he found that LSD and marijuana use tripled between 1969 and 1970.

Two large-scale studies of drug use among adolescent students have been conducted at least at two points in time. These allow some assessment of changes in patterns of use, but they are of minimal predictive value. A study of drug use conducted in Halifax in 1969 (Whitehead, 1970) was repeated 1 year later in 1970 (Whitehead, 1971). Marked increases in the use of some drugs were found, e.g., marijuana, 162%; LSD, 238%; and other hallucinogens 168%; while only small increases characterized such drugs as tobacco, alcohol, stimulants, and tranquilizers.

Surveys were conducted in Toronto in 1968 (Smart and Jackson, 1969) and again in the same schools in 1970 (Smart, Fejer, and White, 1971) and 1972 (Fejer, Smart, and White, 1973). This study found that there was a doubling or more in the percentage of students using marijuana, opiates, LSD, and other hallucinogens such as STP. The percentage of students using marijuana was 18.3, compared to only 6.7 in 1968. Use of opiates also increase (1.9 to 4.0%) as did LSD (2.6 to 8.5%) and other hallucinogens (2.0 to 6.7%). The percentage of students reporting the smoking of cigarettes dropped slightly from 37.6 to 35.5%. The use of psychoactive drugs such as barbiturates, stimulants, and tranquilizers appear to be relatively stable, although the use of stimulants and tranquilizers has decreased slightly. However, the prevalence of illicit drug use increased substantially between 1968 and 1970.

The survey in 1972 showed that the use of illicit drugs such as marijuana, LSD, opiates, speed, other hallucinogens, glue, and other solvents had not changed very much since 1970. Marijuana use increased very slightly during 1970–1972, but the use of other illicit drugs decreased or stayed the same. This is in contrast to the large increases between 1968 and 1970. The largest increase was in alcohol use: alcohol users increased from 60 to 71% of the high school population. Much of this change would have been due to the change in the law allowing 18 year olds to drink in Ontario (formerly it has been 21). This raises the possibility that greater availability of alcohol for young people helped to reduce the use of illicit drugs such as marijuana.

Plans are underway to repeat this study at approximately 2-year intervals in order to assess changes in the extent of use as well as changes in its character. For example, great concern exists about the importation of a wave of youthful heroin use into Canada. Some relief has been expressed (Zsoter, 1971) about a reduction in the prescription of amphetamines in Canada. However, establishing the real fact of historical trends will be contingent upon in-depth epidemiological studies, especially if the reasons for these trends are to be explained. This means that some studies of drug use in large populations should be established so as to be replicated at regular intervals.

The existence of such data on different populations at about the same time also makes it possible to search for large-scale epidemiological regularities and differences across widely spaced communities.* For instance, one such study (Smart, Laforest, and Whitehead, 1971) found that rates of marijuana and LSD use were quite similar among students in Halifax, Toronto, and Montreal, while another identified regularities in the patterns of multiple drug use among marijuana smokers in these same communities (Whitehead, Smart, and Laforest, 1972). Yet another study (Fejer, Smart, and Whitehead, 1972) made possible the distinction between some trends in drug use in different communities over time that appear to be general ones (e.g., increases in the use of hallucinogens) and those that are much more localized (e.g., rates of solvent sniffing).

DIAGNOSE THE HEALTH OF THE COMMUNITY

A variety of studies have been made of the extent of drug use among high school students and adults as well as of special populations of heavy multiple drug users. For the most part, they are studies of the extent of usage, but a variety of researchers has established that where per capita use is high, abuse is also likely to be more common (cf., Whitehead and Smart, 1972; Smart and Whitehead, 1973). Some studies (e.g., Annis, Klug, and Blackwell, 1971; Smart and Jones, 1970) have been concerned with unpleasant drug effects and recurrences in large untreated populations. Much of this work has been concerned with identifying vulnerable groups among both students and adults.

The most frequently studied type of population is the high school student. Surveys have been conducted from coast to coast in cities of varying size and composition. At least six studies have been made in Ontario alone during the past 2 years, including such diverse communities as Toronto (two studies), North Bay, Timmins, Haldimand County, and the Niagara Counties. Table 1 shows the extent of use of drugs such as alcohol,

* Some surveys have been conducted that are national in scope, but in the case of one (Kucharsky, 1969) the methods by which provinces, schools, and respondents were selected are not yet available while in the case of the others—one dealing with secondary school students (Lanphier and Phillips, 1971a) and one focusing on university students (Lanphier and Phillips, 1971b), and a third involving a household survey (Lanphier and Phillips, 1971c)—no systematic reports on the data are generally available.

Table 1
A Comparison of the Prevalence of Drug Use in North Bay with Toronto, Timmins, Niagara Counties, and Haldimand County

Drug	% using in last 6 Months					
	North Bay[a]	Timmins[b]	Haldimand[b]	Niagara Counties[b]	Toronto,[c] 1970	Toronto,[d] 1972
Tobacco	47.7	49.3	44.8	40.6	35.5	38.3
Alcohol	70.9	62.5	57.2	70.3	60.2	70.6
Marijuana	21.2	24.6	10.4	12.4	18.3	20.9
Glue	1.8	2.4	5.2	7.6	3.8	2.9
Solvents	3.5	5.3	9.7	—	6.3	6.5
Barbiturates	8.2	5.8	7.6	5.8	4.3	18.2[e]
Opiates	3.5	3.1	2.8	3.6	4.0	4.0
Speed	4.3	4.1	4.4	5.6	4.5	3.3
Stimulants	4.6	4.1	8.7	9.0	6.7	6.4
Tranquilizers	7.0	6.6	8.8	10.1	8.8	10.2
LSD	10.5	8.2	5.3	8.0	8.5	6.4
Other hallucinogens	6.5	9.9	4.7	5.6	6.7	7.2

[a] Sample in North Bay includes students in Grades 9, 11, and 13.
[b] Sample in Haldimand County, Niagara Counties, and Timmins includes students in Grades 9, 10, 11, 12, and 13.
[c] Sample in Toronto (1970) includes students in Grades 7, 9, 11, and 13.
[d] Sample in Toronto (1972) includes students in Grades 7, 9, 11, and 13.
[e] Change from 1970 to 1972 due to change in the wording of the question.

tobacco, psychoactives, and illicit drugs in the various areas of Ontario. It can be seen that the most commonly used drugs everywhere are alcohol, tobacco, and marijuana, in that order. The extent of use of other drugs and their rank order in importance varies with the community. These studies show that illicit use occurs in both urban, rural, and semirural areas, and that probably few areas will be immune from the effects of drug use. Studies in Toronto showed that about 20% of students used some drug other than alcohol and tobacco, but only 10.4% had used an illicit drug.

A large amount of information has been collected on the most vulnerable populations. Background and environmental factors such as area of residence, sex and grade are important. It has been shown that students from broken homes have significantly higher rates of drug use than those who live with both their parents (Whitehead and Laforest, 1971). It was originally thought (Fejer and Smart, 1971) that the use of illicit drugs increased with population density (Haldimand, Niagara Counties, and Toronto). However, the studies in low-density areas such as Timmins and North Bay show far higher rates of use of marijuana and equal or higher rates for LSD, speed, and other hallucinogens. Although the northern studies were done somewhat later than the other, there appears to be no close relationship of illicit use to population density. However, a study in the Niagara Counties showed that cities contained higher proportions of users of alcohol and marijuana, but lower proportions of glue users.

A relationship of drug use to sex has always been found. In all high school studies in Ontario there are consistently more males than females who are users of drugs such as alcohol, tobacco, marijuana, speed, and the hallucinogens. Usually there are two or three times as many male as female illicit users, and the ratio is even higher for heavy users. However, there are indications that this ratio has been decreasing in the past few years (Smart, Fejer and White, 1971). Several studies have found little sex difference in the use of drugs such as stimulants and barbiturates (cf., Smart, Laforest, and Whitehead, 1971; Fejer, Smart, and Whitehead, 1972) while tranquilizer use tends to be more characteristic of females than males (Whitehead, Smart, and Laforest, 1971). Essentially the same results were found in a study of drug use among adults (Smart and Fejer, 1971b).

THE WORKING OF HEALTH SERVICES

Epidemiology usually deals with general populations and not with treated or hospitalized patients, consequently its relationship to health services is likely to be indirect. Epidemiological studies are rarely concerned with outcomes of treatment but with how treatment facilities are used by the population at risk. A further concern relates to the way in which knowledge about health services is received and utilized.

No studies have systematically dealt with the general knowledge about the availability of health services. Several studies of drug use among young people have shown that they frequently receive psychiatric treatment for problems unrelated to drug use. The study in Haldimand Country (Fejer and Smart, 1971), for example, inquired about previous treatment of drug users. All drug users had more treatment for psychological problems than did nonusers, and they typically had more visits. The rate of treatment was four times greater for users of marijuana, barbiturates, tranquilizers, and other hallucinogens than for nonusers of these drugs, and five times greater for opiate, speed, and LSD users. More than 20% of users of opiates, speed, tranquilizers, LSD or other hallucinogens had been treated for psychological problems, compared to less than 6% of nonusers of these drugs. The reasons for treatment also varied in that nonusers were most frequently treated for family or school problems but illicit drug users were most frequently treated for depression. Studies of heroin, speed, and LSD users (Smart and Jones, 1970; Smart and Cox, 1970; Whitehead and Brook, 1973) also showed that large proportions had been treated for psychiatric problems other than drug use, and that for most of them their problems predated their drug use.

The studies of adult drug use (Smart and Fejer, 1971b, 1972) also indicated that users of marijuana and other drugs often had treatment. Users of marijuana had more treatment for psychological problems, but this occurred mainly in users aged 30 or over. Tranquilizer, barbiturate, and stimulant users had received more treatment than nonusers. For a substantial number of persons, drug use is related to some medical or psychological problem. However, this is not the case for an equally large number. For example, 7% of tranquilizer users rated their health as good or excellent, and over 75% had not been treated for a psychological problem. However, they still had prescriptions for tranquilizers. Stimulant users, especially males, report even fewer medical or psychological reasons for use, but most barbiturate users do have serious medical problems. It appears that much tranquilizer and stimulant use by males is engaged in by basically healthy persons. Special study would probably be required to discover the reasons for their drug use. Speculations as to the role of fad, fashion, and social influence in creating some psychoactive drug use are tempting but probably premature.

A further area of research on health services concerns the credibility of different sources of drug information. Several studies (e.g., Fejer, Smart, Whitehead, and Laforest, 1971) have shown that mass media is the most influential and trusted source of information for the general population of students and adults. However, drug users, especially illicit drug users, tend to rely on and most trust their friends or own experience for their knowledge about drugs (Fejer and Smart, 1971). These studies have implications for education programs about drug use and services for drug users. They strongly suggest that educational and treatment intervention that focus upon drugs should be carried on by former drug users, if they are designed for users of illicit drugs.

INDIVIDUAL RISKS

Epidemiological studies involve a departure from clinical or case-history studies in dealing with large populations of users, not merely those being treated for ill effects. This makes them particularly important in assessing what Morris (1964) has called "individual risks and chances, on average, of disease, accident and death." Such risks are usually estimated for cases seen in treatment, which of course are highly selected in terms of pathology.

The problem of "risks" from drug use is important since so many possibly dangerous drugs are used. However, many risks are reduced by the infrequent and exploratory nature of drug use (Smart, Laforest, and Whitehead, 1971). Many student users take drugs so infrequently that any chronic risks are unlikely to be experienced by any but a few. Nonetheless, a study of high school students in Timmins (Annis, Klug, and Blackwell, 1971) found that over half of students who had used solvents, speed, or hallucinogens reported confusion, anxiety, or other unpleasant drug effects on at least one occasion. About one-third of the marijuana users reported the same effects. With all types of users unpleasant effects were more commonly reported by frequent rather than infrequent users. Smart and Jones (1970) found that 63% of heavy LSD users had unpleasant effects from LSD at least once. The most common complaint was an overwhelming state of fear or panic, sometimes involving terrifying hallucinations.

Annis, Klug, and Blackwell (1971) also investigated the frequency of recurrences. Over half of the students who had taken LSD or other hallucinogens reported one or more recurrences of drug effects. However, of students who used LSD seven or more times in 6 months, three-quarters reported recurrences. These data show that drug use persists in the face of many unpleasant drug reactions, and that the deterrent value of these reactions is far from complete.

Whitehead and Brook (1973) found that drug users presenting themselves for treatment during the summer of 1970 usually attributed their problem as related to speed or LSD use. However, their history of drug use included a wide variety of substances whose use was frequently coterminous with the use of LSD or speed.

CLINICAL PICTURE AND NATURAL HISTORY

Epidemiological studies can be of considerable value by making it possible to examine the generalizability of some clinical impressions. Research along these lines has been mentioned in earlier sections of this paper, but it can be briefly noted that the cogency of such factors such as broken homes and previous psychiatric treatment not related to drug use was established by epidemiological studies.

Attempts have also been made to establish the natural history of drug use through the use of epidemiological studies. The literature on the use of drugs contains a well-known hypothesis—the "Stepping Stone Hypothesis" (Cohen, 1971)—on the natural history of drug use, which is that the use of marihuana "leads to" the use of heroin. The existing research on this topic has been summarized and assessed in two studies, and the application of a variety of research methodologies has resulted in very little evidence to support this hypothesis (Loiselle and Whitehead, 1971; Whitehead, Smart, and Laforest, 1972). A third study (Whitehead and Cabral, 1971) used data from the 1970 Halifax survey which asked students to indicate the order in which they first used a variety of drugs. There was considerable uniformity in the order in which the first fiive drugs in the sequence were used. Specifically, the first used drug is tobacco, followed by alcohol, solvents are third, marijuana fourth, and speed fifth. There is only slightly more than chance ordering of tranquilizers, opiates, LSD, other hallucinogens, and barbiturates.

The sequence of drug use among persons seeking treatment for drug use in London, Ontario has also been examined. While there are some differences in the sequence of these patients and the students in the Halifax survey, both groups have generally used a number of drugs in a similar order (Whitehead, 1972).

Such findings suggest that some drugs may have more etiological significance than others insofar as drug-using behavior is concerned. They also allow for empirical definition of the "natural history" as it has developed to date. Its predictive value is, of course, extremely limited, but it has heuristic value in terms of generating hypotheses about the future. Such epidemiological studies also allow us to monitor whether the natural history of drug-using behaviors varies in response to changes in social policy or other factors.

IDENTIFY SYNDROMES

One of the purposes of epidemiology is to identify syndromes, i.e., recurrent patterns of symptoms and signs, regularities of onset, course, and prognosis (Morris, 1964). Work on the nature of syndromes of drug use has typically been concerned with the pattern of drug use among various user populations. For example, studies of heavy LSD and speed users (Smart and Jones, 1970; Cox and Smart, 1972; Whitehead and Brook, 1973) indicated that both are essentially multidrug-using groups with preferences for certain drugs. Alcohol was the only readily available drug not used for mood or perceptual modification. It was surmised that

LSD users "own selves are aversive and they aim by drug use merely to change but not to change in any special way" (Smart and Jones, 1970).

A study by Smart and Whitehead (1972a) described a typology of high school drug users involving medicinal usage, mood-modification, and "tripping." This study of 8,503 students found that 19.2% had used some drug other than alcohol or tobacco in the past 6 months. Of these, 43% were users of psychoactive drugs and 57% users of illicit drugs. "Medicinal" users were defined as persons reporting use of only one psychoactive drug—they constitute 36% of all drug users. Those using more than one psychoactive and termed "mood-modifiers" constitute only 7.3% of drug users. Cautious trippers using only marijuana make up 15.1% of the users, and "incautious trippers" using more than one illicit drug constitute 57.1% of the total. It is clear that incautious tripping is the most common form of drug use, and that most psychoactive users confine themselves to a single drug whereas most illicit users do not.

A study of high school marijuana users in three Canadian cities by Whitehead, Smart, and Laforest (1972) found that the rates of tobacco and alcohol use are twice as high for marijuana smokers as for nonusers, and three times as high on tranquilizer use. Six times as many marijuana users have used glue, nine times as many for stimulants, and 11 times for barbiturates. The ratios for LSD, other hallucinogens, and opiates are even more striking. Twenty-four times as many marijuana smokers had used hallucinogens other than LSD and 29 times as many used opiates. The rate of LSD use was 62 times greater among marijuana smokers than nonsmokers. The associations then are closest between marijuana, LSD, stimulant, and opiate use, although weaker associations exist between marijuana and psychoactive drug use.

The studies of adult marijuana use also showed clear typologies (Smart and Fejer, 1971b). Marijuana-using adults were found to be heavier users of alcohol, tobacco, and most psychoactive drugs than were nonusers of marijuana. About nine times as many users as nonusers had taken stimulants, and about twice as many had taken tranquilizers. However, there was no difference in the use of barbiturates. The contingency coefficients showed that LSD and marijuana use were most closely related ($C = .555$); in fact, all LSD users had used marihuana. LSD and stimulant use ($C = .522$) and marijuana and stimulants ($C = .436$) were also associated. Marijuana, LSD, and stimulant use are most closely related. Multidrug use among marijuana users then appears to be common, and there is no indication that marijuana substitutes for the more socially acceptable drugs such as tobacco and alcohol.

SEARCH FOR CAUSES

Rather than merely cataloging events, epidemiological work should search for the causes of health and disease by studying incidence in different groups defined in terms of their experience, behavior, and environment (Morris, 1964). It is hoped that within the knowledge of causes comes the possibility for prevention and control as well as for effective treatment. A variety of searches for causes have been pursued, chiefly along the lines of family patterns of drug use and personality predispositions.

A variety of studies have been made in Canada of the relationships between parental and adolescent drug use. Such a relationship might be predicted from a knowledge that the psychopharmacological revolution of the 1950s preceded the current problems of youthful drug use. This revolution affected mainly adults and has meant that many adolescents were raised by parents who have taken psychoactive drugs. Drug taking as a form of mood modification could be a phenomenon learned within the family environment. Several studies of high school students have shown an apparent positive relationship between reported drug use of parents and their adolescents (Smart, Fejer, and Alexander, 1971). This relationship holds for parental use of psychoactive drugs and alcohol and tobacco, and for adolescent use of psychoactive and illicit drugs. Parents who were reported as frequent users of a psychoactive drug much more often had children who were using a hallucinogenic or psychoactive drug than parents who did not use these drugs. The relationship was very close when both parent and child were using the same drug (i.e., tranquilizers, barbiturates, or stimulants). These studies should be repeated utilizing self-reports from both parents and children as at present a clear causal connection cannot be shown. However, these studies do suggest that students may be modeling their drug use after their parents. In any case much adolescent drug use probably does take place in families where parental pill-use is common. It is possible that much adolescent drug use or abuse cannot be reduced without parallel reductions in parental use. It also indicates that the major target groups for educational efforts should be parents as well as young persons.

As well as looking at modeling, efforts have been made to understand youthful drug use as an aspect of alienation. Alienation may be taken to have three components: normlessness, social isolation, and powerlessness. Much has been made of alienation as a feature of modern life and of its importance in creating the conditions for drug use. The 1970 study of

Toronto high school students compared users and nonusers of various drugs on the Dean Alienation scale, giving scores on the three dimensions. A significant relationship was found between normlessness and the use of all 12 drugs, and between overall alienation scores and all drugs except speed. Powerlessness was related to the use of all drugs except opiates, speed and LSD. Social isolation was related to only half of the drugs, namely alcohol, tobacco, glue, other solvents, barbiturates, and tranquilizers.

Drug use appeared to be most consistenly related to normlessness. Those students whose norms are consistent with those of their parents and the so-called "straight world" are less likely to use drugs than other students. The use of drugs, therefore, may be part of a search for identity and meaningful norms, and students under pressure from conflicting norms may use some drugs as an escape.

While many students with a high sense of social isolation used drugs such as alcohol and tranquilizers which are accepted in the adult world, most users of marijuana, opiates, speed, stimulants, LSD and other hallucinogens did not feel isolated, perhaps because they were members of a "drug subculture."

Powerlessness was associated with the use of all drugs other than opiates, LSD, and speed. Apparently the users of most drugs tend to seek in them for feelings of power which would otherwise be lacking. This is particularly true of the way in which alcohol is sometimes used—to give people "strength" and "courage" to face difficult situations.

While drug use tended to be positively related to alienation, the relationship was not always consistent. Generally, alienation increased as frequency of drug use increased but then decreased among heavy drug users. In effect, the heavy users tended to be less alienated than the moderate users. This suggests that heavy users enter a drug subculture which decreases felt alienation whereas less frequent users do not.

Several personality traits as well as alienation have been examined in relation to drug use. The study in Haldimand compared various types of users on an anxiety scale used to differentiate clinically significant levels of anxiety. All types of drug users had higher anxiety scores than nondrug users. The highest anxiety scores were obtained by users of glue, speed, opiates, and psychoactive drugs and the lowest by users of tobacco, alcohol, and marijuana. Users of LSD and other hallucinogens were intermediate in anxiety level. It would appear that chronic anxiety could be an important antecedent or predisposing variable for the use of psychoactives and some illicit drugs, but less so for the use of the more acceptable drugs.

The study in Timmins (Annis, Klug, and Blackwell, 1971) examined the relationships between drug use and acceptance of self and others. It was expected that drug use would be associated with low levels of acceptance of self and others than did nonusers. The associations between low self-acceptance, low acceptance of others, and use of drugs was especially close for users of barbiturates, tranquilizers, solvents, stimulants, including speed, and hallucinogens. Of course, further studies would be needed to determine whether these personality characteristics predated drug use. However, alienation, high anxiety, and low self-acceptance prior to drug use would be predicted from the knowledge that many illicit drug users have had psychiatric treatment.

The search for causes of drug use is directly related to an interest in prevention. Several epidemiological studies have been applied to the development of preventive principles in Canada. Smart, Whitehead, and Laforest (1971) demonstrated that data on the total drug use of students (taking all their drugs together) in Toronto, Halifax, and Montreal describes a unimodal, log normal curve. This is a curve in which there are many light users, fewer moderate users, and even fewer heavy users. The curve is unimodal in that there is no clear differentiation into "normal" and very heavy users or "abusers" on the basis of consumption alone. This suggests that there will be no way to cut off the heavy or "abusing" end of the curve without reducing the average of the whole curve. Smart and Whitehead (1972b) have also demonstrated the consistency of this drug use distribution curve in various cities (Toronto, Halifax, Niagara Counties), at different times (Toronto, 1968 and 1970) and for different drugs (marijuana, LSD, speed, solvents, stimulants, tranquilizers, and barbiturates). In the only attempt to date to replicate these investigations, it was found that similar patterns characterize the drug use of a sample of British university students (Smart and Whitehead, 1973). In addition, a sizeable correlation ($\rho = .75$) has been demonstrated to exist between average or per capita use and the prevalence of heavy use (Smart and Whitehead, 1973). These epidemiological patterns strongly suggest that the already small number of heavy users cannot be reduced unless average consumption of drugs is decreased.

Other research along comparable lines has examined the distribution of attitudes favorable to intoxication with drugs among students in London (Whitehead and Aharan, 1973). The principal findings are that drug using behaviors and attitudes favorable to intoxication are significantly related to each other ($\gamma = .39$, $p < .001$), and that attitudes favorable to intoxication with drugs are also log-normally distributed. These epidemiological investigations suggest that the reduction of drug abuse should involve efforts at both the behavioral and attitudinal levels, and that in both cases the appropriate target for intervention is not just persons who are at the "extreme" or "excessive" end of the distribution but rather throughout the entire range of the distribution, and that efforts should be directed toward significantly reducing the mean value of the distributions.

This paper has presented a summary of uses and some of the major findings of epidemiological studies of drug use in Canada. Where appropriate, we have mentioned some of the needs for further research along these lines.

According to the criteria outlined by Morris (1964), some of the uses of epidemiology have been served to a greater extent than others, but some work has been conducted on each aspect.

REFERENCES

ANNIS, H. KLUG, R., and BLACKWELL, D. *Drug Use among High School Students in Timmins.* Addiction Research Foundation, Substudy 1–38 and 39 and B1–71, 1971.

BERG, D. The non-medical use of dangerous drugs in the United States: a comprehensive view. *Intern. J. Addictions* 5: 777–834, 1970

CAMPBELL, I.L. *Non-medical psychoactive drug use at Bishop's University: 1965–1970.* Montreal: Sir George Williams Univ., 1970.

COHEN, H. Multiple drug use considered in the light of the stepping-stone hypothesis. *Intern. J. Addictions* 7: 27–55, 1972.

COX, C., and SMART, R.G. Social and psychological aspects of speed use: A study of types of speed users in Toronto. *Intern. J. Addictions* 7: 201–218, 1972.

FEJER, D., and SMART, R.G. *Drug Use and Psychological Problems among Adolescents in a Semi-Rural Area of Ontario: Haldimand County.* Addiction Research Foundation, Substudy 4-Jo and 7–71, 1971.

FEJER, D., SMART, R.G., and WHITE, J. *The Knowledge about Drugs, Attitudes Toward Them and Drug Use Rates of Metropolitan Toronto Students.* Toronto: Addiction Research Foundation, Substudy No. 529, 1973.

FEJER, D., SMART, R.G., and WHITEHEAD, P.C. Changes in patterns of drug use in two Canadian cities; Toronto and Halifax. *Intern. J. Addictions* 7: 467–479, 1972.

FEJER, D., SMART, R.G., WHITEHEAD, P.C., and LAFOREST, L. Sources of information about drugs among high school students. *Public Opinion Quart.* 35: 235–241, 1971.

KUCHARSKY, H. *Progress Report: Use of Drugs and Alcohol by Young People.* National Family Life Committee, The Canadian Home and School and Parent-Teacher Federation, 1969.

LANPHIER, C.M., and PHILLIPS, S.B. *Secondary School Students and Non-Medical Drug Use: A National Survey of Students Enrolled in Grades Seven through Thirteen.* An unpublished research project conducted for the Commission of Inquiry into the Non-Medical Use of Drugs, 1971a.

LANPHIER, C.M., and PHILLIPS, S.B. *University Students and Non-Medical Drug Use: A National Survey*. An unpublished research project conducted for the Commission of Inquiry into the Non-Medical Use of Drugs, 1971b.

LANPHIER, C.M., and PHILLIPS, S.B. *The Non-Medical Use of Drugs and Associated Attitudes: A National Household Survey*. An unpublished research project conducted for the Commission of Inquiry into the Non-Medical Use of Drugs, 1971c.

LOISELLE, P., and WHITEHEAD, P.C. Scaling drug use: an examination of the popular wisdom. *Can. J. Behavioural Sci.* 3: 347–356, 1971.

MORRIS, J.N. *Uses of Epidemiology*. Edinburgh: Livingstone, 1964.

ROGERS, F.B. (ed.) *Studies in Epidemiology*. New York: Putnam, 1965.

SMART, R.G., and COX, C. *Personality and Psychopathological Traits of Speed Users: A Study of MMPI Results*. Toronto: Addiction Research Foundation, Substudy 4–32 and 7–70, 1970.

SMART, R.G., and FEJER, D. The extent of illicit drug use in Canada: a review of current epidemiology. In C. L. Boydell, C. F. Grindstaff, and P. C. Whitehead (eds.) *Critical Issues in Canadian Society*. Toronto: Holt, Rinehart and Winston, 1971a, pp. 508–520.

SMART, R.G., and FEJER, D. *Marihuana Use among Adults in Toronto*. Toronto: Addiction Research Foundation, Substudy 6–7 and Jo–71, 1971b.

SMART, R.G., and FEJER, D. *The Use of Psychoactive Drugs by Adults*. Toronto: Addiction Research Foundation, Substudy No. 461, 1972.

SMART, R.G., FEJER, D., and ALEXANDER, E. *Drug Use among High School Students and Their Parents in Lincoln and Welland Counties*. Toronto: Addiction Research Foundation, Substudy 1–7 and Jo and A1–70, 1974.

SMART, R.G., FEJER, D., and WHITE, J. The extent of drug use in Metropolitan Toronto Schools: A study of changes from 1968 to 1970. *Addictions* 18: 1–17, 1971.

SMART, R.G., and JACKSON, D. *A Preliminary Report on the Attitudes and Behaviour of Toronto Students in Relation to Drugs*. Toronto: Addiction Research Foundation, 1970.

SMART, R.G., and JONES, D. Illicit LSD users: their personality characteristics and psychopathology. *J. Abnormal Psychol.* 75: 286–292, 1970.

SMART, R.G., LAFOREST, L., and WHITEHEAD, P.C. The epidemiology of drug use in three Canadian cities. *Brit. J. Addictions* 66: 293–299, 1971.

SMART, R.G., and WHITEHEAD, P.C. A typology of high school drug use: Medicinal usage, mood-modification, and tripping. *Intern. J. Addictions* 7: 735–738, 1972a.

SMART, R.G., and WHITEHEAD, P.C. The consumption patterns of illicit drugs and their implications for prevention of abuse. *United Nations Bull. Narcotics* 24 (March): 39–47, 1972b.

SMART, R.G., and WHITEHEAD, P.C. The prevention of drug abuse by lowering per capita consumption: distributions of consumption from Canadian adults and British university students. *United Nations Bull. Narcotics*, 25: 49–55, 1973.

SMART, R.G., WHITEHEAD, P.C., and LAFOREST, L. The prevention of drug use among young people: an argument based on the distribution of drug use. *United Nations Bull. Narcotics* 23 (June): 11–15, 1971.

WHITEHEAD, P.C. The incidence of drug use among Halifax adolescents. *Brit. J. Addictions* 65: 159–165, 1970.

WHITEHEAD, P.C. The epidemiology of drug use in a Canadian city at two points in time: Halifax, 1969–1970. *Brit. J. Addictions* 66: 301–214, 1971.

WHITEHEAD, P.C. *The Sequence of Drug Use among Drug Abusers.* London: Addiction Research Foundation, 1974.

WHITEHEAD, P.C., and AHARAN, C. *Drug Using Attitudes and Behaviours: Their Distributions and Implications for Prevention.* London: Addiction Research Foundation, 1973.

WHITEHEAD, P.C., and BROOK, R. Social and drug using backgrounds of drug users seeking help: some implications for treatment. *Intern. J. Addictions* 8: 75–85, 1973.

WHITEHEAD, P.C., and CABRAL, R.M. Sealing the sequence of drug using behaviours: A test of the steppingstone hypothesis. *Drug Forum.* In press.

WHITEHEAD, P.C., and LAFOREST, L. Observations relatives aux foyers desunis et à l'usage deviants des drogues. *Toxicomanies* 4: 199–203, 1971.

WHITEHEAD, P.C., and SMART, R.G. Epidemiological aspects of drug use and implications for the prevention of drug abuse. In C. L. Boydell, C. F. Grindstaff, and P. C. Whitehead (eds.) *Deviant Behaviour and Societal Reaction.* Toronto: Holt, Rinehart and Winston, 1972.

WHITEHEAD, P.C., SMART, R.G. and LAFOREST, L. Les tranquilisants: drogues ou medicaments? *Toxicomanies* 4: 225–241, 1971.

WHITEHEAD, P.C., SMART, R.G., and LAFOREST, L. Multiple drug use among marihuana smokers in Eastern Canada. *Intern. J. Addictions* 7: 179–190, 1972.

ZSOTER, Survey on stimulant-sedative drugs. In Canadian Medical Association, Submission to Commission of Inquiry into the Non-Medical Use of Drugs, 1971.

The International Journal of the Addictions, 9(3), 389–399, 1974

Behavioral Approaches for Problems with Alcohol

John A. Ewing, M.D.

School of Medicine
University of North Carolina
Chapel Hill, North Carolina

INTRODUCTION

Although the psychoanalytic literature contains many references to the dynamics and treatment of the chronic alcoholic, I doubt if anyone today would see analysis as the primary treatment of choice. Psychoanalysts have perceived the alcoholic as having an oral and narcissistic premorbid personality as well as homosexual tendencies (Fenichel, 1945), as being masochistic (Bergler, 1946), depressed and impulse-ridden (Rado, 1933), and self-destructive (Menninger, 1938), to name just a few of the findings which have been published. Knight (1937) reported upon his considerable experience with psychoanalytic work with alcoholics, but in 1954 (Shea, 1954) was quoted as saying he would now emphasize more the early acceptance of abstention. In his earlier work with alcoholics he had the idealistic concept that a thorough-going analysis would result in the capacity to drink socially and normally. However, he had found that "the words involved in psychotherapy or psychoanalysis are pretty weak in comparison with the potent pharmacological effect of alcohol."

* Presented at Winter Meeting of the American Academy of Psychoanalysis, New York, New York, December 8–10, 1972.

Of those of us who have attempted psychoanalytic approaches to the alcoholic, I think that most would agree with Knight and with the idea that insight on the part of the alcoholic is simply not enough when it comes to his acquired habit patterns (Fox, 1967a; Dubourg, 1969). On the other hand, insight may be enormously helpful to the alcoholic once patterns of sobriety have been established and he is beginning to come to grips with reorganizing his life. However, the major conflicts which he typically has regarding dependent needs (Blum, 1966) often lead to a repeated tendency to isolate himself from would-be helpers and to turn instead to pharmacological solace. Thus, as I have described elsewhere (Ewing, 1972), holding the alcoholic in any kind of therapeutic relationship demands great skill and a willingness to titrate the "distance" between therapist and patient against the latter's changing capacity to withstand closeness.

In recent years, therapies based upon learning theory and laboratory experimentation have become increasingly prominent for a series of psychological problems (Franks, 1969). Under the general headings of Behavior Therapy or Reinforcement Therapy, these have begun to offer therapeutic methods which may precede or supplement any insight therapy which is indicated. Various writers (Shoben, 1956; Conger, 1956) have pointed out that there is not necessarily any conflict between reinforcement theory and psychodynamics, but that rather these two approaches may supplement each other. The need for the medical profession to be more concerned about alcoholism and alcohol problems which affect about 9 million Americans has been emphasized in recent times (American Medical Association, 1969, 1972). Even though the psychiatrist or the psychoanalyst may not be the prime therapist of choice in all cases (Ewing, 1972), there is an undoubted role for him in the treatment of some cases of alcoholism and in planning the treatment of many. This, then, would seem to be a good time to review the present status of behavioral approaches to the problem of alcoholism. These can be divided into two types, those aimed at inculcating total abstinence and those seeking to modify alcoholic drinking patterns toward more normal ones.

TOTAL ABSTINENCE APPROACHES

Franks (1967) has stated that behavior therapy is best viewed as a general approach to the beneficial modification of existing behavior and to the prevention of future abnormal behavior. Many approaches such as those of Alcoholics Anonymous, some individual and group psychotherapies, milieu therapy, and Antabuse therapy could be placed under such a wide umbrella. In my experience the use of Antabuse (disulfiram) is probably the single most important thing a therapist can advocate, at least in the early months of contact with the alcoholic. Some therapists fear that blocking the usual avenue of escape (intoxication) will lead to greater complications, but this has not been my general experience or that of Ruth Fox (1967a) who has treated thousands of alcoholics with Antabuse. Indeed, when the alcoholic is prevented from taking what seems at the time to be the easy way out, he may be forced into interpersonal relationships within which some psychological growth is fostered. The use of any type of tranquilizing drug which may make the alcoholic feel "high" is contraindicated, but during the early weeks and months when physiological and psychological tension states may threaten to overwhelm him, the careful use of phenothiazine tranquilizers coupled with Antabuse blockade often proves to be an ideal combination (Ewing, 1972). Other direct approaches to help the alcoholic develop new coping techniques include training in relaxation, the Electrosone relaxation therapy (Rosenthal and Wulfsohn, 1970) and some of us are investigating the potential of alpha wave biofeedback.

Franks (1967) has pointed out that some of the early approaches to aversive conditioning were lacking in scientific rigor, but nevertheless some impressive results were reported. For example, in a follow-up study of up to 13 years, Lemere and Voegtlin (1950) contacted 90% of almost 4,500 aversion treated patients. Following one hospital admission for treatment, 44% had maintained total abstinence, and an overall abstinence rate of 51% was found if the 878 patients who were re-treated were included. A variety of techniques has utilized drugs which create nausea and vomiting (Voegtlin, 1940; Lemere, 1950; Smith, 1971), electric shocks (Hsu, 1965; Blake, 1965 and 1967; Vogler et al., 1970), covert sensitization (Asham and Donner, 1968; Anant, 1968), apneic paralysis produced by curarizing drugs (Laverty, 1966; Clancy et al., 1967; Holzinger et al., 1967; Proaño, 1972), and gases with repulsive smells (Gordon, 1971). Scientific studies of the effects of such methods are beginning to offer improved techniques and understanding (Morosko and Baer, 1970; Chapman, 1972; Hallam et al., 1972). Rachman and Teasdale (1969) have concluded that the chemical form of aversive therapy can be classified as a form of classical conditioning, since repeated associations are made between the stimuli associated with the undesirable activity and an unconditioned nausea reaction provoked by an emetic. However, Hallam, Rachman, and Falkowski (1972) failed to find psychophysiological supporting evidence for the classical conditioning theory of electrical aversion therapy, since the patients did not develop conditioned skin resistance or heart rate responses to the alcoholic stimuli. On the other hand, they did find the development of a repulsion and/or aversion to drink. These workers point out that their findings appear to favor a cognitive explanation of aversive therapy effects, but that a purely cognitive explanation is as unsatisfactory as a purely noncognitive explanation.

To summarize this necessarily sketchy review of aversion therapy, it seems appropriate to emphasize the existence of active research and clinical practice in the area. The research workers must continue their efforts if our understanding and theory are to make progress. On the other hand, even in the absence of the latter, the techniques already offer substantial therapeutic gains for the patient when applied by the clinician. Thus, for the clinician whose patient has decided on a future of total abstinence, I do advocate making every attempt to invoke behavior therapy aimed at creating total aversion to alcohol. Even if the aversive responses eventually become extinguished, the patient may have been given weeks or months of abstinence on which to start building a better future.

ATTEMPTS TO INCULCATE CONTROLLED DRINKING BEHAVIOR

This topic is newer as well as more controversial and should, I think, be regarded as a research issue at the present time. However, the lay press (*Time*, 1971; Zimmerman, 1972) has already carried accounts of at least one technique and psychiatrists are now meeting patients who ask about it.

There is a huge body of professional opinion which says in effect that there is little or no hope of returning to controlled drinking once alcoholism has occurred. Jellinek (1952) applied his "disease concept" solely to the group of alcoholics showing loss of control after many years of excessive drinking. Fox (1967b) stated that none of her 3,000 patients has returned to moderate social drinking, since exposure to alcohol seemingly triggers the craving. Many previous authorities made similar statements such as the need to accept a completely nonalcoholic future (Strecker, 1941), the impossibility of reverting to controlled drinking (Lolli, 1949), the incapacity ever to acquire the ability to handle alcohol as do other men (Lovell, 1951), and the fact that even successful analysis did not permit the individual to become a moderate social drinker (Shea, 1954; Fox,

1967a). However, in 1962 Davies did report a few examples of apparently normal drinking in recovered alcohol addicts and, in so doing, led some professionals to reexamine their established prejudices. In 1966 Merry gave alcohol surreptitiously to alcoholic volunteers who thought they were receiving a vitamin preparation. He used a double blind technique and was unable to detect any evidence for increased craving for liquor when alcohol was being ingested. Another significant consideration is the pioneering work of Mendelson (Mendelson, 1964; McNamee et al., 1968; Tamerin et al., 1970), who undertook to study the drinking of alcoholics experimentally in a clinical setting. Before long he and his co-workers were reporting the absence of much evidence for uncontrolled craving for alcohol and the fact that alcoholics, at least in this experimental setting, did not conform to the established expectations of clinicians. The possibility of conducting scientific scrutiny of the alcoholic while he drinks has opened up enormous research potentials. Thus Sobell, Schaefer, and Mills (1972) have demonstrated differences in drinking behavior between alcoholics and normal drinkers. The alcoholics ordered more drinks, preferred to drink them straight, took larger sips and drank faster, but took a longer time between sips. The same group of workers in an experimental study (Sobell, Sobell, and Christelman, 1972) was unable to produce evidence for loss of control in the vast majority of their alcoholic subjects, either after small or large amounts of alcohol.

One of the earliest attempts to moderate the drinking behavior of alcoholics was that of Lovibond and Caddy (1970), who first trained alcoholics to discriminate their existing blood alcohol level from subjective feelings. Patients were instructed that they were to try to learn to drink in such a way as to maintain low blood alcohol levels, and aversive electric stimuli were administered when they exceeded a threshold of about 0.06% of blood alcohol. This level, incidentally, is just about the average which I find among groups of normal drinkers participating in cocktail parties in a social setting. The results of Lovibond's efforts appear to offer therapeutic promise at least on a relatively short-term follow-up. In a more recent report (Lovibond, 1972), he is utilizing his method to train controlled drinking behavior in persons arrested for driving under the influence of high blood alcohol levels. His results are better in younger people than in older ones, and he is now placing greater emphasis on what he calls "self-regulation training."

Mills, Sobell, and Schaefer (1971) developed a similar program within a California state hospital to try to train social drinking as an alternative to abstinence for alcoholics. In follow-up reports of their work (Schaefer,

1972; Sobell and Sobell, 1972) they found that within the first year the patients treated with behavior therapy functioned better in society than those given conventional therapy, and they indicate that apparently in the second year the controlled drinkers are remaining stable and are probably doing better than the nondrinkers.

From Baltimore comes a series of research and therapy reports which indicate that the drinking of alcoholics can be modified when appropriate incentives are offered (Cohen, Liebson, Faillace, and Speers, 1971; Cohen, Liebson, Faillace, and Allen, 1971; Faillace et al., 1972). A recent paper from the same group (Bigelow et al., 1972) demonstrates that volunteer chronic alcoholics in a hospital setting could drink moderately when offered an enriched environment for so doing and when an impoverished environment was enforced for excessive drinking. These workers point to the great advantage of moderate drinking as a therapeutic goal, since the majority of alcoholics are unsuccessful at maintaining total abstinence, since there is evidence that some do maintain moderate drinking spontaneously, and since the experimental procedures now being tested do offer some success.

From Philadelphia, Gottheil and colleagues (Gottheil, 1972; Gottheil, Corbett, Grasberger, and Cornelison, 1972a, 1972b) report a research method which involves treating the alcoholic in the presence of alcohol and requiring him to make decisions throughout the day as to whether or not to accept an offered drink. This group is now performing follow-up studies on their experimental subjects and exploring the group dynamics involved. Similar drinking opportunities with hospitalized patients have been reported by Paredes (1972), and the results of this work have led him also to question the loss of control hypothesis.

I have reported (Ewing and Rouse, 1972) a similar experimental project, except that this one, unlike the others, has involved alcoholic outpatients. A complication from working in a less controlled setting has been the problem of keeping some impulse-ridden people in such a therapy program. So far I have only accepted those who have failed with Alcoholics Anonymous and with total abstinence goals, or have rejected such approaches for the time being. Needless to say, many colleagues are skeptical of such a goal as developing controlled drinking, and sometimes the comments of professionals or members of Alcoholics Anonymous have led patients to abandon the technique without giving it a fair trial. However, of the few patients who have completed a 3-month exposure, half are still drinking in a controlled fashion during a relatively brief follow-up varying from 8 to 24 months. The technique involves much focus upon drinking behavior and no effort is made to invoke dynamic psychotherapeutic methods, although some patients continue in therapy with other psychiatrists while in the program. Patients come once a week for a 3-hour evening session and whenever possible the spouse comes too. I believe that modifying the view of the spouse is important, since frequently he or she has developed major negative reactions to the drinking of the alcoholic and probably has the capacity to sabotage the acquisition of controlled drinking unless involved collaboratively as a helper and record-keeper. In line with the experiences of Lovibond and the arguments of Bandura (1969), considerable emphasis is put upon the cognitive and self-regulatory aspects of this approach. Teaching patients to discriminate their blood alcohol levels is carried out along the lines described by Lovibond, and major emphasis is put on giving up alcoholic drinking patterns and acquiring patterns identified with social drinking. In this regard the modeling offered by the therapist and medical student assistants who drink, if they wish, along with the patients, adheres to accepted behavioral principles. Aversive electric shock is given for drinking which occurs when the blood alcohol level exceeds a threshold which is usually set at 50 to 60 mg%. Some beer drinkers have voluntarily sought a lower threshold, and we have consistently seen patients become more comfortable and relaxed at lower blood levels after some exposure to treatment. Indeed, I have wondered if, for many alcoholics, the lower levels of blood alcohol may not represent a conditioned stimulus which has repeatedly been associated with unpleasant withdrawal symptoms when descending from much higher levels. This might explain the alcoholic's tendency to gulp down drinks when he starts drinking as if he needs to hurry past that stage of slight intoxication which normal drinkers find pleasurable. In this treatment approach we are trying to reinforce negatively the higher levels of blood alcohol and to encourage the patient to remain at lower levels while feeling relaxed and supported by group approval. Such techniques as we are using are gradually evolving, and necessary improvements may be developed.

DISCUSSION

Recently Verden and Shatterly (1971) have argued for the commonsense view that alcoholism is fundamentally a bad habit, and Szasz (1972) has refuted the claim that alcoholism is a disease on the grounds that bad habits are not diseases. While not denying the habit aspects of excessive drinking, I feel that our present state of knowledge cannot support such a sweeping conclusion as that of Szasz. Personally I prefer to keep an open mind, and my present working definition of alcoholism is "a chronic relapsing condition of unknown etiology." While we hope for future understanding in terms of biology, sociology, and psychology, there is no doubt that we must now do what we can to stem the tide. In this regard any therapeutic measures which offer help to the alcoholic would seem to be legitimate and worthy of trial. That, I think, is the present state of attempts to inculcate controlled drinking behavior. If your patients raise questions about doing this on their own, I think you should be cautious and point out that presently this is a research technique. However, if you can refer appropriate patients to such research programs as are available, they may benefit. For many patients the prospect of decades of total abstinence is basically unacceptable, and this seems even more true today as we see alcoholics coming for help at earlier times of life than formerly. The fact is that it is a rare alcoholic who will remain abstinent indefinitely, and if we can offer him a ray of hope, perhaps we should.

SUMMARY

Many alcoholics are unable to withstand the rigorous requirements of psychoanalysis, and even the completion of a successful analysis does not guarantee the prospect of their being able to drink moderately. Thus this paper argues for a holistic approach to the alcoholic, utilizing all or any methods of therapy that seem appropriate. Behavioral approaches to alcoholism are quite compatible with psychodynamic views of the condition. As presently developed they fall into two categories: (1) techniques aimed at developing aversion or indifference to alcohol coupled with a planned future of total abstinence; (2) techniques aimed at replacing alcoholic drinking patterns with those of controlled drinking. The aversive approaches have already proved themselves and should be considered whenever available and when a total abstinence program has been decided upon by patient and therapist. Current attempts to inculcate moderate drinking are only in the stage of developmental research and, while promising, require much further experience and experimentation as well as longer follow-up.

REFERENCES

AMERICAN MEDICAL ASSOCIATION. Editorial: Alcoholism is a disease. *J. Amer. Med. Assoc.* 222: 699, 1972.

AMERICAN MEDICAL ASSOCIATION COMMITTEE ON ALCOHOLISM AND DRUG DEPENDENCE. Guidelines for admission of alcohol dependent patients

to general hospitals. *J. Amer. Med. Assoc.* 210: 121, 1969.
ANANT, S.S. The use of verbal aversion (negative conditioning) with an alcoholic: a case report. *Behav. Res. Therapy* 6: 395–396, 1968.
ASHEM, B., and DONNER, L. Covert sensitization with alcoholics: a controlled replication. *Behav. Res. Therapy* 6: 7–12, 1968.
BANDURA, A. *The Principles of Behaviour Modification.* New York: Holt, Rinehart and Winston, 1969.
BERGLER, E. Personality traits of alcohol addicts. *Quart. J. Studies Alc.* 7: 356–359, 1946.
BIGELOW, G., COHEN, M., LIEBSON, I., and FAILLACE, L.A. Abstinence or moderation? Choice by alcoholics. *Behav. Res. Therapy* 10: 209–214, 1972.
BLAKE, B.G. The application of behavior therapy to the treatment of alcoholism. *Behav. Res. Therapy*, 3: 75–85, 1965.
BLAKE, B.G. A follow-up of alcoholics treated by behavior therapy. *Behav. Res. Therapy* 5: 89–94, 1967.
BLUM, E.M. Psychoanalytic views of alcoholism: a review. *Quart. J. Studies Alc.* 27: 259–299, 1966.
CHAPMAN, R.F. Electric aversion conditioning to alcohol: individual measurement. Presented at 30th International Congress on Alcoholism and Drug Dependence, Amsterdam, The Netherlands, September 1972. In press.
CLANCY, J., VANDERHOOF, E., and CAMPBELL, P. Evaluation of an aversive technique as a treatment for alcoholism. *Quart. J. Studies Alc.* 28: 476–485, 1967.
COHEN, M., LIEBSON, I., FAILLACE, L.A., and ALLEN, R.P. Moderate drinking by chronic alcoholics. *J. Nervous Mental Disease* 153: 434–444, 1971.
COHEN, M., LIEBSON, I.A., FAILLACE, L.A., and SPEERS, W. Alcoholism: controlled drinking and incentives for abstinence. *Psychol. Rep.* 28: 575–580, 1971.
CONGER, J.J. Reinforcement theory and the dynamics of alcoholism. *Quart. J. Studies Alc.* 17: 296–305, 1965.
DAVIES, D. Normal drinking in recovered alcohol addicts. *Quart. J. Studies Alc.* 23: 94–104, 1962.
DUBOURG, G.O. After-care for alcoholics—a follow-up study. *Brit. J. Addictions* 64: 155–163, 1969.
EWING, J.A. How to help the chronic alcoholic. *Amer. Fam. Physician* 6: 90–97, 1972.
EWING, J.A., and ROUSE, B.A. Outpatient group treatment to inclucate controlled drinking behavior in alcoholics. Presented at 30th International Congress on Alcoholism and Drug Dependence, Amsterdam, The Netherlands, September 1972. In press.
FAILLACE, L.A., FLAMER, R.N., IMBER, S.C., and WARD, R.F. Giving alcohol to alcoholics: an evaluation. *Quart. J. Studies Alc.* 33: 85–90, 1972.
FENICHEL, O. *The Psychoanalytic Theory of Neurosis.* New York: Norton, 1945.
FOX, R. Disulfiram (Antabuse) as an adjunct in the treatment of alcoholism. In R. Fox (Ed.) *Alcoholism: Behavioral Research, Therapeutic Approaches.* New York: Springer, 1967a.
FOX, R. A multidisciplinary approach to the treatment of alcoholism. *Amer. J. Psychiat.* 123: 769–778, 1967b.
FRANKS, C.M. Behavior modification and the treatment of the alcoholic. In R. Fox (ed.) *Alcoholism: Behavioral Research, Therapeutic Approaches.* New York: Springer, 1967.

FRANKS, C.M. (ed.) *Behavior Therapy: Appraisal and Status.* New York: McGraw-Hill, 1969.

GORDON, W.W. The treatment of alcohol (and tobacco) addiction by differential conditioning. *Amer. J. Psychother.* 25: 394–417, 1971

GOTTHEIL, E. Drinking decisions during treatment. Presented at 30th International Congress on Alcoholism and Drug Dependence, Amsterdam, The Netherlands, September 1972. In press.

GOTTHEIL, E., CORBETT, L.O., GRASBERGER, J.C., and CORNELISON, F.S. Treating the alcoholic in the presence of alcohol. *Amer. J. Psychiat.* 128: 475–580, 1971.

GOTTHEIL, E., CORBETT, L.O., GRASBERGER, J.C., and CORNELISON, F.S. Fixed interval drinking decisions: I. A research and treatment model. *Quart. J. Studies Alc.*, 33: 311–324, 1972.

HALLAM, R., RACHMAN, S., and FALKOWSKI, W. Subjective, attitudinal and physiological effects of electrical aversion therapy. *Behav. Res. Therapy* 10: 1–13, 1972.

HOLZINGER, R., MORTIMER, R., and VAN DUSEN, W. Aversion conditioning treatment of alcoholism. *Amer. J. Psychiat.* 124: 246–247, 1967.

HSU, J.J. Electroconditioning therapy of alcoholics. A preliminary report. *Quart. J. Studies Alc.* 26: 449–459, 1965.

JELLINEK, E.M. Phases of alcohol addiction. *Quart. J. Studies Alc.* 13: 673–684, 1952.

KNIGHT, R.P. The psychodynamics of chronic alcoholism. *J. Nervous Mental Disease* 86: 538–548, 1937.

LAVERTY, S.G. Aversion therapies in the treatment of alcoholism. *Psychosom. Med.* 28: 651–666, 1966.

LEMERE, F. Psychological factors in the conditioned-reflex treatment of alcoholism. *Quart. J. Studies Alc.* 8: 261–264, 1950.

LEMERE, F., and VOEGTLIN, W.L. An evaluation of the aversion treatment of alcoholism. *Quart. J. Studies Alc.*, 11: 199–204, 1950.

LOLLI, G. The addictive drinker. *Quart. J. Studies Alc.*, 10: 404–414, 1949.

LOVELL, H.W. *Hope and Help for the Alcoholic.* New York: Doubleday, 1951.

LOVIBOND, S.H. Self regulation and discriminated aversion conditioning in the moderation of excessive drinking. Presented at 30th International Congress on Alcoholism and Drug Dependence, Amsterdam, The Netherlands, September 1972.

LOVIBOND, S.H., and CADDY, G. Discriminated aversive control in the moderation of alcoholics' drinking behavior. *Behav. Therapy* 1: 437–444, 1970.

McNAMEE, B.H., MELLO, N.K., and MENDELSON, J.H. Experimental analysis of drinking patterns of alcoholics: concurrent psychiatric observations. *Amer. J. Psychiat.* 124: 81–87, 1968.

MENDELSON, J.H. (ed.) Experimentally induced chronic intoxication and withdrawal in alcoholics. *Quart. J. Studies Alc.* Suppl. No. 2, 1964.

MENNINGER, K. *Man Against Himself.* New York: Harcourt, Brace, 1938.

MERRY, J. The "loss of control" myth. *Lancet* 1: 1257–1258, 1966.

MILLS, K.C., SOBELL, M.B., and SCHAEFER, H.H. Training social drinking as an alternative to abstinence for alcoholics. *Behav. Therapy* 2: 18–27, 1971.

MOROSKO, T.E., and BAER, P.E. Avoidance conditioning of alcoholics. In R. Ulrich, T. Stachnik, and J. Mabry (eds.) *Control of Human Behavior, Vol 2.* Glenview, Illinois: Scott, Forsman, 1970.

PAREDES, A. A revision of the loss of control hypothesis in alcoholism: experimental findings. Presented at 30th International Congress on Alcoholism and Drug Dependence, Amsterdam, The Netherlands, September 1972. In press.

PROAÑO, A. Psychochemical behavioral treatment of addictions, a report on alcoholism. Presented at 30th International Congress on Alcoholism and Drug Dependence, Amsterdam, The Netherlands, September 1972. In press.

RACHMAN, A., and TEASDALE, J. *Aversion Therapy and Behaviour Disorders: An Analysis*. London: Routledge and Kegan Paul, 1969.

RADO, S. Psychoanalysis of pharmacothymia. *Psychoanal. Quart.* 2: 1–23, 1933.

ROSENTHAL, S.H., and WULFSOHN, N.L. Studies of electrosleep with active and simulated treatment. *Curr. Therapy Res.* 12: 126–130, 1970.

SCHAEFER, H.H. Twelve-month follow-up of behaviorally treated ex-alcoholic social drinkers. *Behav. Therapy* 3: 386–389, 1972.

SHEA, J.E. Psychoanalytic therapy and alcoholism. *Quart. J. Studies Alc.* 15: 595–605, 1954.

SHOBEN, E.J. Views on the etiology of alcoholism: the behaviorist view. In H. D. Kruse (ed.) *Alcoholism as a Medical Problem*. New York: Hoeber, 1956, Chap. 4.

SMITH, J.W. A comprehensive intensive treatment program for alcoholism. Presented at International Conference on Alcoholism and Addiction, Dublin, Ireland, October 1971.

SOBELL, L.C., SOBELL, M.B., and CHRISTELMAN, W.C. The myth of "one drink." *Behav. Res. Therapy* 10: 119–123, 1972.

SOBELL, M.B., SCHAEFER, H.H., and MILLS, K.C. Differences in baseline drinking behavior between alcoholics and normal drinkers. *Behav. Res. Therapy* 10: 257–267, 1972.

SOBELL, M.B., and SOBELL, L.C. One year follow-up of alcoholics treated by the method of individualized behavior therapy. Presented at 80th Annual Convention of American Psychological Assoc., Honolulu, September 1972.

STRECKER, E.A. Chronic alcoholism; a psychological survey. *Quart. J. Studies Alc.* 2: 12–17, 1941.

SZASZ, T.S. Bad habits are not diseases—a refutation of the claim that alcoholism is a disease. *Lancet* II: 83, 1972.

TAMERIN, J.S., WEINER, S., and MENDELSON, J.H. Alcoholics' expectancies and recall of experiences during intoxication. *Amer. J. Psychiat.* 126: 1697–1704, 1970.

TIME. Training to be sober. March 15, 1971, p. 54.

VERDEN, P., and SHATTERLY, D. Alcoholism research and resistance to understanding the compulsive drinker. *Mental Hyg.* 55: 331–336, 1971.

VOEGTLIN, W.L. Treatment of alcoholism by establishing a conditioned reflex. *Amer. J. Med. Sci.* 199: 802–810, 1940.

VOGLER, R.E., LUNDE, S.E., JOHNSON, G.R., and MARTIN, P.L. Electrical aversion conditioning with chronic alcoholics. *J. Consult. Clin. Psychol.* 34: 302–307, 1970.

ZIMMERMAN, D. Teaching alcoholics to drink. *Today's Health* 5: 26–30, April 1972.

The International Journal of the Addictions, 9(3), 401–410, 1974

Drug Use and Achievement

Albert S. Carlin, Ph.D.

Robin Dee Post, Ph.D.

Department of Psychiatry
University of Washington
Seattle, Washington

The marked increase in the use of marihuana over the past few years has been accompanied by an increase in knowledge about the drug and a decrease in myths surrounding its effects. The fear that marihuana use leads to criminal behavior or unbridled licentiousness, that the marihuana user progresses to heroin addiction, or that marihuana use often leads to psychoses, has markedly diminished in the face of evidence that these fears were groundless. However, the passing of these naive blood-and-guts fears has not left a vacuum. In their place a new set of more sophisticated and realistic concerns has materialized.

One of the more worrisome of the new fears stems from the observation of what has come to be called amotivational syndrome. Smith (1968) first described this syndrome after observing individuals who seemed to have lost "the desire to work or compete. Such cases come to the attention of the physician only if the patient becomes anxious over the loss of a drive he deems desirable or if pressures are exerted by important personal associations" (Table 1). McGlothlin and West (1968) and the so-called Le Dain commission report, (Anonymous, 1972) also mentioned amotivational syndrome but cite little data. A review of the literature on amotiva-

* Present address: Veterans Administration Hospital, Seattle, Washington.

Table 1
References Relevant to Amotivational Syndrome

Author	Year	Sample size	Syndrome criteria
Smith	1968	Two case reports	Loss of desire to work and compete loss of drive
McGlothlin and West	1968	No data	Apathy, loss of drive and ambition, diminished capacity to or willingness to carry out complex long term plans
Hogan et al.	1970	148	Does not identify syndrome. Users have higher grade-point average than nonusers.
Mirin et al.	1971	24	Does not identify syndrome. Heavy users have poor work judgment
Le Dain Commission	1972	References to authors listed above plus "personal communication" from other investigators and clinicians.	—

tional syndrome suggests that a number of authors may have begun citing each other, resulting in a growing number of references on the topic, but relatively little new data.

More systematic data relevant to the question of amotivational syndrome is presented by Hogan, Monkin, Conway, and Fox (1970) in a study of 148 students. Their marihuana smokers, as a group, had a higher grade point average than nonusers and were more likely to be in the humanities-social sciences than in the biological-physical sciences. The authors did not, however, provide sufficient information about frequency of marihuana use. The unknown range of use, together with a relatively narrow range of data gathered from successful students, should be taken into account. College dropouts, for example, could not appear in the sample. Further, there have been major changes in the incidence of marihuana usage since their sample was gathered, and it is likely that marihuana smokers presently are less deviant than in 1969 when their data was gathered. Notwithstanding these limitations, the data collected by Hogan et al. appear to be inconsistent with the notion of amotivational syndrome.

Contrary findings were reported by Mirin, Shapiro, Meyer, Pillard, and Fischer (1971) based on a relatively small sample. These authors interviewed 12 heavy and 12 casual marihuana smokers. They found that heavy users were less well adjusted to work and were working at levels discordant with their educational achievements.

Thus far in this country the data gathered on amotivational syndrome have not been consistent (Hogan et al., 1970; Mirin et al., 1971). The clinical cases presented by other authors (Smith 1968) are of value descriptively, but provide no effective validation. In addition to the inconsistent results reported in these studies, a secondary problem is their failure to take into account use of other psychedelic drugs as a potential contributing factor to amotivational syndrome.

Data relevant to the issue of amotivational syndrome were gathered as a part of a screening procedure for an on-going marihuana research project. The information was obtained over a 2-year period from 1970 to 1972. The survey tapped both marihuana and psychedelic drug use.

METHOD

Subjects

The subjects interviewed in this investigation were drawn from university as well as nonstudent populations. Their drug experience spanned a continuum from confirmed nonuse to high frequency drug use. Initial contact was made through advertisements in the university newspaper. The 266 volunteers who responded to the advertisement thus constitute a nonclinical sample whose only common denominator was access to a university newspaper. Since these subjects are self-selected volunteers, the nonrandomness of this selection procedure must be kept in mind as a possible source of bias in the data.

The average age of subjects was 24.5 years and ranged from 20 to 41 years of age. The majority of the subjects who had used marihuana also reported experience with other psychedelic drugs (Carlin and Post, 1971) including mescaline, lysergic acid diethylamide-25 (LSD), peyote, and psilocybin. A contingency coefficient was calculated for the drug-experienced subjects to determine the degree of relationship between marihuana use and other psychedelic drugs (Siegel, 1956). It was found that $C = 0.48$ ($p < .001$). For these subjects it is not possible to partial out the effects of psychedelic use and marihuana use as they relate to motivation, so that in this sample, when frequency of marihuana usage is discussed, it must be remembered that implicit in the frequency of marihuana use is a relatively high degree of psychedelic use also.

Procedure

During the interview, subjects were asked about their goals, educational experiences, and current occupation. Reponses were assigned to a variety of categories relevant to achievement. These included:

Working. Full-time employed men as well as part-time and self-employed workers. The range of work included in this category varied from technical and skilled jobs to menial labor. Students with part-time jobs were not included in this category.

Unemployed. Those subjects who were neither gainfully employed nor enrolled in school. Also in this category were subjects whose part-time work is on an infrequent basis; for example, house painters with no current customers.

In School. Those subjects who were enrolled in a recognized school and attended at least 3/4 time.

Two additional categories relating to school were employed as well as subjects' reported level of education in years.

College Graduate. Subjects who claimed to be graduates of regular accredited colleges.

College Dropouts. Subjects who left college or graduate school and have no immediate plans to complete their education.

All subjects were asked to state their goals or ambitions. Their responses were subjectively judged as:

Vague or Absent. Included in this category were statements like the following: "I've no idea what I want to do or what I will be doing ten years from now;" "I want to be rich enough not to have to work."

Achievement Goals. Relating to career or educational advancement, including such statements as: "I want to teach college and do research in my major field;" "be a social worker and work with alienated youths."

Growth Oriented Goals. Statements articulating a desire to achieve a satisfactory life style, enhance interpersonal relationships, or develop as an individual. For example, "To learn to live better and relate to others better."

For statistical analysis, subjects were categorized according to frequency of marihuana use and extent of experience with other hallucinogenic drugs. With respect to marihuana, five categories were provided, constituting a continuum of current drug involvement. Included are subjects who have never used the drug; those who have discontinued use; subjects who smoke marihuana three times per week or less; those who are using the drug four to six times per week; and, at the end of the continuum, those who smoke marihuana at least once a day. None of our marihuana-naive subjects have had experience with other psychedelic drugs. The data reported for LSD and mescaline use are drawn from the interviews of the experienced marihuana users only. This data is classified according to the number of psychedelic experiences reported by *S*, ranging from no experimentation with the strong hallucinogens, and including use of 10 times or less, 11 to 30 experiences and, finally, those *S*s who have had more than 30 "trips."

RESULTS

The data for marihuana use and achievement are presented in Table 2, and the data for psychedelic use and achievement are presented in Table 3. Actual sample size varies from category to category because of the randomization procedure used in assigning subjects whose responses overlap categories established by the authors. For example, subjects who reported using marihuana three to four times a week could be included in either of two categories and were assigned randomly to one of the categories. Nominal data were analyzed by χ^2 and an analysis of variance was carried out on data based on years of education.

Both marihuana use and hallucinogenic experience are inversely related to employment, successful completion of school, and present enrollment in school. Years of education completed (presented in Table 4) vary inversely with the amount of marihuana used and inversely with previous psychedelic experiences. Subjects who have had no previous exposure to marihuana offer more achievement goals than subjects who have used marihuana and tend to offer fewer vague or absent goals and fewer growth goals, although these latter trends fall short of statistical significance.

DISCUSSION

These data support the hypothesis that a correlation exists between drug use and the decreased levels of achievement associated with "amotivational syndrome." Nothing in these data can be taken to indicate the

Table 2
Marihuana Use and Achievement

	No marihuana experience		Discontinued		$\leqq 2$		3–6		$\geqq 7$		
	N	%	N	%	N	%	N	%	N	%	χ^2
Current occupation											
In school	43	75.5	17	81.0	81	70.4	26	65.0	9	27.3	27.52***
Working	6	10.5	2	9.5	13	11.3	5	12.5	6	18.2	1.51
Unemployed	8	14.0	2	9.5	21	18.3	9	22.5	18	54.5	25.46***
Sample size	$n = 57$		$n = 21$		$n = 115$		$n = 40$		$n = 33$		
Completion of college											
College graduate	18	31.6	7	36.8	37	32.7	11	25.0	8	29.6	1.14
School dropout	4	7.0	2	10.5	17	15.0	9	20.5	11	40.7	16.40**
Sample size	$n = 57$		$n = 19$		$n = 113$		$n = 44$		$n = 27$		
Future aspirations											
Goals vague or absent	10	17.5	7	33.3	28	26.2	19	39.6	11	33.3	7.20
Achievement goals	44	77.2	11	52.4	58	54.2	24	50.0	18	54.6	10.97*
Growth goals	4	7.0	3	14.3	21	19.6	8	16.7	9	27.3	7.18
Sample size	$n = 57$		$n = 21$		$n = 107$		$n = 48$		$n = 33$		

* $p < .05$.
** $p < .01$.
*** $p < .001$.

Table 3
Hallucinogenic Experience and Achievement

	No hallucinogens		≤ 10		11–30		≥ 31		
	N	%	*N*	%	*N*	%	*N*	%	χ^2
Current occupation									
In school	41	91.1	53	71.6	18	48.7	21	39.6	33.52***
Working	4	8.9	9	12.2	2	5.4	11	20.8	5.13
Unemployed	0	0.0	12	16.2	17	45.9	21	39.6	33.63***
Sample size	$n = 45$		$n = 74$		$n = 37$		$n = 53$		
Completion of college									
College graduate	18	42.9	25	33.3	12	29.3	8	17.8	6.70
School dropout	1	2.4	9	12.0	12	29.3	17	37.8	22.81**
Sample size	$n = 42$		$n = 75$		$n = 41$		$n = 45$		
Future aspirations									
Goals vague or absent	15	33.3	18	24.3	14	37.8	18	34.0	2.67
Achievement goals	23	51.1	42	56.8	18	48.7	28	52.8	0.76
Growth goals	8	17.8	15	20.3	9	24.3	9	17.0	0.88
Sample size	$n = 45$		$n = 74$		$n = 37$		$n = 53$		

* $p < .05$.
** $p < .01$.
*** $p < .001$.

Table 4
Mean Years of Education Beyond High School

Marihuana use	Nonusers	Discontinued	≦ 2	3–6	≧ 7	F
	3.94	3.84	3.97	3.64	2.85	3.35*

Hallucinogenic experience						
	No hallucinogens	≦ 10	11–30	≧ 31		F
	4.29	3.94	3.68	2.93		9.94**

*$p < .05$.
**$p < .01$.

causal direction of the relationship. It is not possible to say that drug use precipitates a decline in achievement behaviors, nor that failure to achieve in our society leads to drug use.

With respect to achievement, the data suggest an inverse relationship between motivation and the extent of experience with psychedelics. This relationship is parallel for both marihuana and the stronger psychedelic drugs. Subjects who have had no previous experience with marihuana do not differ in terms of productive activity from those who are currently using the drug at low levels, nor from those subjects who have discontinued marihuana use. Subjects who are extensively involved with drugs are, however, less likely to be engaged in educational activities and have a higher rate of unemployment than either moderate drug users or abstainers.

They are more likely to be involved in a variety of activities that fill time. Obviously they spend more time smoking marihuana and engaging in drug-related past-times—listening to music and sharing drug experiences. These individuals engage in the leisure activities of other subjects, but more extensively; they read, visit with friends, walk, hike, and plan. Occasionally their leisure is interrupted by an odd job, but for the most part they make elaborate plans for the future, which seem to be rarely realized.

A commonly held hypothesis that might account for this decline in achievement is that young people who are using drugs have opted out of the cultural norms and expectations related to achievement. This viewpoint depicts the "amiable hippy" as one who values interpersonal, esthetic, and growth experiences more highly than achievement. The data only partially support this conception of the drug culture, in that the goals and ambitions offered by the drug-experienced group tended to be somewhat different from drug-naive subjects. The drug-experienced group related significantly fewer achievement goals than did the naive group. There was also a trend, though not statistically significant, for drug users to be reluctant to formulate goals and to offer more goals of an experiential, interpersonal nature to a greater extent than the nonexperienced subjects.

However, the relationship between goals and achievement is unclear. In contrast to achievement behavior, which seems to be best predicted by frequency of drug use, goal-setting seems to relate to the decision to use drugs or abstain. With respect to their ambitions, discontinued drug-users and moderately experienced subjects are more similar to high-rate drug-users than they are to people who have never used psychedelics. While there are differences when drug-naive and experienced groups are compared, the differences are typical of only a proportion of the experienced subjects, since many of the drug-users also endorsed conventional ambitions.

Within the various subject groups, the relationship between the type of goals offered by subjects and their actual achievements does not appear to be impressive. While the ambitions cited by low frequency and high frequency drug-users were essentially similar, the productivity of these groups differed sharply. Moreover, the difference in goals that characterized drug-naive and low-rate drug-users was not paralleled by any difference in actual achievements, as these groups were comparable. Thus the hypothesis relating lack of achievement to a subcultural change in values appears to be questionable.

A number of other hypotheses can be formulated to account for an "amotivational syndrome." In all likelihood, any one of the hypotheses is valid for some individual. That is, for some individuals high levels of drug use may lead to a mildly toxic state that interferes with functioning. For other individuals, drug use may allow the person to defend against recognizing the psychological difficulties in his life, or it may allow him to deal with the boredom engendered by massive amounts of free time. For some individuals, heavy drug use and nonachievement may both relate to decisions about our society and their role in it. Finally, there are those that engage in heavy drug use and continue to achieve. Clinical impressions based on the interviews with these subjects lend support to all of these hypotheses. That is, there appears to be no singular relationship between drug use and achievement.

These data alone cannot be taken as a blanket indictment of the nonmedical use of drugs, but they do suggest a complex relationship between drug use and achievement. These data do indicate a need to examine the history and life style of individual drug users in order to determine how the relationship found in the sample came about.

SUMMARY

The relationship between lowered achievement and nonmedical use of drugs has become a concern as drug use increases. Two hundred sixty-six young males, some of whom were marihuana smokers, and some of whom used other drugs also, were interviewed about their levels of achievement and drug use. It was found that lowered levels of achievement were associated with higher rates of drug experience for both marihuana and other psychedelic drugs. Goal setting varied as a function of the decision to use drugs or not, rather than amount of drugs used. These two findings, taken together, suggest that observed lowered achievement is not the result primarily of a change in values, but of perhaps several factors which are discussed.

ACKNOWLEDGMENT

This research was supported, in part, by grant #2 RO1 MH19015 from the National Institute of Mental Health to the senior author.

REFERENCES

ALLEN, J.R., and WEST, L.J. "Flight from violence: hippies and the green rebellion." *Amer. J. Psychiat.* 125: 364–374, 1968.

ANONYMOUS. *Cannabis: A Report of the Commission of Inquiry into the Non-Medical Use of Drugs.* Ottawa, Canada, 1972.

CARLIN, A., and POST, R. Patterns of drug use among marihuana smokers. *J. Amer. Med. Assoc.* 218: 867–868, 1971.

HOGAN, R., MONKIN, D., CONWAY, J., and FOX, M. Personality correlates of undergraduate marihuana use. *J. Consult. Clin. Psychol.* 35: 58–63, 1970.

MIRIN, S., SHAPIRO, L., MEYER, R., PILLARD, M., and FISCHER, M. Casual versus heavy use of marihuana: a redefinition of the marihuana problem. *Amer. J. Psychiat.* 127: 1134–1140, 1971.

McGLOTHLIN, W., and WEST, L.J. Themarihuana problem: an overview. *Amer. J. Psychiat.* 125: 126–134, 1968.

SIEGEL, S. *Nonparametric Statistics for the Behavioral Sciences.* New York: McGraw-Hill, 1956.

SMITH, D.E. Acute and chronic toxicity of marihuana. *J. Psychedelic Drugs* 2: 37–47, 1968.

The International Journal of the Addictions, 9(3), 411–429, 1974

Assisted Covert Sensitization for Drug Abuse*

Barry M. Maletzky,† M.D.

Department of Neuropsychiatry
U.S. Lyster Army Hospital
Fort Rucker, Alabama

Covert sensitization describes a procedure which pairs imagined scenes of behavior with imagined scenes aversive to the patient in an effort to diminish the strength of a given response. The notion that such imagination of scenes might be of some therapeutic benefit springs from two well-defined sources: (1) The discovery that scenes presented in imagination can produce powerful changes in "real life" behavior, and (2) the impressive emergence of aversion therapy as a useful clinical technique.

Wolpe (Wolpe, 1969; Wolpe and Lazarus, 1958), beginning with conditioning experiments on animals in the early 1950s, introduced a technique suggested by his laboratory studies: systematic desensitization. Over the past 15 years, many clinicians have demonstrated the wide applicability of this technique. The patient is first taught a relaxation technique; then a hierarchy of scenes which previously had elicited avoidance or anxiety is presented while the patient is fully relaxed. Wolpe contends that there are two factors of importance in this therapy: (1) The association of a relaxed state with previously fearful stimuli, and (2) the

* Presented to the Fifth Western Institute of Drug Problems, Portland, Oregon, June 1972.

† Present address: 11108 S. W. Collina Avenue, Portland, Oregon 97219.

gradual introduction of increasingly fearful scenes, such that the patient never experiences overwhelming anxiety.

Systematic desensitization has been effectively applied to a variety of conditions, most notably the phobias. For example, a patient fearful of closed-in spaces might be presented with scenes first of large empty rooms, progressing through crowded rooms to those with even smaller confines. As the patient associates the relaxed condition with these imaginations, his real life behavior is seen to change. He gradually can experience closed-in spaces without the discomfort experienced before treatment.

Systematic desensitization attacks a class of conditions called maladaptive *avoidance* behaviors. These include anxiety syndromes which severely constrain a patient's function. There remain, however, a variety of behaviors which produce problems for patients, called maladaptive *approach* behaviors: homosexuality, overeating, smoking, drug abuse, and the like. Because of their active nature, they produce societal, as well as individual, mischief and malaise.

To combat such behaviors, clinicians have amassed a powerful armamentarium of aversive therapies. These usually employ electric shock as the noxious stimulus. However, those working in this medium have discovered that shock yields several side-effects. For one, many patients fear electricity and quite actively refuse to participate (Gold and Neufeld, 1965; Kolvin, 1967). For another, shock can produce a generalized increase in anxiety (Rachman and Teasdale, 1969) and aggression (Morgenstern, Pearce, and Davies, 1963). Then again, not all reports of electric shock aversions have been entirely successful (McConaghy, 1970; McConaghy, 1971; Birk, Huddelson, and Miller, 1971). Morever, shock is cumbersome to use and expensive to employ.

Out of such considerations have emerged attempts to combine the Wolpean principle of imaginal therapy with aversive conditioning against the maladaptive approach behaviors. Cautela (1966, 1967, 1970) stands out among the early explorers of this technique (but also see Lazarus, 1958), variously dubbed aversive imagery or covert sensitization. He has reported successful uses of the technique in the sexual perversions, obesity, and drug and alcohol abuse. For example, an alcohol patient might be asked under relaxation to clearly visualize being in a tavern sipping his favorite cocktail. At the moment of imagined ingestion, Cautela would introduce graphic images of the patient becoming nauseous and vomiting into his drink. Running out of the tavern would produce immediate relief. In other scenes, the patient would imagine himself about to drink, feel nauseous, put his glass down, and hence feel much relieved.

Several authors have now commented favorably upon the use of such techniques in alcoholism (Franks, 1958; Anant, 1967; Ashem and Donner, 1968) and cigarette smoking (Mullen, 1968; Viernstein, 1968; Lichtenstein and Keutzer, 1969; Sachs, Bean, and Morrow, 1970). Moreover, Barlow and his colleagues (1969) have recently demonstrated that introduction of the noxious scenes is the crucial element in this form of therapy.

With such enthusiastic evidence, we were somewhat disappointed when we first experimented with this technique. For example, one homosexual patient complained that the stimuli "were not strong enough . . . I can feel a little nauseous, but no enough to do much good." Another, an older alcoholic, found himself shunning only the specific locations and beverages covered in the scenes with little generalization.

In an attempt to inject strength yet flexibility into this procedure, we borrowed an old idea from several authors (Wolpe, 1969; Kennedy and Foreyt, 1968) and introduced a noxious odor, valeric acid,* at appropriate points during scene presentations. This substance, with an odor benignly termed foul, seemed quite appropriate for many of the scenes because of its almost human fetid properties. The odor not only strengthened verbal suggestions of nausea, it allowed us to treat patients in actual situations which had elicited the unwanted behaviors: an alcoholic could smell the odor in his favorite taverns, a homosexual in the men's rest rooms where he used to solicit partners (Maletzky, In press, a).

Our results using this strengthened or "assisted" form of covert sensitization for homosexuality (Maletzky and George, In press) and exhibitionism (Maletzky, In press, b) have been published elsewhere. Our trials were not strictly controlled. However, the number of subjects involved and the reliance upon objective verification of treatment effects provided support for this new technique. It produced not only elimination of unwanted motor acts, but elimination of the covert behaviors, such as thoughts, urges, and dreams, connected with these acts as well. Table 1, listing a sampling of studies employing covert sensitization to date, provides convincing evidence of this technique's effectiveness and versatility.

In attempting to employ this technique with drug abusers, however, we were confronted with several interesting questions. It appears as if assisted covert sensitization works because it produces autonomic nervous system conditioning: pairing a consummatory sexual response with an

* The author is indebted to Dr. Don Molde for first experimenting with valeric acid in the behavior therapies. This substance is not harmful when sniffed and can be purchased from most chemical supply firms. The author is currently using the smell of rotting meat innoculated with the bacterium *Pseudomonas*.

Table 1
Selected Studies Employing Covert Sensitization

Author(s)	Date	Sample size	Technique	Outcome
Lazarus	1958	Single case study—compulsive behavior	"Aversive imagery," anecdotal	Successful after 16 hr treatment; no follow-up
Gold and Neufeld	1965	Single case study—homosexual adolescent	Covert sensitization, anecdotal	Successful after 10 sessions, successful 12 month follow-up
Cautela	1966	Two case studies, including alcoholism and obesity	Covert sensitization, anecdotal	Successful; no follow-up
Cautela	1967	Review plus five additional cases, including alcoholism and glue sniffing	Covert sensitization, anecdotal	Successful; no follow-up
Anant	1967	26 Chronic alcoholics	Covert sensitization, uncontrolled	All 26 rated "improved"; short follow-up
Kolvin	1967	Teenage fetishist and teenage petrol sniffer	"Aversive imagery," anecdotal	Successful; follow-up at 13 and 17 months; still effective
Ashem and Donner	1968	23 Chronic alcoholics	8 Subjects, covert sensitization; 15 subjects, controls	40% of experimental subjects abstinent; 0% of controls; all at 6 month follow-up
Barlow, Leitenberg, and Agras	1969	Pedophilic patient; homosexual patient	Single cast, controlled design	Imagining the noxious scene is the crucial element in covert sensitization
Sachs, Bean, and Morrow	1970	Three groups of 20 each, cigarette smoking	Group 1, covert sensitization; Group 2, "self-control"; Group 3, "placebo attention"	Covert sensitization significantly more effective
Barlow et al.	1972	Two homosexual patients	Single case controlled design	Therapeutic instructions not crucial in covert sensitization
Maletzky	1973	Two case report; a homosexual and a compulsive eater	"Assisted" covert sensitization, anecdotal	Successful at 12 and 7 month follow-ups

(continued)

Table 1 (continued)

Author(s)	Date	Sample size	Technique	Outcome
Maletzky and George	1973	10 Homosexual patients	"Assisted" covert sensitization; no controls but blind testing employed	Successful at 12 month follow-up in 8 cases
Maletzky and George	1973	10 Exhibitionist patients	"Assisted" covert sensitization; no controls, but frequency data and legal sources checked	All 10 successful at 12 month follow-up

unpleasant gastrointestinal one, such as nausea. Would such a pairing work for the act of ingesting a pill? Moreover, most of our sexual patients approached us for treatment. Would this technique work with drug abusers who are notorious for their lack of interest in therapeutic change?

To answer such questions we have begun a systematic study of assisted covert sensitization in the treatment of various forms of drug abuse. An examination of our present information may be useful in answering the following questions:

1. Is assisted covert sensitization a useful approach to drug abuse?
2. Is it differentially useful among various forms of drug abuse?
3. Which subject variables help us predict for whom it might be most useful?
4. Is this technique a practical approach to the wide spread problem of drug abuse?

METHODS

Subjects

Subjects in the present study were drawn from a military base in the Southeastern United States. Our 20 subjects encompassed a range of parameters in terms of age, sex, and military status, as well as in terms of drugs abused. Most, but not all, of our subjects were treated within the Drug and Alcohol Program's Halfway House. The remainder were treated in the Department of Neuropsychiatry.

Two groups of 10 subjects each were randomly chosen and designated treatment and control. The treatment group was afforded assisted covert sensitization. In other regards, however, both groups received similar handling. As appropriate, both groups were provided with group and individual counseling either at the Halfway House or within the Department of Neuropsychiatry. During the times each treatment subject received assisted covert sensitization, each control subject received individual counseling. Antabuse was used with all alcohol patients in both groups. The single difference was, then, the presence of assisted covert sensitization.

Table 2 lists subjects within each group in terms of demographic, drug use, and treatment variables. Treatment and control groups did not differ significantly on any of these parameters.

Table 2
Demographic, Drug Use, and Treatment Variables for Treatment and Control Groups

Subject	Sex	Age	Military status	Marital status	Major drug of abuse	Therapist[a]
			Treatment Group			
1	M	18	Active	S	Paint	Technician
2	M	22	Active	D	Heroin	Technician
3	F	37	Dependent	M	Alcohol	Psychiatrist
4	M	32	Active medically	M	Alcohol	Technician
5	M	25	Retired	S	Alcohol	Technician
6	F	20	Active (WAC)	S	Valium	Psychiatrist
7	M	41	Retired	M	Alcohol	Technician
8	M	33	Active	M	Cigarettes	Psychiatrist
9	F	27	Dependent	M	Marijuana	Technician
10	F	43	Dependent	M	Alcohol	Technician
			Control Group			
11	M	35	Active	M	Alcohol	Technician
12	F	42	Dependent	M	Cigarettes	Psychiatrist
13	M	20	Active	S	Alcohol	Technician
14	M	19	Active	M	Marijuana	Technician
15	F	27	Dependent	M	Valium	Psychiatrist
16	M	43	Retired	D	Alcohol	Technician
17	M	24	Active	S	Heroin	Technician
18	M	16	Dependent	S	Hallucinogens	Technician
19	M	28	Active	M	Alcohol	Technician
20	F	41	Dependent	M	Alcohol	Psychiatrist

[a] Halfway House treatments were performed by technicians, Neuropsychiatry Clinic treatments by the psychiatrist.

Treatment

Following training in relaxation (Wolpe and Lazarus, 1958), each treatment subject composed a list of his usual drug taking behaviors. A list for a sniffer included:

1. Being in woods behind barracks with other friends at night; squeezing glue into paper bag; passing it back and forth.
2. Sneaking into bathroom alone; spraying paint onto washcloth; sniffing it.
3. Being in friends' trailer; cutting up towel and passing pieces around; spraying paint on towel pieces; sniffing.

Such a list for an alcoholic included:

1. Entering Non-commissioned Officers Club; sitting at table; ordering, then drinking scotch and sodas.
2. Drinking beer with friends in front of television at home.
3. Being in local tavern, drinking beer.
4. At friend's house, in back yard, drinking beer.

Each subject was also asked to compose a list of most feared and disgusting scenes. Typical scenes included vomiting, contact with feces and urine, contact with insects, suffocation, nauseating odors, and discovery of illegal activities. Scenes of drug-taking behavior were then combined with scenes aversive to the patient. An example of a scene presented to a sniffing patient follows. An asterisk marks the introduction of valeric acid; a double asterisk marks its removal.

> Imagine clearly now that you are in your friends' trailer, in the living room. Bill and John are with you and you are all cutting up a towel into small pieces. Each now has a piece. You can see and feel your piece now. You begin to spray that can of white Devoe paint on it—you can see the paint on the towel now as you place it in a plastic bag and begin to inhale those familiar fumes.* But this time something's wrong! The smell of the paint is disgusting and it's making your stomach retch and turn. You want to get away. You are afraid what Bill and John might think, but that odor is making you sick. Food particles catch in your throat; you try to gag them back down but you can't and suddenly big chunks of vomit gush

out of your mouth. Vomit dribbles down your chin and the smell makes you even sicker. Bill and John look disgusted at you. You quickly wipe yourself off and run out of the trailer.** As you do, you notice that smell is gone and you can relax again. You breathe the fresh clean air outside and feel your stomach calming down, relaxing, now that you're away from there.

Scenes presented to other drug abusers might similarly utilize nauseating images or might combine the offensive odor of valeric acid with ideas of suffocation (smoking, glue sniffing) or with apprehension by authorities (pill-taking, self-injection). Scenes were also included in which the patient, confronted with temptations to drink or take drugs, experienced a brief whiff of valeric acid with consequent nausea, and resisted the temptation, thereby feeling relaxed and refreshed, proud of himself for being able to resist.

Each scene was presented twice per session for an average of 12 sessions. Such 30 minute sessions were conducted three times weekly. "Booster" sessions were utilized at 3 and 6 month intervals following treatment to stamp in earlier effects. All scenes were also tape recorded; patients were thus able to practice with the tapes, using their own vials of valeric acid. Moreover, the valeric acid smell was associated with the implements of drug abuse within each session, with the feel and sight of actual beer cans for an alcoholic, or with the bags and paint cans of the sniffer. As a final touch, each subject sniffed valeric acid in trips to the surroundings of his drug abuse. Thus "in vivo" techniques were used to bolster purely imaginal treatment. Treatments were carried out by the author and by psychology and social work technicians trained by the author. A paradigm of treatment is presented in Table 3.

Evaluation

1. *Self Reports*. Reports were collected prior to treatment, immediately thereafter, and at 6 months' follow-up for the following data:

a. Incidents of drug abuse.
b. Urges to abuse drugs.

2. *Reports of Authorities*. Military and civilian police records were scrutinized to determine if drug abuse was a continuing problem. Observers such as spouses and commanding officers were also requested to

Table 3
Paradigm of Treatment for All Treatment Subjects

Treatment phase	Description	Average duration and frequency
I. Data collection	Self-explanatory	One-half of the first hour
II. Education	Explanation of drug abuse as partly a learned behavior, not necessarily a manifestation of personality	One-quarter of the first hour
III. Treatment explanation	Description of treatment technique	One-quarter of the first hour
IV. A. Relaxation training with therapist	Listening to instructions by therapist in office	One-half of three succeeding sessions
B. Relaxation training	Listening to taped instructions at home or in office without the therapist	Fifteen minutes daily for 2 weeks
V. A. Sensitization sessions with therapist	Scene visualizations under relaxation with valeric acid performed by therapist	Thirty minutes, thrice weekly, for an average of 72.1 weeks.
B. Sensitization sessions without therapist	Scene visualizations under relaxation, by tape, self-administering valeric acid	Thirty minutes twice weekly, for an average of 10.7 weeks
VI. A. Sensitization sessions "in vivo"	Sniffing valeric acid in situations previously associated with drug abuse	Several minutes, twice weekly, during the middle 4 weeks of treatment
B. Sensitization sessions "in vivo"	Sniffing valeric acid in office in association with sight and feel of drug paraphernalia	Several minutes, thrice weekly, for an average of 5.6 weeks
VII. A. "Booster" sessions with therapist	Same as V.A	Thirty minutes, given at 3, 6, and to be given at 12 month intervals
B. "Booster" sessions without therapist	Same as V.B. Optional	As required, whenever subject felt it necessary. By report, an average of 2.1 sessions over a 6-month period after treatment

report observations of drug activity. In all cases, such observers had no knowledge of the specific therapies involved.

3. *Objective Tests*. For those abusing drugs amenable to objective evaluation, follow-up urinalyses were utilized at random intervals. All alcoholics submitted to blood alcohol and Breathalyzer analyses, also at random intervals.

RESULTS

Self-Reports

Incidents of Drug Abuse. Across all forms of drug abuse, the use of assisted covert sensitization produced a greater decline in drug use than more conventional therapies alone. Figure 1 depicts weekly pre- and posttreatment incidences of drug abuse for treatment and control groups. Weekly frequencies of drug abuse immediately following treatment averaged 14.3 for treatment subjects as compared to 31.5 for controls. These frequencies averaged 15.1 for treatment subjects at 6 months' follow-up as compared to 44.9 for controls. Table 4 presents these averaged data as well as individual results. Both these differences are significant at the .01 level. The greater spread between groups at 6 months may indicate more lasting benefits with the addition of assisted covert sensitization as well as the efficacy of "booster sessions."

Naturally, weekly frequencies depend upon the type of drug abused; the number of drinks or cigarettes smoked will usually exceed the number of hallucinogens ingested, for example. Because treatment and control groups were evenly balanced in this regard, these data can be equally compared. However, a more meaningful comparison might be numbers of subjects achieving a significant decline in drug use. Among 10 treatment subjects, nine achieved significant decreases in drug use at 6 months' follow-up, as compared to five of the control subjects, again a significant difference. The slight increase in abuse at 6 months in contrast to immediately following treatment probably indicates the need for continuing "booster sessions."

Although the subgroups are small, there appear to be no significant differences in the efficacy of assisted covert sensitization depending upon the nature of abuse. As will be seen in Table 3, even "pill-takers" benefitted, though not to the extent of our alcohol, smoking, and sniffing patients. Moreover, no significant differences emerged in comparing efficacy with sex, age, military status, or therapist involved. It is our impression that, surprisingly, neither did a difference exist whether a client was particularly interested in therapy or not. This has been corroborated by research in the sexual deviations (Maletzky and George, In press; Maletzky, In press, b).

Urges to Abuse Drugs. Again, as demonstrated in Table 5, assisted covert sensitization resulted in a significant decline in urges to abuse drugs

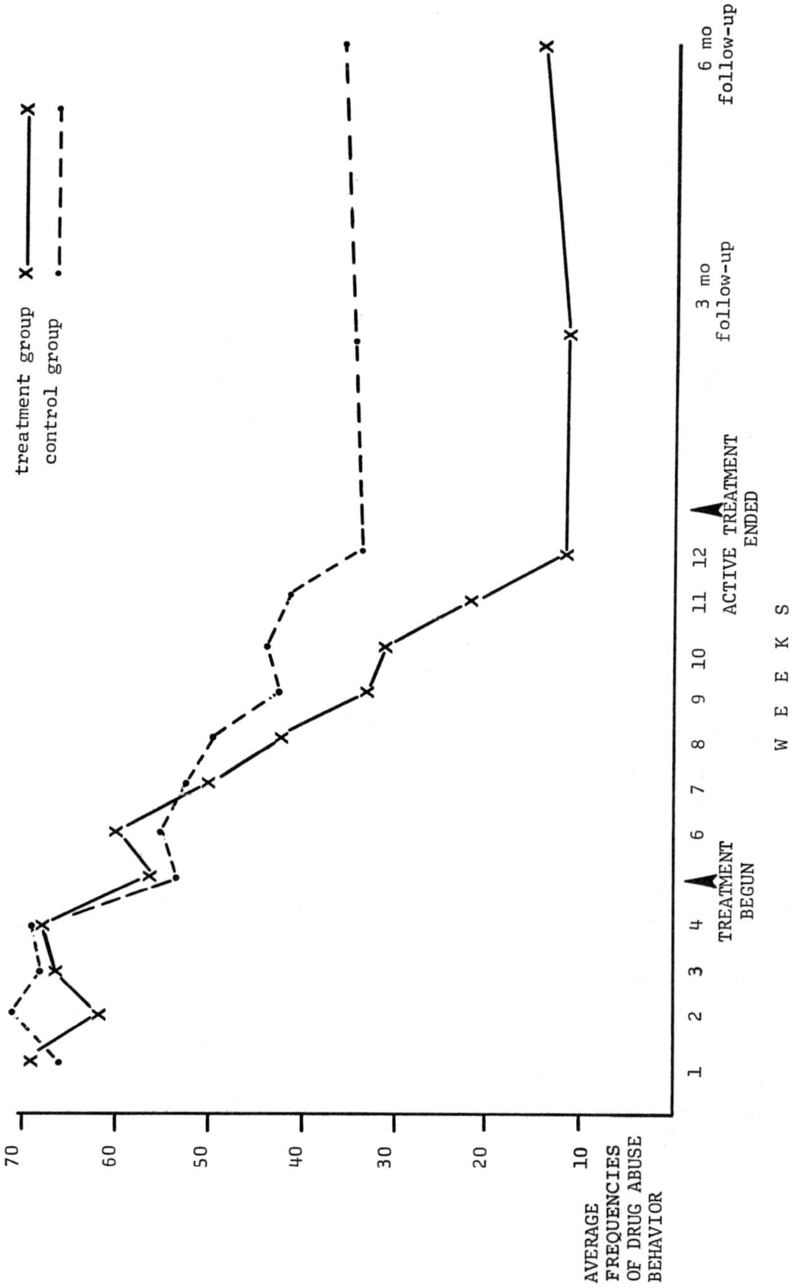

Fig. 1. Pre- and posttreatment weekly incidences of drug abuse for treatment and control subjects.

Table 4
Per- and Posttreatment Weekly Frequencies[a] of Drug Abuse for Treatment and Control Subjects[a]
(Italic values significant to $p < .01$ as compared with pretreatment values)

Subject	Major drug of abuse	Pretreatment	Posttreatment	Six months
		Treatment Group		
1	Paint	4.5	*0*	*0*
2	Heroin	13.2	*0*	*0*
3	Alcohol	27.5	*0*	*5.7*
4	Alcohol	98.7	*4.5*	*10.2*
5	Alcohol	63.2	*15.7*	*14.9*
6	Valium	25.4	*0*	*0*
7	Alcohol	112.0	122.3	120.7
8	Cigarettes	254.7	*0*	*0*
9	Marijuana	8.4	*0*	*0*
10	Alcohol	75.2	*0*	*0*
Average		65.3	*14.3*	*15.1*
		Control Group		
11	Alcohol	58.8	72.4	105.4
12	Cigarettes	207.1	*70.5*	*68.2*
13	Alcohol	43.2	45.7	53.7
14	Marijuana	20.7	*3.2*	*0*
15	Valium	31.5	*0*	*0*
16	Alcohol	105.4	*0*	96.2
17	Heroin	7.0	*0*	*0*
18	Hallucinogens	3.2	5.7	2.6
19	Alcohol	87.6	*0*	*0*
20	Alcohol	111.3	117.5	123.0
Average		67.6	*31.5*	*44.9*

[a] Comparison of treatment and control group means significantly different at the $p < .01$ level at posttreatment and 6 months' follow-up. Frequencies are defined as times per week a drug is abused, computed over a 4-week period at the times specified. Frequencies for cigarettes and alcohol vastly exceed those for paint or hallucinogen abuse, for example.

at both posttreatment and 6 months' periods ($p < .01$). An interesting differential, documented in the table, can be found: successful subjects in both groups who abused physically addictive drugs—alcohol, heroin—experienced craving more often than those who abused drugs such as marijuana. Of additional significance is the fact that a drug not usually thought of as physiologically addicting, tobacco, fit the addicting pattern of craving closely. It is of interest in this regard that evidence (Brown,

Table 5
Pre- and Posttreatment Weekly Frequencies of Urges to Abuse Drugs for Treatment and Control Subjects[a]
(Italic values significant to p < .01 as compared with pretreatment values)

Subject	Major drug of abuse	Pretreatment	Posttreatment	Six months
		Treatment Group		
1	Paint	10.7	*1.5*	*0*
2	Heroin	17.9	*2.3*	*0.7*
3	Alcohol	15.2	*3.1*	7.3
4	Alcohol	37.1	*5.0*	*11.7*
5	Alcohol	31.0	20.5	17.1
6	Valium	17.5	*2.7*	*0*
7	Alcohol	41.3	57.1	46.8
8	Cigarettes	311.4	*62.5*	*7.0*
9	Marijuana	12.7	*0*	*0*
10	Alcohol	37.3	*0.9*	*0*
Average		53.4	*15.6*	*9.1*
		Control Group		
11	Alcohol	92.5	181.3	210.4
12	Cigarettes	222.5	*63.4*	*71.5*
13	Alcohol	80.2	97.3	95.7
14	Marijuana	15.2	*0*	*0*
15	Valium	20.5	*2.7*	*0*
16	Alcohol	32.6	16.5	39.5
17	Heroin	15.2	*0*	*0*
18	Hallucinogens	9.3	7.6	11.5
19	Alcohol	41.0	36.5	24.0
20	Alcohol	55.4	57.6	71.5
Average		59.4	46.9	52.4

[a] Comparison of treatment and control group means significantly different at the $p <$ .01 level at posttreatment and 6 months' follow-up.

1963; Schwartz and Dubitzky, 1968) exists documenting the truly addicting nature of tobacco abuse.

Reports of Authorities

Table 6 compares the frequency of reports of drug abuse by authorities and observers for treatment and control groups. Again, a significant difference favoring the treatment group is clear, and this difference is significant at the .01 level.

Table 6
Pre- and Posttreatment Weekly Frequencies of Reports of Drug Abuse by Authorities and Observers for Treatment and Control Groups[a]
*(*Italic *values significant to* p *< .01 as compared with pretreatment values)*

Subject	Major drug of abuse	Pretreatment	Posttreatment	Six months
		Treatment Group		
1	Paint	7.4	*0*	*0*
2	Heroin	15.2	*0*	*2.5*
3	Alcohol	13.6	*0*	*4.7*
4	Alcohol	34.5	*0.5*	*3.2*
5	Alcohol	23.7	*10.0*	14.5
6	Valium	27.3	*0*	*0*
7	Alcohol	53.5	62.3	62.4
8	Cigarettes	207.7	*0*	*0*
9	Marijuana	5.6	*0*	*0*
10	Alcohol	33.5	*0*	*0*
Average		42.2	*7.3*	*8.7*
		Control Group		
11	Alcohol	41.5	47.3	62.5
12	Cigarettes	116.3	*52.5*	*57.3*
13	Alcohol	19.7	23.4	40.6
14	Marijuana	15.2	*1.0*	*0*
15	Valium	30.7	*0*	*0*
16	Alcohol	123.5	*10.7*	119.4
17	Heroin	7.5	*0*	*0*
18	Hallucinogens	5.4	7.6	7.7
19	Alcohol	80.5	*22.5*	*14.6*
20	Alcohol	87.6	112.5	98.7
Average		52.8	*27.8*	40.1

[a] Comparison of treatment and control group means significantly different at the $p <$ .01 level at posttreatment and 6 months' follow-up.

Objective Tests

Although not entirely reliable, these tests lend some objectivity to our study because of the random yet repeated nature of their use. Table 7 demonstrates a difference favoring the use of assisted covert sensitization as measured by these tests in most subjects at posttreatment and 6 months' follow-up. No tests of significance have been employed due to the small numbers involved.

To summarize, the assisted covert sensitization group demonstrated

Table 7
Pre- and Posttreatment Weekly Frequencies of Positive Blood and Urine Tests for the Presence of Drugs for Treatment and Control Subjects

Subject	Major drug of abuse	Pretreatment	Posttreatment	Six months
		Treatment Group		
1	Paint	0.8	0	0
2	Heroin	3.0	0	0
3	Alcohol	3.0	0	1.0
4	Alcohol	3.0	0	0
5	Alcohol	2.5	1.0	0
6	Valium	Not applicable		
7	Alcohol	3.0	2.5	3.0
8	Cigarettes	Not applicable		
9	Marijuana	0	0.5	0
10	Alcohol	2.5	0	0
		Control Group		
11	Alcohol	2.5	3.0	2.0
12	Cigarettes	Not applicable		
13	Alcohol	1.0	1.0	2.0
14	Marijuana	0.6	0	0
15	Valium	Not applicable		
16	Alcohol	3.0	0	1.5
17	Heroin	3.0	0.5	0
18	Hallucinogens	1.2	1.4	0
19	Alcohol	2.5	0	0
20	Alcohol	2.5	2.5	2.0

a significantly lower incidence of drug abuse, a significantly lower report of suspicions and incidents by observers, and a better record on tests of drug and alcohol levels in blood and urine.

DISCUSSION

Not all investigators experimenting with covert sensitization for drug abuse have reported complete success. Ashem and Donner (1968) claimed abstinence at 6 months' follow-up in six of 15 alcohol subjects. Sachs, Bean, and Morrow (1970) have recently documented some of the difficulties in applying covert sensitization to smoking behaviors.

Our results (Maletzky, In press, a; Maletzky and George, In press; Maletzky, In press, b) with this assisted technique have been somewhat better, perhaps only because of the stronger conditioning involved, but perhaps also due to the use of more "in vivo" conditioning. The strength of this conditioning is impressive: not only were *overt* acts of drug abuse eliminated in most subjects, but *covert* ones, such as urges to abuse drugs, as well. It appears as if a key factor in such conditioning is the association of consummatory responses, such as drinking or smoking, with stimuli designed to produce an aversive gastrointestinal reaction. A typical reaction to treatment was "I just don't think about drinking any more . . . the thought of it doesn't exactly make me sick . . . it's kind of neutral."

The study reported herein is hardly definitive. Small numbers were involved and no double-blind controls were possible. Most seriously, assisted covert sensitization was simply added to other ongoing therapies; an active placebo was not employed. Moreover, objective evaluations of continuing drug abuse were not strictly valied, and in any event are extremely difficult to obtain. One proposal might be a temptation test similar to those described to assess the effects of behavior therapy in the sexual deviations (Maletzky and George, In press; Maletzky, In press, b).

Nonetheless, these results do indicate that assisted covert sensitization can be beneficial when added to a preexisting drug abuse program. In answer to another of our original questions, we must admit that these data do not indicate which forms of drug abuse are peculiarly sensitive to assisted covert sensitization, perhaps because of the small numbers involved. Moreover, no salient subject variables seemed to predict success or failure. Perhaps studies involving larger numbers will be helpful in resolving such issues in the future, as well as indicating criteria for the use of such techniques in widely divergent patient groups.

Further questions concerning this technique abound. Larger, well-controlled studies will probably be forthcoming to compare a number of treatments; however, also needed are studies into the parameters of such behavior techniques. In assisted covert sensitization, for example, the therapist exerts little control over the timing, duration, and intensity of stimulus presentations. Of what importance are such parameters for the efficacy of treatment? A better understanding of the neurophysiologic mechanisms involved, both in addiction and in aversive conditioning, would be of benefit in resolving such issues. Some progress toward this goal has already been made (Villareal, 1972).

It might also be of interest to test which, if any, of the components of assisted covert sensitization are essential to the technique. Recent evidence (Agras, Leitenberg, and Barlow, 1971), for example, casts doubt on the assumption that deep muscular relaxation is necessary in desensitization, a technique that is in several ways the obverse of sensitization. Evidence

(Leitenberg, Agras, and Barlow, 1969) also exists that the type of instructions or "set" given to subjects may be of greater importance than previously imagined, although others disagree (Barlow et al., 1972).

Another kind of question has been suggested by the study of Ashem and Donner (1968), who treated hospitalized alcoholics with covert sensitization. These workers stressed the importance of hospitalization so that drinking could not occur during treatment. Yet most studies, including the present report, have yielded excellent results in outpatients who, at any time during treatment, might have emitted the unwanted behaviors. Studies deliberately requiring some subjects to emit the treated behavior outside the clinical setting might be informative.

Of more immediate relevance is the issue of how practical such a technique, or others like it, can be in the face of a growing realization that drug abuse is not a restricted phenomenon (Maletzky, 1972). "Drugs of the fathers," such as alcohol, minor tranquilizers, and cigarettes, quite probably outweigh, in prevalence and danger, "drugs of the sons," such as marijuana and the hallucinogens (McCracken, 1972). In this regard, assisted covert sensitization may possess several advantages:

1. It is effective against a wide variety of drug abuse behaviors.
2. It lends itself to group techniques. Relaxation and scene presentations can be effected within a group setting, thereby increasing efficiency of treatment.
3. It can be easily learned. Many of the treatments reported here were carried out by technicians taught the technique in a week's time. Their efficiency equalled the author's.
4. It lends itself to self-use. All patients here carried out practice sessions with tape recordings using their own vials of valeric acid; they were also able to smell the acid on their own in surroundings previously evocative of drug abusing behavior.
5. It is inexpensive. While mundane, the ease and cost of applying techniques provide valid bases for their comparison. Group and individual therapies for drug abuse are time-consuming and produce variable results. The use of aversive drugs or electric shock also entails a measure of effort and expense in all cases more costly than the use of imaginal methods. All results reported here were obtained with a single 500-g bottle of valeric acid ($4.50); a tape recorder, if not already on hand, can be inexpensively purchased.

Were assisted covert sensitization merely a less expensive behavioral technique, its use might still be occasionally condoned on grounds of easy availability to virtually all clinicians. That studies have now documented its efficacy is sound argument for its consideration against a host of drug abusing behaviors.

SUMMARY

A novel technique has been described in which a malodorous substance, valeric acid, is used to bolster the behavioral technique of covert sensitization. This "assisted" covert sensitization, applied to a myriad of drug abuse behaviors, including alcoholism, cigarette and marijuana smoking, and paint and glue sniffing, produced beneficial results in helping drug abusers cease not only overt drug abuse, but thoughts and urges surrounding drug abuse as well. Assisted covert sensitization is demonstrated to be not merely effective, but practical as well. The issue of its use in an overall approach to drug abuse and indeed, of all behavioral answers to drug abuse, must, however, await more definitive research for final resolution.

REFERENCES

AGRES, W.S., LEITENBERG, H., and BARLOW, D. Relaxation in systematic desensitization. *Arch. Gen. Psychiat.* 25: 511–514, 1971.

ANANT, S.S. A note on the treatment of alcoholics by the verbal aversion technique. *Can. Psychol.* 8a: 19–22, 1967.

ASHEM, B., and DONNER, L. Covert sensitization with alcoholics: a controlled replication. *Behav. Res. Therapy* 6: 7–12, 1968.

BARLOW, D.H., AGRAS, W.S., LEITENBERG, H., CALLAHAN, E.J., and MOORE, R.C. The contribution of therapeutic instruction to covert sensitization. *Behav. Tes Therapy* 10: 411–415, 1972.

BARLOW, D.H., LEITENBERG, H., and AGRAS, W.S. Experimental control of sexual deviation through manipulation of the noxious scence in covert sensitization. *J. Abnormal Psychol.* 74: 597–601, 1969.

BIRK, L., HUDDELSON, W., and MILLER, E. Avoidance conditioning for homosexuality. *Arch. Gen. Psychiat.* 25: 314–323, 1971.

BROWN, I.A.C. The nature and treatment of smoking. *Med. World* 98: 187–192, 1963.

CAUTELA, J.R. Treatment of compulsive behavior by covert sensitization. *Psychol. Rec.* 16: 33–41, 1966.

CAUTELA, J.R. Covert sensitization. *Psychol. Rep.* 20: 459–468, 1967.

CAUTELA, J.R. Covert reinforcement. *Behav. Therapy* 1: 33–50. 1970.

FRANKS, C.M. Alcohol, alcoholics, and conditioning. *J. Mental Sci.* 104: 14–33, 1958.

GOLD, S., and NEUFELD, I.L. A learning theory approach to the treatment of homosexuality. *Behav. Res. Therapy* 2: 201–204, 1965.

KENNEDY, W.A., and FOREYT, J. Control of eating behavior in an obese patient by

avoidance conditioning. *Psychol. Rep.* 23: 571–573, 1968.
KOLVIN, I. "Aversive imagery" treatment in adolescents. *Behav. Res. Therapy* 5: 245–248, 1967.
LAZARUS, A.A. New methods in psychotherapy: a case study. *S. African Med. J.* 32: 660–663, 1958.
LEITENBERG, H., AGRAS, W.S., and BARLOW, D.H. Contribution of selective positive reinforcement to systematic desensitization therapy. *J. Abnormal Psychol.* 74: 113–118, 1969.
LICHTENSTEIN, E., and KEUTZER, C.S. Investigation of diverse techniques to modify smoking: a follow-up report. *Behav. Res. Therapy* 7: 139–140, 1969.
MALETZKY, B.M. Hidden forms of drug abuse. *Aviation Dig.* 18: 8–11, 1972.
MALETZKY, B.M. "Assisted" covert sensitization. *Behav. Therapy.* In press (a).
MALETZKY, B.M. The treatment of exhibitionism by "assisted" covert sensitization. *J. Consult. Clin. Psychol.* In press (b).
MALETZKY, B.M., and GEORGE, F.S. The treatment of homosexuality by "assisted" covert sensitization. *Behav. Res. Therapy*, In press.
McCONAGHY, N. Subjective and penile plethysmograph responses to aversion therapy for homosexuality: a follow-up stud. *Brit. J. Psychiat.* 117: 555–560, 1970.
McCONAGHY, N. Aversion therapy of homosexuality: measures of efficacy. *Amer. J. Psychiat.* 127: 1221–1224, 1971.
McCRACKEN, S. The drugs of habit and the drugs of belief. *Reflections* 7: 41–62, 1972.
MORGENSTERN, F., PEARCE, J., and DAVIES, B. The application of aversive therapy to transvestism. Paper presented at Annual Meeting of the British Psychological Society, Reading, England, 1963.
MULLEN, F.Y. The effect of covert sensitization of smoking behavior. Doctoral Essay, Queens College, Charlottesville, North Carolina, 1968.
RACHMAN, S.J., and TEASDALE, J. Aversion therapy: an appraisal. In C. M. Franks (ed.) *Behavior Therapy: Appraisal and Status.* New York: McGraw-Hill, 1969, pp. 279–320.
SACHS, L.B., BEAN, H., and MORROW, J.E. Comparison of smoking treatments. *Behav. Therapy* 1: 465–472, 1970.
SCHWARTZ, J.L., and DUBITZKY, M. *Psychosocial Factors Involved in Cigarette Smoking and Cessation.* Berkeley, California: Smoking Control Research Project, 1968.
VIERNSTEIN, L. Evaluation of therapeutic techniques of covert sensitization. Unpublished study, Queens College, Charlottesville, North Carolina, 1968.
VILLAREAL, J. Perspectives of research in the biological aspects of drug dependence. Presented to the Fifth Annual Western Institute of Drug Problems, Portland, Oregon, June 1972.
WOLPE, J. *The Practice of Behavior Therapy.* New York: Pergamon, 1969.
WOLPE, J., and LAZARUS, A.A. *Behavior Therapy Techniques.* New York, Pergamon, 1958.

The International Journal of the Addictions, 9(3), 431–446, 1974

Psychological and Social Variables and Personality Patterns of Drug Abusers

Kenneth B. Stein, Ph.D.

Psychology Department
University of California
Berkeley, California

Vitali Rozynko, Ph.D.

Veterans Administrtion Hospital
Palo Alto, California

The present investigation describes in social and psychological terms a sample of addicted persons voluntarily admitted to a state hospital for detoxification and treatment. The efforts were also directed toward examining the heterogeneity among drug abusers of certain a priori personality dimensions in order to observe whether differentiated empirical patterns could be located among them.

Empirical typological studies of personality have emerged recently. A number of these have been based upon the Minnesota Multiphasic Personality Inventory (MMPI) (Hathaway and McKinley, 1951) or similar type measures (for example, Sutker, 1971; Haertzen et al., 1968). These investigations have often centered on the concept of psychopathy (sociopathy) as a means of understanding the addict. In exploring personality aspects of addicted individuals, we included the MMPI as only one of our procedures in focusing upon four general areas: emotional disturbance, cognitive-intellectual level, expressiveness, and socialization, in order to give the study broad scope. The social background factors were employed in several ways, namely, for a general description of our sample, and for definitional and descriptive characteristics of the empirical psychological types.

METHOD

Within a period of 7 months, 201 randomly selected voluntary male admissions (13.6% of total admissions) to the detoxification ward of a California state hospital were interviewed and tested. A detailed description of the subjects appears below in the Results section.

Subjects were interviewed using a structured set of items. Following are the psychological tests and the order in which they were administered: Future and Past Time Perspective Tests (Stein and Craik, 1965); Motoric Ideational Sensory Test (MIST), (Stein and Lenrow, 1970); Socialization (So) Scale of the California Psychological Inventory (CPI), (Gough, 1957); Hidden Patterns Test -CF-2- (Educational Testing Service, 1962b); Extended Range Vocabulary Test -V-3- (Educational Testing Service, 1962a); MMPI and Tryon-Stein-Chu Scales (TSC), (Stein, 1968) derived from the MMPI. Reliability and validity of these tests can be found in their respective publications.

Table 1
Raw Mean Scores and Standard Deviations for the MMPI and TSC Scales of 201 Hospitalized Drug Addicted Patients[a]

Scale	*M*	SD	Scale	*M*	SD
MMPI Q	1.80	4.14	MMPI Ma	23.54	4.98
MMPI L	3.15	1.93	MMPI Si	30.68	9.83
MMPI F	12.65	6.94	MMPI Es	40.26	7.26
MMPI K	10.66	4.61	MMPI R	14.60	4.94
MMPI Hs	11.40	6.70	TSC Introversion	11.35	6.05
MMPI D	26.96	6.98	TSC Body Complaint	11.64	6.44
MMPI Hy	24.34	6.33	TSC Suspicion	15.47	5.47
MMPI Pd	26.40	4.89	TSC Depression	14.32	5.21
MMPI Mf	27.33	5.14	TSC Resentment	11.01	4.58
MMPI Pa	13.12	4.36	TSC Autism	10.86	4.67
MMPI Pt	22.41	9.59	TSC Tension	16.05	6.97
MMPI Sc	24.65	11.91			

[a] *K*-correction has not been included in the above MMPI means.

Table 2
Means, Standard Deviations, and Intercorrelations of Six Key Cluster Dimensions for 201 Subjects

Variable	Tension	Motoric	Idea-tional	Sensory	So	Voc	M	SD
TSC-Tension	—						16.05	6.97
MIST-Motoric	.01	—					39.59	10.47
MIST-Ideational	.08	.39	—				45.13	14.38
MIST-Sensory	–.03	.34	.34	—			37.74	11.60
CPI-Socialization	–.39	–.05	–.18	.09	—		24.59	5.07
ETS-Vocabulary	–.22	–.06	.28	.14	–.11	—	23.60	7.17

The structured interview schedule was subjected to a reliability study between two interviewers. Ten items of the original 63 were eliminated for low consistency. The remainder yielded perfect agreement in 81 to 100% of the cases.

Statistically, the sample was described with means and standard deviations on the 31 test variables and with frequency distributions for each of the interview variables. Programs from the BC TRY system (Tryon and Bailey, 1970) were utilized for type derivation (OTYPE) and for determining significant relations between types and dependent variables (4CAST).

Six of the more promising psychological variables became the input dimensions for the typological analysis: vocabulary level, socialization, motoric expressiveness, ideational expressiveness, sensory expressiveness, and tension.

FINDINGS

Interview Data

The average age of the sample was 25.52 years. More than one-half had completed high school; 51% had never married and another 26% were either separated or divorced, while only 21% were married. The ethnic or racial composition of the group was mostly White (67%), with 17% Black and 12% Chicano. Occupational level was low; 42% were semiskilled or unskilled persons and another 23% were hustlers, that is, supported themselves by extralegal means. Ninety-one percent of the sample had been using heroin on a regular, daily basis, and 70% used other drugs in addition, mostly marijuana and barbiturates. While 60% started taking

Table 3

Standard Score Patterns of Drug Addicts[a]

Type		TSC Tension	MIST Motoric	MIST Ideational	MIST Sensory	CPI So Scale	Vocab-ulary	$\bar{H}$	*N*
1. Motoric-artist/	*M*	*43*	*55*	50	49	*56*	47	0.82	26
musician	SD	5.8	6.8	5.9	4.9	6.1	4.1		
2. Intellectual	*M*	*39*	48	*57*	50	53	*61*	0.80	19
	SD	4.8	6.5	7.1	6.7	5.4	5.0		
3. Low expressive	*M*	*43*	*42*	*40*	*35*	52	47	0.85	17
minorities	SD	5.8	6.4	5.6	3.7	5.7	3.5		
4. Tense and dull	*M*	*55*	*43*	49	*42*	*58*	*42*	0.79	18
	SD	7.6	4.6	4.6	3.6	5.1	9.2		
5. Low expressive	*M*	49	*42*	*41*	46	*42*	51	0.82	21
Chicanos	SD	5.9	6.2	5.2	6.5	5.8	4.5		
6. Anti social	*M*	53	54	*59*	51	*40*	48	0.76	18
ideational	SD	5.8	8.7	8.1	6.4	4.3	4.8		
7. Low verbal	*M*	54	*59*	*64*	48	*58*	*39*	0.81	10
achiever	SD	4.9	3.5	5.4	7.9	6.4	6.3		
8. Intelligent	*M*	48	52	50	*58*	48	*68*	0.74	11
sensory	SD	6.2	7.8	6.3	5.1	8.5	5.8		
9 Tense-dull	*M*	*64*	*57*	49	53	46	*41*	0.79	18
motoric	SD	4.0	7.7	6.1	6.1	6.8	5.7		
10. Sensory-artist/	*M*	60	51	47	*63*	*41*	*55*	0.77	22
musician	SD	5.8	6.9	7.0	5.2	6.6	6.9		
	η	0.82	0.74	0.79	0.82	0.80	0.82		
N Subjects in types									180
Unique subjects									18
Missing scores									3
Grand total									201

[a] The *italicized* mean scores are the unique high and low values of each type.

drugs of any kind at age 16 and below, about 42% were taking "hard" drugs at this early age. Two-thirds of the sample started using marijuana as their first drug. Many persons who started on methedrine, barbiturates, and LSD later switched to heroin. Fifty-seven percent spent more than $50 a day to sustain their drug use; 30% spent from $15 to $50 per day. (Table 4)

While 35% admitted to only the present addiction, 28% of the sample had been addicted more than three times. Sixty-one percent had been using their principal drug (mostly heroin) for less than 6 months. Almost 60% had been hospitalized because of drug-associated conditions.

The great majority were introduced to various drugs through friends (49 to 72%), while 43% originally took their principal drug of choice, heroin mostly, as an experiment; another 16% wanted to be "part of the crowd," while still another 15% "wanted to get high."

The great majority of the sample had extensive contact with the police, only 7% having never been booked. Thirty-six percent had served jail or prison sentences of less than 1 year, and 23% sentences of 1 year or greater. The offenses for which their sentences were meted out distributed as follows: violence 42%; drug-associated offenses 17%; robbery, theft, and burglary 16%; and misdemeanors 8%. Twenty-three percent had been in either federal or state prison.

Almost three-quarters of those married had wives who also took drugs, mostly marijuana and heroin. Thirty-four percent had no female partner. In relation to female partners, 17% felt they related well, were usually happy; 23% related so-so and sometimes fought; and 25% related poorly.

Seventy percent of the sample were raised by both parents, and 61% of the sample's parents were together (not separated) for 15 or more years during the time they were being raised. However, 50% of the sample did not feel close to either parent, and 54% left home before they were 18.

Although most fathers were employed as laborers, one-third were either professionals or small businessmen. Mothers were largely housewives (44%), 26% were laborers, and 25% were either in small business or in the professions. As to education, 23% of the fathers and 28% of the mothers had some college; 20% of the fathers and 25% of the mothers were high school graduates; the rest failed to complete high school. As for legal difficulties, less than 6% of mothers and 18% of fathers had arrest records, mostly for minor violations. In 68% of the sample, no member of the subject's family had used drugs of any kind; 25% of the sample's siblings had used several drugs, 10% of whom had used heroin.

Table 4

Ten Drug Types and Their Means or Proportions on a Variety of Background and Social Variables

	1	2	3	4	5	6	7	8	9	10	Total
Variable											
Age			28.76**	27.56*	22.62***		28.40*		23.44**	22.82**	25.52
Education		4.26**	3.41**		3.48**			4.36**	3.33**		3.84
Marital status											
Single			0.24***		0.71***						0.57
Married	0.12*		0.41***			0.33*	0.10*	0.09*			0.22
Widowed											
Divorced	0.23**	0.05*									0.14
Separated				0.22*	0.00***		0.30**		0.06*		0.12
Common-law				0.05***					0.06***		0.01
Race-Ethnic											
White		0.84**	0.41***	0.22***			0.40**	1.00***		0.95***	0.67
Black			0.29**	0.61***	0.00***		0.60***	0.00***		0.00***	0.17
Oriental	0.04**			0.06***							0.01
American Indian											
Mexican-American		0.05*	0.24***	0.06*	0.29***		0.00***	0.00***	0.06*	0.05*	0.12
Other			0.06*	0.06*					0.06*		0.03
Occupation											
Professional	0	0.11***	0	0	0	0	0	0.09**	0	0	0.02
Small Business	0.08**	0	0	0	0	0	0.20***	0		0	0.03
Skilled labor			0.12*			0.33**			0.11*	0.09*	0.19
Semiskilled		0.00***	0.35**	0.11*	0.33**			0.36**			0.21
Unskilled	0.11**			0.33**				0.09*	0.33*		0.21
Students			0	0		0	0	0	0.11**		0.04

Artist/music	0.15***		0	0	0	0	0		0	0.18***	0.05
Hustler	0.11**					0.11**					0.23
Main drug											
Heroin			1.00	1.00				1.00	0.83*	0.68***	0.91
Methedrine									0.06***	0.05**	0.02
Marijuana		0.05**			0.05**					0.09***	0.02
Barbiturates									0.06***	0.05***	0.01
LSD						0.06**				0.09***	0.02
Amount drug use	5.00***		4.65*	5.00***			4.50**				4.94
Time using drugs								1.18**			1.63
Second drug											
Methedrine										0.09***	0.04
Marijuana			0.18***	0.17***				0.64**		0.55*	0.63
Barbiturates	0.19*			0.22*				0.00***			0.17
LSD										0.13***	0.04
Other		0.16**			0.14**						0.09
Amount drug use—D2	2.93*		1.18***	1.17***						3.32***	3.43
Cost of drugs				4.61**	4.52*				3.44***	3.50***	4.13
Times addicted	2.58*		1.94*	1.94*					1.83***	2.73***	2.33
How started drugs											
Friend	0.46**	0.47*		0.83***							0.60
Dealer	0.19*	0.21**		0.00***			0.20*		0.06*		0.12
Doctor											0
Spouse			0.18*				0.00***	0.00***			0.11
Other		0.26*	0.24*	0.06**				0.27*			0.17
Why started drugs											
Part of crowd	0.04***					0.28*	0.00***	0.00***			0.16

(continued)

Table 4 (continued)

	1	2	3	4	5	6	7	8	9	10	Total
To get high	0.27**			0.06*	0.24*		0.00***	0.00***			0.16
Experiment				0.56*		0.22**					0.43
Kick other drugs		0.26***							0.11*		0.08
Other		0.05*			0.10*		0.50***	0.36**			0.18
When started drugs							4.10**				3.42
First drug—marijuana		0.58*	0.88***		0.81**		0.50*			0.50**	0.68
Age—first hard drug				4.33**				4.18*			3.83
Prior drug hospital	2.15**			1.56**				1.64*			1.91
Police contacts											
Arrests-violence			0.06*		0.10**	0.06*		0.10**			0.03
Robbery	0.04**					0.06**					0.02
Burglary				0.25***			0.10*		0.20***		0.05
Car theft		0.06*						0.10**			0.02
Misdemeanors	0.29*		0.41***	0.31*		0.11*				0.14*	0.21
Marijuana		0.22**	0.00**	0.00**			0.20*			0.24***	0.10
Other drug				0.19*				0.50**			0.29
Deviant sex acts											0.00
Other	0.17**		0.18*			0.44**					0.28
Latest arrest											
Past 6 months	0.54*			0.56*			0.10***	0.30*			0.44
7–12 months	0.08**	0.33*			0.40***						0.23
13–24 months			0.06*		0.05*				0.20*		0.12
25 months or more					0.10**		0.50***		0.07*		0.21
No. of prison sentences			1.65**						1.17*		1.33

Longest prison sentence	1.69*		2.35**	2.28*				1.45**			1.92
Family data											
Amount of spouse drug use					0.00***			3.67**	2.57*	3.00**	1.56
Adequate heterosex		2.17**				1.64*	1.33**		2.17*	2.15*	1.89
Felt close to parents		0.37**		0.33*	0.00***						0.23
Felt close to father	0.19***										0.08
Felt close to mother	0.00***				0.43***						0.20
Not close to parents									0.61*		0.49
Raised by parents			0.88**		0.57*			1.00***			0.70
Mother's education		4.56***			3.21*		3.13*	4.91***			3.70
Father's education		4.33***	2.57***	2.50**		3.00*	2.67**	4.43***		4.11**	3.54
No family drug		0.79*		0.83**	0.47***				0.50**	0.55**	0.68
Father alcoholic		0.11**		0.33*			0.10*		0.33*	0.36**	0.24
Mother alcoholic										0.14***	0.05
Both parents alcoholic	0.08*									0.14***	0.05

* $p \leq .10$.
** $p \leq .05$.
*** $p \leq .01$.

They also used marijuana, methedrine, and LSD. Forty-three percent of the sample's family were reported to use alcohol to excess; 34% had reported either or both parents as using alcohol to excess and approximately 10% had reported excess alcohol use by siblings.

Psychological Test Data

The MMPI clinical scales are generally elevated, five of which are above the critical level (D, Pd, Pt, Sc, Ma). (Table 1) The general intensity of these scales indicates the emotional disturbance experienced by the newly hospitalized addicted group. Anxiety, dysphoric mood, and agitation contribute to the difficulty of these patients to function adaptively and effectively. These clinical features are superimposed upon an antisocial orientation capable of directing aggression outwards as well as inwards (Dahlstrom and Welsh, 1960). This pattern is not unlike the "caged" effect of newly admitted prisoners and neurotic psychopaths incarcerated for drugs (Haertzen and Hill, 1959; Sutker, 1971), as well as newly admitted hospitalized alcoholics (Stein, Rozynko, and Pugh, 1971).

The TSC scales are generally elevated with prominent peaks occurring on depression and body complaints and a lesser one on general tension and anxiety. The personality disorder is also evident. The pattern is somewhat similar to those of enlisted men discharged for ineptitude (Stein, 1968).

On past and future time perspective, the study sample was compared with a mixed group of neurotic and psychotic male patients in an outpatient clinic (Stein and Craik, 1965). (Table 6.) Since the latter group was approximately twelve years older than the addicted sample, the comparison can only be considered very tentative and suggestive. On past time perspective, the psychiatric patients obtained a time length twice that of the addicts (84 to 39 months), which may be a function of age. On future time perspective, the time span again is greater for the psychiatric subjects (33 to 21 months), a result that occurs in spite of the age differential. This latter finding particularly, together with past time, reflects the stimulus bound, constricted time span character of the addicts which is consistent with the presence of immediate pressing drug needs.

The CPI So scale score of 24.6 falls far below the norm of 37 for the general population (Gough, 1957). In Gough's terms these addicts, on the average, are unable to take the role of the other person, to be sensitive to and to empathize with the feelings of others.

A further comparison was made on the motoric, ideational, and sen-

Table 5
Ten Drug Types and Their MMPI Scores and TSC Scales

Variable		1	2	3	4	5	6	7	8	9	10	Total
MMPI	Q	2.35	2.00	1.71	2.67	1.62	1.33	1.30	3.09	0.61*	1.50	1.80
	L	3.35	4.11**	3.88**	2.61*	2.90	2.22***	3.10	3.9	2.61*	2.14***	3.15
	F	9.30***	6.95***	8.12***	13.90	13.57	13.61	13.10	12.73	17.94***	19.45***	12.65
	K	12.19**	14.58***	12.65**	9.17*	10.29	8.39**	8.30	10.91	6.33***	8.14***	10.66
	Hs	8.65***	5.79***	7.47***	14.78**	11.43	11.72	14.00*	9.64	18.06***	15.73***	11.40
	D	24.23**	23.68**	22.59***	28.50	28.42	29.11*	26.30	25.54	30.06***	30.36***	26.96
	Hy	22.92	22.84	20.59***	26.39*	24.38	23.61	24.80	22.45	24.39	29.23***	24.34
	Pd	24.04***	23.53***	24.41**	25.94	27.57	29.39***	25.20	27.09	27.00	31.41***	26.40
	Mf	26.19	27.95	24.29***	27.00	27.52	27.22	26.70	32.09***	25.83*	29.45**	27.33
	Pa	11.04***	10.26***	10.12***	14.39*	12.76	13.11	14.20	13.91	15.72**	17.18***	13.12
	Pt	16.54***	13.21***	15.47***	27.00**	23.52	27.11**	26.50*	19.73	31.89***	31.59***	22.41
	Sc	17.62***	14.05***	14.88***	28.61*	25.33	27.83	27.20	25.00	38.00***	37.41***	24.65
	Ma	22.46	21.05***	21.24**	23.89	23.38	24.56	23.50	23.55	27.39***	27.59***	23.54
	Si	25.81**	24.63***	29.71	31.50	33.14	33.22	30.60	30.45	35.72***	36.05***	30.68
	Es	44.31***	45.58***	45.47***	33.56***	40.62	40.83	37.70	41.36	33.67***	34.64***	40.26
	R	14.38	14.79	16.12	15.06	16.24**	13.67	12.30*	15.64	11.61***	13.23*	14.60
TSC Introversion		9.08**	8.32***	10.00	11.28	11.67	13.67	11.70	12.73	13.50**	14.23***	11.35
Body		8.46***	6.63***	7.82**	15.22***	11.71	12.00	13.50	10.18	18.17***	16.14***	11.64
Suspicion		13.92	11.58***	12.53***	17.39**	16.00	17.33**	17.80*	13.82	20.33***	18.27***	15.47
Depression		10.72***	9.47***	10.94**	15.44	15.71	17.22**	16.30	13.64	18.78***	19.27***	14.32
Resentment		9.19***	6.68***	9.53*	11.50	10.71	13.39**	12.30	10.82	15.72***	14.77***	11.01
Autism		8.54***	7.26***	7.29***	12.72**	11.38	11.67	13.00*	10.18	15.94***	15.27***	10.86
Tension		11.46***	8.68***	11.24**	19.39**	15.57	18.22*	19.10*	14.45	25.61***	23.00***	16.06

* $p \leq .10$.
** $p \leq .05$.
*** $p \leq .01$.

Table 6
Ten Types in Relation to Various Psychological Variables

Variable	1	2	3	4	5	6	7	8	9	10	Total
Past-time perspective	42.08	44.21	45.59	39.11	28.33**	39.00	79.60***	32.55	29.28	28.95*	38.58
Future-time perspective	23.62	19.79	22.53	14.89	24.95	18.00	6.90***	17.55	19.00	16.68	20.73
Motoric	45.12***	37.74	31.24***	32.17***	31.52***	43.83**	48.70***	41.36	47.11***	40.82	39.59
Sensory	45.42	45.74	24.12***	33.89***	39.67**	46.28	42.70	56.73***	49.39*	63.32***	45.13
Ideational	36.08	45.89***	25.76***	36.22	27.14***	47.61***	54.30***	38.27	36.72	34.27*	37.74
Socialization	27.50***	26.00*	25.76	28.78***	20.67***	19.33***	28.60***	23.36	22.67**	20.14***	24.59
Hidden patterns	72.73	81.74**	64.59	50.11**	69.29	71.28	70.10	82.27**	46.67***	75.86*	68.50
Vocabulary	21.12**	31.58***	21.18*	18.11***	24.62	22.50	16.00***	36.64***	17.50***	26.91***	23.60

* $p \leq .10$.
** $p \leq .05$.
*** $p \leq .01$.

sory expressive dimensions between the study group and a college group of males (Stein and Lenrow, 1970). No differences occur. The range of scores, however, tends to be greater for the addicts but short of significance.

Personality Types

The input dimensions for an OTYPE analysis were six a priori personality variables: tension, motoric, ideational, sensory expressiveness, socialization and vocabulary intelligence. A number of these variables served quite successfully as the basis of pattern formation in a previous study of alcoholics (Stein, Rozynko and Pugh, 1971).

The OTYPE analysis resulted in 10 distinctive personality patterns. Considering that the analysis accounted for 180 of the 201 subjects (89.5%), the homogeneities (**H**), that is, the mean partial η's across the six dimensions, are gratifyingly high and indicate very little variability within pattern scores among the subjects within types. Yet the heterogeneity of scores across types is extensive and ranges from one and one-half to three σ. Such a distribution of scores across types and the small variance within types attest to the psychological heterogeneity of those subsumed under the rubric of drug addict. (Table 3.)

The number of significant relationships between each of the discontinuous 10 types on the 104 social and psychological variables greatly exceeds chance expectations at the 10% level. Significant findings range from 19 (18.2%) to 52 (50%), the lowest and the highest number of such findings for the types. Extensive tabular presentation of these results can be found elsewhere (Rozynko and Stein, 1972). The social variables pertain to the categories of age, marital status, education, race, occupation, drug use history, arrest and prison records, and relations with parents and spouse. The psychological variables were previously identified. (Tables 4, 5, and 6.)

The tentative names assigned to the types are: (1) motoric artist/musician; (2) intellectual; (3) low expressive minorities; (4) tense and dull; (5) low expressive Chicano; (6) antisocial ideational; (7) low verbal achiever; (8) intelligent sensory; (9) tense, dull, motoric; and (10) sensory artist/musician. (See Appendix 1.)

SUMMARY

The purpose of the research was to describe drug abusers in social and psychological terms and to discover empirical personality types among them. A random sample of 201 male voluntary admissions to a state hospital detoxification ward was studied using a structured interview and personality inventories. The six personality dimensions which served as the structural basis for a computerized derivation of patterns or types were (1) tension; (2) motoric; (3) ideational; (4) sensory expressive orientation; (5) socialization; and (6) vocabulary intelligence. Computer program OTYPE produced 10 types. Significant relationships between each of these types and a large number of social and psychological variables were found to far exceed chance expectations, and these served as definitional characteristics of the types. The findings have implications for further study, particularly in relation to therapeutic outcome.

APPENDIX I

Types and Descriptions

The tentative names for the types, together with a few of the salient findings are listed below:

1. *Motoric artist/musician type:* Heavy heroin user. Close relationship to father but distant from mother. Parents are alcoholic.
2. *Intellectual Type:* Predominantly white professional who took up principal drug to kick other drugs. Significant number using marijuana. Lowest level of tension of all types. Closeness to parents is expressed.
3. *Low Expressive Minorities Type:* Mainly older, married Blacks, Orientals, and Chicanos. A significant subgroup of these men was started on drugs by their spouse. This group has a large number of arrests for violence as well as for misdemeanors, and a history of state and federal imprisonment.
4. *Tense and Dull Type:* An older group of Blacks and Orientals, all of whom are heavy heroin users. Arrest record mainly for burglary. Father is an alcoholic.
5. *Low Expressive Chicano Type:* Mainly single or in common law arrangement. History of heavy marijuana use. Arrest record principally for violence. This group indicates a closeness to mother and reveals a low past time perspective.
6. *Antisocial Ideational Type:* Criminal record primarily for violence and robbery. Significantly large number use LSD as principal drug.
7. *Low Verbal Achiever Type:* High motoric and ideational interests and low vocabulary suggests a possible overachiever. These men reveal extensive past time but low future time perspective.

8. *Intelligent Sensory Type:* Mainly White professionals as well as a subgroup of semiskilled men whose spouses are heavily into drug use. Violence stands out in their criminal record.

9. *Tense, Dull, and Motoric Type:* Contains subgroups of college students and unskilled workers who are on methedrine and barbiturates. Started current drugs to "kick" other drugs. Burglary arrest record noted. Father is alcoholic. Subjects in this type are likely to be distant from parents.

10. *Sensory Artist/Musician Type:* Highly intelligent, White men who use heroin as their principal drug as well as a variety of other drugs. Parents are alcoholic. This group shows a low time perspective.

ACKNOWLEDGMENT

This research was supported in part by the grant MH 17647 from the National Institute of Mental Health of the U.S. Public Health Service. Our appreciation is expressed to Kathleen Sherman for her invaluable assistance in this research.

REFERENCES

DAHLSTROM, W.G., and WELSH, G.S. *An MMPI Handbook*. Minneapolis, Minnesota: Univ. Minnesota Press, 1960.

EDUCATIONAL TESTING SERVICE. *Extended Range Vocabulary Test-V-3*. Princeton, N. J., 1962a.

EDUCATIONAL TESTING SERVICE. *Hidden Patterns Test CF-2*. Princeton, N. J., 1962b.

GOUGH, H.G. *Manual for the California Psychological Inventory*. Palo Alto, California: Consulting Psychologists Press, 1957.

HAERTZEN, C.A., and HILL, H.E. Effects of morphine and pentobarbital on differential MMPI profiles. *J. Clin. Psychol.* 15: 434–437, 1959.

HAERTZEN, C.A., HILL, H.E., and MONROE, J.J. MMPI scales for differentiating and predicting relapse in alcoholics, opiate addicts and criminals. *Intern. J. Addictions* 3: 91–106, 1968.

HATHAWAY, S.R., and McKINLEY, J.C. *The Minnesota Multiphasic Personality Inventory Manual* (rev. ed.) New York, Psychological Corp., 1951.

ROZYNKO, V., and STEIN, K.B. *Typology of Drug Abusers: A Final Report*. Bethesda, Md.: National Institute of Mental Health, 1972.

STEIN, K.B., and CRAIK, K.H. Relationship between motoric and ideational activity preference and time perspective in neurotics and schizophrenics. *J. Consult. Psychol.* 29: 460–467, 1965.

STEIN, K.B., GOUGH, H.G., and SARBIN, T.R. The dimensionality of the CPI socialization scale and an empirically derived typology among delinquent and nondelinquent boys. *Multivariate Behav. Res.* 1: 197–208, 1966.

STEIN, K.B. The TSC scales: The outcome of a cluster analysis of the 550 MMPI items. In P. McReynold (ed.) *Advances in Psychological Assessment*. Palo Alto, Calif.: Science and Behavioral Press, 1968.

STEIN, K.B., and LENROW, P. Expressive styles and their measurement. *J. Personality Soc. Psychol.* 16: 656–664, 1970.

STEIN, K.B., ROZYNKO, V., and PUGH, L.A. The heterogeneity of personality among alcoholics. *Brit. J. Soc. Clin. Psychol.* 10: 253–259, 1971

SUTKER, P.A. Personality differences and sociopathy in heroin addicts and nonaddict prisoners. *J. Abnormal Psychol.* 78, 247–251, 1971.

TRYON, R.C., and BAILEY, D.E. *Cluster Analysis*. New York: McGraw-Hill, 1970.

The International Journal of the Addictions, 9(3), 447–464, 1974

Group Covert Sensitization with Narcotic Addicts (Further Comments)

G. J. Steinfeld, Ph.D.

E. A. Rautio, Ph.D.

A. H. Rice, B.S.

M. J. Egan

Narcotic Unit
Federal Correctional Institution
Danbury, Connecticut

This paper will describe a program of covert sensitization presently being developed at the Narcotic Unit, Federal Correctional Institution, Danbury, Connecticut. Steinfeld has previously reported work with individual narcotic addicts and with groups using the covert sensitization procedure (1970). The present report is based on further work with groups and is part of a broader therapeutic program consisting primarily of a self-help community. There are two such therapeutic communities at Danbury, each housing approximately 50 residents who spend approximately 14 months in an intensive self-help program for narcotic addicts. These men have been sentenced under Title II of the N.A.R.A. Act of 1966. The covert sensitization program is seen as one adjunct to the basic therapeutic procedure which utilizes various forms of groups, i.e., encounters, seminars, and static group (traditional therapy group), as well as other forms of behavioral approaches and sensitivity workshops. Our hope is to offer the resident several tools to help resist the pull toward drugs once he leaves the protective environment of the institution and returns to his community.

This report details, more precisely than the previous report, the procedures we have used in attempting to reach groups of addicts in the rehabilitation process. The men selected were within a few months of release. This was done so that our behavioral program would not interfere with the major thrust which focuses on the clarification of feelings, the differentiation of thoughts from feelings, the use of groups to help the men achieve insight into their motivations, while at the same time attempting to use the reality of group pressure to facilitate more honest communication and more responsible behavior.

An announcement was made to the residents that an eight session covert sensitization program would be initiated. Covert sensitization was briefly described, it was stressed that participation was strictly voluntary and would have nothing to do with their ultimate parole. The only stipulation was that residents would have to come to all eight sessions. The following describes, in summary fashion, what took place in each of the eight sessions.

SESSION 1

An explanation of the program was again given. The relaxation training and the conditioning process was described, and more detail was gone into about the use of systematic desensitization to decrease maladaptive avoidance responses such as specific fears or phobic behavior, and covert sensitization to decrease maladaptive approach behavior such as alcoholism, overeating, and, more relevantly, the taking of drugs. In our case, the drug focused on was heroin. The group then heard a tape of Dr. Arnold Lazarus of Yale University. These tapes are part of a series entitled "Coping with Tensions and Anxieties" and are produced by Instructional Dynamics, Inc. (1972). The first tape, on the use of relaxation, describes the how and why of relaxation training. The mechanisms of relaxation are explained and Dr. Lazarus describes some of the research on the physiological and psychological aspects of relaxation.

On this tape the process that is involved in relaxation training is stressed, and the listener is given facts to enhance relaxation training. Also discussed is the use of differential relaxation, a procedure which can be used when the person is standing or driving, and which helps him to relax the muscles that are not in use. Lazarus also offers reminders about when to use relaxation. He stresses the confidence that a person gains through training to relax his body, the psychologically constricting effects of high states of tension, and the difference between relaxation and recreation. In the first tape he also summarizes the subsequent relaxation program. In the next tape, Relaxation Training 1, which is the first actual training session, the difference between feelings and sensations during the tension and relaxation stage is stressed, and Dr. Lazarus systematically takes the listener through the relaxation of muscle groups from head to toe. This tape is essentially the procedure described in the literature (Wolpe and Lazarus, 1966) and is based on Jacobson's technique of muscle relaxation (1938). The men were advised to practice at least twice a day. Previous experience indicates that one of the problems during relaxation is that men go to sleep when they listen to the tape. Addicts are generally very willing subjects for this procedure, a phenomenon which is understandable given the history of heroin addiction and the ritual which induces the experience of total relaxation. Another problem we encountered is that people close their eyes too tightly and this becomes painful. The importance of remaining awake and practicing was stressed over and over again. There was some restlessness when the relaxation of the lower part of the back was being worked on. This was hard for our men to do, given the chairs that we were using, but more generally we have found the arching of the back to be somewhat disruptive to some persons who become highly relaxed before reaching this part of the body in the procedure. When this happens we encourage these persons to either pass over this part of their body or to tense the lower back without actually arching it.

In addition to urging the men to practice, they were told to repeat the tensing and relaxation of various parts of their body which still felt tense after the tape had been completed. They were also given inventories to complete which tapped situations in which they felt fearful or anxious. The results of that questionnaire, in terms of categories of stimuli which evoked fear in our group, are described below. The fears they checked would be used to weave a story which could arouse anxiety around the "shooting of heroin." This is, essentially, the covert sensitization procedure as developed by Cautela (1966, 1967) and used by Steinfeld in his previous work (1970).

Another questionnaire was administered by which information was sought to clarify the feelings associated with drug taking, as well as to specify some of the conditions under which the shooting of heroin took place. The results of this questionnaire are also presented below.

One could ask why we train the men in relaxation procedure. Cautela (personal communication) claims covert sensitization can be applied without the use of relaxation. We did this for three reasons. One is that we wanted to offer men the opportunity to learn a procedure that could help them in their lives, regardless of whether or not covert sensitization was effective, and relaxation training can be useful in a variety of ways. We know that we all struggle to cope with the tensions of daily life, and addicts returning to their communities after months in prison will clearly have much to deal with. We invariably see a good deal of this anxiety even before the men leave the institution, let alone in many social situations afterwards. Two, we felt that if the level of anxiety could be reduced, then the difference between relaxation and the increase in tension with the presentation of the aversive scene would be more clear. We would thereby make the procedure more effective. Third, we went into elaborate details on the use of relaxation to lend more credibility to the precedure. There is recent evidence that cognitive processes are important variables even in an automated process of systematic desensitization. In an unpublished thesis, supervised by the senior author (Mark and Genzer, 1972), we found evidence of the effect of cognition on the systematic desensitization of test anxiety. In that study the entire procedure was tape recorded, and subjects were treated over a number of sessions believing that the procedure was "new" vs "tried" and that the therapists were either a professional "doctor" or a graduate student. An interaction was found in that a "tried" procedure used by a "professional" doctor was most effective in reducing reported test anxiety, but that the "tried" variable contributed mainly to the effect. In our work we wanted to enhance the believability in our procedure, and we felt that spending a good deal of time describing the relaxation process itself would contribute to this belief.

SESSION 2

Before engaging in relaxation training, we checked the number of times the men relaxed during the previous week. We also discussed the fear inventory, attempting to clarify what was called for, as well as discussing the general problem of social anxiety. The discussion involved social anxiety as a possible contributing factor to drug addiction, and set the stage for future work with systematic desensitization if people were interested. Relaxation tape 1 was repeated because the men had not practiced as much as they might have. This has been a general problem in that the men seemed to need to be pressed to follow through on their own. Though we started with six men, another joined us the second week, giving us a total of seven. We felt that we could take him into the group without disruption because the men had not practiced as they should have. Therefore, he would not be behind schedule. The same was done on the third week, when another man joined us for a total of eight in our group. In Session 2, during the relaxation training itself, we encouraged men to "let their arms drop" so that they could sense the difference between tension and relaxation in a more heightened fashion. This "looseness of a puppet" idea is based on the thinking that if they slowly brought their arms down, this would be controlling their movements and this implies a state of tension within their arms. In fact, feedback from subjects confirms that letting one's arms drop does heighten the sensation of relaxation. After this relaxation session, a general discussion took place, creating an atmosphere of comfort, acceptance, and positive group cohesiveness. This factor of group cohesion was felt to be increasing at this point and generally lasted throughout all our sessions.

SESSION 3

Relaxation tape 2 was played. This helped the men to achieve deeper levels of relaxation. A question arose of how to clear the "blackboard" image that Lazarus presents to the listener. The importance of getting a clear image was stressed, but it was also conveyed to the men that individuals differ in their ability to image scenes clearly, so as to reduce any feelings of competition during this process. The subject is asked to picture the numbers 1 to 10 on a blackboard, and to increase relaxation by saying to himself phrases such as "more relaxed," "more deeply relaxed," "serene and tranquil," "confident," and "calm" as they moved through the numbers. Additional words were given to the subjects to increase their levels of relaxation. For instance, some people used "more and more relaxed," "profoundly relaxed," or "bathing yourself in relaxation." Men were urged to try to focus their attention on achieving "an inner calmness," "a growing confidence," "a so what," or "a don't care" attitude. Whatever anxious feelings were encountered during relaxation were discussed with the men afterwards. We also discussed what Lazarus calls a "fractionated effect" in which parts of the body are relaxed while others are engaged in some work. The men returned both the fear inventory and the drug experience questionnaires at the end of this session. The results of these questionnaires are presented below.

SESSION 4

In this session both relaxation tapes were played to provide continuity and an extremely deep level of relaxation. After Relaxation 1, the men were asked to image a personal scene, such as "lying on the beach, waves gently breaking on the shore," or "you're under a tree, lying on the grass looking up at the sky, white clouds drifting by, there's a babbling brook nearby," etc. They were advised to create their own personal scene in order to get a complete feeling of serenity. They were reminded that in the next session we would move into the use of aversive imagery, and we discussed, to some extent, what that would be like.

SESSION 5

Relaxation tape 1 was played, ending with a "beach scene" or the particular scene which helped each man relax more deeply. They were advised to indicate the point at which they all achieved a high degree of relaxation (five or less subjective units of discomfort—SUD). All men reached this level at the end of the tape. At this point the group was given the sensitization tape in which the aversive imagery was presented. This tape was derived from Steinfeld's (1970) work with previous groups, and modified in accord with the present group's fears as indicated on the fear inventories. The first sensitization scene was as follows.

Group Sensitization Scene, First and Second Revision

You wake up in the morning and you feel as though you want to get off (high). As you are getting dressed, you sense something funny about the day; you feel kind of edgy (up tight), as if something eerie (bad) is going the happen to you (as if you might get burnt). Still, you get dressed; you go out into the street to cop (get) some dope. You are all alone, even though the streets are full of people and you are going to meet a so-called friend. You feel all sorts of things; underneath your sickness you really feel lonely and afraid. You are trapped; you are ashamed of what you are doing and what is happening to you, and you know that you are on the treadmill to dooming yourself (edge of destroying) and everyone who is supposed to matter to you. Still, you make contact with the man and score (get down). All the time though, you still feel alone and anxious; it is as if death is all around you. As you are walking toward the apartment (joint) where you are going to get off (high), you feel an overwhelming fear and apprehension (insecurity—you wonder if the dope is good). There are strangers all around you, looking at you; even your friend looks different and funny. It is as if he is a stranger also and is just watching you (you wonder if he is going to stick you up). As you approach the door to your home (joint) you hear a slight noise from inside. Something is in there that you are afraid to face. You hesitate (you're suspicious), feeling very nervous, but you open the door and enter anyway. As soon as you enter (are inside) the door locks behind you. There is a small barred window (on the other side of the room), no other door, and you are trapped. The walls are covered with large gray-green insects. In the corner there are snakes, slimy snakes slithering around. You start taking out your works and you hear squeals, as if rats are around somewhere. You are getting more and more frightened (up tight). Suddenly, your friend is a total stranger and he is just watching you start to cook up. His body is deformed and he has an eerie smirk on his ugly face. The clattering noise and the squeals grow louder, so loud now that your ears are suddenly ringing. You start to get dizzy and almost faint; you are afraid to look up because it sounds as if those insects are fluttering (getting) closer to you and the snakes are coming closer and the rats seem right outside the door. You run to the door and fling it open and all you are faced with is darkness. If you take one step outside that door you feel as though you will fall into a bottomless pit and your life would be over (you would die). You shut the door and manage to keep from fainting. You sit down and start rolling up one of your sleeves (and draw the stuff up, lay the needle down), and all of a sudden a large bat is flying around you, a large, dirty, ugly bat with long, sharp teeth and long hairy wings. Now you see the dirty, squealing rats with their long, slimy tails. They are across the room; they are eating all those diseased insects and some of those snakes and some other small animals. Blood is oozing out all over the place. The rats and bats are both hovering in the corner looking at you, waiting for you. Now you are so scared your heart skips a beat and you wonder if it is going to stop. The walls start closing in on you; your heart is racing and you are afraid it is going to burst right outside your chest. Loud sirens are screaming in your head; you feel panicky, as if you are losing control of your mind. You are about to faint; you are not sure if what's happening is real or imaginary. You are wondering if the stuff you copped the night before had some poison (chemical) in it to cause you to go crazy. Still, you continue to tie up (you take off your belt and start), and as you reach for the dropper (works) more rats, flying insects, snakes, and bats enter through a hole in the wall and are swarming all over the place. Now it is getting to be too much; the walls are coming closer and closer and the animals are very near to you. All of a sudden, a closet door opens and a body falls out; a body which is ripped apart with blood all over it. The rats, bats, and snakes start attacking and tearing at it. The flesh is bleeding. There are open gashes all over the body. The eyes have been ripped out. Odors (the smell) of death emanate (comes) from the bodies of all the animals that are partly eaten. You start to vomit; you vomit all over yourself; you vomit all over the works; you vomit all over the stranger (you're gagging, the burning vomit is in your throat); and all of a sudden the door opens and a woman, the woman you care most about, is looking at you. There is scorn (she's terrified) and disgust on her face. She turns and leaves and you know its all over between you. Even if you live through this ordeal, you are really all alone now. You are about to tie up (you're tied up, your vein jumps up), your heart is pounding. The rats and bats start coming at you. As you are about to tap the spike in, the rats are at your feet; they seem to have been waiting for this moment to attack you. The rats start biting into your legs; the bats start landing on your arms. Rats and bats are now biting your entire body. They are at (the vein in) your neck; they are inside your shirt; they are biting at your veins; they are inside your pants (biting your joint); they are at your throat; they are leaping and piercing (tearing) at your body (flesh) and face. You feel as if you are going to die. Your blood and the blood of other animals is all over you. The squealing and squeeking is deafening. You feel that at any moment you are going to be pinned under a herd of clawing and biting rats and bats and you are going to suffocate to death. With one desperate move you pick up the works and fling (throw) them out the window. All of a sudden the rats and bats and snakes follow, as if they were after the stuff all the time. In a little while all the animals are gone. They vanished as quickly as they came (they've disappeared). The room is larger and brighter. The squealing, crashing noises have stopped. The room is more clear. Your perception (vision) is more clear. All the blood is gone and you sit back in your chair (and breathe a sigh of relief). As you do, you feel better and better. Your friend is with you now. Your desperation is gone. You begin relaxation and this calms you even more. You start feeling better and better, more comfortable and more in control. As relaxation proceeds you grow calmer and calmer until you are completely and fully relaxed, completely calm and serene (the door opens, your woman returns, smiling, her arms outstretched. Keep thinking of this scene, you and your woman. You're feeling more and more calm, more relaxed and comfortable together).

At the end of the sensitization tape we attempted to ascertain the level of anxiety which was aroused in each of the men, as well as the level of relaxation that they felt after the sensitization tape was terminated. During the session we also asked men to think about stimuli which they would like to have in future scenes. The additional items mentioned were things like "ticks, leeches, snakes, worms, the rattle of paper, the striking of a match to cook up, footsteps, sirens, and ticking sounds" all of which seemed to enhance the experience. The following are comments made during our discussion period following the sensitization tape.

M.R.: "I felt anxiety, I was scared, I wanted to yell, to break up, as if something was going to come into my mind that I wanted to be rid of, I felt physically nauseous." Several men felt they wanted to cut the scene off. Others said they felt, or actually smelled, the sulfur from cooking up the dope and others felt nauseous. There were additional comments after the sensitization scene. A.R.: "I heard a female voice—a scream." A.D.: "I was more sensitive to the people in the scene, people always trying to get through to you, to get you to stop shooting dope, to extend themselves to you; a brother asks you to do something, but you ignore him to cop. These are the things that kicked up in me as I listened to the tape." M.R. was more threatened by the possible physical harm that he might encounter. W.W. had a feeling that his head was going to burst.

Observations. Leg and thigh twitches were observed, there was itching of the face and subsequent scratching during the presentation of the aversive scene. The itching took place around the face but especially around the mouth area; stomachs started to jump noticeably.

We asked where the tension was felt. D.T.: "I felt it in my stomach." W.W.: "I felt it in my head; I felt like jumping out the window myself; I wanted to cut it off."

We asked who the person in the scene might have been. O.M.: "When the broad opened the door I saw my old lady (wife); when the door opened, I forgot about the guy." G.B.: "The person was my wife." V.P.: "Just a stranger." A.R.: "My girl."

Additional comments: V.P.: "The tension started in my leg, it jumped up to my face, my hands felt tense, I wanted to run." O.M.: "I heard the paper (these were actually sounds in the background interpreted to be the bits of paper which are wrinkled and used to cook up) I almost smelled the sulfur. I was getting nauseous." V.T.: "I almost started to rationalize. I wanted to say something to the person to clean up the fact that she caught me with drugs." A.R.: "I got paranoid—a flash—as soon as the tapes started I thought of my old girlfriend. She was strung out, she was trying to get me strung out. When the works went out the window, I lost the dope and I lost the broad, too. I went to the window and looked out.

I felt I should be scared, I was disappointed in myself." M.R.: "I couldn't get into it. I pictured all those things but I couldn't really feel anxious." A.D.: "I felt the tension in my arm and in the forehead, the pounding at one point, I felt the closing in of the room, growing smaller and the animals were closer, I felt guilty about my wife catching me. Even if I got through all this it would be all over. I really felt she caught me, I really got fucked up when I spit up on myself, that really fucked me up. I felt helpless and trapped." M.R.: "I saw really my girl and my mother. I couldn't see either really well, fuck it. You got to accept this if you shoot drugs. Its part of the package, the person who you care about walks out on you, it's all part of it. Even the people you know, the strangers watching you, the loneliness, you're more susceptable to using drugs if you're alone, you have no one to talk to. Nothing to do. Maybe because I was alone. The part that affected me most was when the person walked out. I felt helpless and hopeless. Self-destructive. There was too much stimulation, it was unreal. I was in fear of getting busted."

SESSION 6

A revision was made in the sensitization tape based on the feedback from the previous session. The men again listened to the relaxation and sensitization tapes. They seemed more tense during this relaxation session (perhaps this was due to other men in the prison yard playing ball right outside the window and the fact that there were a number of interruptions during the relaxation tape, with the door opening to our room several times and our men feeling uncomfortable by this). Nevertheless, they all reported getting extremely relaxed (less than 5 SUDs). We also got a reading on how much anxiety kicked up after the aversive scene was presented. Then an interesting thing happened.

After the sensitization tape, a profound change was noted. The men became very serious, as if a gloom was hanging over the entire room. In discussing what had occurred the men related the following. A.R.: "I felt frustrated, tension in my arms and hands, my wrists, all over, my lower right jaw, a pain kicked up, feelings in my hands as if I was taking off in my hands, my body was tense—I couldn't get it right, the door opening, I wanted to throw a chair, I felt frustrated, after it was all over, I wanted my chick to come back and relax with me." W.W.: "I felt disgusted." G.B.: "I felt frustrated, happy to become really relaxed after the scene, I wanted to continue the relaxation, I didn't want to get up." V.T.: "I felt depression after the scene, all that led me to really feeling depressed. I started feeling sorry form yself, sympathy for that man who threw the works out, all the bats and rats. I was still lost, I wanted the girl back." M.R.: "I wanted to leave the room to get the girl back, but I couldn't go after her. I still have nothing, I still didn't have anything to get off; also I felt empty, what's the use of throwing the spike away, what did I have to show for it. Then I started to realize I'm here in prison, when I started to relax again, I realized I was here and this was depressing in itself." O.M.: "Yeh, disappointment man, still feel it. I related things to events in my life that took place between me and my woman. I had flashbacks, I brought it up to date, anyway, where I'm at now, disappointed, helpless, hopeless, disgusted. I put myself in that position and now I'm paying for it." V.P.: "I'm just glad to get rid of the bats, I hate them, I threw the spike away. It reminded me of the times I said that before, but the next day I'm in the sewer with the hook trying to get my works back. I used to smack girls in the head; they usually came back but this time I felt she'd never come back. Like some of the guys said, I'd like to lay here for the next 10 years. I forgot where I was for a while and then when I realized I was in jail, it was disappointing, depressing." M.R.: "It's depressing being in a place where you have nothing, and you still have nothing after you throw the spike away; its hard to give it up, the guys are trapped, disillusioned. It's better to be a dope fiend then to be nothing, at least you belong to something." O.M.: "Even if it's part of the dope fiend world, you pick up people to relate to, no matter on what level. You go to the corner where everyone is hanging out, strung out, you get a sense of belonging, if I feel down I take off for a while; there's a sense of family, it's like having an individual static group where everyone's getting off; it seems as though everyone understands even though they may not."

Additional comments. "I was irritated today; I saw a giant rat when I opened the door. I got more in touch today. Rats were steadily fucking with me. I was relieved to get rid of the rats but there were more I was in touch with."

We asked if anyone had felt if they actually had taken off since everyone acted as though they might have shot dope. They all said no, that wasn't the feeling; it was more like depression, it was more like disappointment.

SESSION 7

Relaxation tape 1 was played until every man indicated that he was fully relaxed by raising his index finger. This took place very rapidly, about the time the men were relaxing their lower backs. The first revision and the second revision of the sensitization tapes were played. The second revision was based on one of the residents in our program going over the tape and introducing words that were more appropriate to the "dope fiend" world. We also included the woman coming back into the scene after the man threw the spike away so that she could act as a covert reinforcement. Both Cautela and Lazarus (personal communication) recommended this change when I described what had taken place, i.e., the mood change, the depression that took place in Session 6. We felt that the depression was the result of something important being taken away, possibly the frustration of their dependency needs. As the men said, they had to give up the dope and the woman, so that the loss of two vital sources of support were gone and depression would be natural and predicted reaction to these events. We focused on building in covert reinforcement in the next two sessions. After both the scenes were played and the men were fully awake, we gave them some additional self-control measures like thought stopping. We advised them to practice yelling "Stop" when the thought of dope entered their minds or when their bellies flipped (got a yen or craving for dope). We also discussed other reinforcements they could use for the dope and which they could share with their girl friends or wife in the scene. Some of the comments about Revision 2 were: "That was a heck of a contrast, when she came back everything brightened up, I wanted to yell 'Yay'. There was too much noise from the next room." W.W.: "I wanted to throw the works away when the woman originally came in." M.R.: "I was anticipating her coming back, when she didn't, I was really disappointed. The second time the tape was played, I tripped out until she came back, then I fell right into the scene." G.B.: "Rats gave me a fit; I went off my stick; I really got scared; I wasn't really involved with the dope but the animals really got me." O.M.: "I was really nervous, through the second tape my body was reacting, first one side and then the other. I generally felt more of the tension, when the tape stopped, my body jumped."

SESSION 8

As in the previous session, relaxation tapes were played until the men signaled deep levels of relaxation. The aversive scene was presented with covert reinforcement being stressed. At the end of the second tape the men were encouraged to live out the scene with their female companions, focusing on the things they liked to do together. The men fantasied like this till they were ready to waken completely. This lasted for about five more minutes. The rest of the session was used to wrap matters up and to stress with the men that practice was necessary for the effect to really work.

RESULTS, CONCLUSIONS, FUTURE DIRECTIONS

Of the eight men who participated, all have left the institution. The reports from Aftercare Services indicate one has returned to drug criminal activities and is currently in jail under new charges. The other seven are, to date, doing well, involved in school, working, and not, to our knowledge, involved in criminal activities. The one person who returned to drugs (V.P.) said, "Felt good before copping drugs, copped from a friend on the street, got off at home, *alone*, best liked getting off when first got up, preferred heroin, abused his arms, had family problems (played with my head)." All responses except the shooting of heroin *alone* were similar to the others in the group and may provide a lead for further exploration. In terms of our fear arousing stimuli, V.P. checked open wounds, being alone, dead people, failure, high places on land, looking down from high buildings, people in authority, being watched working, dead animals, fire, sick people, witnessing surgical operations, angry people, parting from friends, enclosed places, prospect of a surgical operation, feeling rejected by others, feeling disapproved of, harmless snakes, cemeteries, being ignored, premature heartbeats, people with deformities, making mistakes, losing control. It must be stressed that no matter what our results, we will not be able to test the effectiveness of our procedure until a controlled study is undertaken. Such a study has been proposed to the Bureau of Prisons and is currently awaiting approval. Not only would variations in our procedure be explored, but we would try to control for "Time in the Institution" and "Time in the Therapeutic Community." Thus, to evaluate our procedure we should use:

Experimental Group I. Covert sensitization and therapeutic community.

Experimental Group II. Covert sensitization without therapeutic community (these men are available in that there are "splittees" from the therapeutic community within our prison).

Control Group. Men with drug history, not sentenced under the NARA Act, and not receiving other forms of treatment at the institution.

Future studies might also explore the use of sound effects on the tapes. In our discussions of the procedure with the men, all felt that specific sounds like the screeches, sirens, the door opening, a woman's voice, slitting of the glassine envelope, a match striking to cook up, etc., would increase the anxiety. The introduction of the smell of burning sulfur might also increase the effect.

Future work might explore the antecendent conditions of narcotic addiction and the consequences of stopping. Several factors stand out as contributing to a man beginning his career as an addict, some of which we may be able to deal with through the use of additional behavioral approaches. For example, many men experience a good deal of social anxiety, especially around heterosexual activities. Systematic desensitization of social anxiety, in conjunction with covert sensitization, may make treatment more effective. The "need for approval," or negative identification, also plays a prominent role in a man getting caught up in the drug world. The use of behavioral rehearsal to develop assertive responses may also add strength to a man who others will attempt to suck back into the criminal-drug world after leaving prison.

As far as preventive work to deal with the drug problem is concerned, Elementary and Secondary School programs may do well to stress the use of assertive training for youngsters who are constantly exposed to peer group pressure to enter the drug culture.

Finally, it is clear that people need "substitute highs" if they are to "kick the habit" or not to develop it in the first place. Schedules of reinforcement, to be used overtly or covertly, need to be developed and instituted if we ever expect young people to lead drug-free, responsible lives. How these scedules can be developed, by whom, and at what stage of a person's social and psychological development are questions which need answering if we are ever to stem the tide of the waste of human lives that has currently reached epidemic proportions. (See Appendices A and B.)

APPENDIX A

We attempted to categorize the fears by sensory modality, discreteness of stimuli, whether they were interpersonal, impersonal, or related to "self." Table 1 indicates our findings in relation to these categories, using the "much" and "very much" dimensions. Examples of each category are also included.

APPENDIX B

The questionnaire we used to determine the individual's drug related behavior follows. We are also including the group's responses.

Table 1

	Much	Very much	Total
Auditory inanimate (vacuum cleaner noise)	2	4	6
Visual inanimate (automobiles)	14	2	16
Interpersonal auditory (loud voices)	0	0	0
Interpersonal visual (deformed person)	39	5	54
Animals (rats)	25	14	39
Self-feelings (failure)	36	24	60
Environmental situation (journey by bus)	14	7	21
Interpersonal situation (one person bullying another)	19	14	33

1. Mood: How did you feel before copping drugs?
   a. When first started shooting.
   b. After strung out.
2. Describe person(s) you got drugs from (street pusher, friend, relative, etc.) and places (street, hallway, etc.)
3. Where did you prefer to get off?
4. With whom did you prefer to get off?
   a. Alone.
   b. With other(s) (specify).
5. What time of day?
   When first getting up. Before supper.
   After breakfast. Evening.
   Noon. Before bed time.
   Afternoon. Anytime you felt you needed to.
6. What drugs did you prefer?
   Heroin. Cocaine. Amphetamine. Barbiturate.
   Marijuana. Hashish. LSD. other (specify).
7. Part of the body abused (arm, hand, leg, etc.).
8. What situations or persons get you up tight so that you went to the cooker?

Responses

1. *Mood; a—b*
   - A.R. Good—Nervous
   - A.D. Insecure, depressed—Trapped, useless, inadequate
   - O.M. Excited, anticipation, fear—Lonely, fear, anxiety, unique
   - W.W. Lonely, anxious, victimized, ashamed—Lonely, confused, afraid
   - D.T. Hip, into the real happenings—Foolish, unreal, trapped
   - M.R. Excitement, fear, anticipation—Fear, anxiety, unique, lonely
   - V.P. Good—Nervous, content
   - G.B. Anxious, fearful—Lonely, doomed, ostracized
2. *Drug Source—Place*
   - A.R. Friends, business acquaintences—Apartments, motel rooms
   - A.D. Street pusher—Street, hallways, bars
   - O.M. Street pusher, relatives—Street, hallways
   - W.W. Friend—Street
   - D.T. Friend—Apartment
   - M.R. Street pusher, friend, relative—Street, hallway
   - V.P. Friend—Street
   - G.B. Friend, relative—Street, hallway
3. *Place Got Off*
   - A.R. Bathroom, bedroom
   - A.D. Bathroom
   - O.M. Home
   - W.W. Anywhere
   - D.T. Apartment
   - M.R. At home (in the bathroom)
   - V.P. At home
   - G.B. Home
4. *With Whom*
   - A.R. Alone and with others (girlfriends)
   - A.D. With others
   - O.M. With others
   - W.W. With others
   - D.T. With my friend
   - M.R. With others (my girl)

V.P.	Alone
G.B.	With others

5. *Time of Day*

A.R.	Anytime I felt I needed (wanted) to
A.D.	Anytime I felt I needed to
O.M.	When first getting up, anytime I felt I needed to
W.W.	When first getting up, noon, afternoon, evening, before bed time, anytime I felt I needed to
D.T.	Anytime I felt I needed to
M.R.	Anytime I felt I needed to
V.P.	When first getting up
G.B.	Afternoon, anytime I felt I needed to

6. *Drug Preferred*

A.R.	Cocaine, amphetamine
A.D.	Heroin, cocaine
O.M.	Heroin, cocaine, hashish, marijuana
W.W.	Heroin, cocaine
D.T.	Heroin, cocaine, marijuana, hashish
M.R.	Heroin, barbiturate, cough syrup
V.P.	Heroin, cocaine, barbiturate, marijuana, hashish
G.B.	Cocaine, marijuana, hashish

7. *Part of Body Abused*

A.R.	Arms, foot, hands
A.D.	Arms
O.M.	Arms
W.W.	Arms, hands, things
D.T.	Arms, hands
M.R.	Arms, hands
V.P.	Arms
G.B.	Arms

8. *Antecedent Conditions*

A.R.	Pressure from the law
A.D.	Depressed (frustrating jobs; domestic problems)
O.M.	Association with others (positive and negative)
W.W.	Other addicts, alcoholics, hustling
D.T.	Women, personal family
M.R.	Depends on the circumstances
V.P.	Family playing with my head
G.B.	No particular person, place or thing

REFERENCES

CAUTELA, J.R. Covert sensitization. *Psychol. Rep.* 20: 459–468, 1967.

CAUTELA, J.R. Treatment of compulsive behavior by covert sensitization, *Psychol. Rec.* 16: 33–41, 1966.

JACOBSON, E. *Progressive Relaxation.* Chicago: Univ. Chicago Press, 1938.

LAZARUS, A. Coping with Tensions and Anxieties (tape). Chicago: Instructional Dynamics, 1972.

MARK, J., and GENZER, L. The role of trait structuring in the systematic desensitization of test anxiety. MSW dissertation, Univ. Connecticut, 1972.

STEINFELD, G.J. The use of covert sensitization with institutionalized narcotic addicts. *Intern. J. Addictions* 5: 225–232, 1970.

WOLPE, J., and LAZARUS, A. *Behavior Therapy Techniques*, Oxford: Pergamon, 1966.

The International Journal of the Addictions, 9(3), 465–473, 1974

Some Descriptive Measures on 100 Consecutive VA Hospital Drug Abuse Admissions

Don Wallace, Ph.D.

Darlene Hiner, Ph.D.

VA Hospital
Houston, Texas

The phenomenon of drug abuse has a long history (Brill, 1969). Its evolution took a dramatic turn (Berger and Potterfield, 1969) in this country within the last decade when the misuse of nonsanctioned drugs underwent a dramatic increase among the White middle class. As the problem touched more and more lives, and particularly since the revelation of drug abuse by American servicemen, there soon developed increased activity in the areas of research and treatment. As a part of this overall activity the Veterans Administration has been developing treatment programs of its own, but research describing the population being treated has been absent. The present study is designed to describe one such treatment population. It is concerned with the presentation of certain demographic characteristics, drug history, and certain personality traits and symptoms present at admission.

* Requests for reprints should be sent to either author at the VA Hospital, 2002 Holcombe Boulevard, Houston, Texas 77031.

METHOD

Subjects

The subjects (*S*s) were 100 consecutive admissions to the Houston VA Hospital's Drug Abuse Unit. All *S*s were voluntary admissions except 13 active duty servicemen detected as drug abusers by urinalysis tests and sent to the VA by the military.

The *S*s were divided into three groups: (1) Group A—60 *S*s whose present admission was related to opiate abuse (predominately heroin); (2) Group B—13 active duty servicemen; and (3) Group C—27 *S*s whose admission related to drug abuse other than opiates.

The procedure involved a structured interview using a rating instrument adapted from the VA Psychiatric Evaluation Project (PEP) and studies by the alcoholic unit of the Houston VA Hospital (Pokorny, Miller, and Cleveland, 1968). These questions were further modified to be applicable to a drug population. Each *S* was interviewed individually by a staff psychologist, and afterwards each *S* took a vocational interest inventory (Kuder DD) and a personality questionnaire (Sixteen Personality Factor Questionnaire).

RESULTS

The results are presented for the total 100 *S*s. However, significant differences between the subgroups are also presented. An important negative finding was an inability to discriminate on the basis of the questionnaire and the other data collected (via regression analysis) those *S*s placed on methadone maintenance from those *S*s not addicted to an opiate.

Demographic and Social Variables

The *S*s in the study were between 18 and 54 years of age with an average of 25.90. The 13 active duty *S*s were much younger than the other subjects ($M = 20.7$ years for the active duty *S*s as compared with 27.3 and 26.1 years for Groups A and C, respectively). Fifty-eight percent were reared in an unbroken home. Twenty-two percent had a parent or sibling hospitalized for psychiatric treatment. While the majority were Caucasian

* Tables containing statistical information are available on request.

(66%), 23% were Black and 11% were Latin American. The average grade completed was 11.34.

Family Characteristics

Half of the sample were living in households with a spouse or parents at the time of admission. Groups B and C reported an increase of 69 and 26%, respectively, in living with parents after hospitalization. Since Group B averaged only 20 years of age and were just returning from military service, this is not unexpected. However, almost half of the subjects in Group C and over a fourth (28%) of the subjects in Group A stated they planned to live with parents after hospitalization.

Exactly half of the sample had married. Not quite one-half of these marriages (44%) ended in divorce.

Vocational Measures

A look at the employment data for the 12 months previous to admission reveals the mean number of months worked was 6.0, but this included 13 *S*s on active duty. Considering only the remaining 87% who had greater freedom regarding vocational choices, 18 (29%) were unemployed the full year, another 32 (37%) were unemployed at least 6 months, leaving only 30 (34%) employed more than half the time period. Eighty-six were last employed on a full-time basis, with the job lasting an average of 38 weeks; $99.90 was the average weekly income.

Measures of Criminal-Legal Involvement

At the time of admission, *S*s reported past or present criminal charges: 54% of the sample reported felony charges; 5% reported three or more misdemeanor charges; 18% one or two misdemeanor charges, and 23% no legal involvement since age 18. Thirty-four *S*s had actually been convicted of a felony. The mean number of days incarcerated was 76.81 with a range of from 1 to 999. Ninety-two percent of Group A reported a criminal record (23% for Group B and 70% for Group C).

Drug Use

The *S*s reported the frequency and types of drugs they had used previous to hospitalization. The *S*s started with alcohol, then marijuana and the "soft drugs" (i.e., barbiturates, amphetamines, and hallucinogens, in that order). Next came use of various opiates (codeine, heroin, Demerol, morphine, and Dolophine). There are some differences between groups. The groups do not differ regarding the frequency of drug use, except for Group A having extensive opiate use. Group B's opiate use was limited mainly to heroin, and Group C had some opiate use that was not extensive.

Mood Level and Affectivity

Fourteen of the *S*s reported never feeling anxious or tense, while 21 reported feeling anxious most of the time. However, nearly half (44) stated that they had been extremely anxious in the week preceding hospitalization. This degree of anxiety was not apparent at the time of the interview in that only two *S*s were judged as exhibiting an extreme amount of anxiety.

The same pattern was reported for feelings of depression. Sixty-two stated that they rarely felt depressed. However, 52 asserted that they had been moderately or extremely depressed in the last week. Some degree of depression was observed in 60 *S*s during the interview.

These *S*s also tended to deny feelings of inertia and apathy (65) and sleep difficulties (48) as typical of their life style, but reported an exacerbation of these symptoms preceding hospitalization.

Fifty *S*s reported feelings of extreme isolation from other people as a life style, while 29 said this was not a problem. The *S*s were asked to assess if they were withdrawn in the week before hospitalization. Thirty-nine said not at all, 27 admitted to moderate withdrawal, and 34 stated they were extremely withdrawn in this time period.

Cognitive Functioning

Memory impairment, hallucinatory behavior, and disorientation were not significant factors in this population; being present in 15, 22, and 6 *S*s, respectively. Paranoid behavior was more common; 12 *S*s manifested slight paranoid behavior and 11 exhibited moderate to severe paranoid ideations. Twelve *S*s were judged to show deficient reality testing and 23 a disruption of communication.

Approximately one-fourth (23) of the *S*s showed odd behavior; i.e., behavior that would likely be judged unusual by a layman. Twenty-seven *S*s appeared somewhat sloppy in their physical appearance and 23 were judged to be evasive.

Self-Concept

Mental Status. Nearly three-fourths of the *S*s (72) denied ever being mentally ill, 13 stated they would rate themselves as mentally ill presently, while 19 rated themselves as having been mentally ill sometime in their life. However, 73 declared they were nervous or emotionally ill, 50 moderately, and 23 extremely so.

Drug Activity. Eighty-three *S*s said they were extreme drug abusers. This is close to the examiners' rating of 72 *S*s as extremely involved with drugs. Seventy *S*s reported that their life was at least moderately affected by drug use (31 said somewhat and 39 said moderately to markedly). Despite admitting excessive use of drugs, most of these *S*s tended to deny any need for external controls. The *S*s were asked if they intended to continue treatment on an outpatient basis. While 78% of Group A and 74% of Group C said yes, almost one-half (54%) of Group B either said no or were ambiguous about this.

Adequacy with Problems. The *S*s were asked to rate how well they felt they could handle their problems compared to the average man. Approximately one-third (32) generally felt overpowered by problems, while 10 stated they almost always felt able to handle problems. Nineteen thought they handled work-related problems better than the average man, and 30 rated their ability as below average. Twenty-three rated themselves as above average in handling family problems, and 37 rated themselves below average.

Feelings about Self. When asked about feelings of guilt, 23 reported that they generally felt guilty, while 24 replied they never felt guilty. Approximately the same proportion were reported as manifesting some feelings of inferiority (28) during the interview. Over one-third felt they had more self-confidence (36) and more self-understanding (37) than the average man. Forty-five *S*s felt their life was more meaningful than the average person. Conversely, 26, 33, and 24 felt they had less than the average person in the above three attributes.

Group B consistently rated themselves, and were rated by the investigators, as "healthier" on most items. Group C admitted to feeling very isolated from others and to being extremely nervous or even mentally ill. Concurrently the investigators rated this group as showing more inferiority and paranoid feelings. Group A was seen as the most severe drug addicts and as manifesting communication difficulties and being evasive.

Personality and Interest Tests

16 PF. When interpreting the results according to the 16 PF manual (Cattell and Eber, 1954), the *S*s appear slightly deviant regarding being apprehensive and strongly deviant in being quite affected by feelings and being tense. *T* tests for single means (Winer, 1962) were significant at the .01 level for the first two variables and .05 for the latter.

Considering individual profiles, no *S* has all his scores in stens 5 or 6 or even 4 or 7. Every *S* had at least one score that was strongly (46) or extremely (53) deviant. Thus these *S*s show some deviance as a group on three traits, and individually they had at least one score that was strongly or extremely deviant.

While the mean profiles for the three groups were similar, there was a difference in the number of deviant scores in each group. An analysis of variance with unequal cells (Winer, 1962) was carried out to investigate if the three groups differed regarding the number and degree of deviant scores. The analysis yielded *t* test comparison of means (Winer, 1962) of 2.48 ($p < .02$) for Groups B and C. Group B had significantly fewer scores in the more deviant range (i.e., healthier) while Group C had more deviant scores.

Kuder. Kuder (1966) views the *V* score as a mark of sincerity or test taking ability. In these *S*s 21 had a *V* score below the critical value of 45, which strongly suggests faking or carelessness. It would appear that the first interpretation is more likely to be correct as the MBI score (also a mark of insincerity) was higher than *M* in 18 *S*s.

The Kuder interprets a profile of low correlations (below .40) as a sign of immaturity. In this sample 32 *S*s had no correlation at or above this score (22 had no correlation above .31 and 10 had all correlations between .32 and .39).

This inventory also provides an S score (determined from scores of 250 high school boys) and F scores (scores from the fathers of these boys). Comparisons of these scores gives an index of maturity also. Fifty-one *S*s had $F > S$. However 44 had $S < F$ and three had $S = F$. Thus nearly half of the *S*s had a pattern of interests more similar to a high school boy than to an adult male. Similarly an *M* score (from adult women) can be

* The Kuder data are for 98 *S*s. One Kuder was not scorable as the *S* had not completed it properly and one *S* left the hospital before completing the Kuder. The 16 PF data are for 99 *S*s. One *S* left the hospital without completing the 16 PF.

compared with the *F* score to determine whether interests are more like those of a male or female. In the present study $F > M$ in 68 *S*s, $M < F$ in 25 *S*s, and $F = M$ in five *S*s. Thus over two-thirds of the *S*s had interests more like females than males.

The groups differ most strikingly regarding the *M* and MBI scores. While only 8% of Group B and 7% of Group C had higher MBI than *M* scores, 26% of Group A had higher MBI than *M* scores. Thus scores designed to measure insincerity indicate that almost one-fourth of the opiate-addicted *S*s were answering the questions less than honestly.

DISCUSSION

There has been interest in studying the various subgroups of drug addicts based on the drug of choice (Hekimian and Gershon, 1968; Henriques, Cutter, Arsenian, and Sumaraweera, 1972; Greden and Morgan, 1972). The present study found very little difference between the groups when demographic variables were considered. Perhaps the variables which differentiate these groups, if they exist, were not explored. Or it could be that choice of drug does not depend on various demographic factors but is fortuitous (i.e., based on whatever drug the person encounters). Another possibility is that certain personality characteristics, not demographic factors, lead an individual to choose one specific drug. While the subjects in this study did differ regarding personality variables, the personality measures were obtained after the subject had used drugs quite extensively. In a retrospective study it is not possible to determine if such personality characteristics existed before the drugs were used or if they resulted from the drug use itself.

There are some differences in symptom patterns of the groups. The heroin addicts, more frequently than the other subjects, present symptoms related to faulty interpersonal relationships based on lack of trust and sincerity. These symptoms seem similar to those listed by Bursten (1972) when he described what he calls the manipulative personality. Those subjects who used amphetamines, barbiturates, and hallucinogens exhibited more symptoms relating to disturbances in thinking. These persons presented feelings of inferiority and isolation from others and paranoid ideation, all of which would lead one to consider a psychotic diagnosis. Hekimian and Gershon (1968) came to similar conclusions when they diagnosed the majority of their heroin addicts as sociopathic personalities and the amphetamine, LSD, and marijuana users as schizophrenic.

The present study also had 13 active duty servicemen. They differed from the other subjects in that they were not voluntary admissions to the program, but were sent by the armed forces. These subjects differed from the other subjects in other ways as well. They tended to deny experiencing symptoms commonly associated with psychological discomfort and were rated as exhibiting fewer pathological symptoms. Concomitantly, they were much more optimistic about their future vocationally and interpersonally, seeing themselves as moving toward a more independent life style. This difference between military personnel involved in drugs and the "street addicts" was noted also by Zinberg (1972) who stated that he felt the heroin addicts among servicemen stationed in Vietnam were not similar to the heroin addicts in the United States. Since these subjects seem to be experiencing little psychological discomfort, they would seem less motivated to seek treatment. As a matter of fact, this group indicated much less interest in treatment or much of a desire to continue treatment even as outpatients.

One personality factor, that of immaturity, has been discussed as characteristic of the drug addict (e.g., Seldin, 1972; Vaillant, 1966). The addicts in this study could also be characterized as immature, not only on personality test measures but also in their tendency to still be living within the family constellation. Excluding the 13 active military who at age 20 could be expected to show more immaturity, there is much immaturity manifest in the other subjects. One-third did not even have vocational interests crystallized enough to manifest vocational preferences on the Kuder or manifest interests more characteristic of adults rather than of adolescents. Additionally, many of the drug addicts anticipated returning to live with their parents upon discharge.

One interesting question concerns why the addict seeks treatment when he does, i.e., why that day instead of last week or next week? This study indicates that something is going on in his life in the week preceding hospitalization which results in an increase in psychological stress. The addict is "hurting" and experiencing some crisis that, without intervention, may result in a solution that is even more maladaptive and detrimental than his previous adjustment. It may be at the time of crisis that the addict seeks treatment, and at this time he may be most amenable to intervention. Since addicts have traditionally been difficult to involve in treatment, this would seem to point to the need for agencies to be prepared to accept them when they are most ready.

SUMMARY

The study concerned 100 consecutive admissions to the Houston VA

Hospital Drug Abuse program. Drug history and various demographic and personality factors were investigated both in regards to the population as a whole and three subgroups; (1) opiate users, (2) active duty personnel and (3) drug users involved with drugs other than opiates. The subgroups did differ on economic and criminality measures as well as presenting different clinical pictures based on personality and symptomatic factors.

ACKNOWLEDGMENT

This research was supported by the Common Research Computer Facility, Texas Medical Center, under USPHS Grant Number RR 00254.

REFERENCES

BERGER, F.M., and POTTERFIELD, J. Drug abuse and society. In J. R. Wittenborn, H. Brill, J. P. Smith, and S. A. Wittenborn (eds.) *Drugs and Youth. Proceedings of the Rutgers Symposium on Drug Abuse.* Springfield, Illinois: Thomas, 1969.

BRILL, H. Recurrent patterns in the history of drugs of dependence and some interpretations. In J. R. Wittenborn, H. Brill, J. P. Smith, and S. A. Wittenborn (eds.) *Drugs and Youth.Proceedings of the Rutgers Symposium on Drug Abuse.* Springfield, Illinois: Thomas, 1969.

BURSTEN, B. The manipulative personality. *Arch. Gen. Psychiat.* 26: 318–321, 1972.

CATTELL, R.B., and EBER, H.W. *Sixteen personality factor questionnaire. Manual for Forms A and B.* Champaign, Illinois: Institute for Personality and Ability Testing, 1954.

GREDEN, J.F., and MORGAN, D.W. Patterns of drug use and attitudes toward treatment in a military population. *Arch. Gen. Psychiat.* 26: 113–117, 1972.

HEKIMIAN, L.J., and GERSHON, S. Characteristics of drug abusers admitted to a psychiatric hospital. *J. Amer. Med. Assoc.* 205: 125–130, 1968.

HENRIQUES, E., CUTTER, H., ARSENIAN, J., and SUMARAWEERA, A.B. Personality characteristics and drug of choice. *Intern. J. Addictions* 7: 73–76, 1972.

KUDER, G.F. *Kuder DD. General Manual.* Chicago: Science Research Associates, 1966.

POKORNY ,A.D., MILLER, B.A., and CLEVELAND, S.E. Response to treatment of alcoholism. *Quart. J. Studies Alc.* 29: 364–381, 1968.

SELDIN, N.E. The family of the addict: a review of the literature. *Intern. J. Addictions,* 7: 97–107, 1972.

VAILLANT, G. E. Twelve-year follow-up New York narcotic addicts: I. The relation of treatment to outcome. *Amer. J. Psychiat.* 122: 727–737, 1966.

WINER, B.J. *Statistical Principles in Experimental Design.* New York: McGraw-Hill, 1962.

ZINBERG, N.E. Heroin use in Vietnam and the United States. *Arch. Gen. Psychiat.* 26: 486–488, 1972.

The International Journal of the Addictions, 9(3), 475–480, 1974

Drug Use and Fantasy Processes: Criterion for Prediction of Potential Users

Bernard Segal, Ph.D.

Murray State University
Murray, Kentucky

Although much research on drug use has been conducted to date, no predictors, based on psychologically derived criteria, have been developed to identify potential drug users. This lack exists because it is difficult to determine whether the psychological correlates of drug use are antecedents of drug use or if they are a manifestation of drug use. Segal and Feger (in press), in order to overcome this problem, assumed that one aspect of drug use—fantasy processes, which represent internalized states of emotions—is part of one's basic personality; and that drug use seemingly heightens or stimulates fantasy processes. These researchers found that marijuana users, as opposed to nonusers, tended to report significantly more incidences and more varied content of fantasy and daydreaming processes. These results were interpreted by Segal and Feger (in press) to suggest that imagery or fantasy processes, associated with drug use, may not only represent internalized emotions, but that these fantasies might also be able to serve as criteria to predict drug usage.

The study reported herein is the result of an attempt to predict drug use by using a set of 14 predictor variables, derived from Segal and Feger's findings, against two discrete criterion: ever used vs never used drugs. A discriminate analysis of the data was conducted to determine if it would be possible to obtain significantly different discriminant equations for the two criterion groups.

METHOD

Subjects

The subjects were 330 students enrolled at Murray State University who volunteered to respond to two questionnaires. (These questionnaires, a Drug Use Survey and the Imaginal Process Inventory, IPI, are described fully in a previous study, Segal and Feger, in press.) One hundred forty-seven were males; 183 females. Ages ranged from 17 to 47. Of these students, 185 reported no use of drugs; 145 indicated use of drugs (of any type) one or more times.

Predictor Variables

The independent variables were 13 IPI subscales found by Segal and Feger (in press) to be significantly related to marijuana use, plus the addition of one other subscale, Achievement Oriented Daydreams, which was found to be significantly ($p < .01$) related to marijuana use on one of the two analyses conducted by Segal and Feger. The predictor variables were: Absorption in Daydreams; Positive Reactions in Daydreaming; Frightened Reactions to Daydreams; Visual Imagery in Daydreams; Past in Daydreams; Bizarre Improbable Daydreams; Mind Wandering; Achievement-Oriented Daydreams; Hostile Daydreams; Sexual Daydreams; Guilt Daydreams; Curiosity: Interpersonal; Curiosity: Impersonal; and the Self-Revelation Scale.

Criterion

The criterion consisted of two discrete variable groups: (A) Nondrug use (N = 185) and (B) use of drugs (N = 145).

Statistical Analysis

The statistical procedure used was a discriminant function analysis derived from Rao's generalization of the Mahalanobis Distance Function Technique (Anderson, 1958). The analysis was run on Murray State

University's IBM 360/40 computer based on a standard program developed by IBM for use with the IBM 360 computer.

DISCRIMINATION RESULTS

The mean subscale scores and the coefficients of the discriminant functions are reported in Table 1 (Group A = nondrug use; Group B = use of drugs).

The analysis yielded a D^2 value of 56.5092, which was statistically significant at the .001 level ($df = 14$). The profile for the 14 predictor variables in each criterion group were therefore considered to differ significantly. It was concluded that the predictive validity of the 14 selected criteria measures was established for determining drug usage among students from Murray State University.

Inspection of Table 1 indicates that there was a noticable trend for the

Table 1
Selection of Criteria in Determining Marijuana Usage

Predictors scales	Nondrug use $N = 185$ means	Drug use $N = 145$ means	Coefficients of discriminant functions	
Absorption in daydreams	58.06	63.34	−.3007	−.2892
Positive reactions in daydreaming	40.11	40.31	.6328	.6049
Frightened reactions to daydreams	27.72	30.34	.0491	.523
Visual imagery in daydreams	33.72	36.34	.2865	.3110
Past in daydreams	36.22	37.97	.3247	.3354
Bizarre improbable daydreams	28.62	31.03	.2272	.2573
Mind wandering	38.64	40.83	.6768	.6710
Achievement-oriented daydreams	31.93	31.24	−.1158	−.1572
Hostile daydreams	33.47	27.77	.0546	.1115
Sexual daydreams	35.56	40.39	−.0615	−.0391
Guilt daydreams	21.25	21.98	.0274	−.0230
Curiosity: interpersonal	41.04	40.78	.7170	.7193
Curiosity: impersonal	30.46	31.66	.6517	.6750
Self-revelation scale	36.30	38.79	.4654	.5046

$D^2 = 56.5092$ $df = 14$, $p < .001$. Constant: −62.7572, −66.9053.

mean scores of the 14 predictor variables to be higher for the drug use subjects. Thus drug users, on the average, tended to report a greater frequency of the kinds of imagery content assessed on the 14 predictor subscales than did the nondrug subjects. The only exceptions to this trend were found to be with respect to Hostile Daydreams and Curiosity: Interpersonal Daydreams for which the means of Group A were higher.

The profile of the Group B students may be characterized as follows: Drug users tend to reveal a greater frequency of Absorption in Daydreaming; Frightened Reactions to Daydreams; Visual Imagery in Daydreams; Past (Thinking) in Daydreams; Bizarre Improbable Daydreams; Mind Wandering; Sexual Daydreams; Curiosity in Impersonal-Mechanical Events; and an interest in reporting or talking about fantasies (Self-Revelation). The Group A students profile may be characterized as showing less of the tendencies described above, but reporting more hostile daydreams as well as more daydreams indicating a greater focus on interest in interpersonal events.

The above findings, with respect to mean subscale scores for the two groups, tend to contrast, in part, with the results of Segal and Feger (in press) in their study of fantasy processes of marijuana only users and nonusers. Segal and Feger reported that Hostile Daydreams and interpersonal type fantasies were associated more with marijuana users than with nonuse. It would be anticipated, therefore, that all types (multiple) of drug users would continue to reveal the same pattern of daydreaming processes. The present findings, however, indicate that the nondrug group revealed more of these kind of daydreams than did the multiple use group. Apparently, when multiple users were included in the analysis, a dramatic shift occurred in that the nondrug group revealed more hostile and interpersonal imagery processes. Perhaps those who turn to multiple drug use become so involved with the effects of the drugs' stimulation of more intense fantasies that interest shifts away from others to preoccupation with drugs and their effects. In addition, if the drug stimulates or heightens fantasies, some of which may be unwanted, such as hostile content, the user may tend to counter these with other, more pleasing types of fantasy content, such as sexual daydreams. McAree, Steffenhagen, and Zheutlin (1969) reported that such characteristics as schizoid personality, withdrawal, poor interpersonal relationships, aloofness, and inability to express emotions were prominent among gross multiple drug users. A cohort of marijuana only users, in the same study, did not differ from a nondrug group in which the attributes described above were minimal. Both the marijuana and nondrug groups differed significantly from the multiple drug group with respect to the characteristics described above. It may be that with the multiple drug user one is dealing with a more emotionally laden individual in which potentially more disturbed or troubled thoughts are avoided by emphasis being placed on the drug experience. Thus it is possible that those who may initially be disturbed might be attracted to the more exotic and more potent types of drugs. Therefore, there may be a qualitative difference in personality between nondrug users, marijuana only users, and multiple drug users. This is a problem which calls for additional research to answer.

PROBABILITY OF GROUP MEMBERSHIP

One of the advantages of discriminant analysis is that the procedure leads to the calculation of the probability of membership in each of the criterion groups. It is merely necessary, therefore, to compare the probabilities calculated from each of the discriminant equations to select the highest probability. Each subject, then, is predicted to belong to that group whose discriminant equation leads to the highest probability for him. An analysis of hits and misses obtained by solving the discriminant equations for each of the 330 subjects in the study revealed that 129 students (70%) in Group A were predicted correctly as to group membership. The remaining 56 students (30%) were predicted to belong to Group B. Thus the equations predicted that 129 of 185 students at the time of the study would tend to not use drugs. For Group B members, the equations were about equally powerful in predicting group membership. Ninety-six out of the 145 student drug users were predicted accurately as belonging to Group B, resulting in a hit rate of 67%; 49 subjects (33%) were predicted to belong to Group A. On the basis of the predictions of the probability of group membership it appeared that the discriminant equation predicting nondrug use yielded the highest probability for group membership.

This study represents part of a long-range investigation of obtaining predictive validity of selection criteria by using a series of personality dimensions, in addition to imagery processes, to predict (or to discriminate between potential drug users). Primary attention will not only focus on following through to determine the accuracy of prediction of group membership, but also to develop additional predictor variables to the present set and to extend the criterion groups to include abusive drinking in college students. A further objective will be to cross-validate the present set of predictors.

REFERENCES

ANDERSON, T. *Introduction to Multivariate Statistical Analysis*. New York: Wiley, 1958.

McAREE, STEFFENHAGEN, and ZHEUTLIN. Personality factors in college drug users. *Intern. J. Soc. Psychiat.* 15: 102–106, 1969.

SEGAL, B., and FEGER, G. Drug use and fantasy processes in college students. *Altered States of Consciousness*, 1: In press.

The International Journal of the Addictions, 9(3), 481–487, 1974

An Epidemiological and Ecological Study of Risk Factors for Narcotics Overdose: I. Retrospective Study of Psychosocial Factors

Elizabeth E. Force, Ph.D.*

Division of Medical Sciences
National Academy of Sciences-National Research Council
Washinton, D.C.

Jack W. Millar, M.D.

Department of Epidemiology and Environmental Health
The George Washington University School of Medicine
Washington, D.C.

* In partial fulfillment of the requirements for the Doctor of Philosophy Degree, Department of Epidemiology and Environmental Health, The George Washington University School of Medicine, Washington, D.C. 20005.

A study of psychosocial factors associated with narcotics overdose was carried out through interviews of 50 addicts who were participants in the Narcotics Treatment Administrations' (NTA) Program at the D.C. General Hospital in Washington, D.C.

Two hypotheses were tested: (1) there is a relationship between specific social variables such as addict attitudes and behavior and narcotics overdose; and (2) there is a relationship between previous overdose experience and precautionary behavior in drug use.

STUDY GROUP

Ninety-four percent of study group addicts (47/50) were Black, possibly reflecting the predominantly Black population in Washington, D.C., with 46% (23/50) males and 49% (24/50) females. Caucasians made up 6% (3/50) of the study population, two White males and one White female. The average age of Black males was 26.0 years; of Black females, 24.2 years; of two White males, 25.0 years. The one White female was 33 years. The age range for Black males was from 16 to 36 years, with three addicts over 30 years of age; for Black females, 14 to 34 years of age, with two addicts over 30 years of age.

The average length of addiction for White males was 4.0 years; for the White female the length of addiction was 5 years; and for the entire study group, 5.2 years. In Black males the lengths of addiction ranged from 2 to 25 years and averaged 7.6 years; included were five addicts with greater than 10 years of addiction. For Black females, addiction periods ranged from 4 months to 13 years and averaged 4.1 years; only one case had an addiction period greater than 10 years.

Black males were first addicted at an average age of 19.4 years; with four males addicted at age $\leqq$ 16 years. Black females averaged 17.8 years when addicted; 10 females were addicted at age $\leqq$ 16 years. White males averaged 21 years when addicted; the white female was addicted at age 28. Black females seemed to have used narcotics at an earlier age than Black males. No valid statement can be made concerning White addicts.

RESULTS

Knowledge about Narcotics Overdose

As shown in Table 1, 96% (48/50) of the addicts knew of at least one symptom associated with narcotics overdose. Eighty-four percent (42/50)

Table 1
Sources of Knowledge and Known Symptlns Associated with Narcotics Overdose, 50 Cases

	No. addicts indicating
Symptom	
"Falling out" or unconsciousness	42
Body trembling	2
Eyes go back in head	8
Foaming at mouth	5
Fatal	6
Nothing known	2[a]
Source	
Personal experience (self, other addicts)	29[b]
Addict street talk	27[b]
Literature on drugs	6[b]
Medical personnel	9[b]
Other persons (relatives, clergy, police, teachers)	7[b]

[a] Sole answer given by the addicts; multiple symptoms given by all other addicts.
[b] All addicts indicated more than one source of information.

stipulated unconsciousness. Other symptoms were body trembling, foaming at the mouth, eyes going back in the head, and death. Two addicts with short addiction periods (4 to 5 months) claimed no knowledge of overdose. Information about overdose was obtained mainly through personal overdose experience (self or addict friends) and conversations with other addicts.

Overdose was primarily attributed to shooting-up before checking the purity of street heroin. In fact, 72% (36/50) experienced a "deep nod" from unexpectedly pure heroin. Greed for narcotics, defined as wanting to achieve the maximum "high" short of overdose, was believed to be another major cause of overdose. In seeking this type of "high," the addict shoots ever-increasing heroin doses and runs the risk for overdose. Alcohol ingestion together with heroin or methadone was also indicated as a risk factor.

Concern about Narcotics Overdose and Precautionary Behavior

As indicated in Table 2, 60% (30/50) expressed no concern about overdose, while 40% (20/50) were worried. Yet 62% (31/50) took precautions to protect against overdose, while 38% (19/50) did not. The principal

Table 2
Addict Concern and Behavioral Precautions for Narcotics Overdose, 50 Cases

Condition	Answering "Yes"		Answering "No"	
	No.	%	No.	%
Concerned about overdose	20	40	30	60
Take precautions against overdose	31	62	19	38

precautionary measure was checking heroin purity and adjusting the dose before shooting-up. Questioned was: (1) why the addict would or would not worry about overdose; and (2) what precautions were taken by some addicts and why, and why no precautions were taken by others. Data are given in Table 3.

Concern about narcotics overdose and precautionary behavior in drug-use were primarily responses to a fear of death. Fatalistic attitudes were noted in 42% (8/19) of the addicts who took no precautions and 80%

Table 3
Reasons for Addict Concern about and Behavioral Precautions to Protect Against Narcotics Overdose, 50 Cases

Question posed—answers given	No. answering total	%
Concerned about overdose (20 addicts)		
(a) Why do you worry?		
Don't want to die	19/20	95
Relatives/friends have died	1/20	5
Not concerned about overdose (30 addicts)		
(a) Why don't you worry?		
Watch dose taken	6/30	20
"If your number's up, it's up"	24/30	80
Precautions against overdose (31 addicts)		
(a) What precautions?		
Check heroin, control dose	28/31	90
Narcotics abstinence	3/31	10
(b) Why precautions?		
Don't want to die	20/31	65
Relatives/friends have died	11/31	35
No precautions against overdose (19 addicts)		
(a) Why no precautions?		
"Can't help what happens"	8/19	42
Need the "high" or "fix"	11/19	58

(24/30) who presumably did not worry about overdose. Immediacy of a need for a "fix" due to craving a "high" or experiencing withdrawal was indicated by 58% (11/19) of those who did not take precautions.

Previous Overdose Experience and Precautionary Behavior

As shown in Table 4, 40% or 20/50 had a history of narcotics overdose and averaged 2.4 such reactions; 8/20 had one reaction; 12/20 had more than one overdose reaction. Sixty percent or 30/50 had not experienced overdose.

The percentage of Black males with a history of overdose was 48% (11/23); the average number of overdose reactions was 2.2. Thirty-three percent of Black females (8/24) experienced overdose an average of 1.5 times. Since Black males in the study had an average length of addiction of 7.6 years vs 4.1 years for Black females, the greater number of overdose reactions in Black males may be related to the length of addiction rather than to sex differences in drug response. Also, length of addiction did not appear correlated with a history of overdose. No valid comparative data statement could be made for White addicts (three cases).

Data given in Table 5 indicate that of the 20 addicts with a positive history of overdose, 60% (12/20) took no precautions against such a reaction, while 40% (8/20) of the group did. Of the 30 addicts with no history of overdose, 77% (23/30) took positive measures for protection while 23% (7/30) took no precautions. For addicts who took no precautionary measures, the 60% case rate with a history of overdose was

Table 4
Narcotics Overdose Reactions in Study Group Addicts, 50 Cases

Group	Total no. addicts	History of overdose		No history of overdose		Average no. of overdose reactions
		No.	%	No.	%	
Black:						
Males	23	11	48	12	52	2.2
Females	24	8	33	16	67	1.5
White:						
Males	2	0	0	2	(100)[a]	0
Females	1	1	(100)[a]	0	0	2.0
All addicts	50	20	40	30	60	2.4

[a] Percentage cannot be considered as accurately representative of white females (1 case) or white males (2 cases).

Table 5
Relationship between Previous Narcotics Overdose and Attitudes, and Precautionary Behavior, 50 Cases

Category	Precautions against overdose: No./total cases	Precautions against overdose: %	No precautions against overdose: No./total cases	No precautions against overdose: %
Previous overdose	8/20	40	12/20	60
No previous overdose	23/30	77	7/30	23
	Worry about overdose		No worry about overdose	
Previous overdose	10/20	50	10/20	50
No previous overdose	10/30	33	20/30	67
	No worry about overdose, precautions		No worry about overdose, no precautions	
No previous overdose	17/20	85	3/20	15

statistically significantly greater ($p < .01$) than the 23% case rate with no previous overdose experience. Thus failure to exercise precautionary behavior seemed a significant risk factor. Apparently, overdose experience did not influence drug-use behavior since the average number of overdose reactions in this group was 2.4.

For addicts who did not worry about narcotics overdose, the 50% case rate with a history of overdose was not significantly different from the 67% case rate with no history of previous overdose. Lack of concern apparently was not a risk factor.

For the 30 addicts with no previous history of overdose (Table 5), the 67% rate (20/30) of addicts who presumably did not worry about overdose was significantly greater than the 33% rate (10/30) who did worry ($p <$ .01). Lack of concern shown by 67% of these addicts could be due to their never having experienced overdose or to assumed protection afforded by precautionary behavior. Precautionary behavior and lack of concern seemed correlated as indicated by the significant 85% (17/20) who took precautions and were not worried about overdose, as compared to the 15% (3/20) who did not take precautions and did not worry ($p < .001$).

DISCUSSION

This limited unsystematic sociopsychological survey employing 50 narcotics addicts suggested that fear of withdrawal and narcotics craving, reportedly associated with perpetuation of addiction and failure at attempts at withdrawal (*American Journal of Psychiatry*, 1972, Bowden, 1971; Brown, 1970; Cameron, 1971; Lindesmith, 1968), are strong motivating factors for narcotics use by addicts despite a clear understanding of the potential danger of overdose and death. Even previous overdose experience did not modify drug-use behavior. The prominent identifiable attitudinal and behavioral risk factors were failure to exercise precautionary behavior, alcohol consumption together with narcotics, and greed for narcotics.

The morbidity and mortality associated with narcotics overdose may possibly be dealt with not only through rehabilitation of addicts, but also through instruction of addicts in the proper medical self-help methods to treat overdose prior to hospitalization.

ACKNOWLEDGMENT

This study could not have been carried out without the cooperation and encouragement of Dr. Robert L. DuPont, Director, Narcotics Treatment Administration, Washington, D.C.

REFERENCES

ANONYMOUS. Narcotics and addiction (Special Section). *Amer. J. Psychiat.* 128: 842–868, 1972.

BOWDEN, C.L. Determinants of initial use of opioids. *Comp. Psychol.* 12: 136–140, 1971.

BROWN, B. Addict's reasons for initiating and withdrawing from heroin. *Trends* 1: 8–11, 1970 (Department of Human Resources of District of Columbia).

CAMERON, D.C. Abuse of alcohol and drugs: concepts and planning. *World Health Organ. Chron.* 25: 8–16, 1971.

LINDESMITH, A.R. *Addiction and Opiates*. Chicago: Aldine, 1968.

The International Journal of the Addictions, 9(3), 489–494, 1974

Research Note

Demographic Characteristics of Black and White Male Alcoholics

Jorge A. Viamontes, M.D.

Barbara J. Powell, Ph.D.

Malcolm Bliss Mental Health Center
and Department of Psychiatry
Washington University Medical School
St. Louis, Missouri

The existing literature on drinking patterns of Black alcoholics is relatively limited; however, most of the data suggest that drinking behavior of Blacks may be different from that of Whites. A summary of recent studies in this area is presented in Table 1. Robins et al. (1968) indicated that heavy drinking is a common pattern among Black urban males and that drinking behavior usually resulted in objective difficulties and personal worry. Maddox and Williams (1968) reported that drinking is twice as common in urban Black men as in urban White men of similar socioeconomic class origins. King et al. (1969), in a study of the social problems of Black men, demonstrated the significance of alcohol abuse in the Black urban ghetto and how this related to broken homes, delinquency, sexual and reproductive irresponsibility, and underemployment.

At least two investigators (Robins et al., 1968; Vitols, 1968) report that Blacks tend to start drinking at a relatively early age. In Robins' study, 84% of the subjects reportedly became heavy drinkers before the age of 19. Vitols found that about one-third of a group of Black high school

Table 1
Summary of Studies Relating to Black Alcoholics

Authors	Date	Sample size	Sex	Sample characteristics	Summary results
Malzberg	1947	616 White, 58 Black	Male and female	First admissions for alcoholic psychoses, New York	More alcoholic psychoses in Blacks
Locke et al.	1960	1,778 Black and White	Male and female	Admitting diagnosis of alcoholic psychosis, state hospital, Ohio	Early onset of alcoholic psychosis and early hospitalization for Blacks
Locke et al.	1964	3,339 Black and White	Male and female	First admissions to state hospital, Ohio	Non-Whites admitted earlier than Whites
Maddox et al.	1968	262 Black	Male	Interview data from college freshmen, North Carolina	Early onset of drinking in Blacks
Robins et al.	1968	235 Black	Male	Records of *S*s attending elementary schools in St. Louis	Earlier onset of alcoholism in Blacks, higher delinquency in drinkers
Vitols	1968	907 White, 132 Black	Male and female	Admitting diagnosis of alcoholism, state mental hospital, South Carolina	Addiction starts earlier in Blacks
King et al.	1969	223 Black	Male	Attended public elementary schools in St. Louis	Drinking begins early in Blacks, causes increased social deviance
Gorwitz et al.	1970	10,376 Black and White	Male and female	Admitting diagnosis alcoholism, Maryland	Non-Whites admitted at earlier ages than Whites

students had become dependent on alcohol between the ages of 12 and 14. Three students reportedly had experienced DT's at age 15.

In an epidemiological study, Gorvitz et al. (1970) found that in the youngest age groups, non-White admissions for alcoholism were substantially higher than White. The greater number of non-White admissions at earlier ages has also been noted by others (Malzberg, 1947; Locke, Kramer, and Pasamanick, 1960; Locke and Duvall, 1964) who suggest that non-Whites tend to be from lower socioeconomic groups and are thus more susceptible to nutritional and health problems which might accelerate the recognition and occurrence of physical symptoms of alcoholism.

Another explanation for earlier admissions of Blacks is that they may be less likely to have family members able and willing to care for them at home, with the result that hospitalization must be sought earlier. It was also speculated that Blacks exhibit more acting-out behaviors at earlier ages and thus tend to be diagnosed earlier.

Another alternative explanation may be that Blacks start drinking earlier in life because the Black culture has a higher tolerance for drinking behavior. Lewis (1955), in a study of Black culture, states that "the seven taverns of Kent rank with the churches as major symbols of Negro community—both churches and taverns are places of regular ritual, like attendance places where one can be somebody."

As noted, the existing literature on the Black alcoholic and on drinking behavior of Blacks suggests that in certain areas they may differ from Whites. The present study was an attempt to amplify and perhaps clarify some of this information by comparing alcohol-related behaviors and problem areas of a randomly selected group of Black and White alcoholics from similar socioeconomic backgrounds.

METHOD

The charts of one hundred Black male and one hundred White male alcoholics hospitalized in Malcolm Bliss Mental Health Center during a 6-month period (January to June 1970) were selected for study. Both groups were from low socioeconomic backgrounds and if employed were engaged in unskilled or semiskilled positions. All the subjects were hospitalized for treatment of alcoholism. Medical complications and poor social performance attributable or related to alcoholism characterized the sample.

The major emphasis of this study was placed upon the exploration of (1) possible demographic differences between Black and White male alcoholics, and (2) possible differences in reported incidence of alcohol-related symptomatology.

RESULTS AND DISCUSSION

The mean educational level was comparable, 9.3 for Blacks and 9.6 for Whites. Marital status among the groups was also similar with the exception that approximately twice as many Blacks (28%) were single. Subsequent data suggest that this result might be attributed to the overall younger age of the Black patients.

Blacks reported earlier drinking behavior than Whites and also earlier "loss of control" over drinking. On the average, drinking reportedly began for the Blacks at 15.7 years while for Whites it was 19.0 years or approximately 3.5 years later. While these data are not significant (t = 1.62, $p > .10$), the relatively earlier onset of drinking in Blacks is consistent with Lewis' notion that the Black culture has a higher tolerance and/or greater permissiveness for early drinking. Blacks reported an average loss of control at 28.5 years, while for Whites the mean age when loss of control was reported was 32.9. The loss of control over alcoholic consumption occurred for both groups approximately 13 to 14 years after the onset of drinking. In our random sample of patients, the mean age of the Blacks was 37.0 years while that of Whites was 46.2. Thus, at the time of our survey, the average White patient was approximately 9 years older than the average Black.

Several explanations for these findings are suggested. It can be speculated that Black alcoholics are motivated to seek treatment for their condition *earlier* than Whites. On the other hand, it may be that alcohol-related problems in Blacks attain a greater magnitude earlier in life than they do in Whites. Thus Blacks may be "forced" into treatment earlier. If this is true, Blacks should demonstrate a greater number of alcohol-related symptoms or problems than Whites. To investigate this, data pertaining to alcohol-related arrests, blackouts, hallucinations, DT's, and convulsions were tabulated.

In terms of alcohol-related arrests, there was virtually no difference between the groups. Roughly one-half of each group (55% of the Blacks and 58% of the Whites) indicated that they had been arrested one or more times because of behavior or actions associated with excessive use of alcohol; however, when *age differences* between the two groups were taken into account, the mean age of Blacks reporting arrests was 34.5 while that of Blacks reporting *no* arrest record was 40.5 years, or 6 years older. Among Whites, there was only an average age difference of 1.25 years between arrested and nonarrested alcoholics. This result suggests that "trouble" associated with alcohol may explain, in part, our finding that, as a group, Blacks were seen in treatment earlier in life than Whites.

In the reported incidence of alcohol-related symptoms, *t* tests revealed significant race differences for convulsions and hallucinations, but not for blackouts and DT's. Sixteen percent of the Blacks reported convulsions compared to 7% of the Whites ($p < .05$). Seventy-nine percent of the Blacks reported experiencing one or more hallucinations compared to 57% of the Whites. This difference was significant beyond the .01 level. The groups did not differ in reported incidence of blackouts. Of the Blacks, 82% reported experiencing one or more alcohol blackouts while 89% of Whites reported blackouts. A few more Blacks than Whites (48% as opposed to 38%) reported DT's; however, this difference was not significant.

CONCLUSION

Our results are consistent with those of Robins in that our sample of Black alcoholics began drinking at an earlier age than a comparable group of Whites. We also found, as did Locke and Malzberg, that the Black population was younger on admission. However, since our groups were of comparable socioeconomic background, our interpretation of this finding is related more to alcohol-related problem areas (arrests, debilitating symptoms, etc.) than to nutritional problems. Their speculation of less reliance on family as contributing to earlier admission of Blacks could also apply to our data since a greater proportion of the Blacks were unmarried, divorced, etc.

The finding that Blacks report significantly more hallucinatory behavior and convulsions than Whites clearly merits further investigations. It may be speculated that cultural factors play an important role in the hallucinatory phenomena. Genetic differences may also possibly account for the observed variations. The observation that the Black alcoholic started drinking at a relatively early age may explain the high incidence of convulsions through an increased vulnerability of the central nervous system.

REFERENCES

GORVITZ, K., BAHN, A., WARTHERN, F.J., and COOPER, M. Some epidemiological data on alcoholism in Maryland. *Quart. J. Studies Alc.* 31: 423–443, 1970.

KING, L.J., MURPHY, G.E., ROBINS, L.N., and DARVISH, H. Alcohol abuse: a crucial factor in the social problems of Negro men. *Amer. J. Psychiat.* 125: 1882–1890, 1969.

LEWIS, H. *Black Ways of Kent*, Chapel Hill, North Carolina: Univ. North Carolina Press, 1955.

LOCKE, B.Z., and DUVALL, H.J. Alcoholism among first admissions to Ohio public mental hospital. *Quart. J. Studies Alc.* 25: 231–234, 1964.

LOCKE, B.Z., KRAMER, M., and PASAMANICK, B. Alcoholic psychosis among first admission to a public mental hospital in Ohio. *Quart. J. Studies. Alc.* 21: 457–474, 1960.

MADDOX, G.L., and WILLIAMS, J.R. Drinking behavior of Negro collegians. *Quart. J. Studies Alc.* 29: 117–129, 1968.

MALZBERG, B.A. Study of first admissions with alcoholic psychosis in New York State, 1943–1944. *Quart. J. Studies Alc.*, 8: 274–295, 1947.

ROBINS, L.N., MURPHY, G.E., and BRECKENRIDGE, M.B. Drinking behavior of young Negro men. *Quart. J. Studies Alc.* 29: 657–684, 1968.

VITOLS, M.M. Cultural patterns of drinking in Negro and White alcoholics. *Diseases Nervous System* 29: 391–394, 1968.

A Statement of Purpose

INSTITUTE FOR THE STUDY OF DRUG MISUSE, Inc.

The Institute for the Study of Drug Misuse, Inc. (formerly the Institute for the Study of Drug Addiction) was established in 1965 as an international organization to develop clear channels of communication and to encourage research in the field of drug abuse. To fulfill its goals, the Institute participates in research, professional training, and education. In addition, it serves as a consulting agency in the establishment of treatment programs in the United States and abroad. As professional, government, and lay concern increases in the field of drug abuse, the Institute has been called upon to serve as a resource agency for the dissemination of scientific materials through the press, television, radio, and other media.

In order to achieve its purposes, the Institute for the Study of Drug Misuse:

Sponsors the INTERNATIONAL JOURNAL OF THE ADDICTIONS, published by Marcel Dekker, Inc.

Sponsors national and international conferences and workshops in cooperation with universities, medical teaching centers, governmental agencies, and private industry.

Sponsors a lecture series "The Use and Misuse of Drugs and Alcohol," for professionals and interested lay people.

Sponsors international awards for significant research reports focusing upon various aspects of drug abuse.

The expanding programs of the Institute have been dictated by the present crisis in drug abuse. It is apparent that in the United States and in the world at large, certain social forces are at work which have magnified the scope of the problem. In order to insure that the Institute reaches the broadest group of interested individuals, it has become necessary to establish several categories of membership.

Membership in the Institute for the Study of Drug Misuse is tax exempt.

For membership information, write:

Institute for the Study of Drug Misuse, Inc.
111 Fifth Avenue
New York, N.Y. 10003

INFORMATION FOR AUTHORS SUBMITTING MANUSCRIPTS

Send a clear double-spaced typewritten original and two duplicate copies to the Editor, *International Journal of the Addictions*, Institute for the Study of Drug Misuse, Inc., 111 Fifth Avenue, New York, N.Y. 10003. DOUBLE-SPACE the entire manuscript; do not use single spacing anywhere.

Include authors' academic degrees and present affiliation. If applicable, cite auspices under which work being reported was done. Specify address to which requests for reprints should be sent.

Begin your TITLE with a word useful in indexing. Put news of your finding or a statement of the problem first. Major and minor headings may be used in the text; indicate major headings by typing in capitals. Provide a 100-word SUMMARY at the end.

Use METRIC UNITS of measure. If measurements were made in English units, give metric equivalents.

Cite all TABLES and FIGURES in the text. Tables should have titles, and figures should have brief legends. In tables, give each column a heading. Indicate units of measure in parentheses in the heading for each column. Do not use vertical rules. Do not use horizontal rules other than those in the heading and at the bottom. Submit PHOTOGRAPHS as glossy prints, untrimmed and unmounted; identify each with pencil lightly on the back and indicate top.

ARTWORK will not be returned unless specifically requested, and will be disposed of three months after publication.

REFERENCES in the text should be enclosed in parentheses and include the author's surname and the date of the item cited. Keep footnotes to a minimum.

The BIBLIOGRAPHY (double-spaced) should be given at the end of the article in alphabetical order. Journal references should include authors, title, name of journal abbreviated according to *Chemical Abstracts List of Periodicals,* inclusive page numbers, and date. Book references should include authors, title, place of publication, publisher, and date.

THE INTERNATIONAL JOURNAL OF THE ADDICTIONS

Published by Marcel Dekker, Inc., New York
Sponsored by The Institute for the Study of Drug Misuse, Inc., New York

INTERNATIONAL EDITORIAL BOARD

THE INTERNATIONAL JOURNAL OF THE ADDICTIONS

Volume 9 Number 3 1974

CONTENTS

Mortality in an Alcoholic Cohort: Raymond M. Costello and Sandra Lee Schneider 355

International Issues in Drug Abuse: David E. Raskin 365

The Uses of an Epidemiology of Drug Use: The Canadian Scene: Reginald G. Smart and Paul C. Whitehead 373

Behavioral Approaches for Problems with Alcohol: John A. Ewing 389

Drug Use and Achievement: Albert S. Carlin and Robin Dee Post 401

Assisted Covert Sensitization for Drug Abuse: Barry M. Maletzky 411

Psychological and Social Variables and Personality Patterns of Drug Abusers: Kenneth B. Stein and Vitali Rozynko 431

Group Covert Sensitization with Narcotic Addicts (Further Comments): G. J. Steinfeld, E. A. Rautio, A. H. Rice, and M. J. Egan 447

Some Descriptive Measures on 100 Consecutive VA Hospital Drug Abuse Admissions: Don Wallace and Darlene Hiner 465

Drug Use and Fantasy Processes: Criterion for Prediction of Potential Users: Bernard Segal 475

An Epidemiological and Ecological Study of Risk Factors for Narcotics Overdose: I. Retrospective Study of Psychosocial Factors: Elizabeth E. Force and Jack W. Millar 481

Demographic Characteristics of Black and White Male Alcoholics: Jorge A. Viamontes and Barbara J. Powell 489

Cover illustration courtesy of the Picture Collection, The Branch Libraries, New York Public Library

MARCEL DEKKER, INC., New York

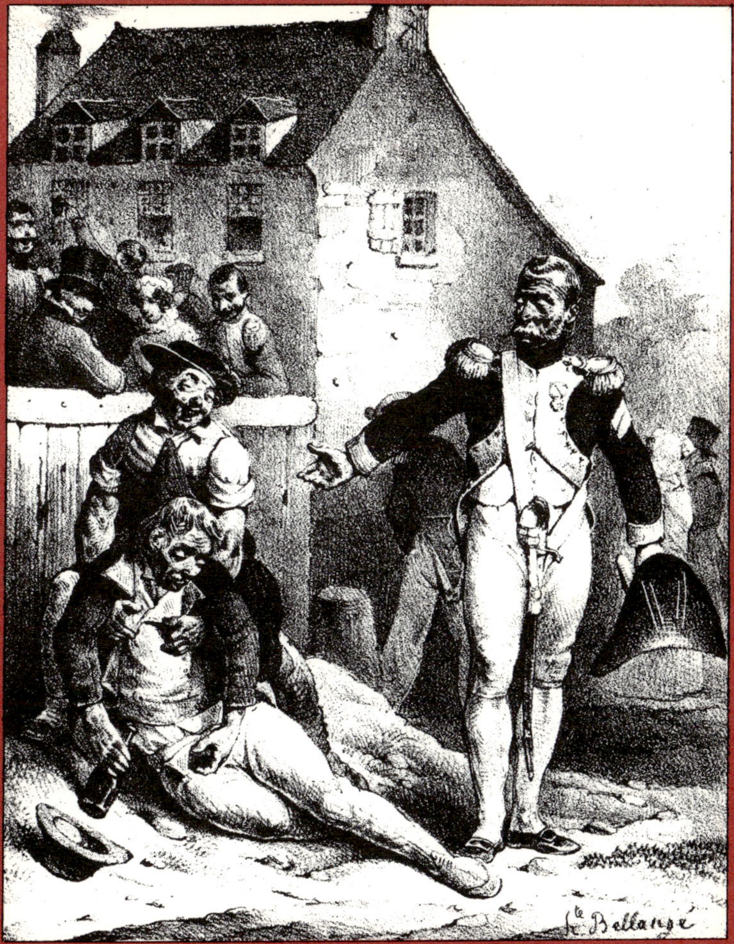

THE INTERNATIONAL JOURNAL OF THE Addictions

Volume 9 Number 4 1974

THE INTERNATIONAL JOURNAL OF THE ADDICTIONS

The International Journal of the Addictions, August 1974

Published six times annually—February, April, June, August, October, December—by Marcel Dekker, Inc., 270 Madison Avenue, New York, N. Y. 10016. The subscription rate for Volume 9 (1974), containing 6 issues is $40.00 (prepaid). Postage outside the United States is $5.10 per volume for all subscriptions. The special discounted rate for individual professionals and students is $20.00. Back volume prices will be sent on request. Please *mail payment with order* to the following address: Marcel Dekker Journals, P. O. Box 11305, Church Street Station, New York, New York 10249.

Second-class postage paid at New York, N. Y., and at additional mailing offices.

Contributions to This Journal Are Published Free of Charge

The International Journal of the Addictions, 9(4), 495–502, 1974

Sweating Function in the Heroin Withdrawal Syndrome of Neonates

Marvin Green, M.D.

Carl Zelson, M.D.

Hans Behrendt, M.D.

Department of Pediatrics
New York Medical College–Metropolitan Hospital Center
New York, New York

Pediatric interest in drug addiction is not confined to the approach and methods most suitable for treating young addicts, particularly adolescents. The pediatrician also faces the unique problem of dealing with addicts whom he first sees when drugs have suddenly been withheld and symptoms of withdrawal are beginning to appear. This is the situation in neonates who are born to heroin-addicted mothers dependent on the drug throughout pregnancy. Their offspring become "physically" addicted during fetal life and, after birth, are prone to develop the withdrawal syndrome.

Since some of the first observations on addicted neonates were reported from this institution in the 1950s (Cobrinik et al., 1956, 1959), the prevalence of drug abuse and the number of infants born to addicted mothers have drastically increased (85% of addicted women are in the child-bearing age). As a result, the ill-effects of fetal addiction are now much better known, although not yet satisfactorily explained. In a recent review article (Zelson, 1971), one of us has dealt with the progress made in recognition and treatment of the neonatal withdrawal syndrome and has presented his personal experience on 384 addicted neonates observed from 1960 through 1969. A conservative estimate puts the number of addicted neonates born annually in New York City at 700 to 800 (Yerby, 1966).

With general supportive therapy and drug treatment (chlorpromazine, phenobarbital, paregoric, or valium), improvement occurs rapidly and most infants recover. Data on the mortality rate among neonates presenting with the withdrawal syndrome are ambiguous. The mortality rate for all neonates born to heroin-addicted mothers, regardless of presence or absence of neonatal withdrawal, has been reported as low as 3.6% by Zelson (1971) and as high as 34% by Goodfriend (1956).

As in adults, many signs of withdrawal are manifestations of a hyperstimulated autonomic nervous system, although responses in the neonate show some peculiar clinical characteristics. The most frequently observed signs are irritability, tremors, vomiting, high pitched cry, sneezing, and respiratory distress. Sweating as a sign of neonatal withdrawal has attracted our particular attention because we have found it not only in full-size, but also in low-birth-weight neonates* who constitute almost 50% of all infants born to addicted mothers. In a recent study (Behrendt, 1972) performed under controlled conditions, we determined the incidence of spontaneous generalized sweating in neonates by means of the starch-iodine reaction or by sweat prints on bromphenol blue paper applied to several body sites. During an observation period of 2.5 hr, we found sweating to be present in 30 of 131 healthy full-size but only in two of 108 healthy low-birth-weight babies, aged 2 to 8 days. In contrast, among heroin-addicted low-birth-weight infants of the same postnatal age range, the proportion of those showing sweating (8/20) was significantly higher than among healthy low-birth-weight infants (2/108), and even higher than in healthy full-size neonates.

The high incidence of spontaneous sweating in addicted prematurely born infants is difficult to reconcile with the established evidence (Behrendt, 1969; Green, 1969, 1970, 1973) that most prematurely born low-birth-weight infants have sweat glands that are physiologically not

* "Low-birth-weight" ($\leq$ 2,500 g) and "premature" ($<$ 37 completed weeks of gestation) are used interchangeably in this paper.

operative, i.e., unresponsive to local and general thermal stimulation as well as to intradermally applied adrenergic and cholinergic stimuli. In order to clarify this paradox, we subjected a series of prematurely born neonates presenting with the withdrawal syndrome to sudorific stimulation tests with acetylcholine, epinephrine, and nicotine, and compared their responses to the reaction of healthy premature neonates.

Exogenous acetylcholine evokes local sweating by a dual mechanism: by direct muscarinic action on the glands (the process through which natural sweating is induced) and by indirect nicotinic action via the sudomotor axon reflex (which does not occur physiologically). Our observations concern only the muscarinic type of response. The action of exogenous epinephrine on the sweat gland is a direct one; a similar endogenous action is probably lacking. Nicotine evokes a sweating reaction via the sudomotor axon reflex.

For our tests, all babies were left in their incubators and the test procedure was carried out through the portholes. Ambient temperature was continuously adjusted by means of the automatic control unit to maintain abdominal skin temperature at 36°C. As a result, forearm (test site) temperature ranged from 33.4 to 35.5°C for the healthy infants, and from 34.2 to 35.6°C for the addicted babies. Relative humidity in the incubators ranged between 40 and 70%. We sought comparable temperatures at the test site since local sweat gland reactivity to pharmacologic stimulation has been found to correlate more closely to this thermal parameter than to environmental temperature in adults (Bronow, 1958; Ogawa, 1970). All babies showing spontaneous (background) sweating were excluded from this series. Since these pharmacologic stimulation tests are being performed on all infants born to drug-addicted mothers in our institution, the present discussion is based on a greater number of observations than our first report (Behrendt, 1972) on these comparative tests.

We determined minimal effective doses contained in 0.02 ml of intradermally injected drug solutions according to the method described previously (Behrendt, 1969). A number of serial dilutions in 0.9% saline were made for each drug, each consecutive dilution being 10 times higher than the preceding one. The strongest permissible concentrations (w/v) were 10^{-3} for acetylcholine and epinephrine and 10^{-4} for nicotine.

The local sweating reaction was visualized by the Wada method

(Wada, 1950). The response was considered as positive if at least five sweat spots were discernible within 10 min. Subjects failing to react to the maximal permissible dose were recorded as negative reactors.

As shown by the proportions of infants with positive sweating reactions, the responsiveness to all three drugs is significantly greater in prematurely born neonates with the withdrawal syndrome than in healthy controls: When tested with epinephrine, 17 of 24 neonates suffering withdrawal had positive responses, while only seven of 23 controls were positive; for acetylcholine, 15 of 21 infants with withdrawal reacted with sweating, while only four of 26 healthy controls showed positive reactions. Ten of 16 addicted neonates and only two of the 15 healthy babies were positive reactors to nicotine. These differences in reactivity are highly significant with a confidence coefficient $>.95$ for multiple comparisons involving hypotheses on three drugs ($\chi^2 = 7.815$ with three degrees of freedom).

The hyperhidrotic responses of babies suffering from withdrawal are most clearly illustrated by the graphs of Fig. 1, in which threshold values are plotted against gestational age. In both addicted and healthy premature infants there is a trend for the threshold concentrations to decrease with increasing gestational age, but the minimal effective doses for addicted subjects are far below those for healthy babies throughout the range of gestation.

Although therapeutic doses of morphine have been found to induce sweating in adults (Goodman, 1967), persistent hyperhidrosis is more characteristic during acute withdrawal. We are inclined to consider the addicted neonate's increased sweat gland reactivity as a manifestation of changes associated with heroin withdrawal. It is unlikely that fetal exposure to heroin alone produces the hyperhidrosis persisting throughout the first few weeks after birth. Indeed, in a number of premature addicted neonates who failed to show withdrawal, we could not elicit positive responses to stimulation with drugs.

We believe that the physiologic deficiency of the sweating mechanism of prematurely born infants is not necessarily due to incompetence of the end-organ but is at least in part caused by immaturity of the sweating centers. We assume that the premature infant's sweat glands are potentially functional but remain unreactive because the centers fail to supply: (1) the tonic innervation that renders the end-organ susceptible to direct pharmacologic stimulation (Rothman, 1954), and (2) the actual nerve impulses which produce reflex sweating. This concept is supported by the

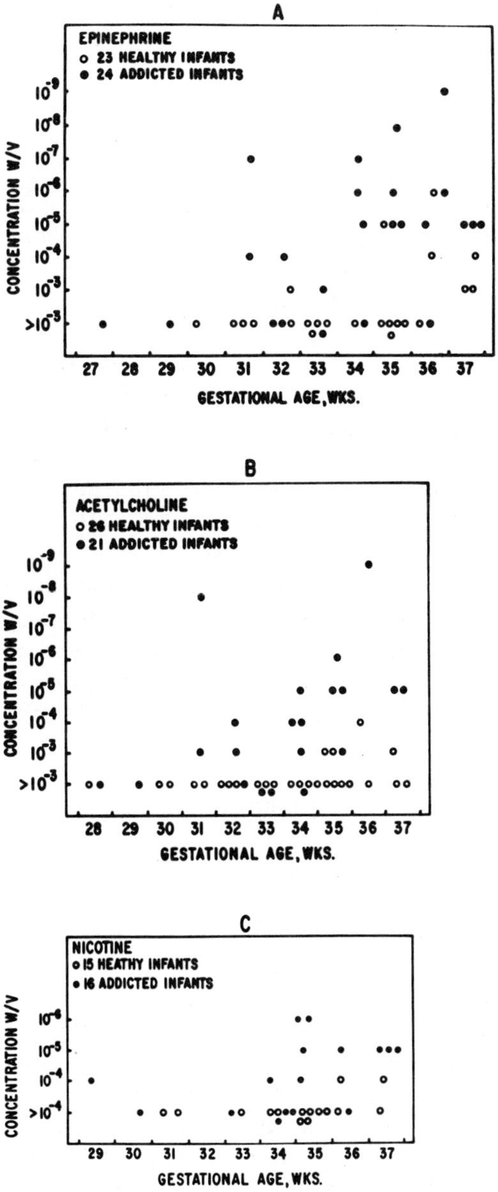

Fig. 1. Hyperhidrotic responses of babies suffering from withdrawal.

altered sweating function associated with neonatal withdrawal. It appears that only a potentially functional sweat gland can be activated by the abnormally increased autonomic output.

Thus far the diagnosis of the neonatal withdrawal syndrome has to be based on clinical manifestations. Presence of morphine or quinine in the urine of the infant is evidence of recent intake of heroin by the mother but not related to the development of signs of withdrawal. Spontaneous generalized sweating, if present in a prematurely born neonate, is almost pathognomonic of the withdrawal syndrome.

Unlike hyperhidrosis, physiologic jaundice (Zelson, 1971) and the hyaline membrane syndrome (Glass, 1971) have a lower incidence in addicted than in healthy prematurely born neonates. Both conditions can be considered as due to physiologic metabolic immaturities: the former to a deficit in hepatic glucuronyl transferase activity, the latter perhaps to incompetence of alveolar cells to produce tension-lowering lipids. One may speculate that early maturation of both functions is promoted during fetal exposure to heroin. Liver homogenates from morphine-treated mice indeed show increased transferase activity (Cohen, 1971).

Finally, a word about methadone. Addiction to this drug is becoming more common and may lead to an increased incidence of neonatal addiction as well. Methadone is of slower action than heroin, and its withdrawal in adults causes less intense clinical signs. As yet, we are not able to say whether this applies also to methadone withdrawal in the neonate and its effect on the sweating mechanism.

SUMMARY

Offspring of heroin-addicted gravidae frequently show narcotic withdrawal after birth. Many clinical signs are indicative of hyperactivity of of the autonomic nervous system, generalized hyperhidrosis being one example. Since many of these infants are prematurely born, their capacity for reflex sweating is very unusual. Still, they show generalized sweating with significantly greater frequency than do healthy premature controls and even mature neonates. In response to local stimulation tests with sudorific drugs (epinephrine, acetylcholine, and nicotine), a significantly greater proportion of these addicted premature babies show sweat gland responsiveness than do controls, and minimal effective doses are lower.

Accelerated development of sweating function in neonates ill with heroin withdrawal shows that the sweating deficit of healthy premature babies cannot be due to refractoriness of the sweat gland, but is, at least in part, attributable to immaturity of autonomic centers.

ACKNOWLEDGMENT

Supported by a research grant (MC-R-360049-02-0+1) from the Maternal and Child Health and Crippled Children's Services, U.S. Department of Health, Education and Welfare.

REFERENCES

BEHRENDT, H., and GREEN, M. Drug-induced localized sweating in full-size and low-birth-weight infants. *Amer. J. Diseases Child.* 117: 299–306, 1969.

BEHRENDT, H., and GREEN, M. Nature of the sweating deficit of prematurely born neonates. *New England J. Med.* 286: 1376–1379, 1972.

BRONOW, R.S., DESILETS, D.T., and SONNENSCHEIN, R.R. Influence of environmental and skin temperature on threshold for nicotine axon reflex sweating in human. *Proc. Soc. Exp. Biol. Med.* 97: 272–274, 1958.

COBRINIK, R.W., HOOD, Jr., R.T., and CHUSID, E. The effects of maternal narcotic addiction on the newborn infant. Review of the literature and report of 22 cases. *Pediatrics* 24: 288–304, 1959.

COBRINIK, R.W., HOOD, Jr., R.T., CHUSID, E., and SLOBODY, L.B. The effects of maternal narcotic addiction on the newborn infant. *Amer. Med. Assoc. J. Diseases Child.* 92: 504, 1956.

COHEN, M.I., NATHENSON, G., McNAMARA, H., and LITT, I.F. The mitigating effect of addiction to heroin on neonatal jaundice. Eighty-first Annual Meeting, The American Pediatric Society, April 28 to May 1, 1971.

GLASS, L., RAJEGOWDA, B.K., and EVANS, H.E. Absence of respiratory distress syndrome in premature infants of heroin-addicted mothers. *Lancet* 2: 685–686, 1971.

GOODFRIEND, M.J., SHEY, I.A., and MILTON, D.K. The effects of maternal narcotic addiction on the newborn. *Amer. J. Obstet. Gynec.* 71: 29–36, 1956.

GOODMAN, L.S., and GILMAN, A. *The Physiologic Basis of Therapeutics.* New York: Macmillan, 1967, p. 247.

GREEN, M., and BEHRENDT, H. Sweating capacity of neonates: Nicotine-induced axon reflex sweating and the histamine flare. *Amer. J. Diseases Child.* 118: 725–732, 1969.

GREEN, M., and BEHRENDT, H. Drug-induced localized sweating in neonates: Responses to exogenous and endogenous acetylcholine. *Amer. J. Diseases Child.* 120: 434–438, 1970.

GREEN, M., and BEHRENDT, H. Sweating response of neonates to local thermal stimulation. *Amer. J. Diseases Child.* 125: 20–25, 1973.

OGAWA, T. Local effect of skin temperature on threshold concentration of sudorific agents. *J. Appl. Physiol.* 28: 18–22, 1970.

ROTHMAN, S. *Physiology and Biochemistry of the Skin*. Chicago: Univ. Chicago Press, 1954, p. 165.

WADA, M. Sudorific action of adrenalin on the human sweat glands and determination of their excitability. *Science* 111: 376–377, 1950.

YERBY, A.S. Problems of neonatal narcotic addiction. *New York State J. Med.* 66: 1248–1249, 1966.

ZELSON, C., RUBIO, E., and WASSERMAN, E. Neonatal narcotic addiction: 10 year observation. *Pediatrics*, 48: 178–189, 1971.

The International Journal of the Addictions, 9(4), 503–512, 1974

Asthmador: A Legal Hallucinogen

Keith W. Jacobs

University of Southern Mississippi
Hattiesburg, Mississippi

During the past 10 years scattered reports have reached the medical literature pertaining to the use of Asthmador as a hallucinogenic agent. Historically, the abuse of this compound appears to have been very sporadic with a local "outbreak" of usage in various areas being followed by a period of relatively little publicity given to its effects and abuse potential. A recent local increase in the abuse of this product has prompted closer attention to its availability and its effects.

Asthmador is a nonprescription product available in many pharmacies throughout the country, primarily in the older and low income areas, and by mail from the manufacturer. It is furnished as a relatively inexpensive green powder (costing $1.40 for a 3-oz container) which is intended to be burned with the inhalation of the fumes providing relief from acute asthmatic attacks. It has been manufactured for more than 100 years by the same firm and is apparently a popular asthma medication with older Americans. At the request of the FDA, the manufacturer has placed a label on the container advising pharmacists of its abuse potential and requesting that it not be openly displayed or sold to potential abusers, even though it is an over-the-counter drug. The effectiveness of this voluntary restriction requires that pharmacists and health professionals be informed about this product, and about several similar products which contain the same ingredients.

The OTC forms of Asthmador contain from 0.23 to 0.31% alkaloids of stramonium and belladonna, both of which contain hyoscyamine as the principal alkaloid. The pharmacological properties of the belladonna alkaloids are well documented (see Cutting, 1969; DiPalma, 1971; Goodman and Gillman, 1970; Krantz and Carr, 1965; Solloman and Gill, 1956). Stramonium is the crude drug present in *Datura stramonium* (Jimson weed) and contains atropine (*dl*-hyoscyamine) as the principal alkaloid. Belladonna is the crude drug form of *Atropa belladonna* (deadly nightshade) and contains 1-hyoscyamine as the principal alkaloid. The structure of these alkaloids is presented in Fig. 1. This group of drugs (the belladonna alkaloids) has a very colorful history, including being instilled in the eyes to increase pupil size to make medieval damsels more attractive, and being used by sorcerers to produce hallucinations. Schultes (1969) has suggested that stramonium, which is native to the northeastern United States, may have once been used by the American Indians of the area for its pain relieving properties, presumably by inducing hallucinations. The modern forms of the belladonna alkaloids have a wide range of legitimate medical applications including preanesthetic uses to reduce secretions and relax smooth muscles, to dilate the pupils and reduce visual accommodation for opthalmic examinations, as an adjunct in the treatment of acute diarrheal disease, as antidotes in nerve gas poisoning, and other medical uses, in addition to the asthma relief attributed to Asthmador.

While the intended route of administration of Asthmador is the inhalation of the fumes from burning the product, the abuse pattern appears to be by oral ingestion of the compound, either alone or mixed with beverages such as tea and soft drinks. The medical literature contains several cases of patients hospitalized after consuming from one-half to three teaspoons of Asthmador (Keller and Kane, 1967; Muller, 1967). There apparently have been no cases of Asthmador abuse reported in the last several years. The present cases observed were the result of oral administration of the powder after it had been placed in empty gelatin capsules. This method of administration appears to reduce the gastric upset which follows other methods of oral administration.

The general pattern for Asthmador abuse appears to resemble a "fad" which occurs sporadically in limited geographic areas, rather than as an abuse problem which accelerates in any area with the passage of time. The three cases reported by Muller (1967) were seen in a hospital setting in the course of 3 days and the cases recently observed by this author occurred in a much different nonhospital setting in the course of a week. It is interesting that a similar local outbreak of "accidental" atropine injections was observed by this author in the Army where several soldiers

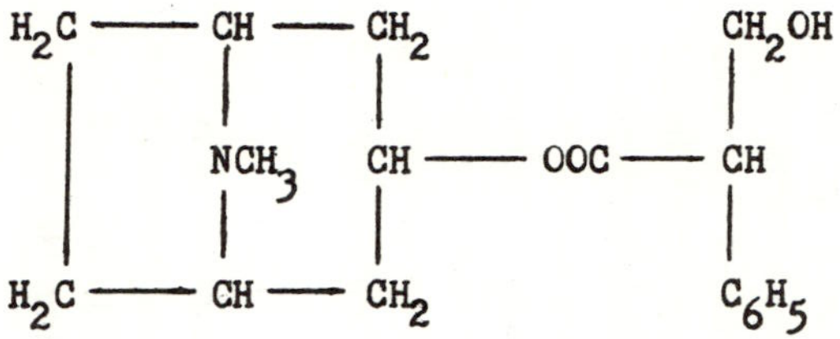

Hyoscyamine

($\underline{l}$-tropyl-tropine)
($C_{17}H_{23}NO_3$)

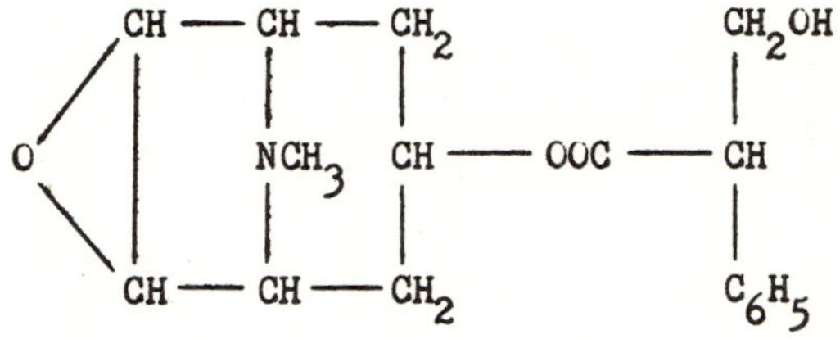

Scopolamine

($\underline{l}$-tropyl-$\underline{a}$-scopine)
($C_{17}H_{21}NO_4$)

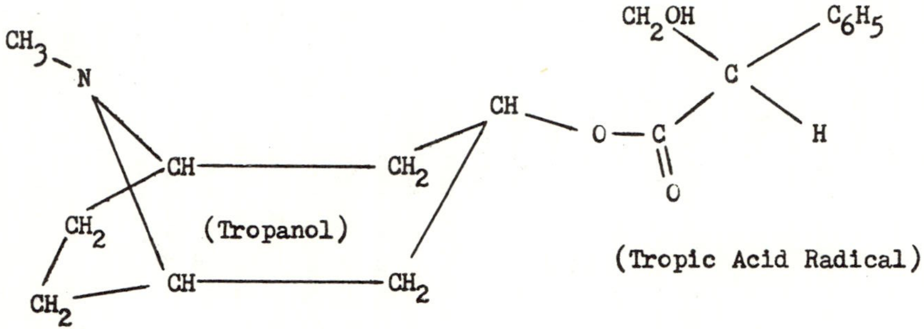

Fig. 1. Structure of active ingredients contained in Asthmador: hyoscyamine and scopolamine. The structure shown for hyoscyamine is identical to the structure of its racemic form *dl*-hyoscyamine (atropine). Racemization occurs in the tropic acid radical on the right.

on guard duty in one unit self-injected themselves with atropine which was provided to them as an emergency antidote for nerve gas poisoning. Due to the adverse effects which accompany the belladonna alkaloids, their abuse is generally self-limiting.

CASES OBSERVED

It recently became possible to observe the local abuse of Asthmador after a group of students contacted the author to discuss the effects of the drug and indicated that they were already experimenting with the product. Relatively unobtrusive observations were made over the course of the following week, and these subjects were later questioned to confirm the observations. Undoubtedly the majority of such Asthmador use is not reported in the literature or well explored since it is not necessarily seen in legal or medical settings. The following observations resulted from this experience as an observer.

The group of users initially consisted of a young married couple and some of their friends, all of whom apparently were experienced and knowledgable in the use of several abuse drugs including marijuana, LSD and other hallucinogens. Several had tried amphetamines and depressants, and none had any experience with the opiates. The age range for the group was estimated to be from 17 to probably the late 20s, and all were either college students or were employed near the college community. The students represented several areas of study, were above average in their grades, and demonstrated attitudes toward drugs which included both concern over the effects and the safety of the drug. The experimentation with Asthmador occurred during a time of increased local law enforcement efforts to control marijuana and other illegal drugs, which had an effect of somewhat decreasing the availability of those drugs. This group of subjects appeared to be experimenting with a group of drugs which was both legal and "organic" (naturally occurring), including such drugs as nutmeg, wild mushrooms, and morning glory seeds, even though the illegal drugs were still available. It was possible to observe five of these subjects during various parts of their Asthmador experience.

One day prior to consulting with this author, one member of the group had experimentally consumed one-quarter of a teaspoon of Asthmador and after several hours, during which no effects were observed, he consumed an additional one-half teaspoon of the product, followed by the effects of a dry mouth, headache, and difficulty in walking. He reported very mild hallucinations and planned at that time to continue to experiment with increased dosages of the drug after a passage of time and in the company of his friends. The headache and dry mouth reportedly persisted for some 12 hr after consuming the drug.

Prior to this author's first appearance with the group, a second member of the group, a male of approximately 150 lb and 21 years, had consumed one and a half teaspoons of Asthmador which he had placed in empty gelatin capsules. During the first hour he reported a dry mouth and began to experience difficulty walking and impairment of voluntary movements. During the next 2 hr he gradually began experiencing visual distortions of reality and was hallucinating real objects which were difficult for him to distinguish from reality. As the "peak experience" approached at 3 to 4 hr, this subject was playing with objects which were not present, talking to persons who were not present, and visually distorting many of the objects which were present. For example, he insisted that the rim of his water glass contained bubbles of melted plastic which came off in his mouth and possessed an odor characteristic of burning plastic; he insisted that small white bugs were present on another person's face and that he was able to pick up these bugs and examine them; and he observed a full-sized automobile drive through a nonexistant crack under a door. It is interesting that he was able to carry on conversations with people who were present, identify them by name, even though he was not fully oriented to time or place. For example, he called his wife by name and told her that he had to pick up his wife at work, but when she explained that she was his wife he decided that he wanted to pick up his other wife who must have the same name. This state lasted for at least 4 hr, during which time the subject was awake, cooperative, and insisted that what he was experiencing was real. He was well oriented to his present surroundings and was able to move from room to room (with some difficulty in walking) to obtain drinks of water, blankets, and other objects he desired.

This subject was next seen at 9 hr after taking the compound and was still experiencing mild visual hallucinations but was able to differentiate them from reality. He was totally oriented to time, place and person. He could not, however, remember many of the events which occurred during the peak experience. After 24 hr this subject was continuing to report headache, lack of appetite, widely dilated pupils, a dry mouth, and blurred vision. At 48 hr after taking the compound his vision had returned to normal but a mild headache persisted. During the questioning, the subject reported that Asthmador produced a more complete break with reality than the other hallucinogenic drugs and that the hallucinations were indistinguishable from reality. In comparison with other hallucinogenic drugs, the Asthmador experience was of longer duration, more intense, and had a marked "hangover" period. He indicated that it would be some time before he tried the product again, if ever.

However, as knowledge of this subject's experience with Asthmador spread among his friends, several individuals not present during his "trip" decided to try the drug. Approximately 48 hr after the first subject tried Asthmador, one of his friends telephoned to say there were several other people at his home who had consumed similar quantities of the drug. The invitation to observe them was accepted and the observations appeared to parallel the earlier observations but with a wider range of individual reactions to the drug. On this occassion, three subjects, a male and two females, had each consumed approximately one and a half teaspoons of the drug and 2 hr after ingesting the drug (the earliest observation made) they were able to relate well to the observer. It should be noted that when they were later questioned they were unaware that the observer had been present. When first seen these subjects all were experiencing dry mouth and skin, widely dilated pupils, and increased pulse rate (pulse rate between 100 and 150). One subject was having difficulty walking, to the extent that he chose to crawl on all fours to the bathroom.

During the peak experience of the drug, the wide variability in effects included one subject withdrawing from the group and apparently falling asleep, another showing fairly mild hallucinogenic effects and generally appropriate behavior, with the third subject reacting to the drug in a fashion that was more exaggerated than the subject observed several days previously. She was the smallest of the subjects and had consumed probably just less than one and a half teaspoons of the drug. She was highly mobile, experiencing difficulty in her overt coordination and frequently bumping into furniture and other people. Her attention span was extremely short, to the extent that when she got up to do something she would look puzzled in a few seconds and not be able to recall what she was going to do. She was verbal but when answering questions only the first sentence of her answer was appropriate, with her word usage becoming unique and the idea being lost. The volume of her voice was considerably reduced. Some of her more meaningful communications were with persons who were not present, and at times she appeared to be carrying on both sides of conversations. Her visual hallucinations could frequently be related to distortions of reality (such as examining a speck of dust and replying to questioning that it was a "four of clubs") or hallucinating objects that were normal parts of her behavior (such as smoking nonexistant cigarettes).

She appeared to be preoccupied with her personal appearance and the application of make-up (spending large amounts of time in front of a mirror applying both real and nonexistant cosmetics). It was interesting that whenever she saw a comb lying on the floor or when handed a comb, she immediately began to comb her hair. On one occasion she exited the bathroom without completely fastening her jeans and with her belt hanging from one belt loop, but for some time she could not percieve anything other than her usual well-kept appearance when told to fasten her jeans. Other inappropriate behavior during this time included attempting to drain the water from a pot of soup on the stove (later being able to recall the experience and reporting that she thought it was a meal she prepared the previous day). Her behavior toward other people was exceptionally polite, excusing herself when she would walk on someone or when she would bump into furniture.

All three of the subjects using the Asthmador on this occasion appeared to be well oriented to their familiar environment, were responsive to questions, appeared to relate fairly well to other persons present at the time and to call them by name, and were capable of following simple directions that did not exceed their attention spans. They were generally unable to differentiate the unreal from the real persons and objects. For these three subjects the "peak experience" was considerably shorter than for the first subject observed, with the complete loss of reality contact lasting only 2 to 3 hr. Mild hallucinogenic effects were still reported at approximately 8 hr after consuming the drug, and the unpleasant side effects (headache, dilated pupils, etc.) persisted for approximately another 18 hr.

SUMMARY

The physical and psychological effects observed in these subjects are reported in Table 1, along with an indication as to the time span associated with the effects. Based on the review of the Asthmador literature and the cases observed, there are several conclusions which can be drawn.

1. The physical effects of Asthmador abuse correspond well with the effects reported in the literature for the belladonna alkaloids and include (generally in the order of appearance): dry mouth, widely dilated pupils, increased heart rate, difficulty in visual accommodation (with the eyes focusing well only at a fixed distance), muscular incoordination and difficulty walking, and headache. The pharmacological literature suggested

Table 1
Physical and Psychological Effects of Asthmador

Effect	Occurence of effect		
	Early	Peak	Late
Dry mouth and skin	×	×	×
Mydriasis (widely dilated pupils)	×	×	×
Tachycardia (increased heart rate)	×	×	
Paralyzed visual accommodation (inability to focus) with accompanying blurred vision	×	×	×
Muscular uncoordination and difficulty walking	×	×	
Headache		×	×
Loss of appetite		×	×
Sedation		?	?
Mild visual hallucinations		×	×
Vivid visual hallucinations indistinguishable from reality		×	
Auditory hallucinations indistinguishable from reality		×	
Disorientation to time		×	
Shortened attention span		×	
Meaningless verbal behavior		×	
Inability to recall experiences during peak experience			×
Inappropriate behavior		×	

that urinary retention might accompany the use of Asthmador, but changes in urinary frequency were not reported. The physical effects may persist for more than the 24-hr period previously reported and include a marked "hangover" effect.

2. The psychological effects of Asthmador occur only during the middle or "peak" period and include: varying degrees of visual and auditory hallucinations which are very vivid and indistinguishable from reality, shortened attention span, a reduction in inhibition, and apparently a personality during this time which closely parallels the person's normal personality. Evidence of partial amnesia for events during the peak experience was observed as was amnesia for the presence of persons who entered during the peak experience. During the peak experience the general behavior pattern quite closely agrees with what would be observed in a schizophrenic reaction, including inappropriate behavior, meaningless verbalization, and hallucinations. This inappropriate behavior requires that the subject be closely observed during the drug experience to prevent

harm to himself and damage to property. The duration and intensity of the psychological and hallucinogenic effects exceeds what is expected with the other hallucinogenic drugs, lasting from 4 to 12 hr.

3. The abuse pattern for Asthmador appears to suggest that it is not a preferred drug for continued use by most individuals who are using hallucinogenic drugs. Even though it is not likely to be repeated by most users, the novelty of the experience contributes greatly to experimental usage by other persons who hear about the drug from their peers. Usage across the country would be expected to be sporadic with a number of persons using the drug in any location within a short period of time. Such usage may frequently not be made public.

4. The intensity and duration of the experience may frighten drug users even though they are experienced with other drugs; quite possibly frightening the observers more than the users. This fright or panic may itself contribute to an acute situation which leads to hospitalization. A contrast between the manic or violent hospitalized patients reported in the literature and the observations made of the five subjects in their homes suggests that the familiarity of surroundings may contribute to the tranquil behavior observed and the pleasant return to normality. It might be suggested that acute Asthmador experiences should be hospitalized only as a medical emergency with "on-site" crisis intervention being preferred for the less severe emergencies.

5. Due to the little attention given to Asthmador in the literature, most physicians have no plan for the treatment of acute Asthmador "poisoning." Of the physicians contacted in this area during the local increase of Asthmador abuse, none had seen any Asthmador patients and most were unaware of its abuse potential. The treatment approach anticipated by most physicians was limited to "observation" of the patient. The medical community needs to recognize the similarity between Asthmador abuse and poisoning from belladonna alkaloids. For medical emergencies a treatment approach similar to atropine overdose would appear to be indicated, to include supportive medical therapy and possibly intervention with a cholinesterase inhibitor (neostigmine or phyostigmine). Krantz and Carr (1965) note that hyoscyamine itself is more potent than atropine or the other cholinergic blocking agents with which physicians may be more familiar. In large dosages the products containing belladonna alkaloids may produce coma, decreased respiration, and death.

6. Considering the intensity and duration of the physical and psychological effects of the drug, there is evidence that Asthmador may

constitute a greater danger to life than the other hallucinogens. Individuals involved in programs of drug education and in acute or crisis treatment must be aware that the effects of Asthmador differ from other hallucinogens and include potentially dangerous effects.

REFERENCES

CUTTING, W.C. *Handbook of Pharmacology*, 4th ed. New York: Appleton-Century-Crofts, 1969.

DiPALMA, J.R. (ed.) *Drill's Pharmacology in Medicine*, 4th ed. New York: McGraw-Hill, 1971.

GOODMAN, L.S., and GILLMAN, A. (eds.) *The Pharmacological Basis of Therapeutics*. New York: Macmillan, 1970.

KELLER, M.H., and KANE, F.J. The use of hyoscyamine as a hallucinogen and intoxicant. *Amer. J. Psychiat.* 124: 852–853, 1967.

KRANTZ, J.C., and CARR, C.J. *The Pharmacologic Principles of Medical Practice.* Baltimore: Williams and Wilkins, 1965.

MULLER, D.J. Unpublicized hallucinogens: The dangerous belladonna alkaloids. *J. Amer. Med. Assoc.* 202: 650–651, 1967.

SCHULTES, R.E. Hallucinogens of plant origin. *Science*, 163: 245–254, 1969.

SOLLOMAN, C., and GILL, E.S. *Pharmacology and Therapeutics.* Philadelphia: Lippincott, 1956.

The International Journal of the Addictions, 9(4), 513–529, 1974

Narcotics-Related Deaths Decrease in 1972 from the Number of Narcotics-Related Deaths in 1971*

William I. Barton, M.A.

Special Action Office for Drug Abuse Prevention
Executive Office of the President
Washington, D.C.

A survey of medical examiners/coroners offices in the United States conducted by the Special Action Office for Drug Abuse Prevention shows that there was a lower number of narcotics-related deaths in 1972 than had occurred the previous year. For 25 areas in the United States, there were 1,853 narcotics-related deaths in 1971; however, there were 1,738 narcotics-related deaths in 1972 for these same areas. This is a decrease of over 6%.

The decrease in narcotics-related deaths in 1972 does not necessarily mean that drug abuse is becoming less of a problem in the United States since this is only one of a number of indicators being studied by the Special Action Office. However, in view of the vast amount of money and manpower being applied to this problem, that less people are dying from narcotics abuse could be interpreted as a positive sign that these applications are paying off.

*Requests for reprints should be sent to the author's present address: Drug Enforcement Administration, Department of Justice, 1405 I Street, N.W., Washington, D.C. 20537.

SURVEY METHODOLOGY

The sampling method used to contact medical examiners/coroners was purposive. Guiding criteria to including an area in the sample were: (1) relatively large population (i.e., over 500,000) and/or (2) estimated sizable drug problem. Other areas were included if, for example, *within* a state the area had a relatively large population (i.e., at least over 100,000). While an attempt is being made to survey at least one area within each state, it is very doubtful that meaningful and reliable data on narcotics-related deaths can be obtained from the areas not yet contacted.

The selection of areas already contacted was greatly influenced by the size of the population in an area because (1) drug abuse is primarily an urban problem, occurring for the most part in the larger cities and counties of the United States, and (2) the medical examiner/coroner system is more highly developed in terms of diagnosing a cause of death in the larger population areas. In the larger areas, for example, it is more likely that the person serving the function of medical examiner/coroner will be a full-time licensed physician and that better toxicological facilities will be available. It is quite possible, for example, that in smaller areas the coroner has no medical training at all and may only function in office part of the time. In some areas the person who serves as coroner also serves other functions as, for instance, justice of the peace. For these smaller areas it was discovered during the course of the survey that not only was there less reliable data, but it was often the case that no statistical tabulation of data had ever been made. In some states, for not a single large city or county contacted was it possible to obtain any kind of statistical data on cases of death coming under purview of the coroner or medical examiner. This does not mean, however, that data on drug-related deaths was necessarily more reliable when gathered from larger population areas or even that it was always possible to collect statistical information of this sort. Rather, the possibility of gathering statistical information which was more or less reliable was greater when larger population areas were contacted. [A breakdown by States shows that eight have statewide, formal medical examiner systems; nine have such systems in most or all of their large jurisdictions; and the remainder have isolated medical examiners or none at all. See "Accident or Murder" in *Med. World News*, 14 (1), 41, 1973.]

The survey was carried out by means of a telephone call to some 45 areas, selected on the basis of the criteria mentioned above. The 25 areas for which there is data on narcotics-related deaths for 1972 represent over one-half of the areas which have been contacted. Telephone data on narcotics-related deaths for each of these areas were confirmed by a written letter from the medical examiners/coroners. The areas for which no data are presented were primarily excluded for at least one of the following reasons: no statistical tabulation of data for the time periods desired; poor reliability of data (as judged by the medical examiner/coroner contacted); relative inefficiency in producing data; data tabulated on a fiscal year basis which was not immediately convertible to a calendar year basis;* a change had occurred from a coroner system to a medical examiner system in mid-1972; toxicological capability had been added in mid-year, which meant that prior cases did not receive an identical amount of analysis in determination of cause of death; the medical examiner/coroner did not keep statistical data at all but rather relied upon vital statistics offices to tabulate the data;† or, for some areas, it was even the case that upon leaving office a medical examiner or coroner was reluctant to have the incoming official view the prior case records. In some areas, while statistical data was kept, data was not immediately available on the number of drug-related deaths (much less narcotics-related overdose deaths) as apart from other types of deaths. In order to minimize expended effort on the part of the officials contacted in the survey, if the desired data was not immediately available or could not be obtained with little effort, a request was not made for this information at this time.

It is apparent that there are more than a minimum of restrictions to obtaining statistical data on narcotics-related deaths from medical examiners/coroners. At the present time, no truly national statistics are available nor has a sampling plan been effected which would allow for national estimates to be made with little variance. Nonetheless, this aggregate decrease in narcotics-related deaths for these 25 areas can probably be interpreted as applying nationwide. The raison d'être is that included in the 25 areas are those cities or counties in which it is believed most of the nation's drug abuse problem is located. For example, in-

* Such was the case for Los Angeles County which only began tabulating data so that it could be shown on a calendar year basis in 1972.

† Cause of death data as tabulated by vital statistics offices is not comparable with data tabulated directly from medical examiners/coroners case records. Vital statistics data differ from case record data since vital statistics data on cause of death are tabulated according to the World Health Organization's *International Classification of Diseases.* See W. I. Barton, "Drug-Related Mortality in the United States, 1963–71" (unpublished paper done for Special Action Office for Drug Abuse Prevention).

cluded among the 25 areas are New York City; Philadelphia; Washington, D.C.; Dade County (Miami); Cook County (Chicago); Essex County (Newark); Cuyahoga County (Cleveland); Dallas County (Dallas); Harris County (Houston); and San Francisco County. The 25 areas included in this paper accounted for 21% of the continental United States population in 1970.

That the data shown in this paper refer to narcotics-related deaths, and not all drug-related deaths, is an example of an additional restriction levied upon the data collector. Prior research into the type of data on drug-related deaths that was generally available from medical examiner/coroners offices brought forth the finding that in terms of drug-related deaths, it was most likely that statistics were kept on narcotics-related deaths ("overdoses"),* rather than on all types of drug-related deaths. In most cases the data shown here refer to narcotics-related "overdose" deaths since this was the type of information asked for in the telephone survey. In most cases the data refer to *accidental* narcotics-related "overdose" deaths involving heroin and/or methadone. If a medical examiner/coroner did not actually state this, it is nonetheless felt that there are few persons who intentionally commit suicide through the use of narcotics. In some cases the data shown in this paper include, in addition to "overdose" cases, cases of death due to "narcotic addiction"—however it is defined by the medical examiner/coroner collecting the data. It is assumed that homicide cases in which narcotics are found in the body of the deceased are not included in these data. Since some medical examiners/coroners find it a difficult task to determine whether the narcotics-related death was an accident or suicide, the statistical category into which they classify the death is "narcotics-related death, with undetermined reason."

Thus, while the sampling units included in this paper did not allow for collection of data under a standardized and agreed-upon definition, for each data source the deaths were related to narcotics use. For all data sources taken individually the definition under which the data was gathered remained the same for each year. Since "different" data were not gathered from the same source for the period of time under consideration, it is possible to aggregate the information obtained from each source for a particular point or interval in time and make a comparison with data

* The term "overdose death" is used in quotation marks in this paper to indicate that attributing a death to an "overdose of heroin" is a controversial matter—not agreed upon by all medical sources. In Philadelphia and New York, for example, the term "adverse reaction" is used, rather than "overdose." See Edward M. Brecher, *Licit and Illicit Drugs*, Boston: Little, Brown, 1972, pp. 101–114.

aggregated from the same source for another point or interval in time. It is the findings of just such a comparison of data that are reported here.

FINDINGS

Table 1 shows the number of narcotics-related deaths for 1971 and for 1972 for 25 areas in the United States.

As shown in this table, for 1971 there was a total of 1,853 narcotics-related deaths occurring in the 25 areas. For the same areas, there were 1,738 narcotics-related deaths in 1972—a decrease of over 6%.

Although not all areas within a region were contacted (nor, if they were contacted, would data necessarily be available), it is nonetheless possible to classify each area contacted into one of the four regions of the country to gain some insight as to what might be occurring on a regional basis. As Fig. 1 shows, the decrease occurred for three of the four regions of the country. The decrease was greatest in the North Central region (a 31% decrease) and least in the Northeast (a 4% decrease). In the West there was about a 23% increase in narcotics-related deaths.

On a statewide basis, there were only two states contacted which had statewide medical examiner systems and which were not excluded for one of the reasons mentioned at the beginning of this paper. These states were Maryland and North Carolina. In Maryland there occurred a 26% decrease in narcotics-related "overdose" deaths (heroin/morphine, methadone) in 1972. In North Carolina the number of narcotics-related "overdoses" (heroin and/or methadone) was slightly more in 1972 than in 1971 (18 deaths in 1972 compared to 15 in 1971).

Although a statewide trend cannot be arrived at, for not one of the three areas contacted in Texas was there a decrease in narcotics-related "overdose" deaths in 1972. For Harris County there was about a 94% increase in narcotics-related "overdoses" in 1972 over the previous year, for Dallas County there was a 67% increase in heroin and/or methadone "overdose" deaths in 1972, and in Bexar County there occurred a 34% increase in narcotics-related "overdoses." The three areas contacted in Texas accounted for about 35% of the population residing in Texas in 1970.

On a county basis, the largest county contacted was Cook County (Chicago), Illinois. In 1970 there were an estimated 5.492 million persons residing within this county. In 1971 there were 190 narcotics-related "overdoses" in Cook County. In 1972 there were 137 narcotics-related "overdoses," a decrease of about 28%.

Table 1
Number of Narcotics-Related Deaths According to Selected Areas in the United States by Year of Death

Area	1970 Population	Calendar year 1971	Calendar year 1972	Cause of death
Arizona				
Maricopa County (Phoenix)	967,522	9	11	Heroin (morphine) and/or methadone "overdoses"
California				
Sacramento County	634,190	5	7	Heroin and/or methadone "overdoses"
San Diego County	1,357,854	29	46	Narcotics-related deaths
San Francisco County	715,674	56	65	Narcotics-related "overdoses"
Colorado				
Denver County	514,678	12	7	Heroin and/or methadone "overdoses"
District of Columbia	756,510	82	71	Narcotics-related "overdoses"
Florida				
Dade County (Miami)	1,267,792	35	26	Narcotics-related "overdoses" (heroin/morphine, methadone, opiate NEC)
Georgia				
Fulton County (Atlanta)	607,592	18	14	Narcotism deaths
Illinois				
Cook County (Chicago)	5,492,369	190	137	Narcotics-related "overdoses"
Indiana				
Marion County (Indianapolis)	792,299	19	11	Narcotics-related "overdoses"
Louisiana New Orleans (Orleans Parish)	593,471	25	16	Narcotism (narcotism nec and "overdoses")
Maryland (State of)	3,922,399	105	78	Narcotics-related "overdoses" (Heroin/morphine, methadone)
New Jersey				
Essex County (Newark)	932,526	53	25	Narcotic-addiction deaths
New York				
New York City	7,894,862	916	942	Deaths "directly" due to narcotic addiction

(continued)

Table 1 (continued)

Area	1970 Population	Calender year 1971	1972	Cause of death
Erie County (Buffalo)	1,113,491	15	10	Heroin (morphine) and/or methadone "overdoses"
Monroe County (Rochester)	711,917	11	11	Narcotics-related deaths
North Carolina (State of)	5,082,059	15	18	Heroin (morphine and/or methadone "overdoses"
Ohio				
Cuyahoga County (Cleveland)	1,720,835	25	22	Narcotics-related "overdoses"
Hamilton County (Cincinnati)	924,018	13	4	Heroin and/or methadone "overdoses"
Lucas County (Toledo)	483,594	4	0	Accidental poisonings (heroin)
Pennsylvania				
Philadelphia City and County	1,949,896	100	113	Adverse reactions (narcotics)
Allegheny County (Pittsburgh)	1,605,133	61	15	Narcotics-related "overdoses"
Texas				
Bexar County (San Antonio)	830,460	21	28	Narcotics-related "overdoses"
Dallas County (Dallas)	1,327,695	18	30	Heroin and/or methadone "overdoses"
Harris County (Houston)	1,741,912	16	31	Narcotics-related "overdoses"
TOTAL		1,853	1,738	

Three other large counties contacted were Cuyahoga County (Cleveland), Ohio; Allegheny County (Pittsburgh), Pennsylvania; and Harris County (Houston), Texas.

For Cuyahoga County, Ohio (1970 population: 1.721 million persons) there were 25 narcotics-related "overdoses" in 1971. There were 22 narcotics-related "overdoses" in all of 1972, a 12% decrease.

For Allegheny County, Pennsylvania (1970 population: 1.605 million persons) there were 61 narcotics-related "overdose" deaths in 1971. There

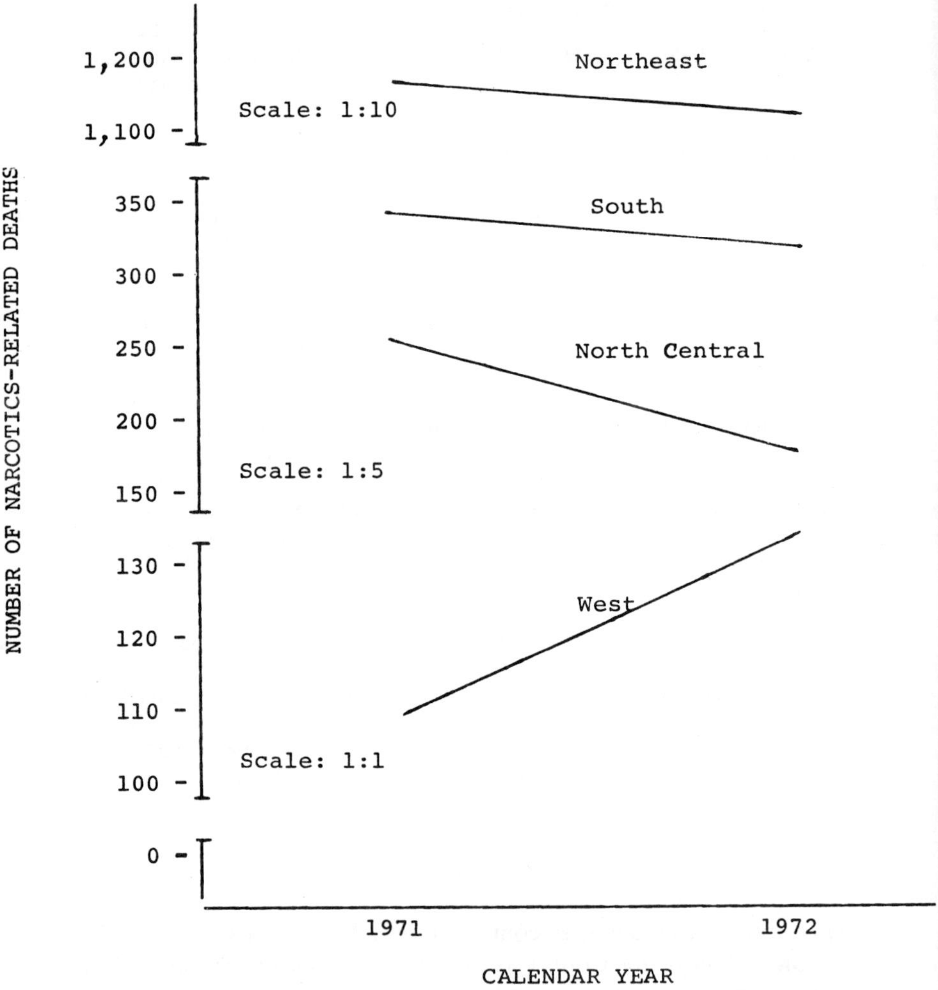

Fig. 1. Number of narcotics-related deaths in selected areas of the United States, 1971–1972.

were only 15 narcotics-related "overdose" deaths in 1972, an amazing decrease of 75%.

The decreases in narcotics-related deaths for the above two counties are contrasted with the increase which occurred within Harris County, Texas (1970 population: 1.742 million persons). The number of narcotics-related "overdose" deaths occurring in 1971 for this county was 16. A year later, there were 31 narcotics-related "overdose" deaths, an increase of 94%.

On a city basis it is obvious that New York City (1970 population: 7.896 million persons) was the largest city contacted. New York City also accounted for close to one-half of the deaths occurring in the 25 areas in 1971 and for about 54% of the narcotics-related deaths in 1972 in these same areas.

In New York City there occurred in 1972 some 942 deaths "directly" due to narcotic addiction. This is about a 3% increase from the previous year. For New York City, deaths "directly" due to narcotic addiction refer to deaths from infections as well as adverse reactions. Figure 2 shows deaths "directly" due to narcotic addiction, subclassified by these two categories for 1969–1972.

Another city contacted was the District of Columbia, which had about 757 thousand persons in 1970, where 82 narcotics-related "overdose" deaths occurred in 1971 compared to 71 in 1972, a decrease of about 13%.

The Period 1970–1972

For 19 of the 25 areas having data presented in this paper, it was possible to obtain data for the entire period 1970–1972.* Thus, six of the original 25 areas were rejected for this period of time because of one of the reasons mentioned at the beginning of this paper.

Table 2 shows narcotics-related deaths for these 19 areas for this period of time. As can be seen in this table, there were 1,433 narcotics-related deaths for these areas in 1970; 1,573 narcotics-related deaths in 1971; and 1,454 narcotics-related deaths in 1972. Thus, there was a 10% increase in narcotics-related deaths for these areas between 1970 and 1971, countered by an 8% decrease in such deaths between 1971 and 1972.

Of the seven areas shown in Table 2 having more narcotics-related deaths in 1972 than in 1971, for three of these areas the increase in deaths

* In Table 1, data for Maryland pertain to the entire state. In Table 2, data pertain to Baltimore City only. This was in accordance with using data *available* in the Office of the Chief Medical Examiner in Maryland.

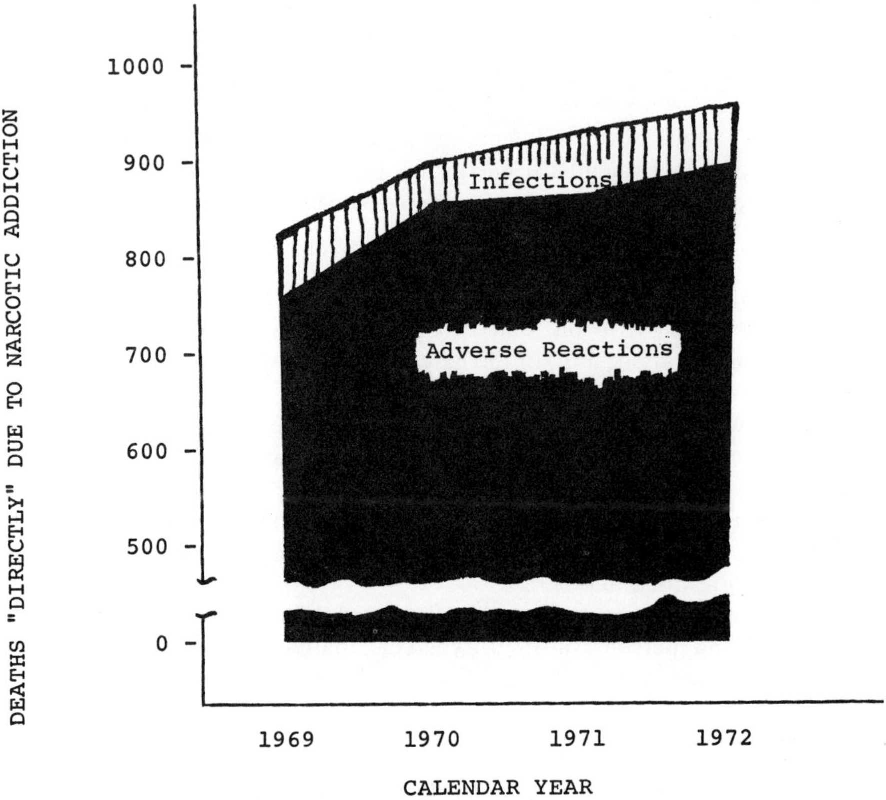

Fig. 2. Deaths "directly" due to narcotic addiction according to cause of death in New York City, 1969–1972.

represents only another point in a continuum—that is, for these areas there was also an increase in narcotics-related deaths occurring in 1971 over the number occurring in 1970.

For seven of the 11 areas showing a decrease in narcotics-related deaths in 1972 from 1971, the downturn represents a reversal of events occurring between 1970 and 1971.

The Period 1969–1972

Four of the 19 areas which are shown in Table 2 were rejected for the period 1969–1972 because of one of the reasons mentioned at the begin-

Table 2
Number of Narcotics-Related Deaths According to Selected Areas in the United States by Year of Death

Area	1970 Population	Calendar year 1970	1971	1972	Cause of death
Arizona					
Maricopa County (Phoenix)	967,522	9	9	11	Heroin (morphine) and/or methadone "overdoses"
California					
Sacramento County	634,190	8	5	7	Heroin and/or methadone "overdoses"
San Francisco County	715,674	56	56	65	Narcotics-related "overdoses"
Florida					
Dade County (Miami)	1,267,792	31	35	26	Narcotics-related "overdoses" (heroin/morphine, methadone, and opiate nec)
Illinois					
Cook County (Chicago)	5,492,369	142	190	137	Narcotics-related "overdoses"
Indiana					
Marion County (Indianapolis)	792,299	20	19	11	Narcotics-related "overdoses"
Louisiana					
New Orleans (Orleans Parish)	593,471	41	25	16	Narcotism (narcotism nec and "overdoses")
Maryland					
Baltimore City	905,759	53	81	55	Narcotics-related "overdoses" (heroin/morphine, methadone)
New Jersey					
Essex County (Newark)	932,526	42	53	25	Narcotic-addiction deaths
New York					
New York City	7,894,862	893	916	942	Deaths "directly" due to narcotic addiction
Monroe County (Rochester)	711,917	9	11	11	Narcotics-related deaths
North Carolina (State of)	5,082,059	24	15	18	Heroin (morphine) and/or methadone "overdoses"
Ohio					
Cuyahoga County (Cleveland)	1,720,835	21	25	22	Narcotics-related "overdoses"
Hamilton County (Cincinnati)	924,018	13	13	4	Heroin and/or methadone "overdoses"

(continued)

Table 2 (continued)

Area	1970 Population	Calender year 1970	1971	1972	Cause of death
Lucas County (Toledo)	483,594	0	4	0	Accidental poisonings (heroin)
Pennsylvania					
Allegheny County (Pittsburgh)	1,605,133	27	61	15	Narcotics-related "over-doses"
Texas					
Bexar County (San Antonio)	830,460	13	21	28	Narcotics-related "over-doses"
Dallas County (Dallas)	1,327,695	12	18	30	Heroin and/or methadone "overdoses"
Harris County (Houston)	1,741,912	19	16	31	Narcotics-related "over-doses"
TOTAL		1,433	1,573	1,454	

Table 3

Number of Narcotics-Related Deaths According to Selected Areas in the United States by Year of Death

Area	1970 Population	Calendar year 1969	1970	1971	1972	Cause of death
Arizona						
Maricopa County (Pheonix)	967,522	3	9	9	11	Heroin (morphine) and/or methadone "overdoses"
California						
Sacramento County	634,190	3	8	5	7	Heroin and/or methadone "overdoses"
San Francisco County	715,674	40	56	56	65	Narcotics-related "overdoses"
Florida						
Dade County (Miami)	1,267,792	22	31	35	26	Narcotics-related "overdoses" (heroin/morphine, methadone, opiate nec)
Indiana						
Marion County (Indianapolis)	792,299	8	20	19	11	Narcotics-related "overdoses"

(*continued*)

Table 3 (continued)

Area	1970 Population	Calender year 1969	1970	1971	1972	Cause of death
Louisiana						
New Orleans (Orleans Parish)	593,471	36	41	25	16	Narcotism (narcotism nec and "overdoses")
New Jersey						
Essex County (Newark)	932,526	37	42	53	25	Narcotic-addiction deaths
New York						
New York City	7,894,862	817	893	916	942	Deaths "directly" due to narcotic addiction
Monroe County (Rochester)	711,917	4	9	11	11	Narcotics-related deaths
Ohio						
Cuyahoga County (Cleveland)	1,720,835	12	21	25	22	Narcotics-related "overdoses"
Hamilton County (Cincinnati)	924,018	3	13	13	4	Heroin and/or methadone "overdoses"
Lucas County (Toledo)	483,594	1	0	4	0	Accidental poisonings (heroin)
Pennsylvania						
Allegheny County (Pittsburgh)	1,605,133	17	27	61	15	Narcotics-related "overdoses"
Texas						
Bexar County (San Antonio)	830,460	4	13	21	28	Narcotics-related "overdoses"
Harris County (Houston)	1,741,912	6	19	16	31	Narcotics-related "overdoses"
TOTAL		1,013	1,202	1,269	1,214	

ning of this paper. This left 15 areas for which data could be studied for the period 1969–1972.

Table 3 shows that the total number of narcotics-related deaths for these 15 areas in 1969 was 1,013; in 1970 the number was 1,202; in 1971 the number was 1,269; and there were 1,214 narcotics-related deaths in 1972. Thus there occurred a 19% increase in narcotics-related deaths between 1969 and 1970 and another 6% increase between 1970 and 1971. These increases were countered by a 4% decrease in narcotics-related deaths between 1971 and 1972.

DISCUSSION

It is important to look at not only a decrease or increase in narcotics-related deaths when comparing two or more time periods, but also the rate of increase or decrease in narcotics-related deaths. Thus, for example, if these 25 areas were to show an increase in the number of narcotics-related deaths in 1972 over the number occurring in 1971, but the rate of increase was less than had occurred when comparing two time periods in the past, this would also be a significant development—depending on the degree to which the rate had declined. In this paper it is possible to obtain information of this sort for 19 areas (if one wishes to compare the time period 1970–1971 with 1971–1972) or for 15 areas (if one wishes to compare the time periods 1969–1970, 1970–1971, and 1971–1972).

By comparing the period 1970–1971 with the period 1971–1972 it can be seen that there was a 10% increase in narcotics-related deaths between 1970–1971 for the 19 areas so included. In order to bring about an identical 10% increase in narcotics-related deaths for these same areas in 1972, there would have had to occur around 1,731 narcotics-related deaths. As can be seen in Table 2, however, rather than there being an identical increase in narcotics-related deaths for 1971–1972 as had occurred for 1970–1971, there was in fact an 8% decrease—bringing the number of narcotics-related deaths in 1972 almost down to the 1970 level. It can be assumed that this drop in deaths is somewhat significant.

There was a 19% increase in narcotics-related deaths for the 15 areas between 1969 and 1970. For these same areas, there was only a 6% increase in narcotics-related deaths in 1971 compared to 1970. Since there appeared to be a declining rate of increase in narcotics-related deaths for these 15 areas, it would be expected that, if one assumes the decline in the rate of increase in narcotics-related deaths occurs in a hyperbolic manner,* there would be 1,300 narcotics-related deaths in 1972. The 1,214 narcotics-related deaths which actually occurred in 1972 thus represent 7% fewer deaths than might be expected to occur.

Figure 3 shows narcotics-related deaths for the areas discussed in this paper according to the three time periods for which data were available.

By looking at Table 1 in which a comparison is made between two

* Data for 1969, 1970, and 1971 were used to estimate the number of expected narcotics-related deaths in 1972. The method of estimation was curve fitting. The curve $[y = A + (B/X)]$ had a standard error of estimate of 2.35339. This curve is a hyperbolic function and was one of two curves found to be best fitted for these data.

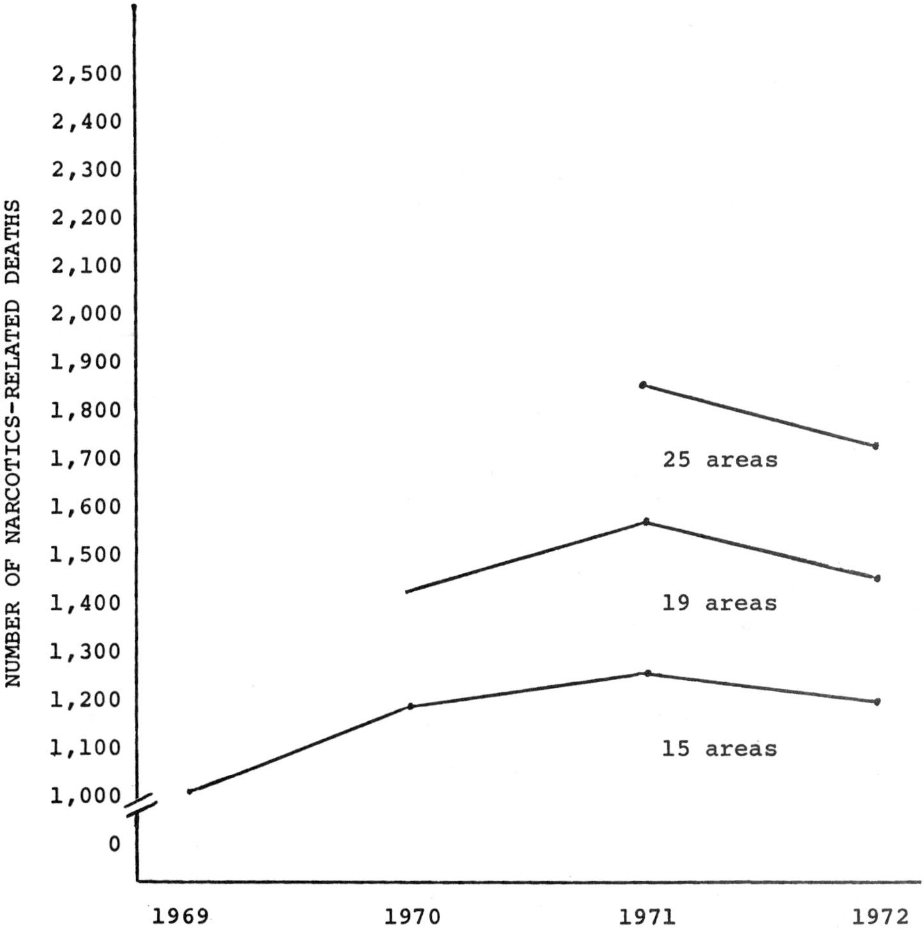

Fig. 3. Number of narcotics-related deaths in selected areas of the United States, 1969–1972. Source of data: SAODAP survey of medical examiners/coroners.

time periods for at least 25 areas in the country, it is possible to arrive at the interpretation that some *x* factor or factors were responsible for bringing about the decrease in the number of narcotics-related deaths. Speculation about the responsible factors leads to the following: (1) increase in the number of clients in treatment programs, (2) increased efforts on the part of law enforcement officials to "reduce the flow" of narcotics in the United States, and (3) increased effectiveness of prevention materials and efforts—materials and efforts which warn of the dangers of misuse of drugs. This is certainly not the total sum of factors which could be responsible for bringing about a decrease in narcotics-related deaths in 1972—indeed, there is probably a myriad of factors which could be utilized. Whatever factor or factors are responsible for bringing about the decline in narcotics-related deaths in 1972, the occurrence is a "welcome" indication that America's "Public Enemy Number 1" may be weakening.

This interpretation is somewhat diluted by the increase in narcotics-related deaths which occurred in some areas in Texas and California as well as in New York City and Philadelphia. For these areas, it is possible that only a small proportion of the drug-dependent population is enrolled in treatment programs, or that while more than a small proportion may be so enrolled, the programs are not always effective in curbing drug misuse;* or it may be that the supply of narcotics in these areas, particularly California and Texas, is greater now than in the past. It additionally may be that prevention efforts are not especially effective in these areas, or are overcome by such factors as more permissive lifestyle, relative poverty and deprivation, or lack of employment opportunities.

CONCLUSION

This is merely a formative paper on the subject of narcotics-related deaths. To date, while there have been quite a few papers written on the subject from a case-study viewpoint, there have not been as many papers as might be expected from a statistical stance—particularly in terms of

*It is also possible that it takes longer for the effects of adequate treatment programs to show beneficial results in larger population areas. The effect of treatment efforts in New York City and in other large metropolitan areas established in 1972 may not be readily apparent until about mid- or late 1973. This interpretation employs the "push-pull" theory of personality. In larger metropolitan areas, due to a number of factors, addicts may be "pushed" into seeking treatment; however, a host of negative influences may be exercising even greater "pull."

gathering data from more than one city or county. Probably one reason for this is that there are varying degrees of reliability and validity of data for the areas involved. This is not just between areas, but also within areas. Whenever there is a changeover from a coroner system to a medical system; when one medical examiner leaves and is replaced by another; when additional toxicological equipment is brought to bear on the diagnosis of cause of death; or when more cases are given toxicological analysis one year than the previous year, the resulting statistics on deaths by cause may be more reflective of these occurrences than of differences in the occurrence of events over time. Hopefully, by aggregating the data received from the 25 areas, the influence of some of these biases is cancelled out.

The 25 areas selected for inclusion in this paper were chosen from 45 areas which were contacted. These 25 areas were chosen because they did not satisfy the criteria established for exclusion. This may be a rather negative manner by which to select sample units; however, the establishment of rigid positive criteria for inclusion would have resulted in only a small number of the areas being so included.

The data shown for the 25 areas in this paper are exactly the data being reported by each area individually. There thus should be no difference between the reporting of narcotics-related deaths shown in this paper and the reporting of such deaths within a particular community.

In conclusion, as shown in this paper, for these 25 areas there occurred over a 6% decrease in narcotics-related deaths when data from all areas were aggregated. It is felt that, as far as indications of the seriousness of the drug problem go, this may be one of the more "firm" indications to date that efforts on the part of federal, state, and local governments—not to mention private individuals and organizations—to control and reduce the drug abuse problem may be working.

The International Journal of the Addictions, 9(4), 531–540, 1974

Drug Use and Social Integration

Jens J. B. Winsløw

Bronchitis Screening Center
Aalborg, Denmark

In earlier papers the author, among others, has attempted to view the increasing nonmedical use of various drugs from a diffusion theory point of view, with reasonable empirical success. It has been repeatedly found that young drug users resemble other groups of innovators or introducers on variables such as sex, socioeconomic background, educational level, and self-reported level of interaction in peer groups of many kinds (Ulff-Møller, 1971; Winsløw, 1972, 1972b). It has also been repeatedly demonstrated that the recent diffusion of cannabis use has followed a more or less S-shaped cummulative curve, while both the time of the onset of the diffusion process and its speed have been seen to be dependent upon the level of urbanization of the community in which the spread took place (Holstein in Winsløw, 1972c).

Another guiding approach for the empirical study of drug use in recent years has been the subculture theory in its Beckerian form (Becker, 1963; Ulff-Møller et al., 1971; Ulff-Møller and Jørgensen, 1971). While this approach appears to have met with less clear empirical success than the diffusion approach, it has the advantage of explaining the generalizations which it has given rise to—i.e., it is a "theory"—which is more than can be said about the many and varied hypotheses that make up what is called the "diffusion approach" above.

The purpose of this paper is to present data from a study which rejects two hypotheses; one from the diffusion approach, the other from the subculture theory. This study is a direct continuation of the results published earlier (Winsløw, 1972).

The diffusion hypothesis may be stated as follows: (1) Hash users, being innovators or introducers of a new mode of recreation into their social environments, are better integrated in their school classes than their noninnovating peers (cf. Coleman, Katz and Menzel, 1966; Rogers, 1962), while the subculture hypothesis may be formulated as (2) hash users, engaging in recreational activities that are regarded as deviant by the majority of their immediate peers, tend to form subgroups within their school classes.

In the section to follow, the procedure adopted in connection with the study mentioned above is described while the subsequent section contains the results relevant to the two hypotheses.

METHOD

The data stem from a questionnaire administered among students in their ninth school year in the municipal schools of Hjørring, Denmark, conducted between the 22nd and 24th of February 1972. The sample comprised all the students present in school from 14 of the 18 classes of students in their ninth year in the nine schools of the municipality. The four classes not included in the study were left out for practical reasons (vide infra). The sample thus consisted of 251 students, which corresponded to 92% of the students enrolled in these 14 classes.

The questionaire consisted of 23 questions on:

(1) The students' own use of hash, amphetamines, opiates, and "strong" hallucinogenes (LSD, STP and mescalin).

(2) The students' sex, department in school, age, and filing number.

(3) Their interest in the establishment of a municipal counseling center for the young.

(4) Their participation in youth club, sports, and night school activities during the first 7 weeks of 1972.

(5) Their objective as well as subjective integration in their classes.

Of these 23 items, only four questions concerning hash use and sociometric integration will be utilized in this paper. For a translation of these questions, see the Appendix.

The fact that the distribution of answers to questions such as (3) above appears to be influenced by whether or not drug questions occur in the same questionnaire will not be given attention here, although it is feasible that an interference from counseling questions to the distribution of answers to drug use questions might exist as well (Winsløw, 1972a). Unfortunately, neither the present inquiry, nor any other study known by the author, has yielded any hard and fast answer to this question.

The study was arranged by the author with the assistance of the municipal school authorities of Hjørring, who selected a teacher in one of the schools to act as the local administrator of the study. The questionnaires were completed by the students themselves. This was accomplished as follows: The class that was to fill out the questionnaires was assembled in the school's gymnasium during an ordinary teaching period. Each student was seated at a table at such a distance from all other students that he or she could fill out the questionnaire in full privacy. In all classes the questionnaires were administered by the same teacher, who also took care of the formal introduction of the study to the respondents. These were told:

(1) That participation in the study was voluntary.

(2) What measures had been taken to safeguard the anonymity of their answers.

(3) That the purpose of the study was "scientific."

Apart from the survey administrator, the only other school official present during the administration of the questionnaires was the school principal. He had been previously instructed to:

(1) Provide the administrator with a list of those students in the class who were to be surveyed (i.e., those present in the school on the day of the study), giving information about each student's filing number, sex, age and recent grades in different subjects, as well as the number of days each student had been absent from school during the academic year 1971–1972 up to the day of the study. (This list did not contain the names of the students in the class, and was not to be handed over to the administrator until the questionnaires had been collected).

(2) Issue the students with lists of their names and filing numbers. These lists were to be used by the students in answering the sociometric questions, and were to be destroyed by the students themselves after they had returned the questionnaires.

During the half-hour allotted for the completion of the questionnaires in each class, the survey administrator and the school principal were to remain in the corner of the gymnasium farthest from the students.

As mentioned above, only 14 out of the 18 classes in the cohort were included in the study, the reason for this being that in two out of the nine schools there were more than two classes of students in their ninth year, while two was the maximum number of classes that could be handled by one administrator within one ordinary period. The four classes to be left out were chosen at random from the two large schools by the author.

On three questions it was possible to compare the students' answers with information from the school, viz., sex, age and department. The "reliability index" on no variable was less than .96, with no response from a student counted as an inconsistency. No questionnaire was completely blank, but one person had not given his filing number, while another had given a "wrong" one. Both these errors were corrected by comparing the two students' sex-age-department answers with the schools' lists of students. As the question of the reliability of drug studies of this kind is more problematic than students of the subject generally acknowledge (see, for instance, Parry et al., 1971), it is left to the reader to make whatever inference concerning the validity of the data presented below he or she feels justified in making from the information supplied above.

The sociometric data presented in the next section are based on the relative status on each of the three dimensions "interaction," "best like," and "leadership" as measured by the three questions translated in the Appendix. Relative status has been used instead of raw scores because the 14 classes varied in size from 6 to 25 students, which meant that the number of classmates a student could choose, or could be chosen by, varied from 5 to 24. On the "interaction" and "best like" dimensions, each student's raw scores were divided by the average raw score of his class, so that "average status" in the following is always about 1.00. On the "leadership" dimension, where each student was asked to name at most two of his classmates, the relative status of each student is expressed as the percentage of the total number of choices given in his class that he or she received.

RESULTS

In Tables 1–3 the results relevant to the diffusion hypothesis are set out. The base numbers have been subjected to the chi-square test with the categories "hash triers" and "hash users" collapsed into one, while the means presented in Tables 1 and 2 have been subjected to analyses of variance. The significance level is .05, except where otherwise is stated.

Table 1
Hash Use by Relative Status on the "Interaction Dimension (see Appendix)[a]

Status group	Never tried hash %	Never tried hash n	Hash triers %	Hash triers n	Hash users %	Hash users n	Total %	Total n
No mutually reported interactions with classmates	84	91	7	7	9	10	100	108
One or more, but fewer mutually reported interactions with classmates than the class average	90	27	7	2	3	1	100	30
More mutually reported interractions with classmates than average in the class	76	81	15	16	9	10	100	107
ALL	81	199	10	25	9	21	100	245
Mean relative status on the "interaction" dimension	0.93		1.45		1.12		1.00	

[a] One of the fourteen classes was excluded from this analysis due to lack of mutually reported interactions.

Table 2
Hash Use by Relative Status on the "Like Best" Dimension (see Appendix)

Status group	Never tried hash %	Never tried hash n	Hash triers %	Hash triers n	Hash users %	Hash users n	Total %	Total n
No reciprocal choices on this dimension	82	23	18	5	0	—	100	28
One or more, but fewer reciprocal choices on this dimension than class average	83	91	8	9	9	10	100	110
More reciprocal choices on this dimension than class average	80	90	10	11	11	12	101	113
ALL	81	204	10	25	9	22	100	251
Mean relative status on "like best" dimension	0.99		0.86		1.28		1.00	

Table 3
Hash Use by Relative Status on the "Leadership" Dimension (see Appendix)

	Never tried hash		Hash triers		Hash users		Total	
Status group	%	*n*	%	*n*	%	*n*	%	*n*
Isolates	88	128	6	9	6	9	100	146
Nonisolates	72	76	16	16	12	13	100	105
ALL	81	204	10	25	9	22	100	251
Mean percent of the choices given in each class received by those who received one or more choices on this dimension (i.e., nonisolates)	13.8		11.5		14.6			

From Table 1 it can be seen that the hash triers and users do not differ significantly from those who have not tried hash with respect to their relative sociometric status on the "interaction" dimension. The data presented in the table are only those for mutually reported interactions, but the picture was the same for all interactions reported, whether mutually reported or not.

In Table 2 the corresponding data for the "like best" dimension are given. Also on this dimension there was no significant difference between hash triers and those who had not tried hash. As on the "interaction" dimension, there was no appreciable difference between the reciprocal results and the results for all choices given and received.

In Table 3, however, there can be seen a significantly higher proportion of hash triers and users among those receiving one or more choices on the "leadership" dimension than among the "isolates"; i.e., those receiving no choices on this dimension. The difference is significant ($p < .01$). But when the analysis is confined to the "nonisolates," it turns out that there is no statistically significant difference in the mean percentage of the choices given in a class which individual students received between hash triers and users on one hand and those who had not tried hash on the other.

Summing up Tables 1–3, the data, with one exception, reject the diffusion hypothesis stated in the introductory section.

The results pertaining to the subculture hypothesis are seen in Tables 4 and 5. These may be summed up as follows:

Table 4

Mutually Reported Interactions between Hash Users, Hash Triers, and Others During the Three Days Preceding the Survey[a]

Of the mutually reported interactions reported by	% Involved							
	Nontriers		Triers		Users		Total	
	%	*n*	%	*n*	%	*n*	%	*n*
Nontriers	73	72	10	10	17	17	100	99
Triers	63	10	0	—	37	6	100	16
Users	59	17	21	6	21	6	101	29
ALL	69	99	11	16	20	29	100	144

[a] Only five of the original 14 classes were included in this analysis. In the nine remaining classes, there were no possibilities for interactions between users and triers.

Table 5

Choices on the "Like Best" Dimension Given by Hash Users, Hash Triers, and Nontriers to Hash Users, Hash Triers, and Nontriers, Respectively[a]

Of the choices given by	% Went to							
	Nontriers		Triers		Users		Total	
	%	*n*	%	*n*	%	*n*	%	*n*
Nontriers	72	350	13	64	15	73	100	487
Triers	62	34	18	10	20	11	100	55
Users	75	79	14	15	11	12	100	106
ALL	71	463	14	89	15	96	100	648

[a] Only five of the original 14 classes were included in this analysis. In the nine remaining classes, there were no possibilities of choices between users and triers.

(1) Hash users did not choose, and were not chosen, disproportionately by other categories in the material on the "interaction" dimension.

(2) Hash users did not choose, and were not chosen, disproportionately by other categories in the material on the "like best" dimension.

The evidence of relevance to the subculture hypothesis is less satisfactory than the evidence available in connection with the diffusion hypothesis. In Tables 4 and 5, nine out of the original 14 classes surveyed had to be excluded because only in five classes was it possible for hash users and hash triers, as well as nontriers (cf. the definitions given in the

Appendix) to choose equally among, and be chosen equally by, other hash users, hash triers, and nontriers, respectively. The 144 mutual choices represented in Table 4 thus represent only 72 relations distributed over 102 persons, minus 47 students in these five classes who were not involved in mutual choices on this dimension, while in Table 5 the 648 (not necessarily mutual) choices on the "like best" dimension only involved the same 102 persons, of which seven gave no choices (but received some), and one received no choices (but gave one). The χ^2 test was not applicable to the data in Table 4, and for the data in Table 5 it gave no significant results.

In sum, the outcome of the present study must be said to be highly negative for both the diffusion and the subculture approaches. But, on the other hand, it must be added that as long as no more convincing sociological alternative(s) to the study of nonmedical or recreational drug use has been offered, these two approaches will have to suffice unless one is satisfied to continue doing empirical sociology on this subject with no more then one's more or less explicit hunches about "what would be interesting to know" as a guide.

APPENDIX

Translation of Four Questions from the Questionnaire Used in the Present Study

Hash trying and use:

Question 15. Have you tried hash? (yes, no)
If yes: When did you try hash for the first time? (state month and year)
Have you used hash during the past four weeks? (yes, no)
If yes: How many times have you used hash during the past four weeks?

Definition of "hash users:" "those reporting to have used hash during the four weeks preceding the survey."
Definition of "hash triers:" "those reporting to have tried hash, but not having used it during the four weeks preceding the survey."

The "interaction" dimension:

Question 5. Have you spent any time together with any of your class-

mates outside school hours during the past three days? (yes, no)
If yes: With which of your classmates have you been together during the past three days? (State the filing numbers of the persons in question.)

The "like best" dimension:

Question 20. Mention the one or those of your classmates that you like best (you may mention as many as you wish) ["mention" meaning "give the filing number(s) of"].

The "leadership" dimension:

Question 22. Mention the one or two of your classmates whom you would consider most fit to direct your class in the performance of a joint task ["mention" meaning "give the filing number(s) of"].

REFERENCES

BECKER, H. *Outsiders.* New York: Free Press, 1963.

COLEMAN, I.S., KATZ, E., and MENZEL, H. *Medical Innovation.* Indianapolis: Bobbs-Merrill, 1966.

PARRY, H.I., et al., Primary levels of underreporting psychotrophic drug use. *Public Opinion Quart.* 34: 582–592, 1971.

ROGERS, E.M. *Diffusion of Innovations.* New York: Free Press, 1962.

ULFF-MØLLER, B. Drug use among youth in Denmark in the spring of 1968. *Danish Med. Bull.* 18: 105–111, 1971.

ULFF-MØLLER, B., and JØRGENSEN, F. To modeller for udviklingen af stofbrug blandt skoleelever i Danmark, *Socialt Tidsskrift.* 47: 427–438, 1971.

ULFF-MØLLER, B., et al., *Udbredelse af stofbrug blandt danske skoleelever.* Copenhagen: The Government's Inter-Ministerial Committee on the Drug Abuse among the Young, 1971.

WINSLØW, J.J.B. *Hash Use/Trying and Social Participation.* Paper presented at the First International Student Drug Survey Conference, Newark, New Jersey, September 1971. Published in *Proceedings of the First International Student Drug Survey Conference.* New York: Baywood, 1972.

WINSLØW, J.J.B. *Om rådgivningsundersøgelsen i Hjørring.* Hjørring, Denmark: Municipality of Hjørring (mimeo), 1972a.

WINSLØW, J.J.B. Drug use in Denmark, *Intern. J. Addictions.* 7: 305–319, 1972b.

WINSLØW, J.J.B. (ed.). *Ungdom og stofbrug.* Copenhagen: Palndan, 1972c.

Note Added in Proof. Since the submission of this article in January 1973, it has dawned on the author that a certain prudence, perhaps not exhibited in the article, is necessary for the inferences to be made regarding the diffusion hypothesis from the data presented above. The hypothesis, on the author's interpretation, presumes social integretation to be the "cause" of innovative behavior (i.e., drug trying), that is, it should not be interpreted as saying either (1) that social integration in the concrete case is the effect, and drug use the cause, or (2) that there is some kind of reciprocal relationship between drug use and social integration. A not unreasonably complex form of interpretation (2), however, cannot be rejected on the basis of the cross-sectional data presented in the article, for which reason it must be strongly emphasized that the lack of association between integration and self-reported innovative behavior must not be interpreted in terms of cause and effect in the present data.

A general discussion of this question can be found in the author's *Two Problems of Time in Prevalence Studies*, recently submitted to an American journal. The manuscript can be obtained on request.

The International Journal of the Addictions, 9(4), 541–567, 1974

Teach Me What I Want to Know about Drugs for Junior High School Students

Russell N. Cassel, Ed.D.

University of Wisconsin
Milwaukee, Wisconsin

Gail Zander, M.S.

Milwaukee Public Schools
Milwaukee, Wisconsin

This is the report of a study involving upwards of 300 junior high school students that was designed to assess their relative interest for varying areas of drug abuse information. It sought to make meaningful comparisons among 7th, 8th, and 9th grade pupils concerning their degree of interest for varying areas of such information.

Personal Interest Essential to Motivation

The study was based on the notion that human development and the personal interest of individuals are highly related phenomena, and that learning activities and experiences pertinent to dangerous drugs is no exception to this general principle. If significant and meaningful differences exist among 7th, 8th, and 9th grade pupils in relation to their degree of interest for varying areas of dangerous drug information, it is essential that such differences be carefully identified and defined. Learning activities congruent with the personal interests of students are much more likely to secure their motivation than those that violate this critical relationship.

Attitude Development is Critical

Expected outcomes for students involved in drug abuse education programs deal more with attitude of students than with the acquisition of factual information. Attitude change and development is largely a product of the environment in which the experience takes place, and learning programs based on student interest serve to foster attitude change much more effectively than those imposed from teacher or parent interest. The concept of "Teach me what I want to know" in the area of dangerous drugs seeks to make students members of a teacher–student "team" concept for purposes of developing effective drug abuse education programs.

STUDENTS INVOLVED

This study was planned and conducted with the cooperation of Mr. Paul C. Bauman, Principal, Alexander Graham Bell Junior High School, Milwaukee, Wisconsin. It involved three classes in each of the 7th, 8th, and 9th grade levels of the school, with approximately 100 students for each of the different grade levels. These 300 students represented the total population of students taking "home room" or " study hall" for the period when the study was planned to be accomplished. The completed records for a total of 221 students were used in the study: 82 7th graders, 77 8th graders, and 62 9th graders. Guidance counselors had first priority on students' time for the period of the study, and because counselors and others were continuously calling such students during the period of the study, many of them failed to complete all three questionnaires. Only those student records were included for individuals who had satisfactorily completed all of the records during the time period allotted for the study.

The students were almost entirely Caucasian, from middle class families, generally living in single family dwellings several miles from the central core of Milwaukee.

PSYCHOLOGICAL INSTRUMENTS USED

Three separate and quite different psychological instruments were used in this study: (1) The Internal-External Scale, (2) The Ego Development Scale and (3) Teach me what I want to know drug questionnaire.

The Internal-External Scale

This is a 29-item scale developed by Rotter (1966) where six of the items are "filler" items and 23 of them assess the characteristic internal or external control of subjects. The 23 items, then, from a "face validity" point of view deal with the subject's belief about the nature of the world or his expectations of that world. Based on "construct" validity, the I-E scale purports to provide an objective index of a subject's preference or generalized expectancy about how reinforcement is controlled. For objective data on validity, Rotter reports correlations of from $-.12$ to $-.41$ for varying populations against scores on the Marlowe-Crowne "Social desirability scale," and scores of from .03 to $-.22$ against scores on a variety of intelligence tests. In a wide variety of studies reported by Rotter, the I-E scale scores show little or no relationship with such variables as social class, political affiliation, religious affiliation and sex, but significant correlation with measures depicting an individual's attempt to control his own environment. In terms of reliability, for internal consistency scores for a wide variety of populations the r's range from .65 through .79; and for test-retest from .49 through .78. Because the abuse of dangerous drugs represents "inner" control of the subject, it was hypothesized that persons displaying "internal orientation" on the I-E scale would tend not to become involved in excessive dangerous drug abuse. The instrument is included in Appendix 1.

The Ego Development Scale

This is a 60-item scale designed by Cassel to assess the ego development of both elementary and secondary school students, and is presently published by Psychologists and Educators, Inc., Jacksonville, Illinois. Each of the 60 items is rated by the subject taking it on a five point Likert-type scale ranging from "yes," with a value of "1," through "2," "3," and "4" to a position marked "no" and which is valued "5." The first 20 items deal with personal elements and seek to assess personal development; the second 20 items deal with social development; and the third 20 items deal with educational development. The total score is the sum of the three part scores. Cassel maintains that the "ego" represents the basic attest of one's existence, serves as the real anchor for self-awareness, is the substance that guarantess unity to one's life, and serves as the real basis for self-identity of an individual. He maintains that the primary function of the ego in man is to bring about reduction in tension and gratify personal needs; with a secondary function to project and anticipate future needs. Because of this function of the ego, the abuse of dangerous drugs is hypothesized to be an ego function and would be directly related to low ego development as measured by scores from The Ego Development Scale (EDS).

Six different levels of ego development are depicted by the scores on the EDS. First Stage: stable world of objects where integrated wholeness and decentering of Piaget are completed. Second Stage: impulse stage with the advent and completion of basic personallity formation. Third Stage: self-protection where confrontation serves to forge more precisely personality functioning. Fourth Stage: conscientious stage involving motives and consequences with decision making. Fifth Stage: autonomous with complete sense of individuality, and with independence for emotions and inner conflict. Sixth Stage: transcending conflict with the reconciling of polarities and with the sensitivity for self-actualization. Of the three ego areas assessed by the EDS, for all three levels of schooling—elementary, junior high school, and senior high school—the ego development is most neglected and least developed. This finding, indeed, appears to have important significance for drug abuse education because dangerous drug abuse is an ego function of the personal type (Cassel, 1973a–f; Benfield, 1971; Ludwig, 1972). Internal consistency type of reliability indices for a wide variety of populations ranged from .73 to .91, with test-retest reliability indices ranging from .72 to .87. For construct validity purposes (from Benfield and Ludwig studies), scores on the EDS appear to be independently organized (based on principal component factor analysis with varimax rotations) and significantly different from such factors as intelligence, teacher ratings of expected school success, and student attitude toward school. Similarly, scores on the EDS appear to be unrelated to such variables as height, weight, age and number of siblings in family, but significantly related to intelligence. The latter suggests that the ego function in an individual is intellectual in nature. The EDS is illustrated in Appendix 2.

Teach Me What I Want to Know About Drugs Questionnaire

This instrument contains 103 items distributed in 13 different categories on drug abuse information or education. Each separate item on the *Teach*

Me What I Want to Know About Drugs Questionnaire (DQ) contains a five point Likert-type scale ranging from "low" with a value of "1," through "2," "3," and "4" to "high" with a value of "5." Each one of the 103 items contained in the DQ represent units of study contained in *The Computerized Drug Abuse Education System* (PLUDRUG) developed by Cassel, and presently available from Psychologists and Educators, Inc., Jacksonville, Illinois (Cassel, 1973c). Based on findings reported in this and other studies, PLUDRUG contains 10 separate modules which are designed as a one semester course in a secondary school or college: (1) Dangerous drug information, (2) Drug abuse causes, (3) Drug addiction and dependence, (4) Drug treatment programs, (5) Drug control laws, (6) Drug abuse prevention, (7) Research findings, (8) Dialogue with ex-drug users, (9) Teach me what I want to know about drugs concept, and (10) Decision making for drug abuse prevention. PLUDRUG is based squarely on the principles of humanistic psychology where the traditional concept of "knowledge about" is replaced through the use of computer-based gaming and simulation with "experience with" through surrogate role playing of participants.

The DQ contained the 103 items arranged in 13 related groupings, presumed to be independently organized categories, and with varying numbers of items in each ranging from 3 to 13: (1) Nature of dangerous drugs, (2) Critical examination of select dangerous drugs, (3) Genealogy and causes of dangerous drug abuse, (4) Drug addiction and dependence, (5) Major types of dangerous drug abuse, (6) Messages from experienced drug abusers, (7) Drug treatment programs of note, (8) Drug control laws and programs, (9) Dangerous drugs research facts, (10) Drug abuse prevention and education, (11) Select national drug abuse activities, (12) Gaming and simulation-computer based, and (13) Psychological basis for drug prevention. To permit a valid or equal basis for comparing scores for the 13 different categories, all scores were weighted to reflect the same number of items so that the maximum attainable score was equal for all parts as well as for the total score. The total score was the weighted sum of the 13 part scores. The scores for the 221 subjects are contained in Table 4. Internal consistency reliability for the DQ as reported in Table 6 was .984 for the 221 subjects involved. From a status validity point of view, the data contained in Table 3 depicts a statistically significant difference in interest for the 221 subjects involved both among the 13 different categories and among the three class levels of students involved, i.e., 7th, 8th, and 9th grades. The DQ is illustrated in Appendix 3.

ADMINISTRATION OF INSTRUMENTS

All three of the psychological instruments were administered by counselors and school psychologists as a portion of the regular school offerings. All work was accomplished during about the middle of the second semester of the 1971–1972 school year and over about a 2-week period. All completed records where three identifiable results for the same student were evident were used in the study.

FINDINGS

Rotter I-E Scale

The data contained in Table 1 suggest no significant difference among students from the three separate school levels, or school classes, i.e., 7th, 8th, and 9th grades. From Table 4, Variable 2, we observe that the mean I-E score for all junior high students (221 of them) was 12.4. Based on Rotter's previous research, this suggests that they are generally externally oriented. Data contained in Table 5 for Rotter's I-E Score suggests a significant positive correlation between interest in drug information in general and internal-type orientation on the Rotter I-E Scale. Variables 8, 9, and 17 contribute significantly to this relationship, with 8 (Nature of drugs) and 17 (Drug abuse education) having positive values, and 9 (Examination of drugs) being negative related. Thus the evidence in this study suggests that persons who are internally oriented based on Rotter's I-E Scale prefer information related to 8 (Nature of drugs) and 17 (Drug abuse education), while students who are externally oriented prefer, in contrast, 9 (Examination of drugs).

Ego-Development Scale

From Table 2 it is clear that there is a significant difference in ego development, as measured by this instrument, and in relation to areas depicted by the three Part Scores: 1 (Personal), 2 (Social), and 3 (Educational). From Factor B of Table 2 we observe that there is a significant difference among the three grade levels (7th, 8th, and 9th) in relation to ego development. The interaction suggests that the differences contained in A, which are statistically significant cannot be explained in terms of a discernible pattern from the three scores contained in Factor B. Since the differences in Factor A, ego-development scores, were significantly

Table 1
Analysis of Variance for Scores on Rotter I-E Scale Among 7th, 8th, and 9th Grade Pupils

Source of variance	Sum of squares	Degrees of freedom	Mean squares	*F*-test	Significance level
Between groups: 7th, 8th, and 9th grades	5.41	2	2.70	0.25	n.s.
Within groups: 7th, 8th, and 9th grades	2,409.52	218	11.05		
Totals	2,414.93	220			

Table 2
Two-Way Analysis of Variance for Three Scores on Ego-Development Scale and Three Junior High School Grade Levels of Students

Sources of variance	Sum of squares	Degrees of freedom	Mean squares	*F*-levels	Significance levels
Factor A: Three scores on E-D	4,029.68	2	2,014.84	18.66	.001
Factor B: 7th, 8th, and 9th grade levels	1,234.14	2	617.07	5.72	.05
Interaction: A × B	342.15	4	85.54	.79	n.s.
Within sets	70,605.29	654	107.96		
Totals	76,211.26	662			

different, Fig. 1 was drawn to depict those differences. The strong pattern for educational elements related to ego display a clearly discernible relationship with grade level, and which is also depicted in the total score, it suggests that school experiences related to educational aspects of ego development are quite effective, while the same effectiveness is not clear for either personal or social development, i.e., social development for the 9th grade is much less than for the 8th grade, suggesting a regressive movement. Similarly, the lack of progressive personal development in the 9th grade suggests that personal and social areas may be seriously neglected in junior high school experiences.

Teach Me What I Want to Know About Drugs Questionnaire

Data contained in Table 3 suggest that the junior high school student's interest in drug abuse information varies significantly in degree for the 13 areas depicted by the 103 items for the Drug Questionnaire (Factor

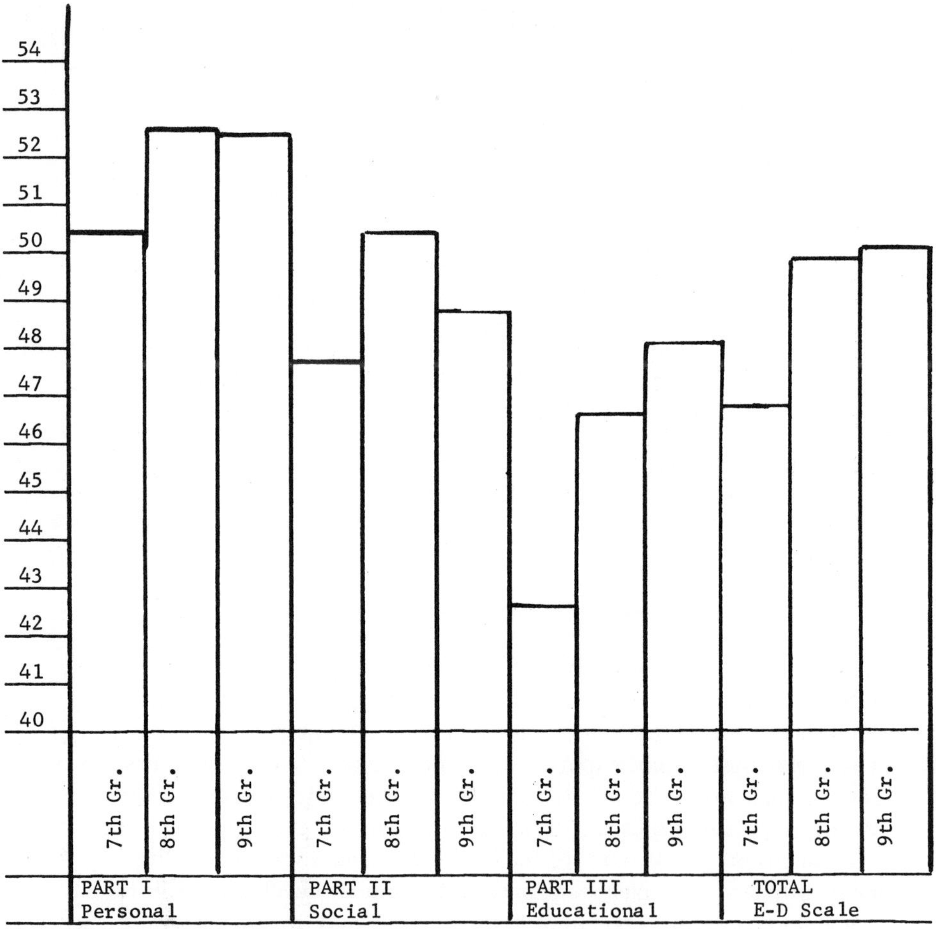

Fig. 1. Comparison of the scores from the Ego-Development Scale for 7th, 8th, and 9th grade students.

Table 3.
Two-Way Analysis of Variance for Thirteen Scores on Teach Me What I Want to Know About Drugs and 7th, 8th, and 9th Grade Students

Source of variance	Sum of squares	Degrees of freedom	Mean squares	*F*-tests	Significance levels
Factor A: The 13 scores on PLUDRUG	2,467.46	12	205.62	8.78	.001
Factor B: 7th, 8th, and 9th grade levels	2,647.59	2	1,323.80	56.50	.001
Interaction: A × B	375.97	24	15.67	.67	n.s.
Within sets	66,399.40	2,834	23.43		
Totals	71,890.42	2,872			

A). Factor B for that table suggests that there is a significant difference for students of the different grades in junior high school (7th, 8th, and 9th). The interaction effect depicted in this table suggests that there is no stabilized pattern that might explain the relationship between grade level and varying degrees of interest for the 13 drug areas. Six of the 13 drug areas might be classed as "high interest," three as "moderate interest," and four as "low interest" areas.

High interest areas:

1. Nature of dangerous drugs.
2. Examination of select drugs.
3. Causes of drug abuse.
5. Major types of drug abuse.
6. Messages from drug abusers.
9. Research facts on drugs.

Moderate interest areas:

4. Addiction and dependence.
8. Drug control law programs.
12. Drug abuse gaming-simulation.

Low interest areas:

7. Drug treatment programs.
10. Drug abuse education.

11. International facts on drugs.
13. Psychological basis drug use.

Figure 2 illustrates the level of interest for the various drug areas for junior high school students in general.

School Level and Drug Information Interest

Figure 3 depicts the pattern for level of drug interest in relation to the 13 areas of the drug questionnaire by grade level (7th, 8th, and 9th grades). Factor B in the two-way analysis of variance contained in Table 2 shows that there is a significant different interest in drug information by grades at the .05 level of confidence, and Fig. 3 depicts that difference. From Fig. 3 we observe that there are a total of 39 "matched-pairs" for the 13 drug information areas to test the hypothesis that the higher the grade level of students, the lower the interest in drug abuse information, i.e., 8th grade is higher than 7th grade level, but 9th grade is higher than both 7th and 8th grades. By use of the Wilcoxon's Matched-Pairs Signed-Ranks Test, we find a statistically significant trend for students in the higher grades to indicate a lower interest in drug abuse information. From Table 5, Column 2, we observe a significant multiple correlation, corrected for shrinkage, in support of the same hypothesis (pupils in the higher grades in junior high school depict lower interest in drug abuse information). It is of considerable interest to note that the only regression coefficient with significant relationship is 12 (Drug abuse gaming-simulation).

Sex Differences

For 12 of the 13 different areas on the drug questionnaire, from Table 4, it may be observed that girls exhibited a greater interest than boys. It should be noted from Table 5, Column 3, that the only two variables receiving significant regression weights were 16 (Drug research facts) and 20 (Psychological basis drugs).

Reliability of Instruments

Data contained in Table 6 suggest that all three of the instruments used in the study have high coefficients of reliability in relation to internal consistency and as measured by the K-R Formula 20.

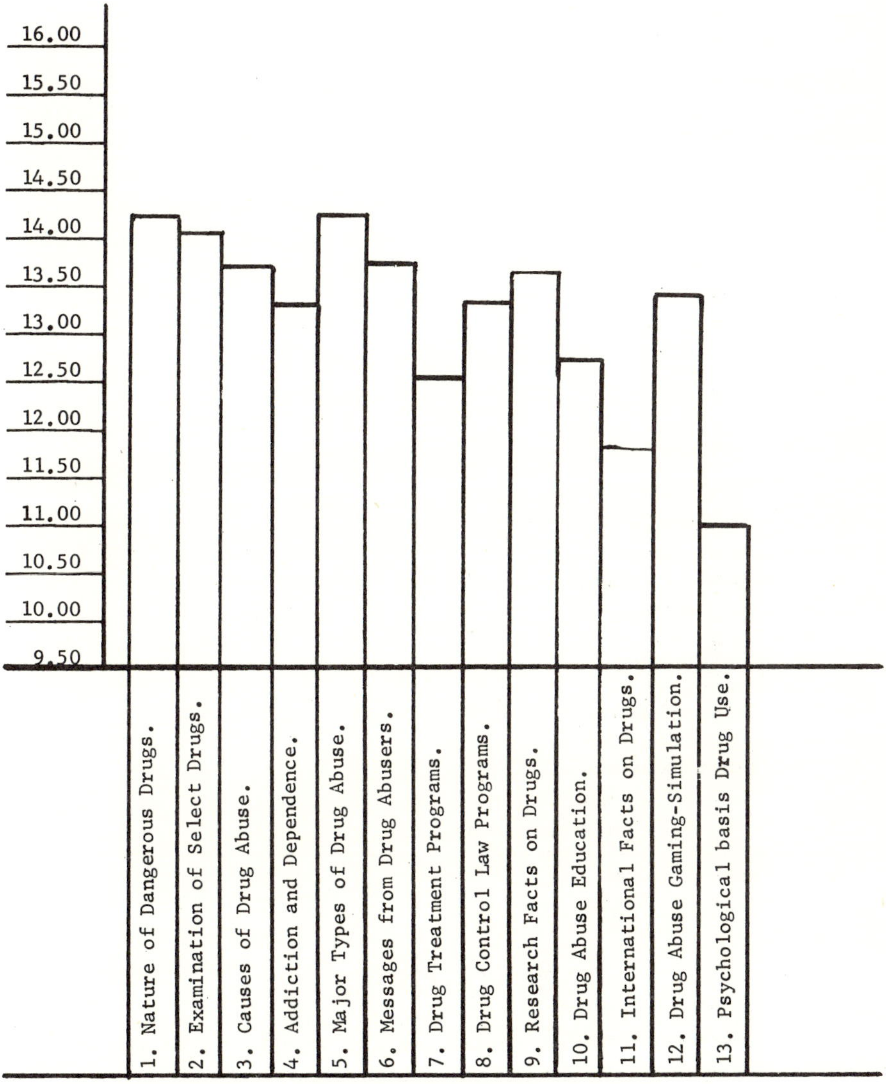

Fig. 2. Comparison of the relative degree to which junior high school students are interested in different areas of drug information.

Table 4
Intercorrelation Matrix of the 21 Variables

Variables	1	2	3	4	5	6	7	8	9
1 Class levels		006[a]	001	091	059	194	187	−095	−115
2 Rotter's I-E score			−011	−203	−156	−305	−311	−003	−111
3 Sex (0 = M, 1 = F)				135	−170	−078	−089	221	211
							Ego-Development		
4 Part I- Personal					488.	529	610	−161	−118
5 Part II-Social						493	653	−320	−302
6 Part III-Educational							978	−265	−223
7 Total score								−273	−233
					Drug Interest Questionnaire				
8 Nature of drugs									834
9 Examination of drugs									
10 Drug abuse causes									
11 Addiction/dependence									
12 Types of drug abuse									
13 Messages from abusers									
14 Drug treatment programs									
15 Drug control laws									
16 Drug research facts									
17 Drug abuse education									
18 International drug									
19 Drug gaming-simulation									
20 Psychological basis drugs									
21 Total of drug questionnaire									
Mean	7.9	12.4	0.5	51.7	48.9	45.5	19.5	14.2	14.0
SD	0.8	3.3	0.5	10.4	9.6	11.2	4.0	5.4	5.1

[a] Decimal point eliminated.

CONCLUSIONS

It is readily admitted that valid conclusions should not be drawn based on the data or findings from 221 junior high school students. However, it is suggested that meaningful hypotheses may be made for the purpose of further testing from such data. It is in this light that the following implications are cited:

Involved in the Study (N = 221)

	10	11	12	13	14	15	16	17	18	19	20	21
	−068	−161	−285	−198	−175	−140	−185	−203	−255	−238	−223	−254
	−040	040	−019	−027	−089	−036	015	015	−142	−042	−124	−037
	196	186	197	134	122	158	217	156	068	188	188	215
Scale												
	=187	069	114	133	141	001	098	063	093	088	070	084
	−327	−059	−026	−027	010	−122	−056	−068	−074	−042	−058	−102
	−249	−128	−090	−063	−013	−121	−147	−094	−062	−120	−023	−131
	−262	−126	−084	−060	−008	−118	−133	−091	−062	−105	−027	−129
(PLUDRUG)												
	777	354	359	325	295	601	425	391	280	348	352	539
	839	482	457	424	377	643	518	501	342	446	406	639
		424	340	380	319	630	436	512	285	360	408	573
			791	734	641	598	694	644	361	543	463	811
				713	630	585	686	612	416	543	501	804
					690	628	725	662	410	596	532	821
						733	768	765	585	567	716	844
							766	726	522	623	596	835
								736	513	663	572	870
									625	650	759	871
										576	695	671
											598	767
												767
	13.6	13.3	14.2	14.0	12.5	13.3	13.6	12.6	11.8	13.4	11.1	17.1
	5.7	4.5	4.5	4.5	4.3	4.4	4.8	4.7	5.2	5.5	5.0	4.8

1. No significant difference exists among the 7th, 8th, and 9th grade students in relation to their inner-outer orientation based on Rotter's I-E Score.

2. There is wide disparity among junior high school students in relation to three areas of ego development (personal, social and educational), and with educational receiving greatest attention.

3. There is a clear difference in degree of interest among junior high school students with greatest interest in relation to nature of drugs, causes

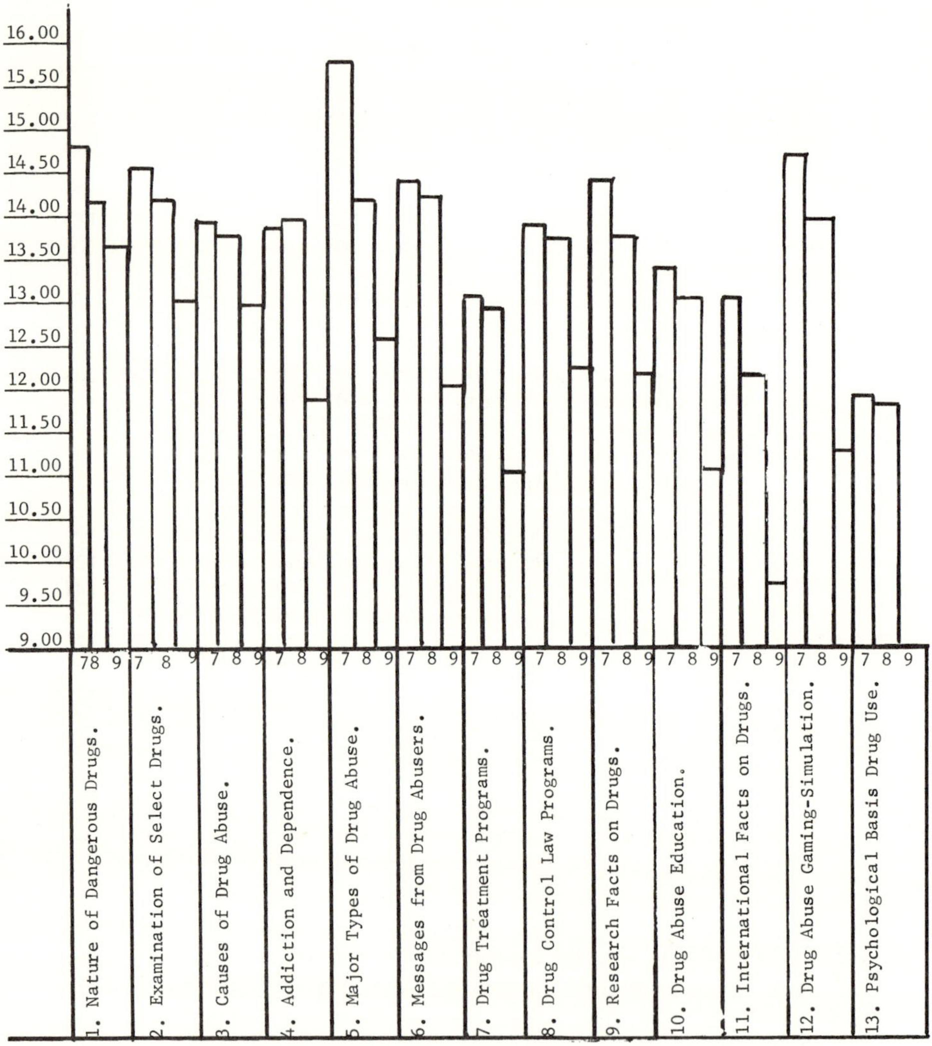

Fig. 3. Comparison of the relative degree of interest in different areas of drug information by grade for junior high school students.

Table 5
Multiple Regression Analysis for Drug Interests of the Junior High School Students (N = *221*)

Regression analysis data	Rotter's I-E score	Grade level index	Sex of students	Other data against 13 drug items
Multiple R_c	.293	.275	.240	.339
Significance level of R_c	.002	.005	.019	.001
Significant regression coefficients	8, 9, and 17	12	16 and 20	1, 3, 5, and 7
Significant partial correlation coefficients	8 = .194 9 = −.228 17 = .190	12 = .207	16 = .136 20 = .139	1 = −.243 3 = .163 4 = .161 7 = −.120

Table 6
Internal Consistency Reliability for Rotter I-E Score, Total Score on Ego-Development Scale, and Total Score on Drug Questionnaire (N = *221*)

Reliability measure	Rotter's I-E Score	Ego-Development Scale, total	Total score for drug questionnaire (PLUDRUG)
Kuder-Richardson Formula-20 coefficient	.608	.866	.984

of drug abuse, types of drug abuse, messages from drug abusers, and research facts. Lowest interest deals with treatment, education, international facts, and psychological basis.

4. Students in the 8th grade express a generally lower interest in drug abuse information that those in the 7th grade, and students in the 9th grade express a lower interest than those in either the 7th or 8th grades. Generally, the higher the grade, the lower the student interest in drugs.

5. There is a significant relationship between the "inner-outer" orientation of junior high students and their degree of interest in drug information, with the inner-oriented students expressing the greatest degree of such interest.

6. Girls generally tend to express greater interest in drug information than boys during junior high school years.

Table 7
Equating the 13 Part Scores on the Drug Questionnaire to Permit Interest Assessments or Comparisons

13 Different areas on the drug questionnaire	Number of items	Weights for each item	Maximum score
1. Nature of dangerous drugs	6	0.67	20.10
2. Examination of select drugs	13	0.31	20.15
3. Causes of drug abuse	5	0.80	20.00
4. Addiction and dependence	5	0.80	20.00
5. Major types of drug abuse	11	0.37	20.35
6. Messages from drug abusers	9	0.45	20.25
7. Drug treatment programs	11	0.37	20.35
8. Drug control law programs	10	0.40	20.00
9. Research facts on drugs	7	0.57	19.95
10. Drug abuse education	9	0.45	20.25
11. International facts on drugs	9	0.45	20.25
12. Drug abuse gaming-simulation	3	1.34	20.10
13. Psychological basis drug use	5	0.80	20.00
Total score on drug questionnaire	103 (262)	0.10	26.18

RECOMMENDATIONS

This study sought to deal with three factors believed to be highly related to the problem of dangerous drug abuse: personal development from both the I-E Scale and the EDS, social development from the EDS, and drug abuse information and decision making from the DQ. Based on the findings contained in this and other studies over the past 5 years, three computer-based programs have been developed for dealing with critical factors pertinent to the present drug abuse problem, and they are presently available from Psychologists and Educators, Inc., Jacksonville, Illinois 62650:

I THE COMPUTERIZED PERSONAL DEVELOPMENT PROGRAM — PERSDEV — Development of competency in individuals for scientific decision making.

II THE COMPUTERIZED HUMAN RELATIONS PROGRAM — HUMRELAT — Development of effective competency for getting along with others—social aspects.

III THE COMPUTERIZED DRUG ABUSE EDUCATION SYSTEM — PLUDRUG — Computer-based drug abuse education—teach me what I want to know concept.

APPENDIX 1

ROTTER INTERNAL-EXTERNAL CONTROL SCALE

Instructions for the I-E Scale

This is a questionnaire to find out the way in which certain important events in our society affect different people. Each item consists of a pair of alternatives lettered a or b. Please select the one statement of each pair (and only one) which you more strongly believe to be the case as far as you're concerned. Be sure to select the one you actually believe to be more true rather than the one you think you should choose or the one you would like to be true. This is a measure of personal belief: obviously there are no right or wrong answers.

Your answers to the items on this inventory are to be recorded on the separate answer sheet provided. Is there any person who does not have the I-E Scale and the separate answer sheet? It is important that you use a soft lead pencil and not a ball-point pen to mark this answer sheet, as it will be scored by use of the computer. A number 2 pencil works best, but any regular lead pencil will do alright. Please print your name on the separate answer sheet at this time. Also, indicate your age to nearest six months, your date of birth, and sex.

Please answer these items carefully but do not spend too much time on any one item. Be sure to find an answer for every choice. Find the number of the item on the answer sheet and black-in the space under the a or b which you choose as the statement more true.

In some instances you may discover that you believe both statements or neither one. In such cases, be sure to select the one you more strongly believe to be the case as far as you're concerned. Also try to respond to each item independently when making your choice; do not be influenced by your previous choices.There is no time limit to the inventory.

I-E SCALE

* *

1. a. Children get into trouble because their parents punish them too much.
   b. The trouble with most children nowadays is that their parents are too easy with them.
2. a. Many of the unhappy things in people's lives are partly due to bad luck.
   b. People's misfortunes result from mistakes they make.
3. a. One of the major reasons why we have wars is because people don't take enough interest in politics.
   b. There will always be wars, no matter how hard people try to prevent them.
4. a. In the long run people get the respect they deserve in this world.
   b. Unfortunately, an individual's worth often passes unrecognized no matter how hard he tries.
5. a. The idea that teachers are unfair to students is nonsense.
   b. Most students don't realize the extent to which their grades are influenced by accidental happenings.
6. a. Without the right breaks one cannot be an effective leader.
   b. Capable people who fail to become leaders have not taken advantage of their opportunities.

GO ON TO NEXT PAGE

7. a. No matter how hard you try some people just don't like you.
   b. People who can't get others to like them don't understand how to get along with others.
8. a. Heredity plays the major role in determining one's personality.
   b. It is one's experiences in life which determine what they're like.
9. a. I have often found that what is going to happen will happen.
   b. Trusting to fate has never turned out as well for me as making a decision to take a definite course of action.
10. a. In the case of the well prepared student there is rarely if ever such a thing as an unfair test.
    b. Many times exam questions tend to be so unrelated to course work that studying is really useless.
11. a. Becoming a success is a matter of hard work, luck has little or nothing to do with it.
    b. Getting a good job depends mainly on being in the right place at the right time.
12. a. The average citizen can have an influence in government decisions.
    b. This world is run by the few people in power, and there is not much the little guy can do about it.
13. a. When I make plans, I am almost certain that I can make them work.
    b. It is not always wise to plan too far ahead because many things turn out to be a matter of good or bad fortune anyway.
14. a. There are certain people who are just no good.
    b. There is some good in everybody.
15. a. In my case getting what I want has little or nothing to do with luck.
    b. Many times we might just as well decide what to do by flipping a coin.
16. a. Who gets to be the boss often depends on who was lucky enough to be in the right place first.
    b. Getting people to do the right thing depends upon ability, luck has little or nothing to do with it.
17. a. As far as world affairs are concerned, most of us are the victims of forces we can neither understand, nor control.
    b. By taking an active part in political and social affairs the people can control world events.
18. a. Most people don't realize the extent to which their lives are controlled by accidental happenings.
    b. There really is no such thing as "luck".
19. a. One should always be willing to admit mistakes.
    b. It is usually better to cover up one's mistakes.
20. a. It is hard to know whether or not a person really likes you.
    b. How many friends you have depends upon how nice a person you are.
21. a. In the long run the bad things that happen to us are balanced by the good ones.
    b. Most misfortunes are the result of lack of ability, ignorance, laziness, or all three.
22. a. With enough effort we can wipe out political corruption.
    b. It is difficult for people to have much control over the things politicians do in office.
23. a. Sometimes I can't understand how teachers arrive at the grades they give.
    b. There is a direct connection between how hard I study and the grades I get.
24. a. A good leader expects people to decide for themselves what they should do.
    b. A good leader makes it clear to everybody what their jobs are.
25. a. Many times I feel that I have little influence over the things that happen to me.
    b. It is impossible for me to believe that chance or luck plays an important role in my life.

GO ON TO NEXT PAGE

26.a. People are lonely because they don't try to be friendly.
b. There's not much use in trying hard to please people, if they like you they like you.

27.a. There is too much emphasis on athletics in high school.
b. Team sports are an excellent way to build character.

28.a. What happens to me is my own doing.
b. Sometimes I feel that I don't have enough control over directions my life is taking.

29.a. Most of the time I can't understand why politicians behave the way they do.
b. In the long run the people are responsible for bad government on a national as well as on a local level.

END OF I-E CONTROL SCALE

APPENDIX 2

THE EGO DEVELOPMENT SCALE

-by-

Russell N. Cassel

Published by
PSYCHOLOGISTS AND EDUCATORS, INC.
Jacksonville, Illinois 62650

Name______________________________
Address____________________________
School_____________________________
Age______ Grade________ Sex__________

GENERAL INSTRUCTIONS

This rating scale is designed to assess the ego development of persons in grades 3 through 12 in three specific areas of the life-space: (1) personal, (2) social, and (3) educational. Pupils with average and better reading competency at the 4th grade level should be able to accomplish the form with a minimum of help. People lacking such reading competency will need additional assistance both in understanding the items and in the mechanics for marking their answers. Always, however, The Ego Development Scale (EDS) is to be accomplished based on the view of the subject involved. If the answer is clearly "yes", the check mark (✓) is placed in the column marked "yes". If it is "no" in the column marked "no". If the answer is neither "yes" nor "no", but somewhere in between, it is placed on the appropriate position on the scale, as per example.
There is no time limit.

Example: Harry is often sick

SCALE				
1	2	3	4	5
yes		✓		no

EGO DEVELOPMENT PROFILE

T - Score	Personal Development			Social Development			Educational Development			TOTAL Ego Development			T - Score
	Elm	JrH	SrH	Elm	JrH	SrH	Elm	JrH	SrH	Elm	JrH	SrH	
80	81	90	99	88	95	99	75	80	99	24	27	30	80
75	76	85	96	83	91	96	70	77	97	23	26	29	75
70	71	80	93	78	86	94	65	73	95	22	25	28	70
65	66	75	88	73	82	90	60	70	93	21	23	27	65
60	61	70	84	67	77	88	56	66	89	18	21	26	60
55	57	65	79	62	72	84	55	62	85	16	20	25	55
50	52	60	73	56	67	80	47	58	81	15	19	23	50
45	44	56	68	51	62	75	43	54	78	13	18	21	45
40	43	51	62	45	57	70	38	50	74	12	16	20	40
35	38	43	57	38	45	65	35	40	68	11	14	19	35
30	33	35	51	30	33	60	31	30	62	10	11	18	30
25	29	29	36	26	27	45	26	25	45	8	9	11	25
20	20	20	20	20	20	20	20	20	20	6	6	6	20

THE EGO DEVELOPMENT SCALE

* *

PERSONAL DEVELOPMENT	1	2	3	4	5	
1. I often giggle when nothing is really funny	yes				no	xx
2. People consider me good natured	yes				no	x
3. I usually get along well with my parents	yes				no	x
4. I usually play fair with my friends	yes				no	x
5. I usually change when I know I am wrong	yes				no	x
6. I am usually careful about things	yes				no	x
7. I often do things wrong without thinking	yes				no	xx
8. I usually figure things out for myself	yes				no	x
9. I often feel I am left out of things	yes				no	xx
10. Often I can hardly wait to get out of bed	yes				no	x
11. Often I feel like crying about nothing	yes				no	xx
12. Often I feel tired in the middle of the day	yes				no	xx
13. My feelings are often easily hurt	yes				no	xx
14. I often have trouble controlling my temper	yes				no	xx
15. Often I am on the go and can't seem to stop	yes				no	xx
16. Often I day dream a lot, and my mind wanders	yes				no	xx
17. Often I lack self confidence in myself	yes				no	xx
18. Often I feel unwanted and disliked	yes				no	xx
19. People often consider me the quiet type	yes				no	xx
20. I often like to start new things	yes				no	x
TOTAL SCORES WITH *						
VALUE OF SCORES WITH *	5	4	3	2	1	
TOTAL VALUE OF SCORES WITH * (Multiply X *)						
TOTAL SCORES WITH **						
VALUE OF SCORES WITH **	1	2	3	4	5	
TOTAL VALUE OF SCORES WITH ** (Multiply X **)						
TOTAL VALUE PERSONAL DEVELOPMENT SCORES						

SCALE

PERSONAL DEVELOPMENT SCORE_____ (Add all scores TOTAL VALUE)

SOCIAL DEVELOPMENT	SCORE 1	2	3	4	5	
21. Most of my friends are in my class	yes				no	x
22. Classmates miss me when I am absent	yes				no	x
23. People usually think I am friendly	yes				no	x
24. I go out of my way to be with friends	yes				no	x
25. I think I am important to my classmates	yes				no	x
26. Often I am aggressive and mean to others	yes				no	xx
27. Often I get into fights with others	yes				no	xx
28. I am often a poor sport when I lose	yes				no	xx
29. Often I play mean tricks on others	yes				no	xx
30. Many friends are much younger than myself	yes				no	xx
31. I have many very bad manners	yes				no	xx
32. I usually enjoy meeting new people	yes				no	x
33. Often I show-off in front of friends	yes				no	xx
34. It is easier for me to talk to the class	yes				no	x
35. My friends often come to see me	yes				no	x
36. Many friends are much older than myself	yes				no	xx
37. I am very popular with boys my own age	yes				no	x
38. I am very popular with girls my own age	yes				no	x
39. Often I have trouble keeping my friends	yes				no	xx
40. I can usually carry on a good conversation	yes				no	x
TOTAL SCORES WITH *						
VALUE OF SCORES WITH *	5	4	3	2	1	
TOTAL VALUE OF SCORES WITH * (Multiply X *)						
TOTAL SCORES WITH **						
VALUE OF SCORES WITH **	1	2	3	4	5	
TOTAL VALUE OF SCORES WITH ** (Multiply X **)						
TOTAL VALUE OF SOCIAL DEVELOPMENT SCORES						

SOCIAL DEVELOPMENT SCORE______

SCORE

EDUCATIONAL DEVELOPMENT	1	2	3	4	5	
41. Usually I like to go to school	yes				no	x
42. When school work is hard, I usually give up	yes				no	xx
43. Arithmetic is easy for me	yes				no	x
44. I usually get along well with the teacher	yes				no	x
45. I usually get good grades from the teacher	yes				no	x
46. Doing well in school is important to me	yes				no	x
47. I usually get my school work done on time	yes				no	x
48. Often I answer before other pupils do	yes				no	x
49. Often I annoy other students at work	yes				no	xx
50. My parents always "nag" me about homework	yes				no	xx
51. Often I read the funny papers	yes				no	x
52. Often I watch TV at home	yes				no	x
53. Often I forget what and where the lesson is	yes				no	xx
54. Often I am sleepy and restless in school	yes				no	xx
55. Often I help others with school problems	yes				no	x
56. Often I have trouble remembering things	yes				no	xx
57. I often read books not in my lessons	yes				no	x
58. I usually do my school homework	yes				no	x
59. I usually do well on school tests	yes				no	x
60. My parents are interested in how well I do	yes				no	x
TOTAL SCORES WITH *						
VALUE OF SCORES WITH *	5	4	3	2	1	
TOTAL VALUE OF SCORES WITH * (Multiply X *)						
TOTAL SCORES WITH **						
VALUE OF SCORES WITH **	1	2	3	4	5	
TOTAL VALUE OF SCORES WITH ** (Multiply X **)						
TOTAL VALUE OF EDUCATIONAL DEVELOPMENT SCORES						

PERSONAL DEVELOPMENT SCORE________

SOCIAL DEVELOPMENT SCORE ________

EDUCATIONAL DEVELOPMENT SCORE________

EGO DEVELOPMENT TOTAL SCORE

____

(Per. Dev.+ Social Dev. + Educ. Dev./10)

APPENDIX 3

DRUGS: TEACH ME WHAT I WANT TO KNOW QUESTIONNAIRE

This questionnaire is designed to assess the degree of interest people have in various aspects of drug abuse education, and based on that evaluation to teach them what they want to know. There are no right or wrong answers on the questionnaire, but a five point rating scale to determine your degree of interest for each of the items included.

General Directions

Each item on this scale is to be read carefully, and then to be answered on the separate answer sheet provided. Do not write on the questionnaire. The interest scale at the top of each column contains five points ranging from "LOW", which is a "1" on your answer sheet, to a "HIGH", which is a "5", and with intervening positions of 2, 3, and 4 as shown.If you have little or no interest, mark the "1" or "LOW"; if you have high interest, mark the "5" or "HIGH". If you have only moderate interest, mark the apropriate position in between the "1" or "5". Always be sure in marking your answer sheet that you have the correct number on the answer sheet for the item you are answering. If you make a mistake, erase and mark the right one. Please complete each and every item on the questionnaire.If you are not familiar with the words on the item, or if you really don't have an interest one way or another, mark the "3" position: so that it does not change your score for the particular category. Please use a regular soft lead pencil on the answer as the computer will be used in scoring. There is no time limit, but you should finish in about 30 minutes of time.

	INTEREST SCALE				
I. NATURE OF DANGEROUS DRUGS:	LOW	2	3	4	HIGH
1. Critical stages in history of dangerous drugs...					
2. Nature of present drug abuse epidemic...........					
3. Classes and categories of dangerous drugs.......					
4. Stages of effect for dangerous drugs............					
5. Trend towards use of drug combinations..........					
6. Purity and strength of dangerous drugs..........					
II. CRITICAL EXAMINATION OF SELECT DANGEROUS DRUGS:					
7. Amphetamines....................................					
8. Antidepressants.................................					
9. Psychic-energizers..............................					
10. Marijuana.......................................					
11. Lysergic acid (LSD-25)..........................					
12. Other hallucinogens.............................					
13. Cocaine...					
14. Tranquilizers...................................					
15. Antihistamines..................................					
16. Barbiturates....................................					
17. Volatile solvents...............................					
18. Alcoholic beverages.............................					
19. Opiate products (Heroin,Morphine,etc.)..........					
III. GENEALOGY AND CAUSES OF DANGEROUS DRUG ABUSE:					
20 Drug using world we live in......................					

GO ON TO NEXT PAGE

	INTEREST SCALE				
III. GENEALOGY AND CAUSES OF DANGEROUS DRUGS (Cont-):	LOW	2	3	4	HIGH
21. Critical stages to drug dependence.............					
22. Sociological causes for drug dependence.........					
23. Psychological causes for drug dependence........					
24. Grouping of drug dependents by causes...........					
IV. DRUG ADDICTION AND DEPENDENCE:					
25. Alcoholic type of addiction....................					
26. Opiate (Heroin) type of addiction..............					
27. Barbiturate type of addiction..................					
28. Dependence and addiction.......................					
29. World Health Organization (WHO) on dependence...					
V. MAJOR TYPES OF DANGEROUS DRUG ABUSE:					
30. Cigarette smoking (Tobacco use)................					
31. Coffee drinking................................					
32. Drinking habits of teenagers...................					
33. Glue sniffing(Cleaning fluid, gasoline,etc.)....					
34. Alcoholic beverage drinking....................					
35. Amphetamine jag (Uppers).......................					
36. Ether jag (Mostly of the 1800's)...............					
37. Pot (Marijuana) smoking........................					
38. LSD (Acid) trips...............................					
39. Barbiturate use (Downers)......................					
40. Opiate (Horse or Heroin) users.................					
VI. MESSAGES FROM EXPERIENCED DRUG ABUSERS:					
41. Short statements from many different ones.......					
42. Commune living.................................					
43. Harry and Girl, users of Heroin................					
44. Art Linkletter's second thoughts on drugs.......					
45. Marina McGuire and her drug life...............					
46. Run-away teenage girls and drugs...............					
47. Marjorie talks about her addiction.............					
48. Typical life of a real drug dependent..........					
49. Mary's first trip on acid at 14................					
VII. DRUG TREATMENT PROGRAMS OF NOTE:					
50. California high school "crash" pads............					
51. Methadone treatment programs...................					
52. U.S.Federal Prison programs....................					
53. California half-way houses.....................					
54. Synanon (Family unit approach).................					
55. Alcoholics Anonymous...........................					
56. Phoenix house (New York City)..................					
57. Underground switchboard........................					
58. Yale alcoholic clinic..........................					
59. Methadone primer...............................					
60. Trends in dangerous drug treatment philosophy...					
VIII. DRUG CONTROL LAWS AND PROGRAMS:					
61. Dangerous drugs availability...................					
62. French research on "alvolar" (Breath test)......					
63. U.S.Overseas drug control efforts..............					

GO ON TO NEXT PAGE

INTEREST SCALE
LOW 2 3 4 HIGH

VIII. DRUG CONTROL LAWS AND PROGRAMS (Cont-):
64. Wisconsin drug control laws
65. U.S. Federal drug control laws
66. Shop lifting
67. Alcohol as a dangerous drug
68. Drinking driving laws in the U.S.
69. High profits-Mafia in Drug Traffic
70. 1 in 50 drivers are drunk

IX. DANGEROUS DRUGS RESEARCH FACTS:
71. Research data on drug effects
72. Harmless marihuana
73. Killer heroin
74. Medical personnel and drug abuse
75. Medication and drug dependence
76. Barbiturate deaths
77. Marijuana causes heart beat to race

X. DRUG ABUSE PREVENTION AND EDUCATION:
78. Drug abuse education program philosophy
79. "Trigger films" to incite drug discussions
80. World Health Organization on drug abuse
81. World Health Organization on drug education
82. World Health Organization on community programs
83. New York program for drug prevention
84. Selected school drug abuse education programs.
85. Can love steer kids from drugs
86. Children of change-Social revolution

XI. SELECT NATIONAL DRUG ABUSE ACTIVITIES:
87. Sweeden
88. Hong Kong
89. France
90 Turkey
91. India
92. Canada
93. The Netherlands
94. Other countries
95. England

XII. GAMING AND SIMULATION--COMPUTER PRESENTED:
96. High school age gaming-drug exposures
97. Junior high school age gaming-drug exposure
98. Adult age gaming with drug exposure

XIII. PSYCHOLOGICAL BASIS FOR DRUG PREVENTION:
99. Use of persuasion-lectures
100. Use of religion
101. Conscience and ego-ideal development-scientific
102. Development of scientific decision competency.
103. Psychological-functional autonomy-cognitive dis.

(Please turn over answer sheet and indicate other areas your are really interested in, not mentioned)

END OF QUESTIONNAIRE

REFERENCES

BENFIELD, K. *Comparing Fifth Grade Pupils' Attitude and Ego-Development Ratings With Teacher Performance Ratings.* Unpublished Master's Thesis, University of Wisconsin, Milwaukee, Wisconsin, 1971.

CASSEL, R.N. *The Ego Strength Q-Sort Test and Manual.* Munster, Indiana: Psychometric Affiliates, 1958.

CASSEL, R.N. *Drug Dependency and Addiction.* Jacksonville, Illinois: Psychologists and Educators Press, 1970.

CASSEL, R.N. *Drug Abuse Education.* North Quincy, Massachusetts: Christopher Publishing House, 1972.

CASSEL, R.N. Systems analysis approach to computer-based counseling for addiction treatment (SCNRCO). *Intern. J. Addiction.* 6(3): 493–495, 1971.

CASSEL, R.N. *The Computerized Personal Development Program-PERSDEV.* Jacksonville, Illinois: Psychologists and Educators, Inc., 1973a.

CASSEL, R.N. *The Computerized Human Relations Program-HUMRELAT.* Jacksonville, Illinois: Psychologists and Educators, Inc., 1973b.

CASSEL, R.N. *The Computerized Drug Abuse Education System-PLUDRUG.* Jacksonville, Illinois: Psychologists and Educators, Inc., 1973c.

CASSEL, R.N. *The Psychology of Decision Making.* North Quincy, Massachusetts: Christopher Publishing House, 1973d.

CASSEL, R.N. *The Ego Development Scale and Manual.* Los Angeles, California: Western Psychological Services, 1973e.

CASSEL, R.N. Fundamentals of humanistic psychology. *World J. Psychosynthesis* 5(4): 21–25, 1973f.

LUDWIG, J. *Comparison of Attitudes and Ego-Development of Fifth Grade Pupils for Two Grouping Methods.* Unpublished Master's Thesis. University of Wisconsin, Milwaukee, Wisconsin, 1972.

ROTTER, J. Generalized expectancies for internal versus external control of reinforcement. *Psychol. Monographs.* 80(1): No. 609, 1966.

The International Journal of the Addictions, 9(4), 569–583, 1974

A University System Drug Profile

Jerry L. Strimbu, Ph.D.

National Bank of Detroit
Detroit, Michigan

O. Suthern Sims, Jr., M.A.

Furman University
Greenville, South Carolina

Abstract

This study was undertaken to determine current patterns of drug usage and related behavior of college, university, and junior college students in the University System of Georgia. A maximum saturation survey technique, utilizing a 112-item questionnaire as the primary research tool, resulted in a usable sample of 24,609 student respondents. The focus of attention was on student usage patterns of tobacco, alcohol, marijuana, LSD, glue, narcotics, stimulants, hallucinogens and depressants. An attempt is made to determine patterns of drug use (estimates of current use, history of use, and plans for future use); attitudes, beliefs, and drug use (attitudes toward drug use, and legal controls, and informed sources about drugs); and demographic variables and drug use (sex, age, religion, marital status, spending money, race, parental drug use and attitudes, student living group, and class standing). If one were inclined to construct a profile of a typical university system drug user from the relative frequencies of drug use reported in this paper, it would appear as follows. The student would be a Caucasian, senior male, 21 years of age or older, divorced, Jewish, residing in a commune or on-campus married housing/Greek housing, with access to more spending money than his average peer.

The value of the University System of Georgia drug study lies in the representativeness and size of the sample, number of items in the questionnaire, and the resulting base-line data which enables the system to know the level of usage among its current student population. Before programs can be generated based on these data, it is recommended that a followup of this survey be conducted within the next 12 months.

INTRODUCTION

In the past few years there has been a steadily increasing concern about the use of drugs by student populations. The data indicating that drug abuse is a serious problem in many college populations are accumulating at an alarming rate, with usage estimates of this group ranging from 31 to 62% (Sievert, 1972). The report of the National Commission on Marihuana and Drug Abuse states that in 14 drug surveys conducted between 1965 and 1967, the mean percentage of those who had ever used marijuana was 14%. A review of 26 surveys conducted during 1968 and 1969 showed the mean percentage of student use as 27%, and of the 11 surveys conducted between 1970 and 1971, the mean for use was 45%, more than three times as great as that for the first group.

There have been numerous surveys of college population drug use since 1965 (Anker et al., 1971; Dvorak, 1972; Garfield, Boering, and Smith, 1971; Greenwald and Luetgert, 1971; Grupp, McCain, and Schmitt, 1971; Harris, 1971; Hogan et al., 1970; Milman and Anker, 1971; Smith, 1970; Toohey, 1971), but only one, conducted in 1968 in the Denver-Boulder, Colorado area (Barter, Mizner, and Werme, 1971) is equivalent to the number of students surveyed in the University System of Georgia in the spring of 1972. However, the Denver-Boulder study was a mail survey and not a supervised questionnaire. It also did not have the diversified number of institutions and environmental backgrounds available to the Georgia project.

The Georgia System survey was similar in the scope of its approach to other college level questionnaires, with the drug-related questions designed to estimate the use of alcohol and tobacco besides that of marijuana and "hard drugs," but the number of items in the Georgia survey questionnaire (112) was significantly larger than most of the other college level questionnaires, and thus allowed a greater flexibility in the interpretation of responses in terms of individual institutions within the system.

METHOD

The Subjects

This study was performed at the request and under the direction of the Board of Regents of the University System of Georgia, thus making available the entire student population ($N = 103{,}000$) of the system as potential subjects (*S*s). To obtain the largest number of *S*s, to assure anonymity, and to preclude the possibility of an individual receiving more than one questionnaire, a single exposure maximum saturation sampling technique was implemented. Each of the 28 system institutions designated the class hour and day during which the largest number of students were in attendance, including a breakdown of student allocation by instructor sections. Based on this data, each institution was then provided the appropriate number of survey material packages divided by instructor-classroom segments. The survey was administered to all voluntarily participating students during the specified hour in all classes during the spring of 1972, and returned to a central collection point on campus. Supervision of the member institution surveys was carried out by local test coordinator's office for coding and analysis. Utilization of this approach resulted in a sample of 24,609 respondent answer sheets acceptable for analysis.

The Survey Instrument

The questionnaire used in this survey was composed of 112 multiple-choice items of three general types: (1) classification items (age, sex, race, religious affiliation, housing arrangement, etc.); (2) biographical information items (Schoenfeldt, 1970); and (3) items concerning drug abuse and attitudes toward drugs (Louria, 1968; Strimbu and Schoenfeldt, 1973; University of Georgia Drug Abuse Advisory Committee, 1971). Previous editions of the final questionnaire were administered to two pilot groups to determine completion time and to identify and subsequently revise items producing contradictory results or interpretive difficulty. Completion time of the final questionnaire was approximately 20 min.

PATTERNS OF DRUG USE

The primary purpose of the project was to provide more information concerning the amount of drug usage in the system in order to establish a solid basis for determining the scope of the problem and plans for combating the problem. The focus of attention was on student usage patterns of tobacco, alcohol, marijuana, LSD, glue, narcotics, stimulants, hallucinogens, and depressants.

Estimate of Current Use

Item analysis of the 24,609 subjects responding to the questionnaire indicate that 26.3% ($N = 6{,}477$) were currently using tobacco, 46.3% ($N = 11{,}385$) alcohol, 15.5% ($N = 3{,}804$) marijuana, 1.5% ($N = 359$) LSD, .5% ($N = 128$) glue, .9% ($N = 212$) narcotics, 3.8% ($N = 935$) stimulants, 2.3% ($N = 560$) hallucinogens, and 2.4% ($N = 579$) depressants. Thus the most frequently used substance is still alcohol at all of the institutions surveyed, with all other substances, with the exceptions of tobacco and marijuana, being indicated as having relatively lower levels of current use.

Based on currently acceptable and scientifically enlightened sampling techniques, the results obtained in this study are useful for an accurate inference of current student drug usage on a state-wide basis. Based on this survey's results the following estimates of state-wide student use are possible to establish approximately the number of individuals currently using particular substances: tobacco, 25,908; alcohol, 45,540; marijuana, 15,216; LSD, 1,436; glue, 512; narcotics, 848; strong stimulants, 3,740; hallucinogens, 2,240; and depressants, 2,316.

History of Use

In the total sample of 24,609 students, those who had reportedly at least "tried" one of the drugs was 57.9% for tobacco, 80.2% for alcohol, 38.5% for marijuana, 9.3% for LSD, 4.2% for glue, 6.6% for narcotics, 22.0% for strong stimulants, 11.2% for hallucinogens and 17.0% for depressants.

Generalization of these results to the current student population allows an estimate of the number of students in the state who have at least tried the drugs investigated in this study. These estimates for the entire student population follow: tobacco, 57,072; alcohol, 78,920; marijuana, 37,876; LSD, 9,144; glue, 4,152; narcotics, 6,372; strong stimulants, 27,135; hallucinogens, 11,060; and depressants, 20,885.

Plans for Future Use

Of the students who had never tried any of the substances surveyed, 1.7% said they "might like to try" tobacco in the future, 2.1% said the same for alcohol, 7.6% expressed a possible interest in trying marijuana, 2.6% for LSD, 1.0% for glue, 1.6% for narcotics, 2.8% for strong stimulants, 3.5% for hallucinogens, and 3.1% for depressants.

ATTITUDES, BELIEFS, AND DRUG USE

The second major purpose of the drug usage survey of the University System of Georgia was an attempt to determine some of the factors that lead to drug abuse. The significant variation in usage patterns between the various institutions in the system would indicate that both environmental and biographical variables play a part in the choice of whether or not to experiment with drugs, and that some understanding of these variables may lead to a greater ability to predict, on an a priori basis, those persons most prone to use drugs.

Attitudes toward Drug Use and Legal Controls

Although there was a difference in response between drug users and nonusers to questions concerning family attitudes, parental drug use, and personal attitudes toward the legal and social issues pertaining to drug use, a sizeable percentage of the nonuser group felt that drug usage was a social problem, not a moral-ethical or legal one, and almost 30% of those responding to the question felt that the use of drugs was an individual decision. On the question of legal controls of marijuana, 16.5% of the nonuser group replied that they thought possession of marijuana should be legalized, while only 30% felt that someone caught possessing marijuana should be severely punished.

A larger number of the user group felt that drug usage was an individual decision (45.5%), and a substantial portion of the users (34.5%) agreed with 40.4% of the nonusers that drug usage was a social problem. The user group, however, advocated an extreme relaxation of the legal strictures governing the use of marijuana, with 50.2% responding that marijuana should be legalized, and 23.5% that penalties for possession should be eliminated. It is perhaps significant that neither in the user nor the nonuser group did a substantial percentage of respondents feel that drug usage was a legal problem, but emphasized the social or individual aspects of the problem.

Information Sources about Drugs

Most of the students who used drugs reported that they learned most of their information about drugs either from friends and acquaintances or from the news media, approximately equal sources of information (31.8% from the news media, 31.9% from friends). A substantial portion of the nonuser group (60.8%) reported that the news media was their source of information. In neither group did family, church, or school play a predominant part in their lives as an informational referent. Thus it would appear that the news media plays a very important part in shaping attitudes toward drug usage, and that an approach to the problem of disseminating information on drug usage should recognize that the dominant attitudes in both user and nonuser groups are that drug usage is a social or individual problem, not a legal or moral-ethical one.

DEMOGRAPHIC VARIABLES AND DRUG USE

The third major focus of the questionnaire was directed toward an attempt to gain information about the personal backgrounds and current living conditions of the students in order to understand if there were significant indicators that could establish the characteristics of a person

Table 1

ANOV F-Ratios, Means, and Relative Rank

	Usage item:	Tobacco		Alcohol		Marijuana		LSD	
	F-Ratio:[a]	117.695*		139.726*		83.45*		20.208*	
N	Age group	Mean	Rank	Mean	Rank	Mean	Rank	Mean	Rank
3,932	17–18	2.65	5	3.53	5	2.16	4	1.27	4
10,471	19–20	2.72	4	3.77	4	2.32	3	1.28	3
5,453	21–22	2.89	3	4.07	3	2.52	2	1.33	1
1,792	23–24	3.31	2	4.20	1	2.58	1	1.32	2
2,894	25 or older	3.35	1	4.12	2	1.95	5	1.16	5

[a] All *F*-ratios designated * significant at $p < .01$.

more prone to experiment with drugs. The personal background variables investigated were sex, age, religious background, marital status, racial group, amount of spending money, and parental drug use and attitudes. The student status variables were class standing and student residence.

Sex

On the 14,744 males and 9,731 females who responded to the questionnaire, 44.9% of the males and 29% of the females reported that they had tried marijuana, while 18.3% of the males and only 11.3% of the females reported current usage. In all of the other drugs investigated, with the exception of depressants, male drug usage was higher than that of the female. Thus, contrary to the data gathered by other studies, it would appear that the sex of the respondent bears some relation to the history of drug usage (Strimbu, Schoenfeldt, and Sims, 1973a).

Age

The 25 or older group of students reported the highest usage level of tobacco and the second highest of alcohol (Table 1). On use of other substances, however, the 25 or older group manifests an extremely low level of use, having the lowest use level in five of the seven remaining drug comparisons. Of notable interest is that this older group ranks second in reported use of depressants. There exists a strong relationship on all other substances (except tobacco) and age group up to 25, with the younger groups exhibiting the lowest levels of usage, increasing proportionally by groups to age 25, then abruptly declining to very low levels of usage.

of Age-Groups on Drug Items

Glue 2.329		Narcotics 5.530*		Stimulants 56.344*		Hallucinogens 31.808*		Depressants 13.075	
Mean	Rank	Mean	Rank	Mean	Rank	Mean	Rank	Mean	Rank
1.12	2	1.18	4	1.52	5	1.36	4	1.47	4
1.10	4	1.19	3	1.63	3	1.38	3	1.48	5
1.11	3	1.22	2	1.86	1	1.43	1	1.55	3
1.14	1	1.23	1	1.80	2	1.40	2	1.62	1
1.10	5	1.15	5	1.59	4	1.19	5	1.60	2

Table 2
ANOV F-Ratios, Means, and Relative

	Usage item:	Tobacco		Alcohol		Marijuana		LSD	
	F-Ratio:[a]	33.680		173.273		436.688		335.745	
N	Group	Mean	Rank	Mean	Rank	Mean	Rank	Mean	Rank
2,180	Catholic	2.99	2	4.31	2	2.53	3	1.32	4
15,540	Protestant	2.80	4	3.81	4	2.09	5	1.66	5
596	Jewish	2.90	3	4.09	3	3.17	2	1.42	2
3,725	Other	2.79	5	3.53	5	2.29	4	1.36	3
2,479	None	3.18	1	4.32	1	3.39	1	1.78	1

[a] All *F*-ratios were significant at $p < .001$.

Table 3
ANOV F-Ratios, Means, and Relative

	Usage item:	Tobacco		Alcohol		Marijuana		LSD	
	F-Ratio:[a]	63.958		23.616		76.354		38.917	
N	Group	Mean	Rank	Mean	Rank	Mean	Rank	Mean	Rank
19,061	Single	2.77	5	3.83	4	2.38	3	1.29	4
4,642	Married	3.09	4	3.97	3	1.98	5	1.19	5
448	Divorced, single	3.54	2	4.33	1	2.87	1	1.55	2
176	Divorced, remarried	3.66	1	4.26	2	2.69	2	1.69	1
77	Widowed	3.16	3	3.73	5	2.23	4	1.45	3

[a] All *F*-ratios were significant at $p < .001$.

Religion

The students who reported they had no religious beliefs exhibited the highest usage level in eight of the nine drug substances (the exception was glue), while the Protestant group reported the lowest usage level on seven of the nine drugs, and the second lowest on the two remaining substances (alcohol and tobacco) (Table 2). Those students who had Jewish backgrounds reported either the first or second highest usage levels of seven of the nine drugs, and the third lowest on the items concerning alcohol and tobacco. Those students who responded Catholic or "Other" to the religious preference item generally fell between the highest usage groups (Jewish and None) and the lowest usage group (Protestant).

Rank of Religious Groups

Glue 72.11		Narcotic 162.136		Stimulants 210.801		Hallucinogens 3.66.381		Depressants 111.361	
Mean	Rank	Mean	Rank	Mean	Rank	Mean	Rank	Mean	Rank
1.16	4	1.29	3	1.73	3	1.42	4	1.58	3
1.07	5	1.12	5	1.57	5	1.24	5	1.43	5
1.23	1	1.30	2	1.94	2	1.59	2	1.78	2
1.18	3	1.28	4	1.61	4	1.43	3	1.55	4
1.21	2	1.47	1	2.32	1	1.97	1	1.91	1

Rank of Groups by Marital Status

Glue 52.866		Narcotic 33.790		Stimulants 33.242		Hallucinogens 52.271		Depressants 46.417	
Mean	Rank	Mean	Rank	Mean	Rank	Mean	Rank	Mean	Rank
1.11	4	1.09	4	1.68	4	1.40	4	1.51	4
1.09	5	1.15	5	1.58	5	1.21	5	1.47	5
1.24	3	1.42	3	2.16	2	1.66	2	2.09	1
1.60	1	1.60	1	2.27	1	1.75	1	2.06	3
1.41	2	1.53	2	1.73	3	1.49	3	2.07	2

Marital Status

The two divorced groups (divorced, single and divorced, remarried) are consistently among the highest on reported mean levels of drug abuse, while the married group is consistently lowest (Table 3). The single group ranks third on reported marijuana use, fifth on tobacco, and fourth on mean usage level of all other drugs.

Spending Money

The group which reported less than $2 spending money per week reported the highest use level on the glue and narcotic items, but were generally among the lowest on the remaining seven drugs investigated

Table 4
ANOV F-Ratios, Means, and Relative Rank

N	Usage item: F-Ratio:[a] Group	Tobacco 158.771 Mean	Rank	Alcohol 307.129 Mean	Rank	Marijuana 126.451 Mean	Rank	LSD 22.356 Mean	Rank
983	Under $2	2.35	5	3.21	5	1.91	5	1.31	3
3,981	$2 to $5	2.47	4	3.38	4	1.95	4	1.20	5
7,443	$5 to $10	2.73	3	3.76	3	2.24	3	1.25	4
4,141	$11 to $16	2.98	2	4.13	2	.2.60	1	1.35	1
7,953	$17 or more	3.16	1	4.17	1	2.47	2	1.31	2

[a] All F-ratios were significant at $p < .001$.

Table 5
ANOV, F-Ratios, Means, and Relative Rank

N	Usage item: F-Ratio:[a] Group	Tobacco 8.885 Mean	Rank	Alcohol 116.469 Mean	Rank	Marijuana 37.711 Mean	Rank	LSD 48.062 Mean	Rank
18,254	White/Caucasian	2.87	3	3.99	1	2.34	3	1.28	4
1,955	Black/Negro	2.67	4	3.26	4	1.94	5	1.22	5
76	American Indian	3.12	1	3.81	2	3.16	1	2.15	1
117	Oriental	2.41	5	2.97	5	2.09	4	1.44	3
145	Other	2.99	2	3.61	3	2.73	2	1.95	2

[a] All F-ratios were significant at $p < .001$.

(Table 4). The two groups having more than $11 per week to spend reported the highest usage level on six of the nine drug items.

Race

The American Indian sample, though small, reported the highest usage level of all drugs investigated with the exception of alcohol (Table 5). The Black group differed from the White group on reported mean usage level of four drugs (alcohol, marijuana, stimulants, and hallucinogens), with the White students' usage greater than the Blacks' in all four comparisons. Those students reporting "Other" to the racial classification question reported the second highest drug usage level on all substances except alcohol and significantly differed from the American Indian group *of Groups by Weekly Spending*

Glue 7.574		Narcotic 16.497		Stimulants 117.708		Hallucinogens 44.309		Depressants 37.328	
Mean	Rank	Mean	Rank	Mean	Rank	Mean	Rank	Mean	Rank
1.18	1	1.26	1	1.41	4	1.31	4	1.46	3
1.09	5	1.14	5	1.40	5	1.24	5	1.39	5
1.10	4	1.16	4	1.59	3	1.32	3	1.46	4
1.12	3	1.22	3	1.82	2	1.49	1	1.57	2
1.13	2	1.23	2	1.84	1	1.42	2	1.62	1

of Groups by Race

Glue 130.887		Narcotic 77.154		Stimulants 57.632		Hallucinogens 48.942		Depressants 26.694	
Mean	Rank	Mean	Rank	Mean	Rank	Mean	Rank	Mean	Rank
1.09	5	1.18	5	1.71	3	1.38	4	1.53	4
1.19	4	1.21	4	1.31	5	1.18	5	1.38	5
1.82	1	2.08	1	2.38	1	2.19	1	2.31	1
1.53	3	1.57	3	1.68	4	1.65	3	1.56	3
1.73	2	1.87	2	2.15	2	1.93	2	2.08	2

only on the use of narcotics. The Oriental group ranked lowest on use of tobacco and alcohol, second lowest on marijuana and stimulants, and third in usage of all other drugs investigated (Strimbu, Schoenfeldt, and Sims, 1973b).

Parental Drug Use and Attitudes

In the responses to the questions regarding parental drug usage, it was evident that parents who used prescription or legal drugs, like tranquilizers, sleeping pills, tobacco, or alcohol, were more likely to have children who had at least tried one or more illegal drugs. These findings seem to support the contention that parental drug use patterns influence the use patterns of their children. It was also evident from the data gathered

Table 6
ANOV F-Ratios, Means, and Relative Rank

N	Usage item: / F-Ratio:[a] / Living arrangement	Tobacco 124.29 Mean	Rank	Alcohol 241.08 Mean	Rank	Marijuana 86.60 Mean	Rank	LSD 40.77 Mean	Rank
6,782	Parents	2.64	5	3.52	5	2.09	5	1.24	5
7,557	Dormitories	2.70	4	3.78	3	2.23	4	1.23	4
8,531	Apartment	3.17	1	4.17	2	2.50	3	1.33	2
1,201	Other on campus	2.78	3	4.32	1	2.68	1	1.29	3
467	Commune	3.00	2	3.77	4	2.53	2	1.66	1

[a] All F-ratios were significant at $p < .001$.

Table 7
ANOV F-Ratios, Means, and Relative

N	Usage item: / F-Ratio:[a] / Class standing	Tobacco 17.443* Mean	Rank	Alcohol 129.551* Mean	Rank	Marijuana 16.230* Mean	Rank	LSD 8.028* Mean	Rank
7,211	Freshman	2.76	5	3.62	5	2.23	4	1.29	1
6,321	Sophomore	2.81	4	3.80	4	2.33	3	1.28	2
5,258	Junior	2.88	3	3.97	3	2.34	2	1.27	4
4,378	Senior	3.01	1	4.15	2	2.42	1	1.26	3
1,364	Graduate	2.95	2	4.25	1	2.13	5	1.15	5

[a] All F-ratios designated * significant ($p < .01$).

on parental attitudes toward drug use that parental approval or disapproval of the use of drugs, including tobacco and alcohol, bears a relationship to the student's membership in either the user or nonuser group.

Student Living Group

A communal type of living arrangement generally supported a high level of drug use; however, this group did not report the highest usage of tobacco, alcohol, or marijuana (Table 6). The communal group was exceeded on alcohol consumption by the other on-campus housing group, off-campus housing or apartments, and university dormitory residents. The usage level of communal residents was exceeded in tobacco use by students living in off-campus houses or apartments, and exceeded in marijuana use by those living in other on-campus housing (Strimbu, Sims, and Schoenfeldt, 1973).

of Groups by Living Arrangements

Glue 28.03		Narcotic 40.47		Stimulants 1.34.44		Hallucinogens 35.67		Depressants 42.35	
Mean	Rank	Mean	Rank	Mean	Rank	Mean	Rank	Mean	Rank
1.11	4	1.17	4	1.46	5	1.31	5	1.45	4
1.10	5	1.15	5	1.58	4	1.32	4	1.45	5
1.11	3	1.23	2	1.89	2	1.43	2	1.63	2
1.13	2	1.20	3	1.85	3	1.38	3	1.47	3
1.36	1	1.53	1	1.94	1	1.74	1	1.81	1

Rank of Class-Standing Groups

Glue 4.592*		Narcotic 6.057*		Stimulants 39.67*		Hallucinogens 11.308*		Depressants 2.93	
Mean	Rank	Mean	Rank	Mean	Rank	Mean	Rank	Mean	Rank
1.13	1	1.20	3	1.55	5	1.37	3	1.50	5
1.12	2	1.21	2	1.65	3	1.38	2	1.52	3
1.10	4	1.17	1	1.74	2	1.39	1	1.51	4
1.09	5	1.19	4	1.83	1	1.35	4	1.57	1
1.11	3	1.12	5	1.63	4	1.20	5	1.56	2

Class Standing

The graduate student usage of alcohol is significantly higher than all other class divisions; however, on the LSD, narcotic, hallucinogen, and marijuana comparisons the graduate student group is significantly lower than all other classes (Table 7). The senior class group reported the highest usage level of tobacco, marijuana, strong stimulants, and depressants. Generally, the class standing comparisons of drug usage corresponded to those derived from the age group-drug use responses.

SUMMARY AND CONCLUSION

If one were inclined to construct a profile of a typical university system drug user from the relative frequencies of drug use reported in this paper, it would appear as follows. The student would be a Caucasian, senior male,

21 years of age or older, divorced, Jewish, residing in a commune or on-campus married housing/Greek housing, with access to more spending money than his average peer.

The value of the University System of Georgia drug study lies in the representativeness and size of the sample, number of items in the questionnaire, and the resulting base-line data which enables the system to know the level of usage among its current student population. Before programs can be generated based on these data, it is recommended that a followup of this survey be conducted within the next 12 months.

ACKNOWLEDGMENT

This research was supported in part by a research grant from the Law Enforcement Assistance Administration, United States Department of Justice, under Discretionary Grant #72-DF-04-0037. The study was undertaken while the authors were affiliated with the University of Georgia, Athens, Georgia, and this article is abstracted from the final project report by Jerry L. Strimbu entitled "University System of Georgia Drug Education Program," March 1973.

Copies of the questionnaire booklet are available upon request from O. Suthern Sims, Jr., Vice President for Student Affairs, Furman University, Greenville, South Carolina 29613.

REFERENCES

ANKER, J.L., MILMAN, D.H., KAHAN, S.A., and VALENTI, C. Drug usage and related patterns of behavior in university students; i. general survey and marihuana use. *J. Amer. College Health Assoc.* 19: 178–186, 1971.

BARTER, J.T., MIZNER, G.L., and WERME, P.H. *Patterns of Drug Use among College Students in the Denver–Boulder Metropolitan Area.* Washington, D.C.: Bureau of Narcotics and Dangerous Drugs, U.S. Department of Justice, 1971.

DVORAK, E.J. A logitudinal study of nonmedical drug use among university students —a brief summary. *J. Amer. College Health Assoc.* 20: 212–215, 1972.

GARFIELD, E.F., BOERING, M.L., and SMITH, J.P. Marijuana use on a campus: spring, 1969. *Intern. J. Addictions.* 6: 487–491, 1971.

GREENWALD, B.S., and LUETGERT, M.J. A comparison of drug users and non-users on an urban commuter college campus. *Intern. J. Addictions.* 6: 63–78, 1971.

GRUPP, S.E., McCAIN, M.J., and SCHMITT, R.L. Marijuana use in a small college: a midwest example. *Intern. J. Addictions.* 6: 463–485, 1971.

HARRIS, E.M. A measurement of alienation in college student marijuana users and non-users. *J. School Health.* 41: 130–133, 1971.

HOGAN, R., MANKIN, D., CONWAY, J., and FOX, S. Personality correlates of undergraduate marijuana use. *J. Consult. Clin. Psychol.* 35: 58–63, 1970.

LOURIA, D.B. *The Drug Scene*. New York: McGraw-Hill, 1968.

MILMAN, D.H., and ANKER, J.L. Patterns of drug usage among university students: iv. use of marihuana, amphetamines, opium, and LSD by undergraduates. *J. Amer. College Health Assoc.* 20: 96–105, 1971.

NATIONAL COMMISSION ON MARIHUANA AND DRUG ABUSE. *Marihuana: A Signal of Misunderstanding*. Appendix I, March 1972.

SCHOENFELDT, L.F. *Life Experience as a Moderator in the Prediction of Educational Criteria*. Paper presented at the meeting of the American Educational Research Association, Minneapolis, March 1970.

SIEVERT, W.A. The campus drug scene: a milkman routine. *Chronicle Higher Educ.* 16: 1–4, 1972.

SMITH, B.C. Drug use on a university campus. *J. Amer. College Health Assoc.* 18: 360–365, 1970.

STRIMBU, J.L., and SCHOENFELDT, L.F. Life history subgroups in the prediction of drug usage patterns and attitudes. Accepted for publication in *J. Selected Abstr. Psychol.* 1973.

STRIMBU, J.L., SCHOENFELDT, L.F., and SIMS, O.S., JR. Sex differences in college student drug use. *J. College Student Personnel* 14(6): 507–510, 1973a.

STRIMBU, J.L., SCHOENFELDT, L.F., and SIMS, O.S., JR. Drug usage in college students as a function of racial classification and minority group status. *J. Res. Higher Educ.* 1(3): 263–272, 1973b.

STRIMBU, J.L., SIMS, O.S., JR., and SCHOENFELDT, L.F. College student drug use as a function of place of residence, *J. College Univ. Student Housing*. 3: 38–41, 1973.

TOOHEY, J.V. An analysis of drug use behavior at five american universities. *J. School Health*. 41: 464–468, 1971.

UNIVERSITY OF GEORGIA DRUG ABUSE ADVISORY COMMITTEE. Unpublished paper, School of Pharmacy Student Questionnaire, 1971.

The International Journal of the Addictions, 9(4), 585–592, 1974

Concepts of Life Style in the Treatment of Alcoholism*

William Warren Garitano, M.D.

Ruth E. Ronall, M.S.

New Jersey College of Medicine
Newark, New Jersey

In recent years the term "life style" has become increasingly popular in the general literature and especially in the social sciences. As noted by Ansbacher (1967) in his comprehensive review, its meaning ranges from that of culture or subculture to one that is quite similar to Adler's. In the former it denotes the characteristic mode of living of an individual or group (for example middle-class or jet-set life style), and as such is a useful concept for the description of the *observable common characteristics* of any group, including alcoholics, who may be considered a subculture. In contrast, Adler's concept of life style refers to the individual's *inner consistency*, unity and goal directedness.

In order to distinguish between these two concepts, this paper will refer to the currently popular concept, as it describes clearly observable characteristics, as "cultural life style" and to Adler's concept as "individual life style."

Adler himself defined life style variously, his definitions ranging from

* This is an expanded version of a paper read at the Alfred Adler Centennial Conference, New York, July 1970.

"self or ego" to "life plan" (Lebens Schablone) (Ansbacher and Ansbacher, 1956). For the purpose of this paper, we shall define "individual internal life style" as "a person's characteristic way of moving within his subjective world—i.e., his manner of structuring his life, based on his subjective experience (biased apperception) of himself and of the world around him in relation to himself."

APPLICATION TO ALCOHOLISM

As we considered these two concepts, it seemed to us that they were particularly useful in understanding the dynamics of alcoholism, alcoholism being a complex phenomenon which in the past has tended to be oversimplified. It has too often been reduced to being "only a symptom" of an underlying emotional disorder, or—conversely—to an "illness in itself" to which some persons are susceptible whereas others are immune.

In our view the alcoholic syndrome is the most readily observable aspect of a pathological process. In this process the alcoholic syndrome interacts in a mutually reinforcing fashion with psychopathology of varying degrees, resulting in severe dysfunctioning of the total person. In its extreme manifestations, alcoholism may even submerge the psychopathology to such an extent that it is often difficult to diagnose psychiatrically an active alcoholic even in a state of temporary sobriety.

In other words, alcoholism presents the picture of specific interlocking cultural and individual life styles. These, as well as the processes leading to their development, will be discussed in this paper.

ALCOHOLISM

There are numerous types and typologies of alcoholism. We have confined ourselves in this paper to the most frequent symptomatic type of alcoholism found in this country, described by Jellinek as "gamma alcoholism" (Jellinek, 1960). This is characterized by the definite progression from psychological to physical dependence with concommitant behavioral and physiological changes. Increased tissue tolerance to alcohol, with adaptive cell metabolism withdrawal symptoms and "craving" resulting from physical dependence, and loss of control are part of the syndrome. It passes through several stages: from occasional, to frequent, to daily "relief drinking" (not necessarily excessive in quantity) through daily excessive drinking, daily drunkenness or frequent binge drinking, resulting in decreasing effectiveness and activity in all spheres of living and functioning until, in its final stage, the alcoholic's life revolves around obtaining and consuming alcohol.

Usually it takes several years to develop fully. If recognized, it can be arrested at any stage. Its arrest depends on total abstinence, in most known cases for life.

INDIVIDUAL LIFE STYLE

It is generally assumed that predisposing factors in the personality must be present in order for alcoholism to develop. These factors have so far been described in the literature mostly in psychoanalytic terms. We, however, wish to describe them in terms of typical individual life styles as they were found in the course of evaluating large numbers of patients for treatment.

In the evaluations, specific methods of interviewing were employed: for example, patients were asked to describe themselves in terms of their most outstanding personality characteristics. These were compared with what could be objectively observed about them in the interview situation and what could be inferred from the case history. Earliest memories were elicited and discussed in an effort to determine the individual's earliest perceptions of his mode of interaction. Earliest memories about drinking were also considered in order to determine the meaning a person gave to alcohol.

When the question of common characteristics was discussed with groups of patients, there was a high incidence of agreement among them, so that three essential character traits emerged as representative of this population. These were:

1. A deeply felt sense of inadequacy
2. Hypersensitivity
3. Immaturity

The deeply felt *sense of inadequacy* seems always present in alcoholics. While often confused with guilt over drinking and its secondary effects (such as unmet obligations, monetary losses resulting from excessive drinking, or aggression and violence expressed in a stage of drunkenness), it inevitably antedates the actual drinking period. Earliest childhood memories frequently center on themes of being damaged or abandoned, with accompanying feelings of helplessness. Often enough, there are real physical defects, congenital or arising from illness or injury. Just as often the history reveals the loss of significant persons at an early age or the actual experience of brutal treatment.

The *hypersensitivity* is most noticed in the area of interpersonal relationships, but also in specific areas of talent. When accompanied by high intelligence, this quality is often related to creativity. Yet achievement is often not experienced as success or fulfillment of real ambitions.

By *immaturity* as a character trait is meant not only low frustration tolerance, but also a disturbed sense of time that confines all interest to the present, with little left to the future, resulting in a demand for "instant solutions." With this we find an intolerance to any sort of interference. Conflicts with authority—even of the most benign sort—assume great importance. And even genuine concern is often interpreted as an effort to control and is resisted.

The individual life style is, therefore, typically one in which the person sees himself as abandoned or damaged—helpless in a hostile world. He compensates by ascribing to himself special qualities or talents and by setting grandiose goals for himself to prove that he is worth more than the others think. However, vaguely aware of the discrepancy between these goals and his ability to perform, he is self-critical and easily discouraged. He is hypersensitive to criticism by others which he easily interprets as hostility, thereby proving to himself that others are against him. He suspects even praise and genuine concern, thus creating an ever-growing distance between himself and others, and between his wish to be acceptable to and accepted by others and the possibility of its being fulfilled. He becomes less and less able to tolerate tension or to work steadily toward a goal. To insure himself against failures, he becomes increasingly passive. In short—it is a life style of flight: from tasks, from others, and eventually from oneself.

CULTURAL LIFE STYLE

The question arises now as to why some persons with these particular experiences and individual life styles resort to alcohol as a solution while others do not. It is here that environmental forces and influences come into play, creating the conditions for the development of the "cultural life style" by fostering and encouraging drinking not only for pleasure but for relief.

Ours is a drinking society in which alcohol is used not only as a necessary ingredient on almost any social occasion but also is presented to the public practically as a panacea for any kind of discomfort—although there is much ambivalence, contradiction, and confusion in the ways alcohol use is taught and learned, sanctioned or prohibited, with considerable variations not only between subcultures but within subcultures as well. And yet, only a fraction of drinking Americans become alcoholics. We present the hypothesis, therefore, that it is the preexisting "individual life style" that predisposes a person to alcoholism by producing an affinity to the use of alcohol as a "cultural life style." (We shall mention here physiological predisposition as a possible *additional* factor in the etiology of alcoholism, although none of the numerous theories so far advanced have as yet been validated.)

INTERACTION OF INDIVIDUAL AND CULTURAL LIFE STYLES

We assume, then, that what distinguishes alcoholics as a group is the discovery in themselves of the compatibility of alcohol—which is made available to them and sanctioned by their environment—with their individual life style: as its effect is immediate, it offers instant relief; it presents escape from pain and from the need to deal with tasks; and through its anesthetizing quality it also provides emotional distance. Initially, the alcoholic becomes aware that alcohol enables him—at least for some time—to maintain a facade of coping and personal effectiveness, thereby protecting his secret feelings of inadequacy from discovery. Then, from using alcohol to cope with the life tasks of love, work, and community, he moves toward using alcohol as a substitute—a substitute for performance, for sex, and for people—and lives in increasing isolation and passivity.

With this, the need for neurotic or psychotic symptomatology is gradually reduced, as it may become displaced by purely alcoholic symptoms, including alcoholic psychosis. Alcoholism assumes a momentum of its own and, because of its observability, becomes the focus of the alcoholic's life as well as that of his environment, such as family, friends, employers, and of the caretaking and therapeutic facilities.

IMPLICATIONS FOR TREATMENT

This has important implications for treatment: the alcoholism must be seen as the patient's primary problem, and not—as is so often the case—"only" as the presenting complaint and as a cover-up for the essential underlying pathology. This failure to give the alcoholism its proper weight has been one of the most frequent pitfalls of therapy. Only when the therapist himself is deeply convinced that the alcoholism is not "just a symptom," which somehow will disappear as the underlying neurotic problems are dealt with, can he hope to convey this to the patient.

However, he must also be aware of the threat that giving up alcohol presents to the patient because of the fear it engenders in him of the reemergence of his symptoms. Therefore, the therapist must be prepared to help his patients face their symptomatology and to offer some substitute for the pain-relieving quality of the alcohol.* This necessitates considerable ingenuity and flexibility and is an additional requirement for the therapist of alcoholics.

When this intitial stage of therapy has begun to take effect, i.e., when the patient begins to experience himself as an alcoholic, a second stage must be initiated: preventing the alcoholic from taking refuge in the identity with the problem. For once their identity with the cultural life style has been established, patients will tend to accept as irreversible the limitations and handicaps typically associated with the alcoholic cultural life style. Thus the alcoholic derives on the one hand the benefit of the increased sense of communality—increased social interest—but, on the other hand, he tends to resign himself and those around him to the limits and handicaps stereotypically ascribed to alcoholics such as forgetfulness, lateness, and inability to keep appointments. His attitude can be summed up in the rhetorcial question: "What do you expect from an alcoholic?": a question which can be applied with great flexibility to a vast range of life tasks and responsibilities, be they in therapy, marriage, or business.

We can then begin the third stage which is to confront the patient with the contradictions and self-defeating aspects of his individual life style. Having stressed and encouraged the awareness of communality, we can then stress the uniqueness of each individual without equating this with isolation.

This can be strikingly observed in group therapy where the individual first experiences, often as a revelation, that his capacity for relatedness is so much greater when sober than when drinking or drunk. The traditional joviality, the detached bonhomie, the superficiality which arises from being emotionally anesthetized, and thereby well insulated, no longer suffices once the individual has come to experience genuine relatedness.

* This is what AA provides through their numerous group meetings, systems of sponsors, "telephone therapy," etc., and what hospitals provide through their protective environment in which medication can be used safely.

And, as the individual becomes aware of himself in interaction and subjects himself to honest peer criticism, he is able to drop the façade and accept what he is able to recognize in himself and that to which others respond. Gradually, patients come to define and reveal their "deep secrets," their underlying deep feelings of inadequacy. When these are revealed and confronted without catastrophic consequences, the individual can with relief begin to reevaluate other aspects of his personality.

While this defines to some extent what occurs in all therapy, the difference lies in the fact that the alcoholic's cultural life style is so deeply ingrained and intertwined with his pathological individual life style that relapses and regressions are almost inevitable and often dramatic, so that it is difficult for the therapist and patient to know to what extent progress is being made. This necessitates frequent repetition, the recognition and acceptance that the stages of therapy will often overlap and sometimes will need to be reversed, and finally the courage of both patient and therapist to begin again seemingly from the beginning as often as needed.

SUMMARY

We have discussed two concepts of life style as they relate to the syndrome of alcoholism. Their interrelatedness and interaction are described as a means for the understanding and treatment of alcoholism. Basically, the individual life style is shaped by a person's need for compensating for his deep sense of inadequacy. He compensates with increasingly grandiose goals and schemes. Because of the discrepancy between these goals and his ability to perform, along with his use of alcohol, a downward spiral of discouragement and lessened activity results. He thus moves, without awareness, toward a goal of total safety from failure through increasing passivity. This style may be described as one of flight—from tasks, from people, and from self.

The cultural life style of drinking develops when the individual discovers the compatibility of alcohol—readily available in his environment—with his individual life style. He uses alcohol often at first to cope with tasks, later almost inevitably as a substitute.

In the treatment of alcoholics the therapeutic task is therefore always twofold as it requires the understanding and modification of both the cultural and individual life styles. Alcoholics are viewed as being discouraged to the point where to them survival seems to depend on the use of alcohol. The therapist, therefore, has to encourage them sufficiently so that they can visualize a life worth living without alcohol and are ready to give up drinking. Simultaneously he must promote emotional growth through confrontation with and modification of the individual life style.

REFERENCES

ANSBACHER, H.L. Life style: A historical and systematic review. *J. Individual Psychol.* 23 (2): 191–212, 1967.

ANSBACHER, H., and ANSBACHER, R. *The Individual Psychology of Alfred Adler*. New York: Basic Books, 1956, p. 174.

JELLINEK, E.M. *The Disease Concept of Alcoholism*. New Haven, Connecticut: College and University Press, 1960, pp. 37–38.

The International Journal of the Addictions, 9(4), 593–604, 1974

Treating the Drug-Dependent Veteran—Perspective from a Veterans Administration Hospital

William W. Van Stone, M.D.

Veterans Administration Hospital
and Department of Psychiatry
Stanford University Medical School
Palo Alto, California

INTRODUCTION

This paper attempts to describe some of the lessons learned over the past few years in initiating a drug dependency treatment program at the Palo Alto Veterans Administration Hospital.

Most professionals who have been involved in setting up a drug program in an existing institution have undoubtedly gone through many of our own experiences. The literature on introducing change into any organization and on methods of changing attitudes in groups is useful and pertinent (Bennis, Benne, and Chin, 1969; Blake and Mouton, 1969; Ellsworth, Dickman, and Maronen, 1972; Gardner, 1965; Levinson, 1964; Toffler, 1970; Townsend, 1970).

Starting a drug program before the influx of new federal funding in mid-1971 gave us one distinct advantage at our hospital. We knew that if our programs did not win the support of the director, the chief of staff, the local community, security staff, physicians, and other professionals in the hospital, it would be shut down. There is something comforting in that. We could state factually to our patients that certain forms of misbehavior or lack of self-policing would result in their program being discontinued, and the support it might offer thereby becoming unavailable to them or their peers. They were forced to develop ways of handling problems arising from the programs without calling upon a resident physician, the night nursing supervisor, or a convenient ward for disturbed psychiatric patients. The creative and manipulative skills of our patients were thus directed to preserving this very special unit of theirs rather than toward outwitting a well-meaning but naive staff. Furthermore, as in any competitive enterprise, the rewards of space, personnel, and equipment were appreciated because they were won in fierce competition with other consumers of hospital funds. In contrast, many recent VA drug programs were started when adequate but unsolicited funds were suddenly granted to surprised and wary hospital administrators, with instructions to start a full-fledged drug program immediately. It should not be unexpected then to find that some of the programs so spawned were found using excessive medications or unsolicited love and permissiveness hopefully to bribe their similarly surprised and wary addict patients to "get well." By now, many of these instant programs may have experienced the cleansing and righteous indignation of hospital communities and as a consequence are developing more solidly.

BACKGROUND

Our first entry into the drug dependency field came as an outgrowth of a visit in 1965 to Synanon and to a so-called "character disorder ward" at Oak Knoll Naval Hospital. In the spring of 1968 we opened our "confrontation ward" based on knowledge gained about these programs and about the drug and alcohol units at California's Mendocino State Hospital. Our experience with this peer confrontation approach in a VA setting was surprisingly positive, although we rarely saw heroin addicts at that time (Van Stone and Gilbert, 1972). In the fall of 1970 a group associated with the Stanford Department of Psychiatry and another group at our Menlo Park Division became interested in creating two additional residential rehabilitation programs in our hospital. These were to be more eclectic and hoped to focus on the young, multidrug dependent Vietnam veteran.

Our first prolonged experience with a "hard core" heroin addict was in October 1969. Mr. W. was a 41 year old Black, ghetto-reared, ex-con who was also rated by the VA as 100% disabled due to schizophrenia. He was a rather talented artist, but was unable to solve his severe dependency needs and pull himself together enough to stabilize his life, with or without heroin. At that time the prospect of treating the well-publicized withdrawal syndrome of a certified heroin addict, even on a closed psychiatric ward, was unnerving to our entire staff. However, since we had a big hospital and he was only one small man, and schizophrenic at that, we determined to undertake the experiment. It was anticlimactic when we learned how easy it was to detoxify Mr. W. with methadone; but then we learned how difficult it was to keep him from readdicting himself. We tried him out on the total range of our psychiatric programs without success. We then attempted to place him in a new community methadone maintenance program but they found him ineligible. By the spring of 1971, as more cases like Mr. W. began to come in, we were quite willing and able to get into the detoxification and methadone maintenance business—at least on a small scale. Subsequently, Mr. W. was placed in our methadone maintenance program, and the fact that he has been relatively trouble-free since has been useful in gaining professional support for an enlarged methadone maintenance clinic.

One of the other things we learned from contact with patients like Mr. W. is that probation officers, lawyers, judges, courts, and postponed hearings all play primary roles in the day-to-day anxieties and realities of these veterans. We also discovered the phenomenal influence of street mythology and hysteria regarding illicit drugs, not only among the drug users but within our own staff. For example, Mr. W.'s wife believed that distilled water taken before a urine test would hide any heroin in the urine. In addition, one of our best head nurses is still convinced that cocaine washes evidence of heroin out of the urine in spite of information to the contrary.

As a result of our experiences, we were, therefore, somewhat better prepared than others when in September 1971 we received funding to expand our programs and to treat heroin addicts on a larger scale. After 1 or 2 weeks of waiting, our 15 authorized detoxification beds were suddenly overwhelmed by 30 to 45 admissions per week; and our methadone maintenance programs, both at the hospital and at our San Francisco Satellite, rapidly filled up. By mid-January, in order to maintain even minimal standards of admission and treatment procedures, we were forced to start a methadone maintenance waiting list. Like other methadone programs across the country, we have consistently underestimated the demand for detoxification and maintenance as well as the emotional drain these patients have placed on our staff.

TREATMENT MODALITIES

General Organization

Our current VA drug dependence program consists of a 15-bed, well-staffed detoxification ward primarily dealing with heroin users, a methadone maintenance clinic at our Menlo Park Division and in San Francisco, and three residential settings, one of which offers inpatient methadone maintenance to selected patients. Our overall strategem is to contact drug-dependent veterans where and when we find them, give them a chance to see who we are and what we can offer, then attempt to negotiate a (psychological) contract which will spell out what they can expect and what the program expects from them. A mutual acceptance must be achieved before a man may enter a program. Most veterans come into our detoxification ward where they are withdrawn and then assigned to (or select) a program, negotiate with program representatives, and either transfer to the program or return home when their detoxification is completed.

A smaller number who do not require detoxification enter programs directly; others come from general psychiatric or medical wards or are referred from jails or courts. Transfers from programs to community resources occur when appropriate.

Detoxification Ward

The primary drugs of abuse in our area since 1971 have been barbiturates and alcohol, heroin and methadone, stimulant drugs such as amphetamines and cocaine, and the psychedelics such as LSD.

We found, after consultation with Dr. David Smith at the Haight-Ashbury Clinic in San Francisco, that the only drugs requiring inpatient detoxification, from a medical viewpoint, are our old friends, *barbiturates and alcohol.* Withdrawal seizures and delirium tremens are still life-threatening and dangerous in comparison with withdrawal symptoms from other drugs. We chose to detoxify heroin in the hospital because, frankly, we needed to learn about it; and we excluded alcohol detoxification from this ward because the demand for such service appeared to be so great we feared there would be no beds for drug addicts. One myth that should be dispelled in this regard is that alcoholics cannot also be dope addicts and vice versa. We have found that there is an increasing overlap of alcohol and narcotic use in both the young and middle-aged drug-dependent veteran.

We have found that detoxifying *heroin addicts* using decreasing doses of methadone over a period of a few days to a week is without complication, comfortable, and acceptable to the addicts. We also learned that from a purely medical viewpoint, withdrawal from heroin "cold turkey" is no worse than a bad case of the flu—with sweating, muscle and stomach cramps, diarrhea, nausea, vomiting, and minimal fever. We learned the importance of these symptoms when our Mr. W., who had been temporarily admitted to a local state hospital, was almost operated on for an "acute abdominal infection" before the attending surgeon could be convinced that his patient was undergoing forced withdrawal from methadone because of his incarceration.

As with our Mr. W., we have continued to have very poor results keeping detoxified addicts off heroin once they hit the streets unless they are on methadone maintenance or enter a residential program. During a 7-month period in 1972, 61% of 383 heroin addicts who entered our detoxification ward and expressed some interest in rehabilitation eventually voluntarily entered one of our programs. Most of those who entered had been on our detoxification ward three to six times before they made their decision. Thus it appears that gradual and multiple exposure of the addict to our programs eventually pays off.

We have seen very few *amphetamine* cases in this unit, but those who come respond well to rest, small doses of phenothiazines, and psychological support. We have rarely seen the "speed freak" who presents acutely in a severe paranoid toxic state and is said to be dangerous. These are treated in an acute psychiatric ward rather than on the drug unit. *Cocaine* is reported to be increasing in popularity and we are beginning to see more cases. Acute *LSD* states are also unusual in our setting but are seen occasionally on our psychiatric wards. Regarding LSD, the Haight-Ashbury Clinic strongly urged us against the use of Thorazine for LSD toxicity or "bad trips." Their experience would lead them to believe that peer support and "talking down" leads to a substantially decreased incidence of later flashbacks (Shick and Smith, 1970). We have not seen this confirmed.

Perhaps because our hospital is not in an urban center and receives few acute emergencies, we have seen few narcotic overdose cases. We have, however, seen both kinds of overdoses that are reported: the slower respiratory depression type and the immediate presumably allergic type where the needle may still be found in the addict's vein. Where mixed drug use is common, and where an addict or his friend may not know what he has been taking, the multiple-drug overdose presents difficult diagnostic problems (Sheppard, Gay, and Smith, 1972).

The social ethic on our detoxification ward deserves comment. Although we try to minimize barriers to admission, we have been very strict about our rules once the patient is inside: no visitors, one phone call prior to discharge, hospital greens, and no leaving the ward without accompaniment. No matter what we do in the way of security, however, a supportive attitude by the staff plus partial control of the program by ex-addict counselors seems to us to be very important. The addict coming in for detoxification is invariably suspicious and distrusting, and may carry a "stash" with him or make arrangements for delivery once he is on the ward. However, when he hears from his peers and sees for himself that the program is not degrading and that our detoxification is safe and comfortable, he generally does not bring heroin or other drugs on the ward.

Unresolved problems that seem most pressing at this time on the detoxification ward are primarily medical. A large number of our addicts have enlarged livers and nonspecific abnormal liver function tests not necessarily consistent with acute or chronic serum hepatitis. In addition, we see many cases of early latent syphilis and, for unknown reasons, about one-half of our serological tests for syphilis (VDRL) are false positive as confirmed with the FTA (Fluroescent Treponema Antibody) test. The causes of these phenomena are unclear.

Methadone Maintenance

Our clinic at Menlo Park started under the direction of an ex-addict counselor, himself on methadone, supervised by a part-time psychiatrist with little prior experience in drug abuse. Our early program, characterized as "by addicts, for addicts," was well attended and, for the most part, presented no major problems. However, doses were high, many above 100 mg/day, and no one was coming off drugs. When additional professional staff was added with better funding in 1972, we found increasing conflicts due to inaccurate reporting practices and a supervisory system among the counselors and patients that combined judicious intimidation, giving of favors, and a general belief that psychoactive drugs solve all personal and most physical problems. Our replacement of the original staff has led to better morale both among the new staff and those patients who were interested in abandoning the drug-dependent life.

Our methadone clinic staff, both in Menlo Park and at our San Francisco Satellite, now generally subscribe to the theoretical formulation of Goldstein (1972) regarding the relative benefits of a dose between 40 and 70 mg daily and the eventual goal of withdrawal from all narcotics including methadone. Use of supportive services, teaching nondrug coping skills, and a general attitude that patients on methadone are adults capable of working and managing their lives are now predominant.

Residential Settings

Our earliest residential setting, modeled after programs at Mendocino State Hospital and Oakland Naval Hospital, developed uniquely but maintained the characteristic features of these programs. In the author's opinion, the five important ingredients are (Van Stone and Gilbert, 1972):

1. *An individualized, negotiated treatment "contract" between each potential member and his peers.* An understanding between the neophyte and his brothers generally starts from the first contact and culminates in an intense group intake interview which serves also as an initiation ceremony into the new peer group "fraternity."
2. *A 24-hr-a-day live-in setting away from the previous social milieu of the participants.* The new members are expected to stay relatively isolated for several months before returning home, hopefully having learned a more adaptive set of values and coping skills.
3. *A drug and medication-free environment, strongly oriented toward honesty, personal growth, and learning.* Feelings of loving and being loved, of real concern for each other, and a warm, family-like atmosphere are seen. An intense identification with the total group and its values is encouraged, formation of spontaneous subgroups or "pairing" between members is treated as an immediate threat to the entire program.
4. *A highly authoritarian, yet member-controlled social structure* constantly evolving from within the membership with graduated responsibilities, status, and jobs designated for each member. Paid staff are treated no differently than patients with regard to their responsibility for their behavior in or out of the program, and on more than one occasion a staff member has been expelled by the

membership. Self-esteem is build on daily achievement, and destructive behavior is stringently discouraged at its earliest inception.

5. *Group confrontation sessions, often called "the game."* During these periodic group sessions each member in turn is presented forcefully with candid, personal facts regarding every observable behavior or attitude recognized by the group as being self defeating or dishonest. "Gut language" at high intensity is often heard. Leverage is obtained for changed behavior by the threat of abandonment and ridicule, not from the straight world but from the member's own peer group.

This kind of setting is designed to break down maladaptive character defenses and teach an alternative life style, but in our experience only a minority of patients is motivated or capable of the intensive self-scrutiny required. One is caught in the dilemma that such a "tight program" that is, incidentally, demonstrably safe to have in a community or institution, is best suited for the most highly motivated drug user who is thoroughly fed up with the addictive life style. The man who is still intrigued by the high prestige of the addict in the deviant subculture is rarely willing to enter such a demanding program. Therefore we felt we must experiment not only with such a group confrontation program, but with intermediate or alternative settings that also may attract those less motivated.

One such program at our hospital, based on the peer confrontation model, had modified the social structure by allowing its members occasionally to use certain psychoactive chemicals such as minor tranquilizers or beer away from the hospital. Recent experiences with that program, however, led to a reevaluation of this position and the establishment of a policy forbidding all psychoactive drugs or medications. Hair styles, clothing, and argot consistent with the youth culture still predominate, in contrast to the more conventional appearance and language required in the parent program. This second program places emphasis on reentry of its members into the community in graduated steps. Its leader encourages individual "raps" (discussions) between members and the primarily nonprofessional staff, and attempts to provide "alternative highs" through emphasis on recreation and sports. A modified "attack therapy" is also important.

The third program is modeled more after Maxwell Jones' therapeutic community (Jones, 1953). It employs a high professional staff to patient ratio and uses the full array of dynamic psychotherapies, both individual and group. Emphasis is on negotiated written "contracts," rules, and contingencies regarding ward behavior, but more importantly on a real concern by the entire community for each member. Methadone maintenance for selected addicts may be prescribed after a trial period in the program, and minor tranquilizers are used when indicated.

Because of current controversy regarding the value of residential settings for rehabilitation of drug abusers, both absolutely and vis-à-vis methadone clinics, controlled clinical experimentation and follow-up is important to determine: (1) what kinds of staffing, organization, and beliefs will survive in an institution or in the community; and (2) what system is most successful for what kind of patient at what time in his life. Our hospital is engaged in such research at this time (Bales et al., 1973).

General Issues

The general public has remarkably strong feelings and opinions about drug misuse and drug misusers. Thus drug programs are unusually susceptible to rumors, misunderstandings, and blackmail. We all hope that, as scientific methods and facts replace speculation or uncritical faith in any authoritative opinion, these phenomena will diminish. In our experience, however, public, staff, and patients alike want immediate explanations and seem to turn to rumor and unsubstantiated conclusions almost by preference. The importance of constant education, training, communication, and attempts to create an informed community of which the drug program is an integral part must be stressed. In particular, we cannot overemphasize the importance of working closely with local police and security staff to allay their suspicions.

One technique that has worked in counteracting destructive rumors at our facility is to help the disputants separate concretely (a) objective reality from (b) speculation and from (c) what may be best called "character assassination." The intervention is simply a labeling process. In column "a" list realistic problems, objective facts, or direct observations such as "George appears to be nodding" or "three patients didn't get chest x-rays." In column "b" list speculations and unsupported rumors that attempt to explain the facts. Examples are: "George is dealing" or "our patients are given the lowest priorities." In column "c" identify pure accusations or assumptions about someone else's thoughts, motives, character or paternity, and other items in this general category. Here are examples: "George is a contaminant to our program" or "that prejudiced so-and-so ought to be fired!"

Aside from the problems of introducing a drug program where techniques are known and have precedents into an institution or community, there are other problems in drug rehabilitation that have no sure answers as yet. In the next few years we hope to develop methods for withdrawing addicts from methadone and to help them avoid the addictive life style completely.

A promising approach through psychopharmacology is to find a longer-acting chemical analog of methadone, or better yet, a nonaddictive blocking agent. This field is developing now; however, there is no drug available today that has been proven safe and effective and at the same time is acceptable to the addict population. The use of new drugs in combination with psychosocial approaches may prove more effective than either alone.

Lastly, there is the enormously complicated and unsolved problem of discovering effective techniques for education and prevention with regard to drug dependence and for promoting cooperation between the many agencies involved in controlling and treating drug abusers.

SPECIAL PROBLEMS

Ex-Addict Counselors

We currently employ about a dozen counselors with varied backgrounds and have used them in a variety of settings. We have reluctantly had to abandon the hopeful myth of their incontestable expertise and are now trying to find where they are most useful and where not. We have found that while the ex-addict drug counselor is knowledgable about street culture and language and about his own subjective experience with drugs he has used, he is incredibly naive about the actual pharmacology of drugs, and he is often no better than the rest of us at detecting someone else who is on drugs. He can offer little in the way of a nondrug oriented life style unless he has been through a therapeutic community-type program, in which case, however, he may be a tremendous asset and provide crucial leadership. He is, at any rate, unmatched in creating rapport with new addicts coming into a program and his very presence offers evidence and encouragement that the drug life style can be defeated.

Many of our counselors are still in transition and need either ongoing support from supervisors, a strong peer-group ethic, or both. Our counselors now indicate that they want and need training. We recommend that each man plan his career individually with the assumption that *drug* counseling per se is essentially a vocational dead end. In these rapidly changing times, to build one's professional identity on being an ex-anything is bound, eventually, to cause frustration or at least a feeling of irrelevance. We encourage junior college courses and in-service training in nursing, administration, counseling, business, social science, and psychology so that a career as "drug counselor" may be temporary and eventually lead to a productive life-style free of the drug culture entirely.

Armed Services Medical Regulating Office (ASMRO)

The question of the returning, active duty, drug-dependent serviceman has been with us since mid-1971. As of July 1973 we have seen about 210 of them come through our hospital. These men were found to have had heroin in their urine while on active duty. They were subsequently classified by ASMRO as unsuitable for retention because of a lack of motivation or because they had so few days of their military obligation remaining that rehabilitation in the service was considered inappropriate.

Following a brief detoxification and rehabilitation period in a service hospital, they are transferred to the VA hospital nearest their home for exposure to a VA drug rehabilitation program. Our hope is that they will see the VA as a resource if and when they decide they need help. In our experience they are usually unwilling to acknowledge that they have any drug problem and maintain that their primary motivation is to finish their military obligation and get home. Because they do not see themselves as patients, they do not fit anywhere in our hospital and have, with few exceptions, rejected and been rejected by our residential rehabilitation programs. Once they find out what base they are attached to, who has their pay record, what their expected date of discharge is, and know that they are still subject to military discipline, they seem to cause relatively little trouble although they still tend to reject intensive treatment. Most of these men are primarily interested in finding out: (1) what is left of their relationships back home; (2) what kind of job they are best suited for; and (3) what has happened to the American culture while they were away. We are currently engaged in an outpatient program with these needs in mind.

SUMMARY

Initiating drug dependence treatment programs within a Veterans Administration Hospital poses (1) general problems related to change in any large institution and (2) special problems resulting from mutual suspicions between the hospital staff and the drug-using population. This paper describes knowledge gained over the past 4 years in the course of initiating a detoxification ward, three different residential settings, and two methadone clinics. Experiences with ex-addict counselors and with active military duty personnel sent to the VA for rehabilitation are included. No specific conclusions are drawn other than that effective drug treatment programs can be established in a VA hospital setting.

REFERENCES

BALES, R., ENGELSING, T., KULDAU, J., VAN STONE, W., and ZARCONE, V. *Proceedings of the Fifth National Conference on Methadone Treatment.* New York: National Association for Prevention of Addiction to Narcotics, 1973, pp. 1027–1034.

BENNIS, W.C., BENNE, K.D., and CHIN, R. *The Planning of Change.* New York: Holt, Rinehart and Winston, 1969.

BLAKE, R.R., and MOUTON, J.S. *Building a Dynamic Corporation Through Grid Organizational Development.* Reading, Massachusetts: Addison-Wesley, 1969.

ELLSWORTH, R.B., DICKMAN, H.R., and MARONEN, R.J. Characteristics of productive and unproductive unit systems in VA psychiatric hospitals. *Hospital Community Psychiat.* 23(9): 261–268, 1972.

GARDNER, J. *How to Prevent Organizational Dry Rot.* New York: Harpers, 1965.

GOLDSTEIN, A., The Pharmacologic Basis of Methadone Treatment. In *Fourth National Conference of Methadone Treatment, Proceedings.* New York: National Association for Prevention of Addiction to Narcotics, 1972, pp. 27–32.

JONES, M. *The Therapeutic Community.* New York: Basic Books, 1953.

LEVINSON, H. *Emotional Health: In the World of Work.* New York: Harper and Row, 1964.

SHEPPARD, C.W., GAY, G.R., and SMITH, D.E. Emergency Treatment of Acute Depressant Drug Overdose. *Missouri Med.* 69: 109–111, 119, 1972.

SHICK, J., and SMITH, D.E. Analysis of the LSD Flashback. *J. Psychedel. Drugs* 3(1): 13–19, 1970.

TOFFLER, A. *Future Shock.* New York: Random House, 1970.

TOWNSEND, P. *Up the Organization.* New York: Knopf, 1970.

VAN STONE, W.W., and GILBERT, R. Peer Confrontation Groups: What, Why, and Whether. *Amer. J. Psychiat.* 129(5): 583–589, 1972.

The International Journal of the Addictions, 9(4), 605–617, 1974

Experiences with a Combination of Group Therapy and Methadone Maintenance in the Treatment of Heroin Addiction*

John C. LaRosa, M.D.

Stephen H. Lipsius, M.D.

Judith H. LaRosa, R.N., M.N.Ed.

Drug Dependence Program
The George Washington University Medical Center
Washington, D.C.

Major American urban centers, including the Washington, D.C. area, have recently been experiencing an epidemic of heroin addiction (Dupont, 1971). A variety of therapies for heroin dependence have been proposed. At one extreme are therapeutic communities like Synanon (Markoff, 1969) which reject the use of all drugs and which in essence remove the addict from society. Therapeutic communities allow addicts to share some of their common experiences and feelings and permit the extensive use of

*Reprint requests should be directed to Dr. John C. LaRosa, The George Washington University Medical Center, 2150 Pennsylvania Avenue, N.W., Washington, D.C. 20037.

ex-addicts in the therapeutic process. The major disadvantage of such programs is that they isolate the addict from the community to which he must eventually return. Little data is available, moreover, on the ultimate fate of addicts returning to the community.

At the other extreme are those programs in which psychological support is minimal and in which the replacement of illegal heroin by legal methadone is central. The rationale for such therapy rests on the assumption that the antisocial behavior of many addicts is the result rather than the cause of heroin dependence and that, when such dependence is interrupted, antisocial behavior disappears or is diminished without the need for ancillary psychological support (Dole and Nyswander, 1968). While the effectiveness of methadone maintenance alone for certain subgroups of heroin addicts, especially older addicts who have not been actively abusing multiple drugs (Dole and Nyswander, 1967), is probably high, considerable question exists about its applicability in the treatment of younger addicts and those with a history of multiple drug abuse. Dole, Nyswander, and Warner (1968) have noted that methadone alone is not always sufficient in enabling their patients to withdraw from heroin and have found it necessary to maintain patients for long periods of time on methadone in order to prevent their return to active heroin abuse.

A small program for the treatment of heroin dependent patients who, in addition, have habitually used other drugs has been in operation at The George Washington University Medical Center since July 1971. The program has combined some of the features of both methadone maintenance programs and therapeutic communities. Psychotherapy has been given either by mental health professionals (nurses or social workers with Master's level training) or by ex-addict counselors, all under the supervision of a staff psychiatrist. This report details our experience with this program after approximately 1 year of operation.

METHODS

Patient Selection

All patients selected for the program lived within an arbitrarily defined district surrounding The George Washington University Medical Center and were volunteers. All were interviewed initially by the two individuals who administered the day-to-day program and were then interviewed by both the medical director and psychiatric director. Only patients with a history of at least 1 year of heroin abuse, a history of habitual abuse of at least one other drug (excluding marijuana but including alcohol), and a history of at least one unsuccessful trial of abstinence from heroin were accepted into the program. By selecting only patients with multiple drug experiences it was our hope to develop a program not directed solely to heroin abuse but rather one which would allow us to gain experience with multiple drug abusers. Patients were required to have previously tried abstinence, since all patients in the program were treated initially with methadone (see below).

A subjective judgment of the patient's motivation was made by all the interviewers, and patients who were felt to have a particularly low motivation for engaging in definitive therapy were excluded from admission. Each patient was given a complete medical history and physical examination upon admission to the program and was assigned to an internist in the University Clinic for follow-up of any medical problems. An initial laboratory survey, including a chest x-ray, electrocardiogram, serological test for syphilis, complete blood count, urinalysis, BUN, fasting blood sugar, uric acid, cholesterol, calcium, phosphorus, alkaline phosphatase, bilirubin, SGOT, LDG, total protein, and albumin, was obtained on all patients. A fee of $1/day was required for all patients in the program.

Methadone Therapy

All patients initially accepted into the program were placed on daily methadone therapy. All were begun on methadone dosages between 20 and 40 mg/day. In the beginning of the program, most patients reached a dose of 100 mg/day within the first 2 months and were stabilized at that level. Patients were required to come to the Medical Center and receive their methadone under the supervision of one of the program administrators on a daily basis. Those in the program longer than 3 months were permitted to take home methadone over the weekend, but all were required to take methadone at the clinic on weekdays. Urine specimens were obtained on 2 days/week and analyzed for the presence of heroin, quinine (with which most heroin in the D.C. area is mixed), methadone, and other drugs (including amphetamines and barbiturates). Patients were not observed in the act of urination but were required to give a fresh specimen on the premises. Initially, weekend privileges were curtailed on the basis of urines indicating continued drug abuse. This was discontinued, however, when it became clear that there was widespread attempts to falsify urine samples. Subsequently, patients were told that no privileges would be curtailed on the basis of urine results but rather that these results would help the staff in judging the effectiveness of therapy.

Day-to-Day Program Operations

The day-to-day operation of the clinic was run jointly by two individuals, one an ex-military corpsman with no personal history of drug abuse, the other a young college dropout who lived in the catchment area and who had personally used "soft" drugs (including marijuana and amphetamines) but had never been drug dependent and had never used heroin. These individuals were responsible for dispensing methadone, collecting urine samples, and keeping all records pertinent to those operations as well as recording their own observations on all patient behavior. Methadone was dispensed in a room which was part of the General Medical Clinic and was open only during the clinic working day. Patients were permitted to stay for as little or as long as they wished, and it was considered part of the job of the two program administrators to be available for minor problems or discussions with patients. Major issues between patients and staff were referred either to the group therapy sessions (see below) or to the general staff meeting (see below). In practice, many patients, particularly in the initial stages of their involvement with the program, spent long periods of time in the office talking informally with each other and with the program administrators. In many cases the individual from the community became a kind of ombudsman for the patients, helping them with legal problems, finding them jobs, following up on patients who were missing or dropped out of the program, etc.

Group Therapy Sessions

Group therapy sessions were conducted 3 hr/week, each session lasting $1\frac{1}{2}$ hr. Therapy sessions were not begun until 40 patients had enrolled in the program. At that time, each patient was assigned in random fashion to one of four groups, two led by a mental health professional, two by an ex-addict counselor. Both mental health professionals (MHP) were White females with Master's level training, one with a Master's Degree in Psychiatric Nursing, the other with a Master's Degree in Psychiatric Social Work. The other two groups were led by ex-addict counselors (EAC), both Black females, both of whom had had 18 months training in group therapy techniques at the Psychiatric Institute of Washington, D.C. All four of these individuals met with the staff psychiatrist for 1 hr/week, where issues raised in the therapy sessions and group processes were discussed. In addition, the entire staff met for 1 hr/week at which time administrative matters were discussed and the progress of individual patients were reviewed. In these meetings, requests for detoxification, as well as discussions of special patient problems, were conducted, usually with the patient present.

Attendance at group therapy sessions was mandatory. Patients who missed sessions without an excuse deemed sufficient by the staff were penalized with the loss of weekend take-home privileges, one weekend for each group session missed. Repeated absences from group sessions led to expulsion from the program.

Methadone Detoxification

Patients were permitted to discontinue methadone if they were able to obtain approval for such a course of action both from their group and from their group leader. They were then required to appear before the staff at one of the weekly meetings and explain their position. If the staff approved, the patient was permitted to detoxify from methadone and remain in the program until the staff felt that he was ready for discharge. Remaining in the program meant that he continued to go to group therapy sessions, give urine specimens, and be welcomed in the program office. Patients who wished to leave the program against medical advice were permitted to detoxify from methadone on exactly the same dosage schedules as those whose detoxification had been approved by the staff. They were not permitted, however, to attend further group therapy sessions or to participate in the other activities of the program. Those patients whose detoxification was approved by the staff were asked to commit themselves to at least 6 months of group therapy and urine testing after they were completely detoxified from methadone.

RESULTS

Characteristics of the Patient Population (Table 1)

These are summarized with respect to sex, race, employment, criminal record, and educational level at the time of admission to the program and after the program had been in operation for 1 year. It should be noted that our population was from the outset a rather unusual one in that it

Table 1
Comparison of Patient Population at the Beginning and End of One Year's Operation

	Sex, %	Race, %	Employed, %	Criminal record, %	Educational level (high school or more), %
Initial (N=42)	62 Male 38 Female	86 White 14 Black	60	19	64
After 1 year (N = 23)	69 Male 31 Female	87 White 13 Black	57	17	79

was predominantly White, that the majority of patients had at least a high school education, that relatively few had a criminal record, and that a rather high percentage were employed. It is not completely clear to us how this evolved. It was not our intention to design a program exclusively for White patients. The fact that all but two members of the staff were White, that the university is located in an area adjacent to areas where large numbers of young Whites live, and finally that the Narcotics Treatment Administration (NTA), which is a large multimodality treatment facility run by the District of Columbia largely run by and for Black patients, undoubtedly contributed to this selection process. Many of our patients had had some experience with the NTA and expressed a feeling of alienation in that program because they were White.

Status of the Program at Year End

Tables 1 through 5 summarize the status of the original group of patients after 1 year of the program. The characteristics of the population remaining after 1 year were virtually identical to those of the beginning population (Table 1). Although a slightly higher proportion of the better educated patients remained in the program after a year, the differences did not prove to be statistically significant.

Of the 42 patients who were with the program in September 1971, 23 (or 55%) remained after 1 year (Table 2). Of the 22 patients who were assigned to the therapy groups run by mental health professionals, 15 (or 68%) remained, while eight (or 40%) of the 20 patients assigned to the ex-addict counselor-led groups remained after 1 year (Table 3). Of those patients who remained, five were methadone-free at the end of 1 year (Table 4). Four of those patients came from mental health profes-

Table 2
Program Totals

Total patients in the program September 1971 through September 1972	42
Patients left during the course of the year	19
Patients remaining	23
% Remaining	55

Table 3
Group Totals

Total patients in mental health professional (MHP) groups	22
Patients remaining after 1 year	15
% Remaining	68
Total patients in ex-addict counselor (EAC) groups	20
Patients remaining after 1 year	8
% Remaining	40

Table 4
Status of Those Remaining[a]

Total remaining who have reached detoxifying state or beyond				5
% Total,	5/42 = 11;	MHP,	4	
% Remaining,	5/23 = 22;	EAC,	1	
Total in program who are on methadone maintenance				18
% Total,	18/42 = 42;	MHP,	11	
% Remaining,	18/23 = 78;	EAC,	7	

[a] MHP: Mental health professional groups; EAC: ex-addict counselor groups.

sional-led groups, one from the ex-addict counselor groups. The remaining 18 patients were still on methadone maintenance at the end of 1 year. Eleven of those were from the mental health professional groups, while seven were from the ex-addict counselor groups.

Of the 24 patients who left the group in the course of the year (Table 5), seven moved from the Washington Metropolitan Area and were enrolled in programs in other parts of the country. Three patients left the program for behavioral reasons. One who was enrolled in the program before group therapy sessions began refused to attend any of these sessions when they were started. A second patient was arrested for armed robbery and imprisoned after about 3 months in the program. The third

Table 5
Status of Those Departed

Transferred for geographic reasons				7
% Total,	7/42 = 16.6;	MHP,	2	
% Departed,	7/19 = 36;	EAC,	5	
Transfererred for disciplinary reasons				3
% Total,	3/42 = 7;	MHP,	2	
% Departed,	3/19 = 15;	EAC,	1	
AMA *before* approved detox			9	
% Total,	9/42 = 24;	MHP,	3	
% Departed,	9/19 = 47;	EAC,	6	

patient was hospitalized for prolonged observation after several episodes of acting-out behavior, including brandishing a gun in the clinic on two occasions and threatening his wife (who was also a patient in the program) with violence unless she left the program. Nine patients left the program against medical advice and were detoxified from methadone without staff approval. Some of the reasons given for their departure are discussed below.

DISCUSSION

Fifty-five percent of the patients initially enrolled in the program remained after 1 year. This compares favorably with another program with a similar number of White patients (Perkins and Bloch, 1970) in which 36% of the patients remained after 1 year. It compares less favorably with a program in New York City with a much higher proportion ot Blacks and Puerto Ricans in which only 16% of the initial population was lost in the course of the first year (Delong, 1972).

The reasons given for leaving the program among those who detoxified against medical advice were varied. Most related in one way or another to the group therapy sessions. Some patients complained that the sessions should be only on a voluntary basis and that no loss of privileges should be involved when a patient missed a group session without what was deemed a reasonable excuse by the staff. Many of the patients were dissatisfied with the ex-addict counselor groups and expressed the feeling that they were being cheated by not receiving therapy from a "professional." Patients in the mental health professional groups, on the other hand, complained that the therapists were perceived sometimes as being cold and unteeling, and that since they had no personal experience with drug abuse, they could not possibly understand the problems which the patients presented. Interestingly enough, however, when these patients were brought before the entire staff, they complained of being manipulated in those sessions by the ex-addict counselors and felt that they were not able to express their feelings because of the presence of ex-addicts.

Of interest, too, was the difference in material discussed in the two groups. In both the EAC and MHP groups, the initial discussions centered around the drug life, including methods for obtaining drugs or money for drugs and similar topics. Boasts of the virtues of the drug life and its value in making the patients more attuned to modern living were particularly frequent, as if the patients were trying to convince the group leader that their status as "patient" was unjustified. Also prominent in these early sessions were expressions of anger and distrust of the staff, excessive lying, and attempts at "conning" staff and other group members.

In the MHP groups these themes were prominent for the first 3 months. As it became clear to the patients, however, that this line of discussion was not considered productive by the MHP group leaders, the topics shifted to what might be called more traditional themes. Patients began to discuss the personal problems which had led them into the drug life, particularly concerning their close family and friends. During this period, patients were anxious to have the group leader provide answers for them instead of seeking their own solutions and became angry at the group leaders when they refused to provide such answers. Also, at this time, some difficulties between Black patients and the MHP counselors (both of whom were White) surfaced. The counselors felt that Black patients interpreted all adverse comments as racial slurs, that they were hesitant to deal with their own problems directly (although often helpful in getting other patients to express themselves), and were likely to use or threaten to use physical violence. Black patients, on the other hand, expressed the feeling that the other patients and the MHP group leaders could not understand their problems because they had not lived them and did not have relevant solutions to offer. As the group evolved further, both Black and White patients became more willing to bring their problems to group and to accept group suggestions. Group members began to take pride in their group as an entity different from the other groups and expressed and acted out of concern for fellow group members.

In the ex-addict counselor groups, on the other hand, the theme of the virtues and costs of the drug life was more viable, and in the beginning there was an attempt on the part of the counselors to outdo the patients at their own storytelling. When other more personal themes were discussed the ex-addict counselors often seemed, despite their training, unable to exploit them and often responded with rather stereotyped replies which did not allow the patient to develop the issues further. In general, the evolution of themes as described in the MHP groups was considerably slower in the EAC groups. Despite the fact that both EAC counselors were Black, many of the same difficulties with Black patients arose. Significantly, those Black patients in MHP groups did not express the desire to transfer to EAC groups.

Special note, in fact, should be taken of the role of the ex-addict counselors and of the administrator with an admitted history of drug abuse in this program, because it is our feeling that these individuals revealed both the strengths and weaknesses of involving ex-drug users in the rehabilitation of drug users. All three individuals were particularly useful in the beginning of the program in helping the other staff members, most of whom had little prior experience with drug abusers, in learning the ploys which such patients use to manipulate their surroundings. The ex-addict group counselors viewed their role somewhat differently from the mental health professionals and frequently became involved with patients in a much more personal way, driving them back and forth to clinic, helping them find work, being available to them after hours, etc. The administrator, as mentioned above, saw his role as one of ombudsman for the patients and frequently became personally involved in a similar way, i.e., in helping patients find work and lodgings and in helping them with minor scrapes with the law. The ex-addict counselors, however, seemed less able to hold patients in the program through group therapy sessions than the mental health professionals, and the rate of attrition in the ex-addict counselor groups, as noted, was higher, although the difference between the two groups was not statistically significant. This may have resulted from several factors, including the fact that the two ex-addict counselors were Black and that most of the patients were White, and that many of the White patients had already rejected the Narcotics Treatment Administration as a treatment facility. Perhaps the experiences within the drug culture were sufficiently different to inhibit communication. The reason the patients most often gave for dissatisfaction was that the topic of conversation in the groups for the most part revolved around the drug life and did not involve feelings of other emotional issues and that the patients felt the ex-addicts were not helping them work through their own problems. In a similar way, the patients regarded the administrator (who was White and whose drug history was known to them) with considerable ambivalence. While many of them at one time or another looked to him for support, many also complained that he was inconsistent and that he continued intermittently to use drugs himself and, therefore, set a poor example for the patients in the program. When he decided to leave the program, the patients were informally polled as to whether they would like to see him replaced with another person with personal drug experience, and they were emphatic in their feelings that this not be done but that the person who replaced him be a person with some medical training and without a history of drug abuse. This rejection of ex-drug users on the part of the patients was almost certainly influenced by the aura of "professionalism" which pervaded the program. Patients' prejudice may have been shaped by the fact that the program was run by two physicians and that most of the personnel in the program were medically or psychiatrically trained and had no history of drug abuse.

One other issue which has not received sufficient attention in other literature was that of the dosage of methadone. This was an issue which was second only to those revolving around group therapy in determining whether many patients stayed in the program or not. In the initial portion of the program, most patients were unhappy that methadone doses were too low. Some physicians at that time in the District of Columbia were treating patients with as much as 160 mg of methadone, and patients who received less than 100 mg of methadone continually complained about feeling withdrawal symptoms. Initially, most patients were maintained at a dose of somewhere between 80 to 120 mg of methadone, but after some experience we decided that this dose could be lowered to between 40 or 50 mg/day and was sufficient to keep most patients drug-free and comfortable. Of the 23 patients now remaining in the program at the end of 1 year, 18 are still on methadone maintenance, and all but one are taking between 40 and 50 mg/day. It is of considerable interest that after 1 year of methadone virtually all are anxious to have their dose lowered, and the issue at the end of the year for these patients is not one of wanting more but rather of wanting less methadone. We can offer no explanation for this phenomenon. It perhaps reflects the progress on the part of some patients; on the part of others, it may reflect an impatience after a year of continued addiction to methadone and strong desire to detoxify. Certainly in many patients in our program the desire to have their dose of methadone gradually lowered represents a desire not to directly confront the issue of whether to continue to be maintained or to seek program approval for detoxification from methadone.

A comment concerning the reaction of the local community to the program seems appropriate. The immediate "community" (that is, the other patients in the Medical Clinic) were little affected by the program except as a result of occasional acting out behavior by program patients. Such behavior subsided quickly when patients in the program realized that it might jeopardize the existence of the program. The business community immediately surrounding the clinic was basically unaware of the existence of the program and there were virtually no complaints about real or suspected patient activities. Two businesses, a grocery store and a nearby restaurant, hired program patients from time to time with varying success and with the full knowledge that they were drug abuse patients. Finally, the program has never been large enough or visible enough to attract serious attention from nearby residents (most of whom live in high-rise apartments) and has not been a subject of concern. As far as we know, no program patient has been involved in any street crime in the immediate area of the clinic.

CONCLUSIONS

On the basis of our experience after 1 year, several conclusions are warranted. First, such a program can in fact be run within the confines of a medical clinic without disruption of the other affairs of the clinic and without unduly inhibiting the patients in the program from feeling free to express themselves and to make solid relationships with the program staff. Second, for some patients, at least, the issue of psychotherapy vs methadone maintenance need not be looked upon as an either/or proposition. The combination of the two, in fact, may enable the patient to overcome his addiction to methadone sooner. It is our feeling that in the initial stages the motivation to seek regular psychotherapeutic support is low and methadone may serve as a bridge of support until such time as that motivation is higher. Third, the issue of using ex-addicts must be carefully considered in any drug abuse program. While our numbers are small and our report is predominantly retrospective, there is at least the indication from our experiences that ex-addicts do not work successfully with all kinds of patients and that there are definite limitations to their roles. Before one takes at face value the statement made by many addicts that only another addict can help him, it is important to note that addicts look upon other ex-addicts or ex-drug-dependent persons with a considerable amount of ambivalence and view their rehabilitative skills with skepticism. Even though there are many common experiences in the lives led by all heroin addicts, differences in racial and socioeconomic backgrounds may be enough to inhibit significant communication between disparate groups. It should also be noted that even the appearance of continued drug abuse on the part of an ex-user in such a rehabilitative program can be devastating to the morale of the patients and alternatively can be used as a potent mechanism for manipulating other staff members.

SUMMARY

This report describes the experience of a program for heroin abusers which combines some features of a therapeutic community with methadone maintenance therapy. The program utilized both ex-addict counselors and mental health professionals in group therapy sessions. The ex-addict counselors, while a valuable asset to a drug abuse program, demonstrated definite limitations. Our experience does indicate, however, that such a program can be set up within the confines of a general medical clinic, and that methadone maintenance and psychotherpay need not be looked upon as mutually exclusive but can be used together effectively in a treatment program.

REFERENCES

DELONG, J.V. Drugs and their effects. In *Dealing With Drug Abuse*. New York: Praeger, 1972.

DOLE, V.P., and NYSWANDER, M.E. Rehabilitation of the street addict. *Arch. Environ. Health* 14: 477–480, 1967.

DOLE, V.P., and NYSWANDER, M.E. Methadone maintenance and its implication for theories of narcotic addiction. *Res. Publ. Assoc. Res. Nerv. Ment. Diseases* 46: 359–366, 1968.

DOLE, V.P., NYSWANDER, M.E., and WARNER, A. Successful treatment of 750 criminal addicts. *J. Amer. Med. Assoc.* 206: 2708–2711, 1968.

DUPONT, R.L. Profile of a heroin addiction epidemic. *New Eng. J. Med.* 285: 320–324, 1971.

MARKOFF, E.L. Synanon in drug addiction. *Cur. Psych. Therapy*. 9: 261–272, 1969.

PERKINS, M.E., and BLOCH, H.L. Survey of a methadone maintenance treatment program. *Amer. J. Psychol.* 126: 1389–1403, 1970.

A Statement of Purpose

INSTITUTE FOR THE STUDY OF DRUG MISUSE, Inc.

The Institute for the Study of Drug Misuse, Inc. (formerly the Institute for the Study of Drug Addiction) was established in 1965 as an international organization to develop clear channels of communication and to encourage research in the field of drug abuse. To fulfill its goals, the Institute participates in research, professional training, and education. In addition, it serves as a consulting agency in the establishment of treatment programs in the United States and abroad. As professional, government, and lay concern increases in the field of drug abuse, the Institute has been called upon to serve as a resource agency for the dissemination of scientific materials through the press, television, radio, and other media.

In order to achieve its purposes, the Institute for the Study of Drug Misuse:

Sponsors the INTERNATIONAL JOURNAL OF THE ADDICTIONS, published by Marcel Dekker, Inc.

Sponsors national and international conferences and workshops in cooperation with universities, medical teaching centers, governmental agencies, and private industry.

Sponsors a lecture series "The Use and Misuse of Drugs and Alcohol," for professionals and interested lay people.

Sponsors international awards for significant research reports focusing upon various aspects of drug abuse.

The expanding programs of the Institute have been dictated by the present crisis in drug abuse. It is apparent that in the United States and in the world at large, certain social forces are at work which have magnified the scope of the problem. In order to insure that the Institute reaches the broadest group of interested individuals, it has become necessary to establish several categories of membership.

Membership in the Institute for the Study of Drug Misuse is tax exempt.

For membership information, write:

Institute for the Study of Drug Misuse, Inc.
111 Fifth Avenue
New York, N.Y. 10003

INFORMATION FOR AUTHORS SUBMITTING MANUSCRIPTS

Send a clear double-spaced typewritten original and two duplicate copies to the Editor, *International Journal of the Addictions*, Institute for the Study of Drug Misuse, Inc., 111 Fifth Avenue, New York, N.Y. 10003. DOUBLE-SPACE the entire manuscript; do not use single spacing anywhere.

Include authors' academic degrees and present affiliation. If applicable, cite auspices under which work being reported was done. Specify address to which requests for reprints should be sent.

Begin your TITLE with a word useful in indexing. Put news of your finding or a statement of the problem first. Major and minor headings may be used in the text; indicate major headings by typing in capitals. Provide a 100-word SUMMARY at the end.

Use METRIC UNITS of measure. If measurements were made in English units, give metric equivalents.

Cite all TABLES and FIGURES in the text. Tables should have titles, and figures should have brief legends. In tables, give each column a heading. Indicate units of measure in parentheses in the heading for each column. Do not use vertical rules. Do not use horizontal rules other than those in the heading and at the bottom. Submit PHOTOGRAPHS as glossy prints, untrimmed and unmounted; identify each with pencil lightly on the back and indicate top.

ARTWORK will not be returned unless specifically requested, and will be disposed of three months after publication.

REFERENCES in the text should be enclosed in parentheses and include the author's surname and the date of the item cited. Keep footnotes to a minimum.

The BIBLIOGRAPHY (double-spaced) should be given at the end of the article in alphabetical order. Journal references should include authors, title, name of journal abbreviated according to *Chemical Abstracts List of Periodicals,* inclusive page numbers, and date. Book references should include authors, title, place of publication, publisher, and date.

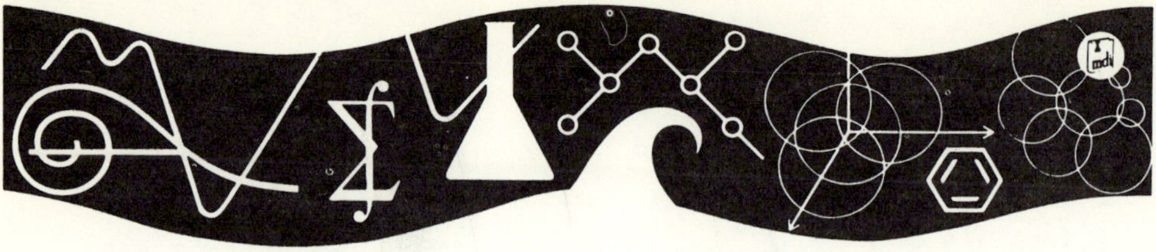

THE INTERNATIONAL JOURNAL OF THE ADDICTIONS

Published by Marcel Dekker, Inc., New York
Sponsored by The Institute for the Study of Drug Misuse, Inc., New York

---

THE INTERNATIONAL JOURNAL OF THE ADDICTIONS

Volume 9 Number 4 1974

CONTENTS

Sweating Function in the Heroin Withdrawal Syndrome of Neonates: Marvin Green, Carl Zelson, and Hans Behrendt 495

Asthmador: A Legal Hallucinogen: Keith W. Jacobs 503

Narcotics-Related Deaths Decrease in 1972 from the Number of Narcotics-Related Deaths in 1971: William I. Barton 513

Drug Use and Social Integration: Jens J. B. Winsløw 531

Teach Me What I Want to Know about Drugs for Junior High School Students: Russell N. Cassel and Gail Zander 541

A University System Drug Profile: Jerry L. Strimbu and O. Suthern Sims, Jr. 569

Concepts of Life Style in the Treatment of Alcoholism: William Warren Garitano and Ruth E. Ronall 585

Treating the Drug-Dependent Veteran—Perspective from a Veterans Administration Hospital: William W. Van Stone 593

Experiences with a Combination of Group Therapy and Methadone Maintenance in the Treatment of Heroin Addiction: John C. LaRosa, Stephen H. Lipsius, and Judith H. LaRosa 605

Cover illustration: "Honneur au Courage malheureux."
Courtesy of the Picture Collection, The Branch Libraries, New York Public Library.

MARCEL DEKKER, INC., New York

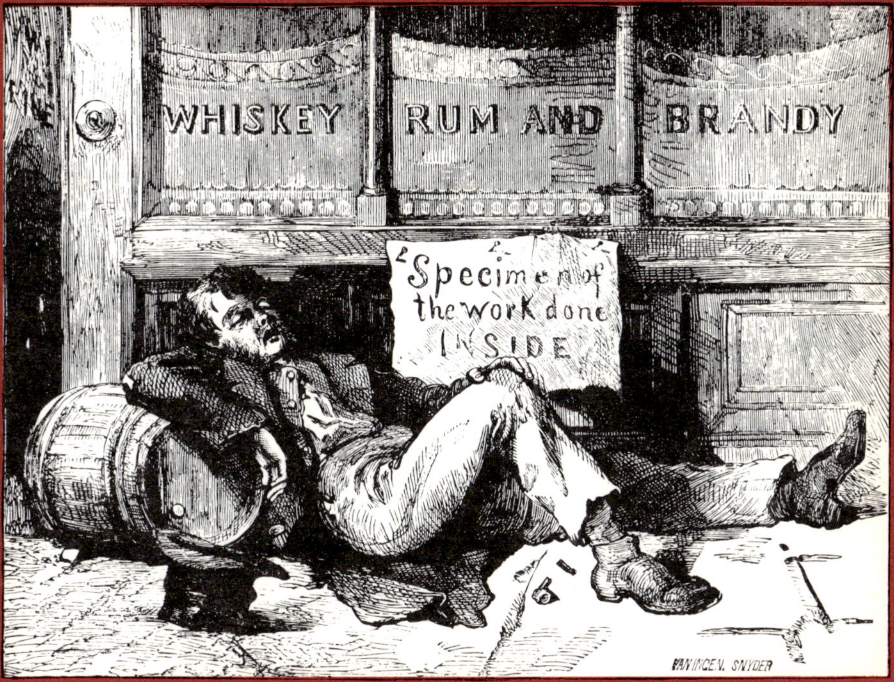

THE INTERNATIONAL JOURNAL OF THE Addictions

Volume 9 Number 5 1974

THE INTERNATIONAL JOURNAL OF THE ADDICTIONS

The International Journal of the Addictions, October 1974

Published six times annually—February, April, June, August, October, December—by Marcel Dekker, Inc., 270 Madison Avenue, New York, N. Y. 10016. The subscription rate for Volume 9 (1974), containing 6 issues is $40.00 (prepaid). Postage outside the United States is $5.10 per volume for all subscriptions. The special discounted rate for individual professionals and students is $20.00. Back volume prices will be sent on request. Please *mail payment with order* to the following address: Marcel Dekker Journals, P. O. Box 11305, Church Street Station, New York, New York 10249.

Second-class postage paid at New York, N. Y., and at additional mailing offices.

Printed in the U. S. A.

Contributions to This Journal Are Published Free of Charge

The International Journal of the Addictions, 9(5), 619–636, 1974

Short- and Long-Term Therapeutic Communities: A Follow-up and Cost Effectiveness Comparison

William S. Aron, Ph.D.

Douglas Daily

Camarillo-Neuropsychiatric Institute Research Program
Camarillo State Hospital
Camarillo, California

Due to the worsening economic situation in the country, it is becoming more difficult to attain public funds to finance long-term drug abuse rehabilitation programs. Recent cutbacks by the federal government in its support of social programs have made the situation even worse. Small local governments, especially, are seeking less expensive and quicker modalities of rehabilitation in an effort to keep up with the growing demand and expense. Pressures are being exerted on existing rehabilitation programs to streamline their efforts to provide greater turnaround at a smaller cost per patient.

The program effectiveness—defined by the number of court convictions in a given cohort after treatment—is compared for two therapeutic community programs whose major difference is the length of treatment:

3 months for the "short-term" program and 10 to 12 months for the "family" program. The findings present evidence that the longer program is more effective, and less costly in the long run, but that both programs serve important needs of different clientele.

HISTORY OF CAMARILLO PROGRAMS

The drug program at Camarillo State Hospital has been in existence for nearly 5 years. It was not until late 1970, however, that it became organized as a coed therapeutic environment. At about this same time the program was divided into two units, one a long-term (10 to 12 months) and the other a short-term (90 day) approach. The long-term program, newly called the Camarillo "Family" Drug Abuse Program, was patterned after the "Mendocino Family" of Northern California (described in Glasscote et al., 1972). After a brief period of functioning as a separate entity, the short-term program was linked to the family and became known as the "Awakening Program." It too was modeled after the Mendocino concept, and served to detoxify addicts, provide a shorter length program, and act as a "feeding" grounds for the long-term family program.

During the $2\frac{1}{2}$-year period since the formation of the family and the short-term program, county politics has considerably influenced the design of both programs. Nearly 100% of the patient population comes from Ventura and Los Angeles Counties. The "home" county of each patient is required to pay 10% of his costs (the rest being paid by the state). For nearly 1 year, however, Ventura County stopped referring people to the program at Camarillo. This occurred for two main reasons: (1) the county budget is much smaller than that of Los Angeles County and (2) the feeling (based on a valid assessment of the situation) that the Camarillo Program does not work well with its large Chicano addict population. (The family program is 86% White and only 5% Chicano). During this period many non-Chicano drug abusers from Ventura County did come into the program by falsifying their home address as Los Angeles County.

In May of 1972, because of its own failing detoxification program, Ventura County decided once again to refer addicts to the Camarillo Program for detoxification and possible short-term treatment. This decision was on condition that the family, whose members had been controlling the short-term unit, be removed and that no one advocate the long-term family approach to the Ventura County people, because Ventura County was unable to pay for long-term treatment.

In the year that has elapsed since that time, the drug program at Camarillo State Hospital has been divided into three separate units, one strictly for detoxification, and the other two for the short-term and family programs. During this time the family and the short-term programs have developed independently of one another, and at times in competition with each other, as to which approach is best. This competition often results in a struggle over prospective members that come into the "feeding" grounds of the detoxification unit. Only 23.2%* of those who leave the detoxification unit go on to one of the two programs, and 86.0% of these are under some kind of legal pressure, be it probation, awaiting court dates, or actual sentences.

The therapy and principles of the two programs are basically the same. In both programs much emphasis is placed on discipline, encounter-type therapy, and peer pressure. The major difference is in the length of treatment. A person completes the short-term program in 90 days, while those in the family remain in the program for 10 to 12 months (sometimes longer) and graduate when their peers and other graduates of the program feel they are ready. Because of its shorter length of treatment, the short-term program is of necessity more professionally run, with the hospital staff taking part in the organization and the running of the group. The family program, on the other hand, is patient-run with the senior members of the program being in charge of its organization.

METHODOLOGY

In an effort to gather immediate data concerning success rates of the two treatment approaches, use was made of the probation files of both Ventura and Los Angeles Counties. As a result, active records were found on 75.3% of the 267 people investigated. Those 267 people that we chose to follow-up consisted of (1) all the people who had completed the short-term program from October 1, 1971 through March 26, 1973 ($n = 117$), a period of nearly 1½ years, and (2) all the graduates and "splittees" (those who left before graduating) from the family from April 1, 1971 through March 26, 1973 ($n = 150$), a period of nearly 2 years.

All those found to have been in legal trouble since leaving the programs were on record in the probation department files for one of two reasons: either they had been in violation of probation (in which case a bench warrant was issued), or they had been found guilty of some infraction of

*From a 33 week population movement study: July 1972 through March 1973.

the law. Those people for whom no records were found (24.7%) were given the "benefit of the doubt" and were considered as not having been in legal trouble since leaving the program. For this reason our figures on "failures" contain only those who have been convicted. The "failure" percentage would, understandably, be higher if information were available on all those arrested (whether convicted or not), or on all those who have started using drugs again.

In addition to the above, a cost effectiveness analysis of both programs is presented (in the Discussion section of this paper). Cost effectiveness is calculated on the basis of the rates of completion, success, and failure actually found to exist with our data. The analysis will also include an estimate of the hypothetical cost of rehabilitating the entire cohorts of both the short-term and family programs. The cost to society of the crime in the streets committed by the failures before reentering the programs is also figured.

FINDINGS

The following discussion focuses on a comparison of the conviction rates of three groups of patients involved in two programs: (1) short-term complettees, (2) family graduates, and (3) family splittees. Short-term splittees are not discussed because most leave before 30 days, and can thus hardly have had much treatment, therapeutic or otherwise.

The differences among the programs are quite apparent. The three groups can easily be ranked: (1) family graduates have far fewer convictions than both the splittees and the short-term complettees—only two out of 40 (5%) family graduates were convicted of an offense (Table 1). In probabilistic terms, individuals in this group have a much better chance of success than those in the other two groups.

(2) Those who left the family program early also did better than those who completed the short term: the overall conviction rate of the family splittees (18.2%) is only two-thirds the size of the short-term's rate (27.4%) (Table 1).

Those in the most recently discharged cohort (10/1/72 to 3/26/73) of all three programs tend to bias the picture because at the time of the study not everyone from this group had been out a full 6 months. If we eliminate from the percentages the people discharged during this period, we find an overall 35.1% conviction rate for the short-term, 24.1% for family splittees, and 7.1% for the family graduates.

Controlling for sex (Table 2) yields a similar distribution pattern: male and female short-term complettees have higher conviction rates than

Table 1
Those Convicted in Each Program by Discharge Cohort

Discharge cohorts	Short-term complettees		Family splittees		Family graduates	
	No. discharged	% Convicted	No. discharged	% Convicted	No. discharged	% Convicted
(1) 10/1/72 to 3/26/73	43	14.0 (6)[a]	31	3.2 (1)	8	0.0 (0)
(2) 4/1/72 to 9/30/72	33	30.3 (10)	32	28.1 (9)	13	7.7 (1)
(3) 10/1/71 to 3/31/72	41	39.0 (16)	26	23.1 (6)	10	0.0 (0)
(4) 4/1/71 to 9/30/71	No information		21	19.0 (4)	5	20.0 (1)
TOTAL	117	27.4 (32)	110	18.2 (20)	40	5.0 (2)

[a] Numbers in parentheses indicate frequencies.

male and female family splittees, respectively (one exception in Discharge Group 2). In considering only those who have been out at least 6 months (that is, eliminating the most recently discharged group), the females from the short-term have nearly twice the arrest record as the females who split from the family (38.9 and 22.2%, respectively).

(3) For the short-term program, but not for the family, it appears that the longer the time since discharge, the higher the conviction rate (Table 1). This pattern is the same when controlled for sex (Table 2): both males and females from the short-term program (but not from the family) exhibit increasing rates over time—that is, the longer the cohort has been out of the hospital, the greater the conviction rate. It is reasonable to expect that the longer the cohort is exposed to the possibility of being arrested and convicted of an offense, the more likely this will happen, thereby raising the conviction rate. The fact that this pattern does not hold for the family indicates that conviction rates do not appear to be a function of increasing time for the family (for the period of this study). Further, the conviction rate for the family splittees seems to be diminishing over time (for the three periods going back in time from 4/1/72 to 9/30/71, while increasing for the short-term—Table 1).

(4) Table 3 deals with the question of how long after release from each program the patient is most likely to be picked up and convicted of an offense (considering only those who have been convicted). The total percentages agree with previous research that the first 6 months out is the most crucial period (Duvall et al., 1963; Bowden and Langenauer, 1972).

Table 2

Those Convicted in Each Program by Discharge Cohort (controlled for sex)

	Short-term complettees				Family splittees			
	Male		Female		Male		Female	
Discharge cohorts	No. discharged	% Convicted	No. discharged	% Convicted	No. discharged	% Convicted	No. discharged	% Convicted
(1) 10/1/72 to 3/26/73	33	15.2 (5)[a]	10	10.0 (1)	20	5.0 (1)	11	0.0 (0)
(2) 4/1/72 to 9/30/72	24	33.3 (8)	9	22.2 (2)	19	26.3 (5)	13	30.8 (4)
(3) 10/1/71 to 3/31/72	32	34.4 (11)	9	55.6 (5)	11	18.2 (2)	15	26.7 (4)
(4) 4/1/71 to 9/30/71	No information		No information		13	30.8 (4)	8	0.0 (0)
TOTAL	89	27.0 (24)	28	28.6 (8)	63	19.0 (12)	47	17.0 (8)

[a] Numbers in parentheses indicate frequencies.

Table 3
Those Convicted in Each Program by Length of Time Conviction Occurred after Leaving the Program (controlled for sex)

Time out of program	Short-term complettees ($N = 32$)			Family splittees ($N = 23$)			Family graduates ($N = 2$)		
	Male	Female	Total	Male	Female	Total	Male	Female	Total
First 6 months	75.0	50.0	68.8	35.7	55.6	43.5	100.0	0.0	50.0
7 to 12 months	20.8	0.0	15.6	43.0	33.3	39.1	0.0	100.0	50.0
13 to 18 months	4.2	50.0	15.6	21.3	11.1	17.4	0.0	0.0	0.0
TOTAL	100.0	100.0	100.0	100.0	100.0	100.0	100.0	100.0	100.0
N	24	8	32	14	9	23	1	1	2

Of those who are convicted of a violation, the majority of the family splittees and two-thirds of the short-term complettees are convicted during their first 6 months out of the program.

Controlling for sex (Table 3) changes the pattern only slightly: (a) of the males convicted, the ones from the short-term tend to be convicted mainly during their first 6 months out, while the family splittees "last" a little longer (the plurality are convicted 7 to 12 months after leaving the family); (b) female short-term complettees tend to be convicted either in the first 6 months or later on, after a year out of the program.

(5) Table 4 presents the classification of convictions for the individuals in the study. (Convicted family graduates, because they only number two, are combined with the splittees). Females in both the family and short-term tend to have probation violations. The males from the family tend to be convicted of the more serious charges (burglary, theft, robbery, or forgery), while the males from the short-term program tend to be convicted of drug-related charges.

DISCUSSION

Before discussing the results, it should be emphasized here that conviction rates are a minimum measure of effectiveness. Arrest rates, were they available, would surely have been much higher. Likewise, it is certain that rates of relapse to drug use would have been still greater. Both authors know several individuals from all three groups who have begun using again, but are still working and have managed to avoid violating parole, arrest, or any court conviction.

Most previous follow-up studies use relapse to drugs as their measure

Table 4
Those Convicted in Each Program by Classification of Charges (controlled for sex)

Charges	Short-term complettees ($N = 31$)			Family splittees and graduates ($N = 20$)		
	Male	Female	Total	Male	Female	Total
Drug related charges (e.g., possession, sales, under the influence, etc.)	41.7	14.3	35.5	38.4	28.6	35.0
Burglary, theft, robbery, forgery	25.0	28.6	25.8	46.2	28.6	40.0
Probation violation only	20.8	57.1	29.0	15.4	42.8	25.0
Vehicle code violations, assault, disorderly conduct	12.5	0.0	9.7	0.0	0.0	0.0
TOTAL	100.0	100.0	100.0	100.0	100.0	100.0
N	24	7	31[a]	13	7	20[a]

[a] *N* is slightly smaller here than in Table 3 because there was no information as to the nature of the sentence on a few of the cases.

of success and are therefore not directly comparable to this study. Some studies, however, do deal with arrest or conviction rates. Trussell et al. (1959) found that in his sample of 49 adolescent patients, 90% had had police trouble, relapsed, or both, 2½ to 3 years after release from the hospital. In Vaillant's (1966) 12 year follow-up study of New York narcotic addicts, he found that 90% had received jail sentences. Levy (1971) found somewhat better results in his follow-up study: 20 out of 50 former patients (40%) were either abstinent or using only occasionally; only nine were actually in jail (18%) at the time of the study, 5 years after release from the hospital. Largenauer and Bowden (1971), in a follow-up of male narcotic addicts treated at Lexington, found that 52% of those for whom information was available had been arrested during their first 8 months in aftercare.

An important finding of this study is that the long-term family program has a good record at keeping not only its graduates, but also its early terminees out of the criminal justice system. In terms of one's chances of avoiding a court conviction, it would be best to be a family graduate (95%), next best a family splittee (81.8%), and third a short-term completee (72.6%) (the figures are the reciprocal percents of the overall conviction rates in Table 1). The pattern of the above previous studies, however, suggest that arrest and conviction rates significantly increase over time. Indeed, such a pattern was found to exist with the short-term complettees. The family exhibits no such patterns as of now (Table 1), but no conclusive statement can really be made until more observation time has lapsed.

Figure 1, on the basis of the available data, illustrates the present findings for the three programs with respect to the total number of convictions in each program over time. It should be noted that the slope of the line representing the short-term complettees continues to rise sharply, over time, while the others taper off in the last time period.

Which program is more effective? The question of effectiveness is obviously a more complex one than is represented by an analysis of conviction rates and the lengths of the programs involved. However, some evaluation of the results of the two programs may be made with the data at hand.

First, what are the completion rates of the two programs? During the year April 1, 1971 to March 31, 1972, 86 individuals entered the family.

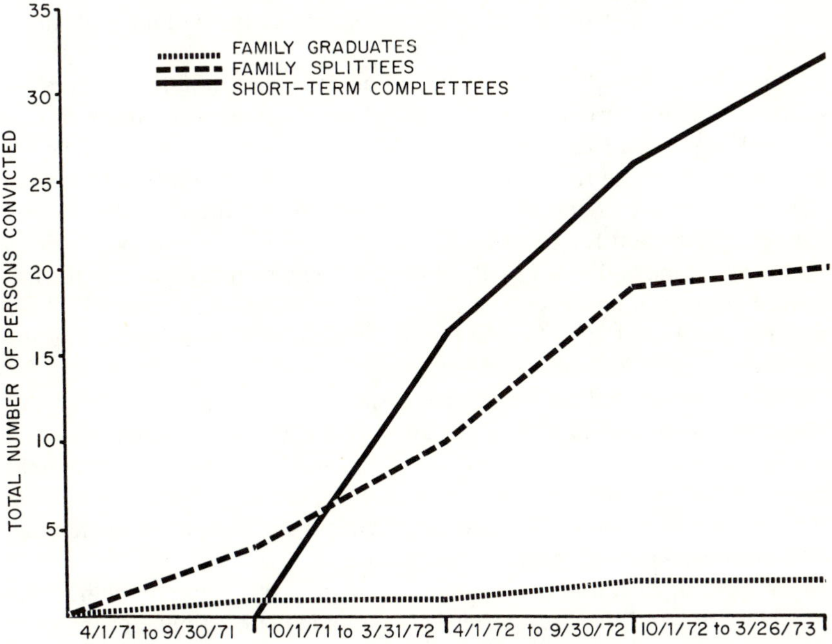

Fig. 1. Total number of convictions over time (cumulative). There is no information available for short-term completees for the 4/1/71 to 9/30/71 time period.

Of this group, 27 eventually graduated producing a completion rate of 31.4%. Because detoxification and the short-term program were combined on the same unit during this period, it was necessary to look at a later time period to compute the total admissions to the short-term for a 1 year period. It was determined in this way that 400 people entered the short-term during 1 year, which produces a graduation rate of 18.5% (74 complettees). Statistically then, the addict, male or female, who enters the family has more of a chance of completing the program than does one who enters the short-term.

In addition to effectiveness in terms of rates of completion and success, cost effectiveness is also an important consideration. Table 5 presents a summary of the program costs.

According to the figures in Table 5, the short-term program is turning out its successes at one-half the cost per success of the family program (Line 18); the ratio of the total program cost to the total number of successes (graduate and splittee) is $1,588 and $3,112 for the short-term and the family, respectively. When other figures in Table 5 are examined, however, the picture becomes more complex. The argument which follows presents evidence that the short-term program is, in the long run, more costly.

The short-term program is able to achieve the number of successes it does at the expense of many failures. The percentage of failures during the first year out of the program is 47.2% for the short-term and 19.7% for the family (these rates are arrived at by obtaining the ratio of the total number of failures—graduates and splittees—to the total number in that cohort: 189 to 400 for short-term and 17 to 86 for the family: Table 5, Line 3 plus Line 6, divided by the cohort N). [To simplify matters, the following discussion on the cost of crime utilizes these failure rates (47% for the short-term and 20% for the family), which are figured by adding the splittee and graduate failures together.]

These failures not only consume a sizeable amount of the program's resources (41.5 and 12.8% of the total budgets for the short-term and family, respectively—the ratio of Line 8 to Line 16), but also incur a great many additional costs: (1) costs to society of crime and stolen goods on the streets, (2) costs to the law enforcement agencies of apprehending and booking, and (3) costs to the courts of trial and commitment to either prison or another rehabilitation program. By combining the rehabilitation and the street crime costs, an adequate estimate of the total cost effectiveness of both programs can be made. (The information needed

Table 5
Summary of Costs for the Short-Term and Family Programs

Item	Short term ($N = 400$)	Family ($N = 86$)
(1) Cost per patient per day, $	20.38	16.86
(2) Average stay for a splittee, in days	30	64.8
(3) Number of splittee failures[a]	163[b]	15
(4) Total cost for all splittee failures (1 × 2 × 3), $	99,658	16,393
(5) Average stay for a graduate, in days	90	330
(6) Number of graduate failures[a]	26	2
(7) Total cost for all graduate failures (1 × 5 × 6), $	47,689	11,128
(8) Total cost for all failures (4 + 7), $	147,347	27,521
(9) Number of graduate successes	48	25
(10) Total cost for all graduate successes (1 × 5 × 9), $	88,042	139,095
(11) Number of splittee successes	163[b]	44
(12) Total cost for all splittee successes (1 × 2 × 11), $	99,658	48,067
(13) Total cost for all successes (10 + 12), $	187,700	187,181
(14) Total cost for all graduates (7 + 10), $	135,731	150,223
(15) Total cost for all splittees (4 + 12), $	199,316	64,479
(16) Total program cost (14 + 15), $	355,047	214,702
(17) Total number of successes (9 + 11)	211	69
(18) Program cost per success, $	1,588	3,112

[a] Those convicted of an offense or who violated parole during their first year out of the program.
[b] Failures (successes) of the short-term splittees were estimated at 50% of that group since no information was available. This was felt to be a conservative estimate, as 35.1% of the complettees were convicted of an offense.

in order to estimate the costs to the law enforcement and criminal justice agencies is not available.)

Rehabilitation Costs. No single program exists in a vacuum; costs do not begin and end with the beginning and completion of any one program. For instance, 49.6% of the family admissions and 46.9% of the short-term admissions said they had been involved in one or more programs before entering the Camarillo Program. Nine and six-tenths percent of the family and 6.1% of the short-term had been in three or more programs prior to coming to Camarillo. When this same group was asked where they were living before coming into the program, 19.3% of the family and 28.6% of the short-term responded that they were "living" in jail. (These figures are based on the results of an interview sample study of members of both programs from July through December 1972: sample size is 83 for the family and 98 for the short-term.) Further, California's Bureau of Criminal Statistics reports that of those individuals who were convicted of offenses related to the use of opiates and other dangerous drugs, 84.2% had prior arrests (Bridges, 1971).

Since the ideal aim of each program is to rehabilitate all admissions, the total costs should then be calculated on the basis of each failure being readmitted to the program until he succeeds (success being here defined as no convictions for 1 year out of the program). Thus the total cost for successful rehabilitation of the entire cohort is equal to the number of each cohort multiplied by the amount of money it takes to produce a program success (400 times $1,588 for the short-term, and 86 times $3,112 for the family). The same amount may be obtained by a longer and more difficult method, that of adding the actual cost of those successes from the original cohorts (53% of 400 in the short-term, and 80% of 86 in the family) to the costs incurred by the failures' returning to the program enough times until the entire cohort achieves success. This total program cost comes to $635,200 for the short-term and $267,632 for the family (see below, and in Table 7).

Street Crime Costs. During the time it takes to achieve success with an entire cohort, failures are constantly returning to their drug habits and criminal activities on the street. With a 47% conviction rate, the short-term cohort of 400 persons would take 752 attempts to achieve 100% success (assuming a constant rate over time); that is, 47% of the original 400, or 188 individuals, would fail the first time; assuming that all these 188 persons return to the program, 47% of them, or 88 would fail the second time, and so on, the total number of attempts being 752. The family cohort of 86 would need 107 attempts to achieve 100% success.

To calculate the amount of crime each failure will commit, it is necessary to know the length of time on the street and the size of the drug habit. According to the results listed in Table 3, the average short-term failure is sentenced 25 weeks after leaving the program; for the family, the average time is 31 weeks. In the interview sample earlier cited, each respondent was asked the most and the least amount of money spent, per week, on drugs during the year prior to entering the Camarillo Program. The average weekly habit was found to be $200 a week (half of these people labeled themselves as heroin addicts). It is assumed that the amount of crime committed by a person is equal to at least the cost of his habit. [Two hundred dollars a week actually represents a conservative estimate

Table 6

Estimated Street Crime Costs for Each Group of Failures until Success Is Achieved with the Entire Original Cohort

	Short term (N = 400)		Family (N = 86)		Hypothetical family (N = 400)	
	No. in or repeating program[a]	Street crime costs for that group of failures,[b] $	No. in or repeating program[c]	Street crime costs for that group of failures,[d] $	No. in or repeating program[c]	Street crime costs for that group of failures,[d] $
	400		86		400	
	188	940,000	17	105,400	80	496,000
	88	440,000	3	18,600	16	99,200
	41	205,000	1	6,200	3	18,600
	19	95,000			1	6,200
	9	45,000				
	4	20,000				
	2	10,000				
	1	5,000				
TOTAL	752	1,760,000	107	130,200	500	620,000

[a] 47% repetition rate.
[b] $200 a week, for 25 weeks, times the number failing the program.
[c] 20% repetition rate.
[d] $200 a week, for 31 weeks, times the number failing the program.

of the amount of crime committed. An accepted procedure is to multiply the cost of the drug habit by a factor of at least 3 (Preble and Casey, 1969; Winick, 1967; O'Connor et al., 1971; Logan, 1972; Stachnick, 1972).]

Table 6 presents the estimates of the amount of crime committed by the family and short-term cohorts for each of the successive subcohorts who become convicted after treatment (e.g., the 188 in the short-term who fail the first time, the 88 who fail the second time, etc.) and must return again to the program. To emphasize: the estimate is based on the average weekly habit of those who attend the Camarillo Programs, and does not include any of the costs related to the criminal justice system; that is, the arrest, booking, trial, and commitment costs.

The total crime costs for the short-term amount to $1,760,000; for the family, they are $130,000. When these costs are added to the program costs, the total costs to society to achieve success (again, in terms of no court convictions for at least 1 year out of the program) amount to $2,390,964 for the short-term cohort of 400 and $394,681 for the family

Table 7
Total Cost to Society Per Success

Item	Short term ($N = 400$)	Family ($N = 86$)	Hypothethical family ($N = 400$)
Program cost,[a] $	635,200	267,632	1,244,800
Crime cost,[b] $	1,760,000	130,000	620,000
Total cost to society,[c] $	2,395,200	397,632	1,864,800
Cost per success,[d] $	5,988	4,624	4,662

[a] N times $1,588 for the short-term program; N times $3,112 for the family program.
[b] From Table 6.
[c] The sum of the crime and program costs.
[d] The total cost to society divided by N.

cohort of 86. The actual cost for each success (total cost divided by the number of successes—in this case, the whole original cohort) then, is $5,988 for the short-term and $4,624 for the family (Table 7).

The difference in the size of the original cohort does not influence the final figures. If the same family rates are applied to a hypothetical cohort of 400, it would take them a total of 500 attempts to achieve complete success. Crime costs for this group amount to $620,000 and program costs ($3,112 per success) to $1,244,800. The total cost to society of $1,864,800 is then divided by 400 to yield an actual cost per success of $4,662 (Tables 6 and 7).

In Figure 2, the total cost to society for each program success is presented and divided proportionately into crime and program costs. It can be seen that while the program costs are higher for the family, the cost to society in subsequent crime is merely one-fourth of the amount for the short-term Program.

In the long run then, the long-term program is less costly to society.

An additional question which must be considered is the contamination effect of having so many individuals go through a program unsuccessfully. In the original short-term program cohort of the 400 admissions, 326 did not finish. Nothing is known of the psychological effect this "failure" has on the addict. If the program has done little more then clean him up and reduce his habit, this could have been accomplished in a much briefer, and less expensive, detoxification program. If we may analogize from the jail experience and speculate that the program has served as a training group for future drug use and crime, what can we say then of program effectiveness? Both programs, of course, are liable to this criti-

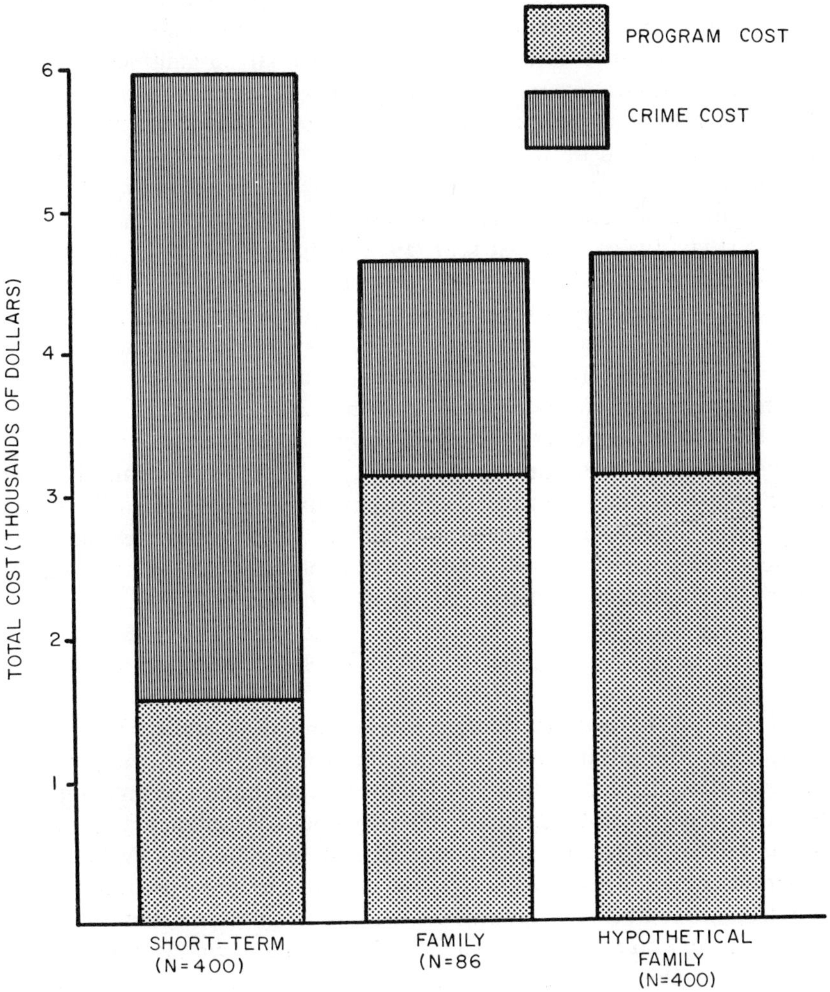

Fig. 2. Total cost to society in achieving each program success.

cism; it's just that much greater numbers are involved in one than in the other.

Finally, it must be understood that the effectiveness of any program is dependent on many variables, not just the length of treatment. Of considerable importance is an individual's personal commitment. By no means is rehabilitation as simple as placing an addict in a long-term treatment program. He must be committed and, in a sense, "ready" to do something about his drug problem.

The family program at Camarillo is regarded as voluntary, allowing no one to be sentenced to it. However, the results of the above cited sample study during this past year (1972) indicate that of the individuals who had entered the family, 54.4% responded that they had been under some kind of pressure, either that of probation, jail, or court, to enter the program. In the short-term program, 73.7% stated they had entered that program under similar law enforcement pressures.

In the Detoxification Unit, where only 23.1% of 1,324 admissions over a 33-week period in 1972 go on to one of the two programs, some individuals have been admitted as many as six times in 6 months. For some people, it does seem to take many failures before they will commit themselves to a serious attempt. In this sense the shorter treatment approaches do serve a vital role in offering people an alternative to jail and, hopefully, in planting in them some seeds of change.

IMPLICATIONS

If our aim is really to do something about drug addiction, then we must begin to think in terms of the entire problem. The growing number of successfully treated addicts is still a drop in the bucket when compared to the currently popular estimate of nearly one-half million active addicts in the United States. By the same token, if we choose to evaluate our programs by simply analyzing the cost of that particular program, it too is a drop in the bucket of the entire costs placed on society that ultimately bring someone to the point of successfully putting down his habit.

It is not enough to analyze the cost effectiveness of a rehabilitation program in terms of that program alone. There are many costs to society involved; we have tried to indicate some of these costs in our analysis. We have also tried to show that cutting costs in one area only raises them elsewhere. This is not meant to convey that there is no place for short-range treatment programs, but rather that there are different consequences to different treatment approaches and we should be aware of what those consequences are.

To conclude, our results indicate that the longer family program is more effective, as determined by a comparison of the completion and the court conviction rates, and by an analysis of the cost effectiveness of the programs.

SUMMARY

The rates of program completion, the rates of court convictions after release from the program, and a cost effectiveness analysis were compared for two therapeutic communities whose major difference is the length of treatment. The longer program was found to be more effective and less costly in the long run, but nonprogram factors were found to emphasize the importance of both the short- and the long-range approaches: the one to provide a long-range and thorough treatment for those who are ready for it, and the other to provide an effective and workable alternative to the criminal justice system.

ACKNOWLEDGMENTS

The authors wish to express their appreciation to the Los Angeles and Ventura County Probation Departments for their cooperation. The authors are also indebted to Steve Nail for his help in collecting the data and to Israela Ettenberg-Aron, Pat Lewis, and Cindy Schersching for their editorial assistance.

This study was supported by funds from the California Council of Criminal Justice, Grant No. 0566.

REFERENCES

BOWDEN, C.L. and LANGENAUER, B.J. Success and failure in the NARA addiction program. *Amer. J. Psychiat.* 128 (7): 853–855, 1972.

BRIDGES, C.K. *Drug Arrests and Dispositions: Reference Tables, 1971: State of California.* Sacremento, California: Bureau of Criminal Statistics, 1971.

DUVALL, H.J., LOCKE, B.Z., and BRILL, L. Follow-up study of narcotic drug addicts five years after hospitalization. *Public Health Rep.* 78: 185–193, 1963.

GLASSCOTE, R., SUSSEX, J., JAFFE, J., BALL, J., and BRILL, L. *The Treatment of Drug Abuse.* Washington, D.C.: The American Psychiatric Association and the National Association for Mental Health, 1972.

LANGENAUER, B.J., and BOWDEN, C.L. A follow-up study of narcotic addicts in

the NARA program. *Amer. J. Psychiat.* 128 (1): 73–78, 1971.
LEVY, B.S. Five years after: A follow-up of 50 narcotic addicts. *Amer J. Psychiat.* 128 (7): 103–106, 1971.
LOGAN, D.G. A pilot methadone program to introduce comprehensive addiction treatment. *Hosp. Commun. Psychiat.* 76–79, March 1972.
O'CONNOR, G., WURMSER, L., BROWN, T.C., and SMITH, J. *The Economics of Narcotics Addiction: A New Interpretation of the Facts.* Paper presented to the 33rd Annual Scientific Meeting of the National Research Council: Committee on Problems of Drug Dependence, 1971.
PREBLE, E., and CASEY, J. Taking care of business—the heroin user's life on the street. *Intern. J. Addictions* 4 (1): 1–24, 1969.
STACHNICK, T.J. The case against criminal penalities for illicit drug use. *Amer. Psychol.* 27 (7): 637–642, 1972.
VAILLANT, G.E. A twelve year follow-up of New York narcotic addicts: I: The relation of treatment to outcome. *Amer. J. Psychiat.* 122: 727–739, 1966.
TRUSSELL, R.E., ALKSNE, H., ELINSON, J., and PATRICK, S. *A Follow-up Study of Treated Adolescent Narcotic Users.* New York: Columbia University School of Public Health and Administrative Medicine, May 1959. Mimeographed.
WINICK, C. Drug addiction and crime. *Curr. History:* 349–354, June 1967.

The International Journal of the Addictions, 9(5), 637–652, 1974

Value Change in Drug Education: The Role of Encounter Groups

Michael Peretz,* M.A.

Drug Education and Training Center
Eastern Pennsylvania Psychiatric Institute
Philadelphia, Pennsylvania

Frederick B. Glaser, M.D.

Department of Psychiatry
Medical College of Pennsylvania and
Eastern Pennsylvania Psychiatric Institute
Philadelphia, Pennsylvania

INTRODUCTION

In the late 1960s the United States, together with other countries, experienced an apparent increase in drug abuse. Public feeling was aroused, and this led to an increased desire to deal with the problem. However, there was a lack of well-qualified personnel to mount an intervention effort, and therefore centers to train such personnel were created. They have now been in operation for some time. One such is the Drug Education and Training Center (DETC) at the Eastern Pennsylvania Psychiatric Institute.

The center trains and educates professionals and paraprofessionals

* Present address: The Al Paul Lefton Co., Philadelphia, Pennsylvania.

in the field of drug abuse. Week-long workshops of approximately 30 people participate in and are exposed to various experiences related to drug abuse: lectures by lawyers, doctors, therapists; site visits to treatment facilities; experiential exercises such as role playing the part of an addict or therapist; films; written material; and encounter groups. It is the philosophy of the center that drug abuse and addiction are complex human problems with roots buried deeply in society as well as in the individual. The workshops focus on honest, straightforward communication as an important way of realizing one's own potential as well as establishing trust, believed to be the first step in reaching an addict.

Early in the course of this project it seemed to us that the staff of the center had a definite and powerful set of values which it communicated to the trainees. We therefore set out to document this. The present paper details the results of our effort.

ENCOUNTER GROUPS

The center's philosophy is best exemplified in the small encounter groups, each led by a staff member. The thirty trainees are divided into four groups which meet for about 2 hours per session for 4 successive days of the 5-day workshop. The content of the encounter groups revolves around the participants' personal feelings toward the issues brought up in the day's presentations, their feelings toward addicts, treatment, one another, and very often, their feelings toward themselves. The nature of DETC groups is similar to the general model of encounter groups described in the *American Psychiatric Association Task Force Report* (Buhler, 1970):

> Despite widely varying formats, most of the groups share some common features: they attempt to provide an intensive group experience; they are generally small enough (six to twenty members) to permit considerable face-to-face interaction; they focus on the here-and-now (the behavior of the members as it unfolds in the group); they encourage openness, honesty, inter-personal confrontation, and total self-disclosure; they encourage strong emotional expression; the participants are not labeled patients; the experience is not labeled "therapy," but nonetheless, the groups strive to increase inner awareness and to change behavior. The goals of the groups vary: occasionally, they are explicitly entertainment—to "turn on," to experience joy, etc.—

> but generally, the goals involve some type of change—a change of behavior, a change of values, a change of being in the world.

Our particular concern with encounter groups is justified by the significance of the groups to participants. A follow-up mail questionnaire confirms our daily observations that the group experience is the most potent aspect of the workshop, providing trainees with their most profound experience. This is not entirely unexpected, since the function of our encounter groups, in part, is not unlike that described in the *APA Task Force Report* (Buhler, 1970):

> Small groups have always served as an important healing agent; from the beginnings of recorded history, group forces have been used to inspire hope, increase morale, offer strong emotional support, induce a sense of serenity and confidence in the benevolence of the universe, all of which serve to counteract psychic and many bodily ills.

A fairly typical written comment from one trainee after the workshop was completed exemplifies the APA description of the functions groups may serve.

> I make a personal commitment to spread the warmth, happiness, love, honesty and trust I have learned to give and to receive at the week's workshop to as many other people as I can. By doing this, I hope they will be able to learn, as I have, that people are really great, no matter what their "stereotype" may be, they can be real if given the chance. I also commit myself to accept and do something about the weaknesses which were pointed out to me in my group training. Lastly, I commit myself to turn to the staff at EPPI for help in dealing with people when I finally find a job in the helping profession. Thank you.

This reaction to the workshop experience is not at all uncommon and appears to be the product of intense feelings, created, in part, by the group experience. The values and attitudes expressed by this trainee are typically those embodied by the staff (group leaders) and are often the collective ideals evolved by each group.

Whether and how such values are adopted by trainees is of primary interest in this paper. Ottenberg (1971) describes a process which might be operating here and calls it the "group high."

> When you get a group of like-minded people together who show mutual interests, extend support for each other, share a common experience, work through problems, there develops a tendency toward suggestibility by hysterical identification to the point of a "group high." You can get a group high the same as you can with any pharmacological agent. With this group high, there is a diminution of inhibition and controls.

The creation of a "group high" may be one of the crucial factors contributing to trainee susceptibility to psychological influence such as a change in values. As Ottenberg says (1971):

> At a time when an individual's defenses are low through excitement, intoxication, and hysterical processes of group identification, there can take place a parasiting of the other members' values and attitudes.

PAST RESEARCH

Experimental evidence bearing on value changes in human interaction exists not in the field of encounter groups directly, but in the related area of therapeutic interaction between patient and therapist. The debate over whether encounter groups are therapy need not be settled here except to agree that there is an overlap between some forms of therapy and some types of encounter groups wherein certain goals and techniques are common to both. In addition, therapists express the same concern over influencing patients' values when they ask the question: "Do patients change their values to agree more with their therapist's values after therapy?" Several studies indicate that the answer may be "yes."

Pentony (1966) reports a study designed to test the hypothesis that patients acquire the values of their therapist. He measured 20 patients' values prior to, during, at termination, and well after the end of therapy. He also measured therapists' values prior to therapy. He concludes that:

> One outcome of psychotherapy is the tendency for the client to express his values in terms corresponding more closely to those of the therapist than was the case prior to therapy.

In a similar study, Parloff (1957a) also reports that patients more closely approach the values of the therapists after therapy. In another study involving 12 patients over a 2-year period, Rosenthal (1955) administered several value measures at the beginning and end of treatment. He also measured therapists' values prior to treatment, hypothesizing that the "patient learns to accept the moral values of the therapist." He found that "patients who improved tended to revise certain of their moral values in the direction of the therapist's, while the moral values of the patients who were unimproved tended to become less like their therapists."

Ortmeyer et al. (1966) found similar results with a slightly different design. He studied 38 psychotherapists and 44 of their patients at two New York City psychoanalytic training institutes. He hypothesized that therapists and their own patients, after interaction (1 to 9 months) in therapy, would be more similar in values than random pairs of therapists and patients. He also hypothesized that there would be a significant relationship between congruence of patient–therapist values and therapists' subjective evaluation of the patients' mental health status. His results support both hypotheses: value similarity between patients and "own" therapists is greater than between therapists and random "non-own" patients; and the value system of "improved" patients (as rated by their therapists) is closer to that of their therapist than that of nonimproved patients.

In addition to this experimental evidence in a situation resembling some of the encounter group dynamics, there are theoretical reasons why trainees might be influenced to adopt staff values.

MODEL OF SOCIAL INFLUENCE

Kelman's theory of social influence (1961) conceptualizes three processes which give rise to social influence: compliance, identification, and internalization. The conditions for at least two of these processes, compliance and identification, are optimal in the DETC group experience. According to Kelman:

> Compliance can be said to occur when an individual accepts influence from another person or group because he hopes to achieve a favorable reaction from the other. . . . The individual may be concerned with gaining approval and avoiding disapproval from the influencing agent in a more general way. For example, some individuals may compulsively try to say the expected thing in all situations and please everyone with whom they come into contact. . . .

In DETC groups, it is not simply the expression of correct opinions which gain approval (although this should not be minimized) but expressing them correctly. For example, "Rap to me" is highly preferred to "What do you think about the subject?" Here, the correct expression of a thought lies in using a certain jargon. More important rules for gaining approval are revealed in the preference for "You're full of shit" over "You don't know what you're talking about." Direct, self-revealing, and often earthy communication couched in a highly specific patois are likely to gain approval.

Trainees also seek approval from the group and the group leader as a way of certifying that the time and energy spent in the workshop has been worthwhile. It seems plausible that being absent from work for a week generates a sense of commitment and a desire to make the week successful. This would motivate the trainee to win the approval of his group and group leader, both of which help define "success" in the group experience.

Compliance also operates when participants want to escape disapproval or punishment. As Ottenberg (1971) says in his paper critical of encounter groups:

> Sanctions are applied overtly and covertly to foster certain expressions of ideas and affects. This gradually builds up a group expectancy toward certain issues. A person who expresses thoughts and behavior contrary to the group-expected norm can be the focus of considerable group attack, punishment, and scape-goating.

A humorous example of this is recounted by Maliver (1971) in a *New York Times* article on the encounter group movement. It suggests that avoidance of disapproval or punishment may be a potent motivator:

> Intelligence, rationality, and thoughtfulness turn out to be negative values in the encounter culture. This is best exemplified by what happened in the Esalen encounter group I described. Taking their cues from Schutz, anyone who asked a question was immediately hissed or shouted down with comments like "Intellectual! Obsessive-compulsive! Sit down! Too cerebral! Get out of your head! Say what your gut says!" Not to respond to someone else's pain or pathos or joy is *verboten*. To be bored or uninterested brings down the group's wrath. Boredom is viewed as "defensiveness" or "unrelatedness," a mask for "re-

> moteness." The response of a group when confronted with such an attitude is generally a litany of "Don't sit there like a dummy!" "You're a cold fish" . . . and perhaps the most effective, because it is the most threatening, "Get out of here if you don't want to be a part of the group."

The dynamics of encounter groups are such that the social and psychological conditions requisite for social influence by compliance are not only present but optimal.

Kelman's second process of social influence is called "identification." He describes the conditions under which it occurs:

> Identification can be said to occur when an individual adopts behavior derived from another person because the behavior is associated with a satisfying self-defining relationship to this person or group. The relationship may take . . . different forms . . . in which the individual takes over all or part of the role of the influencing agent. He attempts to be like or actually be the other person. By saying what the other says, doing what he does, believing what he believes. . . .
>
> An influencing agent who is likely to be an attractive object for such a relationship is one who occupies a role desired by the individual—who possesses those characteristics that the individual himself lacks—such as *control in a situation in which the individual is helpless, direction in a situation in which he is disoriented, or belongingness in a situation in which he is disoriented.* (Emphasis added).

These last three conditions are perfectly met in our encounter groups. Group leaders have control where the trainee is helpless, direction where he is groping, belongingness where he seeks acceptance. The motivation for trainees to seek "control," "direction," and "belongingness" aside from the benefits of general anxiety reduction early in the group, can sometimes be quite compelling. In the view of the American Psychiatric Association (Buhler, 1970):

> Members attend encounter groups not only for affective supplies but for "self-validation"; we are intrigued by and drawn toward an opportunity which permits us, as adults, to expose ourselves, to be examined, and to be approved. A great majority of indivi-

> duals, though they may be functioning competently, nevertheless have some deep concerns about their adequacy; few other institutions offer an occasion for what appears to be a comprehensive final examination of our status as human beings and many individuals attend encounter groups with the hidden agenda of finding out: Am I acceptable, Am I lovable, Do I match up to others?

It is the authors' opinion that at DETC such motives, although they may not be the hidden agenda of trainees, become serious concerns after the groups are under way. If these concerns do not evolve spontaneously within a given trainee himself, other members of the group are likely to share their perspectives on the applicability of these "questions." With psychological stakes as high as these, trainees are apt to be open to influence from a group or person that can shape the final answer. But the group member, more than being just susceptible to influence, seems in a role parallel to the patient in the therapeutic situation. As Parloff (1957b) says:

> The patient becomes a student of what is pleasing and displeasing to the therapist. If the therapist values dreams, the patient dreams; if he values sex material, the patient produces it.

The patient and group member may be in a similar situation in that the therapist or group greatly influence the answers to these ego involving questions: "Am I acceptable? Am I lovable? Do I match up to others?" It is this sort of dynamic that leads Maliver to write:

> Many observers feel that there is in the encounter movement the essence of a profound emotional fascism. Not necessarily a political fascism, but one that elicits emotional conformity, demands the correct behavior and the correct emotion at the designated time, and suppresses criticism.

The experimental evidence presented suggests that the therapeutic situation is conducive to social influence; specifically, influence on patients' values. Kelman's theoretical model of the conditions for social influence seems well fitted to the encounter group situation, and the processes and motives for influence through compliance and identification appear to be operating actively. It seems plausible to hypothesize then, that after training, the values of the DETC trainees will change in the direction of the DETC staff.

RESEARCH METHOD

To test this hypothesis, the authors measured the values of the trainees in a DETC workshop, both before and after training and compared them to the values of the staff measured some months earlier. Correlations between trainee pretraining values and staff, and trainee posttraining values and staff were computed. It was hypothesized there would be a significant increase in the correlation of trainee and staff values after training. The study was replicated in a second workshop.

PROCEDURE

A few months prior to Workshops 16 and 17, staff values were measured using Rokeach's Value Scale. Each staff member who played an important part in the actual day-to-day training activities was asked to complete the scale. No mention was made of the purpose of the study nor that other staff members would be completing the scale. Eventually, the value profile of the six key staff members was completed. A single value profile of the staff was established by choosing the staff's median rank of each of the 18 instrumental values. In determining the final median score for each value, the values of the director of training were counted twice since he was felt to have considerably more exposure to trainees than other staff members.

At the beginning and end of Workshops 16 and 17 the value scales were administered to trainees with the other test materials. Trainees in both workshops were introduced to the evaluation procedures and the nature of the questionnaires to be filled out, including the value scale. They were not told, however, that changes in values were being measured. The staff also was not aware of the study's purpose.

SUBJECTS

Workshop 16 (July 17–21, 1972) contained 32 trainees who took both the pre- and posttest questionnaires. These trainees were primarily female high school students from the Philadelphia area. Most of them were about 17 or 18 years old. From among this group, 20 trainees completed both the pre- and posttest value scale.

Workshop 17 (September 11–15, 1972) contained 27 trainees who took both pre- and posttest questionnaires. These trainees varied in age from 22 to 25 and were primarily drug counselors, social workers, youth workers, teachers, and nurses. All of these 27 trainees completed both the pre- and posttest value scale.

INSTRUMENT

The Value Scale (Form D) published by Rokeach in 1967 (Rokeach, 1968) was used in this study. It asks subjects to rank order 18 instrumental values and 18 terminal values by arranging pressure sensitive labels on a sheet of paper on which a vertical column of 18 blank frames appear beside numbers 1–18. The technique allows subjects to rearrange rankings by peeling off labels if they change their mind so that the final version represents their final value priorities. The most important value should be ranked number 1 and the least important value number 18. In this study, we were interested only in the "instrumental" values, such as "honest," "loving," "logical," etc. We felt that the workshop was relevant to these values as opposed to such "terminal" values as "inner harmony," "wisdom," or "a world at peace."

RESULTS

Shown in Table 1 is the value profile of the staff, the pre- and postvalue profile for trainees in Workshops 16 and 17, plus the amount of change recorded for each value. The Kendall Rank Correlation Coefficient (Kendall, 1956) was used to determine the validity of the hypothesis. Individual scores were constructed by first correlating each trainee's value rankings with that of the aggregate staff, both before and after the workshop. The postworkshop correlation value was subtracted from the preworkshop value. The result of this subtraction was summed across all workshop trainees. In both workshops, the null hypothesis (that there was no change in trainees' values) was rejected at the .05 significance level. Using a one-tailed test, the value change in Workshop 16 was significant at the .03 level and in a replication in Workshop 17 it was significant at the .01 level.

These results support the hypothesis of this study. Analysis of these data revealed another interesting finding: trainees' values and staff values were very highly correlated prior to the workshop. Using the same Kendall Rank Correlation Coefficient and looking only at the pretest correlation with staff, the data show a correlation significant beyond the .001 level for both Workshops 16 and 17.

These data indicate the most important staff values: "honest," "loving," and "helpful." They also indicate values of low priority to the staff: "clean," "obedient," "intellectual," and "logical."

Table 1
Changes in Values

Value	Staff, $N = 6$ median	Workshop #16, $N = 20$ mean Pre	Post	Δ[a]	Workshop #17, $N = 27$ mean Pre	Post	Δ[a]
Honest	1.5	4.8	2.9	* *1.9*	4.4	2.5	* *1.9*
Loving	1.5	5.3	4.2	* 1.1	6.2	4.9	* 1.3
Helpful	3.0	8.3	5.4	* *2.9*	7.2	7.4	- 0.2
Forgiving	5.0	6.4	7.6	- 1.2	9.7	9.4	* 0.3
Courageous	5.0	8.6	6.7	* *1.9*	8.6	7.2	* *1.4*
Responsible	5.0	5.2	6.9	- *1.7*	7.3	7.8	- 0.5
Broadminded	7.0	5.5	6.7	* 1.2	5.0	5.1	* 0.1
Imaginative	8.0	10.9	11.2	* 0.3	7.8	7.7	- 0.1
Capable	9.5	8.5	7.5	- 1.0	7.7	7.0	- 0.7
Self-controlled	9.5	12.0	11.4	* 0.6	12.4	12.1	- 0.3
Independent	11.5	8.1	9.5	* *1.4*	7.7	7.6	- 0.1
Ambitious	11.5	10.8	9.9	- 0.9	12.7	12.5	- 0.2
Polite	13.0	14.8	15.1	- 0.3	14.0	15.3	* 1.3
Cheerful	14.5	10.2	11.0	* 0.8	11.5	10.9	- 0.6
Logical	14.5	10.9	12.9	* *2.0*	9.7	10.6	* 0.9
Intellectual	16.0	10.7	11.5	* 0.8	7.7	9.8	* *2.2*
Clean	17.0	15.2	15.1	- 0.1	14.7	15.4	* 0.7
Obedient	18.0	15.0	15.8	* 0.8	16.5	17.1	* 0.6

[a] An asterisk indicates a change in the direction of the staff. A hyphen indicates change away from the staff. *Italic* numbers designates values showing the most change toward staff.

These data also highlight trainee values undergoing most change. "Honest," "helpful," "courageous" (standing up for one's beliefs), and "loving" rise in importance, as they are more important to the staff. "Logical" and "intellectual" fall in importance, as they are low in importance to the staff.

STAFF AND TRAINEE VALUES COMPARED TO THE NATION'S VALUES

Comparing the values of the staff and the trainees to those of the nation at large may give further insight into the role of values at the Drug Education and Training Center. In 1970, Rokeach published the results of his nationwide survey of adult Americans depicting the nation's value structure (Rokeach, 1970). Shown in Table 2 are the nation's values ranked

Table 2
Comparison of Values

Rank	National values	Staff values	Workshop #16	Workshop #17
1	Honest	1.5	1.0	1.0
2	Ambitious	*11.5*	*12.0*	*15.0*
3	Responsible	5.0	2.0	5.0
4	Forgiving	5.0	5.0	11.5
5	Courageous	5.0	9.0	10.0
6	Helpful	3.0	7.0	4.0
7	Broadminded	7.0	4.0	2.0
8	Clean	*17.0*	*18.0*	*17.0*
9	Capable	9.5	8.0	7.0
10	Self-controlled	9.5	15.0	14.0
11	Loving	*1.5*	*3.0*	*3.0*
12	Cheerful	14.5	10.0	13.0
13	Polite	13.0	16.0	16.0
14	Independent	11.5	*6.0*	7.0
15	Intellectual	16.0	11.0	7.0
16	Logical	14.5	13.5	11.5
17	Obedient	18.0	17.0	18.0
18	Imaginative	*8.0*	*13.5*	*9.0*

from most important to least important. Also shown are the rankings of these values among the staff and the trainees in Workshops 16 and 17.

Using a Kendall Rank order correlation coefficient, we have determined that the values of the staff and those of the nation are significantly different ($p < .05$). The ranks of the four values which account for most of the dissimilarity between staff and nation are in italics in the column titled "Staff values." They are "ambitious," "clean," "loving" and "imaginative." The staff values "loving" and "imaginative" much more than the nation, and "ambitious" and "clean" much less.

DISCUSSION

The main findings of the study show that trainees in two separate workshops shifted their values in the direction of the DETC staff. Specific trainee values most influenced by the staff and which rose in importance were "helpful," "honest," and "courageous" (standing up for one's beliefs). Two values which dropped in importance were "logical" and "intellectual."

What are some of the implications of such a shift in values? Appealing again to the patient–therapist analogy, Buhler (1962) has stated that most therapists agree that "therapists should not try to convert their patient." Since our data demonstrate a conversion in trainee values, one might ask if the same advice applies to DETC. Should the staff not try to convert the trainees, or perhaps the question is more germane when put in the form: "*Can* the staff not try to convert the trainees?" The reasoning behind Buhler's statement when viewed with a knowledge of the DETC staff may answer the latter question.

Most nondirective therapies aim at helping the patient achieve autonomy, which may or may not result in a change in values—depending on the patient's choice. For a therapist to try to "convert" his patients is to bypass one of the chief stated goals of such therapy in favor of counterfeit results. One can ask: "Is the goal at the DETC to encourage autonomy in the sense of freeing trainees from stereotyped ideas and misdirected feelings toward drug addicts?" Or is the goal to replace one blind negative stereotype of the addict and the best way to relate to the addict with another equally blind positive stereotype? Although the center strives for the former goal in theory, there is reason to believe that it may work toward the latter in practice.

If its goal was only to free trainees from those beliefs, feelings, and attitudes toward addicts which they did not choose freely and which were based on inadequate information and irrational conflicts both within themselves and toward addicts, the staff would run the risk of trainees *freely deciding*, after training, to be negative, hostile, and punitive. Such an outcome would be highly undesirable since the personal stake of the staff in the outcome of such a choice is considerable. Most of the staff are themselves ex-addicts or ex-abusers, and if the trainees decide, however freely, to condemn and reject drug addicts, staff members themselves might feel condemned and rejected. It is very difficult, therefore, for the staff to dispassionately encourage autonomy and *not* to try to convert trainees since autonomy can be a double-edged sword.

Another motive making it exceedingly difficult to eliminate staff influence on trainees' values, assuming it is desirable to do so, is that the sense of success and accomplishment the staff feels on completing a workshop is tied to their feeling that they have changed the outlook and the values of the trainees. Bolgar (1962) observes that much of a therapist's success (and indirectly his motivation) may also be dependent on the patients' acceptance of his values:

> Much of what is taught the patient by whatever techniques the

> analyst's skill and tact provide may be unacceptable to the patient. Often what is called "resistance" in psychoanalysis, is rather a conscious rejection of the analyst's values, and conversely, much of the patient's "insight" or "growth" is the direct result of his acceptance of the analyst's values. . . .

For both reasons mentioned—the staff's risk of personal rejection and their job satisfaction—it is likely that the staff cannot *help* but try to convert trainees to their way of thinking.

STAFF, TRAINEES, AND NATIONAL VALUES

When the values of the trainees in Workshop 16 are compared to the nation, one can see the same pattern of dissimilarity as between the staff and the nation. Of the five values which most separate Workshop 16 from the nation, four are the same values which most separate the staff and the nation. The difference in the value hierarchy of Workshop 17 and the nation duplicates exactly the pattern of divergence between staff and nation. Trainees from both workshops and the staff value "loving" and "imaginative" more than the nation, and "ambition" and "clean" less. In sum, trainees and staff are alike in that they share the same dissimilarities from the nation at large. Trainees and staff are also alike in their great similarity in values measured prior to training.

Two questions arise: (1) Are the staff and trainees like "two peas in a pod?" (2) Are government funds being used to further countercultural values? It is impossible to answer the first question, since the data are based on only 2 out of 27 workshops to date. Since many special workshops contained various groups such as policemen, clergy, and mental health administrators, staff and trainees are probably not always alike. The answer to this question may not be as important as the point it serves to make: beware of intentional and unintentional biases in the selection of applicants.

Such biases, if they are operative, may be counterproductive. For example, if the program's objective is to maximize training impact in terms of various changes within the trainees, and if one of these is a change in values, then we should accept trainees whose value priorities allow room for change. If a program accepts trainees with values very similar to its own, there is relatively little room for change. However, trainees with values extremely divergent from the staff may be unreceptive to the entire program. In order to maximize impact, one should accept trainees whose values are *optimally* divergent from the staff, different enough to allow for substantial change, yet not so different as to make persuasive communication impossible.

The implications of government funds being used to support attempts to further what may be countercultural values is a more difficult question. Even though we have shown that staff values *are* significantly different from national values, we must still decide whether or not this is desirable. Perhaps our country's past failure in dealing with drug addiction stems in part from misplaced values in the nation at large. Perhaps, on the other hand, our failure has been due to an insufficient promulgation of essentially valid values. In the first instance, one would be inclined to attempt a change of existing national values; in the second, one might reinforce them. Whatever the case, funding agencies and training centers should recognize that unanticipated effects of training, such as value change, may be operating and should be taken into consideration.

The importance of values pertains also to staff hiring. If trainees acquire staff values, a program director should take into consideration the values of the staff before they are hired. The values of the staff members should probably be compatible with the general philosophy of the program. If there is a mismatch in this regard, it is possible that the overall effect of the staff upon the trainees will be at cross purposes to the goals of the program.

A final point may be made with respect to the mechanism for value change. Although we have focused on the encounter experience as being responsible, it is not possible from this study to rule out other workshop experiences as contributing to the change. Such a study could be done, however, by providing a regular workshop and randomly assigning half the trainees to participate fully in the workshop, the other half to do so except for the encounter groups. Both groups would thereby receive the same didactic material. Subsequent value changes of the two groups would reveal the unique contribution of the encounter groups to value change.

ACKNOWLEDGMENT

This research was supported as part of an NIMH grant #1t15 MH 12822–01 to Dr. Uri Rueveni, Director of the Drug Education and Training Center.

REFERENCES

BOLGAR, H. The role of values in the psychotherapeutic process. In C. Buhler (ed.), *Values in Psychotherapy*. New York: The Free Press of Glencoe, 1962, pp. 9–10.

BUHLER, C. *Values in Psychotherapy*. New York: The Free Press of Glencoe, 1962, p. 11.

BUHLER, C. Encounter groups and psychiatry. *Amer. Psychiat. Assoc., Task Force Report 1*, April 1970.

KELMAN, H.D. Processes of opinion change. *Public Opinion Quart.* 25 (1): 62–65, 1961.

KENDALL, M.G. The Kendall rank correlation coefficient. In S. Siegel (ed.), *Non-parametric Statistics for the Behavioral Sciences*. New York: McGraw-Hill, 1956, pp. 213–223.

MALIVER, B.L. Encounter groupers up against the wall. *New York Times Magazine* 41, January 1971.

ORTMEYER, D., WELKOWITZ, J., and COHEN, J. Interactional effects of value system convergency: Investigation of patient–therapist dyads. In *Proceedings of the 74th Convention of the American Psychological Association*. 1966, pp. 193–194.

OTTENBERG, P. *Critique of Encounter Groups*. Paper read at Hahnemann Medical College Symposium, Philadelphia, June 16, 1971.

PARLOFF, M.B. *Communication of Values and Therapeutic Change*. Paper read at Symposium on Evaluation of Process and Results of Therapies: I. General Problems of Methods and Theory, American Psychological Association, New York, August 31, 1957a.

PARLOFF, M.B., IFLUND, B., and GOLDSTEIN, N. *Communication of "Therapy Values" between Therapist and Schizophrenic Patients*. Paper read at American Psychiatric Association Annual Meeting, Chicago, May 13–17, 1957b.

PETONY, P. Value change in psychotherapy. *Human Relations* 19: 39–45, 1966.

ROKEACH, M. *Beliefs, Attitudes and Values*. San Francisco: Jossey-Bass, 1968, pp. 156–178.

ROKEACH, M. Faith, hope and bigotry. *Psychol. Today* 3 (11): 33–37, 58, April 1970.

ROSENTHAL, D. Changes in some moral values following psychotherapy. *J. Consult. Psychol.* 19 (6): 431–436, 1955.

The International Journal of the Addictions, 9(5), 653–662, 1974

Amphetamines in the District of Columbia. III. Stimulant Abuse in Narcotics Addicts in Treatment, with an Emphasis on Phenmetrazine

Mark H. Greene,* M.D.

U.S. Public Health Service
Department of Heath, Education & Welfare
Health Services & Mental Health Administration
Center for Disease Control
Atlanta, Georgia

Napoleon Turner, Jr.

Narcotics Treatment Administration
Department of Human Resources
Government of the District of Columbia
Washington, D.C.

Robert L. DuPont, M.D.

Special Action Office for Drug Abuse Prevention
Executive Office of the President
Washington, D.C.

* To whom requests for reprints should be addressed at SAODAP, 726 Jackson Place NW, Washington, D.C. 20506.

INTRODUCTION

As the availability and quality of opiates have declined in the District of Columbia, there has been a sharp increase in the use of central nervous system stimulants (Greene and DuPont, 1973). This problem was first documented in Washington during the summer of 1972, when methamphetamine was the drug being abused. In November 1972, patients seen at the central intake facility of Washington's Narcotics Treatment Administration (NTA) began to describe the presence of a new drug in the streets. This drug was subsequently identified as phenmetrazine, a close relative of the amphetamines in both chemical structure and physiologic effects. In December 1972, the Washington Metropolitan Police first began to find phenmetrazine in the possession of addicts arrested. During this same month, phenmetrazine was detected (as an incidental finding) for the first time in the tissues of opiate overdose victims studied by the Medical Examiner of the District of Columbia. By February 1973, urine testing for phenmetrazine was underway at NTA's central intake facility (CMI) and the D.C. Superior Court urine testing laboratory (CJD). In addition, a study of drug use was made on prisoners entering the D.C. Jail. All three sources revealed high rates of phenmetrazine positivity (see Table 1). As of May 1973, this trend was still on the rise, although there were some signs of reaching a plateau. This plateau may be the first reflection of the moratorium on phenmetrazine shipments to the Washington metropolitan area imposed in May 1973 (instituted voluntarily by the drug manufacturer involved). It is hoped that this will curb the phenmetrazine outbreak as effectively as similar measures curbed the amphetamine outbreak.

This new drug problem created the need for an understanding of the

Table 1
Summary of Phenmetrazine Abuse Trends

	D.C. police data			Urine analysis data				Medical Examiner Office	
Month	Buys	Seizures		CMI		CJD		$N+$	% all ODs
December	—	3	1.0%	—	—	—	—	1	33.3
January	—	9	2.4%	—	—	—	—	2	50.0
February	10	25	5.4%	69	28.4%	—	—	2	66.6
March	37	40	6.6%	86	35.2%	70	9.3%	0	0.0
April	59	45	6.9%	86	42.2%	103	11.6%	1	33.3
May	27	20	3.7%	108	40.6%	118	12.5%	0	0.0

extent and nature of phenmetrazine abuse among patients in treatment with NTA. In this report, we will:

1. Document the point prevalence of stimulant use among NTA patients, based on patient self-reporting and urine analysis for illicit drugs.
2. Demonstrate that the phenmetrazine abuse pattern is identical to the amphetamine abuse pattern previously described in Washington.
3. Suggest that there is a subgroup within the treatment population that is at increased risk of being involved in this behavior pattern. In addition, we will discuss the implications of these findings with respect to patient management.

METHOD

Phenmetrazine Surveillance Data

The data presented in the Introduction were collected using the drug abuse surveillance system previously reported (DuPont and Greene, 1973).

Interviews of Active NTA Patients

During April 1973, 50 active NTA patients were interviewed regarding their use of central nervous system stimulants. An interview instrument for this purpose was designed and implemented by NTA's Bureau of Research and Development.

Urine Screening Survey of Active NTA Patients

A random sample of 450 active NTA patients was drawn in April 1973. This sample was restricted to patients who had been enrolled in detoxification modality for at least 1 month (n = 180) or in maintenance modality for at least 1 year (n = 270). Abstinence patients were not studied. The sample was further stratified to include patients in treatment in clinics located in different areas of the city.

During the last 2 weeks of April, an attempt was made to obtain two urine specimens from each patient in the sample. Urines were obtained by diverting specimens from those routinely collected twice weekly from all patients. These samples were analyzed for morphine, quinine, cocaine, codeine (routine), plus amphetamine, methamphetamine, phenmetrazine, and barbiturates. Demographic variables of age, race, and sex were collected on all individuals in the sample.

In order to ascertain the frequency with which specific *drugs* appeared in patients' urine, the number of urine specimens found to be positive for each drug was tabulated. These categories were not mutually exclusive; a patient found to have more than one drug in his urine was counted more than once. The number of samples positive for codeine and cocaine was so small that these drugs were omitted from the analysis.

In order to more accurately describe the drug use patterns of the *patients* in the sample, a second tabulation was done in which each patient was placed in one of eight *mutually exclusive* categories according to which drug or combination of drugs was detected. For those individuals who gave two urine specimens, the presence of a given drug in either specimen was sufficient for that person to be considered positive for that drug. Statistical analysis revealed no significant difference in the distribution of urine test results between those patients who gave one urine and those who gave two. Therefore these groups were combined for purposes of analysis.

Two different point prevalence determinations were made. First, the frequency with which patients were found to be positive for a given drug alone and in various combinations with other drugs was determined (see Table 4). This produced separate prevalence estimates for the number of patients using heroin alone, heroin plus stimulants (stimulants included both amphetamine and phenmetrazine), heroin plus barbiturates, etc. These categories were mutually exclusive. Sccond, prevalence estimates of the number of patients using each drug, whether alone or in combination with other drugs, were determined. These were an index of the number of patients using a particular drug without regard to other drugs found simultaneously. These categories were not mutually exclusive (see Table 5).

Results were tested for statistical significance using chi-square and Student's t-test.

THE PATTERN OF PHENMETRAZINE ABUSE

Questionnaire data obtained from active NTA patients revealed that the pattern of phenmetrazine abuse was identical to that previously described with amphetamine abuse (Greene and DuPont, 1973; Thompson and Brown, 1973). Of those questioned, 42% reported that they were currently using phenmetrazine. Over 90% of the phenmetrazine was administered intravenously (Users crushed phenmetrazine tablets, dissolved them in water, and injected the resulting solution), and in relatively low doses (mean: 12 75-mg tablets weekly). Over 86% of the patients stated that they used phenmetrazine to prolong the effects of heroin and/or methadone. The most common pattern was for phenmetrazine to be used in conjunction with heroin only (38%). Only 14% of those interviewed reported using phenmetrazine alone, not in conjunction with simultaneous opiate administration. Serious side effects reported in association with the use of this agent were uncommon.

URINE SURVEY AMONG NTA PATIENTS

General

Urines were obtained from 379 patients, the majority of whom gave two urines (70.7%). Significantly, 87.8% of the maintenance patients sampled gave at least one urine, as opposed to 78.9% of detoxification patients ($\chi^2 = 5.77$, $p < .02$). In addition, maintenance patients were more likely to give two urines for analysis than were detox patients ($\chi^2 = 7.76$, $p < .01$). Detox patients were more likely to have multiple drugs detected ($\chi^2 = 7.46$, $p < .05$, $df = 2$), and tended to be less likely to have a clean urine (i.e., no illicit drugs detected) than maintenance patients. By definition, all patients should have had methadone in their urines. Of the 697 urine samples analyzed, 87.2% were positive for methadone. Detox patients were less likely to have methadone detected ($\chi^2 = 55.28$, $p < .001$).

Demographic Variables

Age, race, and sex variables are summarized in Table 2. Distribution of race and sex was identical to the overall NTA population. The mean age of the sample was higher than the mean age of the total treatment

Table 2
Demographic Variables for Sample by Modality

Variable		Total sample	Maintenance	Detoxification
Age (mean years)		28.5	30.8	25.1
Race:	Black	94.3%	91.5%	98.5%
	White	5.7%	8.5%	1.5%
Sex:	Male	72.4%	73.3%	71.0%
	Female	27.6%	26.7%	29.0%

population. This resulted from the exclusion of abstinence (young) patients and the emphasis on maintenance (older) patients. The sample was, therefore, very similar to the total NTA population with respect to the demographic variables examined.

Analysis of Individual Urine Samples

A total of 697 urine specimens was analyzed. The drug most frequently detected was phenmetrazine (30.3% of all urines tested). It was detected 8 times more frequently than the amphetamines (3.7%). Heroin (morphine and/or quinine) was detected in 12.6% of the urines tested, and barbiturates in 3.9% (see Table 3).

Analysis of Individual Patients

The 379 patients who gave at least one urine sample were tabulated into eight mutually exclusive categories (see Table 4). Over 40% of the patients studied had no evidence of illicit drugs in their urine.

The largest toxicologic category was comprised of those patients in whom stimulants alone were detected (33.8%). The next largest group had both stimulants and heroin in their urine (11.1%).

Of all patients tested, 48.0% had a CNS stimulant detected, 20.6% had heroin detected, and 6.3% had barbituarates detected (see Table 5). These figures represent the point prevalence of the use of each of the above drugs in the sample studied.

Comparison of urine results to patient modality revealed that maintenance patients tended to be more likely to have clean urines and to abuse barbiturates, although the differences were not statistically significant. Detox patients were more likely to have heroin detected ($\chi^2 = 7.28$, $p < .01$), heroin plus a stimulant ($\chi^2 = 8.78$, $p < .01$), and had a

Table 3
Analysis of Individual Urine Results

Drug detected	Number +	% All urines tested
None	402	57.7
Heroin	88	12.6
Phenmetrazine	211	30.3
Amphetamine	26	3.7
Barbiturate	27	3.9
Methadone	608	87.2%

Table 4
Urine Results on Individual Patients—Exclusive Categories

Urine category	Number	Percent
Clean	153	40.4
Heroin only	30	7.9
Stimulants only	128	33.8
Barbiturates only	12	3.2
Heroin + barbiturates	2	0.5
Heroin + stimulants	42	11.1
Stimulants + barbiturates	8	2.1
Heroin, stimulants, and barbiturates	4	1.0
TOTAL	379	100.0

Table 5
Urine Results on Individual Patients—Nonexclusive Categcries

	Total sample		Maintenance		Detoxification	
Drug detected	*N*	%	*N*	%	*N*	%
Clean	153	40.4	102	43.0	51	35.9
Heroin	78	20.6	39	16.5	39	27.5
Stimulants	182	48.0	105	44.3	77	54.2
Barbiturates	24	6.3	19	8.0	5	3.5

strong tendency to be more likely to have stimulants detected ($\chi^2 = 3.12$, $p < .08$).

Analysis of urine results by geographical distribution of clinics failed to reveal any significant differences. The use of phenmetrazine was equally distributed throughout the city.

Demographically, stimulant users had no unique age, race, or sex characteristics when compared to patients not using stimulants.

DISCUSSION

The results presented support the contention that the use of phenmetrazine in Washington, D.C. follows the same pattern seen with respect to amphetamine abuse (Greene and DuPont, 1973). That is to say, it represents a variant pattern of opiate abuse as opposed to the previously described patterns of CNS stimulant abuse including recreational use of several varieties and high dose debilitating abuse of the "speed freak" type (Blackhouse and James, 1969; Briscoe and Hinterberger, 1968; Black et al., 1971; Morimoto, 1957; Kramer, 1969; Goldberg, 1968). In June 1973 the upward trend in this pattern of abuse showed some signs of leveling off.

Two point prevalence measures of stimulant use have been presented, one (42%) based on addict self-reporting and a second (48%) based on a large random sample of urines. These two independant measures are in remarkably close agreement and document the high prevalence of this type of drug abuse within this heroin addiction treatment population.

Patients enrolled in detoxification modality appeared to be at increased risk for this particular type of drug abuse. Detox patients appeared to be a relatively unstable treatment group in that they were more likely to give none or only one urine sample instead of the two required; more likely to take their methadone irregularly; and more likely to have urine analysis evidence of illicit drug use in general, and heroin and stimulant use in particular (both separately and in combination). Finally, detox patients were more likely to have multiple drugs detected than were maintenance patients. These patients represent a subgroup within the treatment population who appear to require special attention in order to deal with their drug abusing behavior. It should be noted that, by the study design, detox patients were also patients who had been in treatment for a relatively short time (mean: 2 months), whereas all the maintenance patients studied had been in treatment for at least 1 year. The relatively poor performance of the detox group may well relate to their short duration of treatment, rather than to their mode of treatment. These data do not refute the effectiveness of detoxification as a valid treatment technique.

In designing an appropriate programatic response to this phenomenon, one must decide what such behavior means. Is it benign or malignant in its effects upon the patient? Does it represent recreational drug use of little consequence or is it a serious problem?

In a previous study we documented that this pattern of amphetamine abuse was not associated with violent behavior, deteriorating interpersonal relationships, increased criminal activity, or hospitalization for associated medical or emotional problems (Greene and DuPont, 1973). We concluded that this pattern of amphetamine use was relatively benign from both the individual and community point of view. However, *this behavior in an addict undergoing treatment has more serious implications.*

First, there exist the problems associated with intravenous drug abuse in general. Patients using phenmetrazine in this manner continue to expose themselves to the morbidity and mortality of needle abuse. In addition, this pattern represents continued patient reliance on intravenous drug use as an acceptable behavior. From the standpoint of treatment and rehabilitation, giving up intravenous drugs is a primary goal.

Second, this pattern of CNS stimulant abuse is inextricably interwoven with illicit opiate abuse. Patients consistently say that the use of intravenous stimulants is intended to boost the "high" obtained from heroin or methadone. The combination of a stimulant plus heroin was the second most frequent category of drug use in this study. Moreover, finding such a large percent of patients (33.8 %) with a stimulant alone in their urine raises the disturbing possibility that the stimulant was used to modify the effects of therapeutically administered methadone in an attempt to get "high." Those directly involved in the management of patients should be alert to this possibility with regard to stimulants and other drugs as well. This issue needs further study.

We therefore conclude that the use of intravenous central nervous system stimulants by heroin addicts in treatment is undesireable behavior, and should be considered as equivalent to illicit opiate abuse. This finding highlights a new area of patient education. The patients should be reminded of the potential medical hazards to which he is exposing himself: sepsis, endocarditis, hepatitis, pneumonia, arrhythmias, exacerbation of hypertension, etc. Most addicts do not realize that medication tablets are made for oral, not intravenous, use, and that they contain a variety of substances never intended to enter the bloodstream. These substances can produce pulmonary hypertension and chronic pulmonary parenchymal damage.

In conclusion, finding that a patient is using intravenous stimulants should be taken as an indication that his treatment is not optimally successful and that his case needs reevaluation. The same procedures applied to patients found to be using heroin should be applied to those using intravenous amphetamine or phenmetrazine, such as more frequent counseling visits and loss of medication take-home privileges. Other possible treatment alternatives include an attempt to identify an acute source of stress in the patient's life, group sessions, and a more aggressive attempt at vocational stabilization.

REFERENCES

BLACK, S., OWENS, K.L., and WOLFF, R.P. Patterns of drug use: A study of 5482 subjects. *Amer. J. Psychiat.* 127: 420–423, 1971.

BLACKHOUSE, C.I., and JAMES, I.P. The relationship and prevalence of smoking, drinking, and drug taking in adolescent delinquents. *Brit. J. Addictions* 64: 75–79, 1969.

BRISCOE, O.V., and HINTERBERGER, H. Survey of the use of amphetamines by parts of the Sydney community. *Med. J. Australia* 1: 480–485, 1968.

DUPONT, R.L., and GREENE, M.H. Monitoring the dynamics of a heroin epidemic. *Science* 181: 716–722, 1973.

GOLDBERG, L. Drug abuse in Sweden. *Bull. Narcotics* 2: 8–12, 1968.

GREENE, M.H., and DUPONT, R.L. Amphetamines in the District of Columbia. I: The identification and resolution of an epidemic. *J. Amer. Med. Assoc.*, 226: 1437–1440, 1973.

KRAMER, J. An introduction to amphetamine abuse. *J. Psychedelic Drugs* 2: 1–16, 1969.

MORIMOTO, K. Amphetamine abuse in Japan. *Bull. Narcotics* 2: 8–12, 1957.

THOMPSON, R., and BROWN, B. *Survey of Amphetamine and Stimulant Use by Narcotics Treatment Administration Clients.* Unpublished data, 1973.

Note Added in Proof. Following the moratorium on phenmetrazine distribution imposed in May 1973, there ensued a sharp decline in all phenmetrazine abuse indicators. These indicators reached a nadir in September 1973 and then began to rise again, following reinstitution of phenmetrazine shipments into the Washington metropolitan area by the drug's manufacturer. By mid-1974, phenmetrazine abuse reached levels that were considerably in excess of those observed prior to the moratorium. In June 1974, the manufacturer agreed to reduce phenmetrazine shipments to Washington area pharmaceutical wholesalers to preepidemic levels. In addition, the District of Columbia Grand Jury indicted a Washington physician for selling phenmetrazine prescriptions to addicts. It is hoped that these developments will permanently control the problem of phenmetrazine abuse in the District of Columbia. The impact of these actions is being monitored prospectively using Washington's drug abuse surveillance system.

The International Journal of the Addictions, 9(5), 663–672, 1974

Naloxone and the Narcotic Abuser: A Controlled Study of Partial Blockade

Albert A. Kurland, M.D.

Thomas E. Hanlon, Ph.D.

Maryland Psychiatric Research Center
Maryland Department of Health and Mental Hygiene
Baltimore, Maryland

O. Lee McCabe, Ph.D.

Maryland Psychiatric Research Center
Maryland Department of Health and Mental Hygiene and
Loyola College
Baltimore, Maryland

INTRODUCTION

The potential usefulness of narcotic antagonists in the management of the narcotic abuser has made these compounds a subject of increasing clinical investigation over the past several years (Fraser and Rosenberg, 1966; Jaffe and Brill, 1966; Freedman et al., 1968; Martin et al., 1966). Among these compounds, *N*-allylnoroxymorphone (Naloxone) has attracted considerable attention due to its "pure" antagonistic properties (Blumberg et al., 1961; Sadove et al., 1962; Jasinski et al., 1967; Fink et al., 1968; Zaks et al., 1971). A major obstacle to its clinical use, however, has been the relatively large dosage, i.e., 2 to 3 g, required to yield a 24-hr blockade. A dosage of this size, administered for a prolonged period, not only represents a serious financial problem but is likely to be associated with secondary effects.

In seeking more parsimonious methods of utilizing Naloxone clinically, the present authors carried out a pilot study to assess the therapeutic potential of a dosage providing only a partial blockade. For this purpose, 75 parolees with a history of narcotic abuse and attending an abstinence aftercare program were placed on an open trial in which Naloxone was administered on a maintenance basis. The daily oral dosage ranged from 200 to 800 mg, producing a blockade of only 3 to 5 hr duration. The medication was administered in the evening between 6:00 and 9:00 P.M., the time the individual ordinarily reported to the clinic to provide a urine specimen in an ongoing monitoring program.

Over a 2-year study period, no serious side effects or sequelae were observed despite the daily administration of Naloxone over periods ranging from several weeks to 6 months and involving prescriptions in which dosages were rapidly increased, decreased, or stopped abruptly. Also, no dependency reactions were noted following prolonged administration. The main objective of the study, to determine whether the partial blockade approach would result in an increased retention of subjects in the program, was ultimately unattainable because of the possible operation of bias in the decision-making process. The uncertainties that remained led to the following systematic, controlled study.

METHOD OF PROCEDURE

Male parolees from the correctional institutions of Maryland who were between the ages of 17 and 55, resided in Baltimore, and had a history of narcotic drug abuse were selected for the present evaluation. Participation was voluntary, with the understanding that each subject would abide by rules specifically designed for the successful implementation of the study. Those individuals who had a history of chronic brain damage, psychosis, or long-lasting physical illness were not accepted for the program.

Upon release from prison, subjects were required to attend the narcotic outpatient clinic every evening between the hours of 6 and 9 o'clock, at which time they were required to provide a urine specimen under direct supervision.

At the clinic the subjects were randomly assigned to one of three groups and observed for a 9-month treatment period. Individuals in the first group, referred to as the concurrent control group, were assigned to a urine monitoring program which also involved group psychotherapy on a weekly basis. In addition to participation in the basic urine monitoring-group psychotherapy program, members of the two remaining groups received placebo and Naloxone, respectively, with the medication for both groups dispensed orally on a double-blind basis at the time of daily urine collection.

Medication was packaged separately for each patient in individual envelopes containing four tablets. Placebo tablets contained an inactive substance and were identical in appearance. Each tablet of Naloxone contained 200 mg of the drug. Medication envelopes were identified only by subject number, name, and date. At the time medication was administered, special care was taken to see that the subjects swallowed their tablets.

Naloxone was administered in a dosage range of 200 to 800 mg. (Since four tablets were always given on each occasion, dosages below 800 mg required the administration of both active and placebo tablets, e.g., 400 mg = 2 tablets of 200 mg Naloxone and 2 placebo tablets.) Within this range, a flexible dosage was administered which was determined on the basis of urine monitoring evidence of narcotic drug usage.

The criterion for an increase in Naloxone dosage was the presence of at least two narcotic positives and/or unexcused absences in any given 3-day period. Higher dosage levels of Naloxone (i.e., 600 to 800 mg) were utilized as long as urine tests remained positive. Reduced levels were subsequently prescribed whenever urine tests became negative. If, however, a subject continued to use narcotic drugs in spite of the utilization of the maximum dosage, he was discharged from the program and transferred either to a hospital for detoxification or to a correctional institution.

Subjects assigned to the placebo group received placebo throughout their involvement in the project, with the administration of their medication identical to that for subjects in the experimental group, i.e., the prescription of flexible dosages depending upon urine analysis results.

The treating physician was unaware of whether placebo or active drug was involved in the treatment of any individual case. The medication code was known only to the member of the research team responsible for the packaging of the medication and was broken only in those emergency cases in which the health or welfare of a subject was in jeopardy. This occurred on two occasions, and in both instances the individuals were on placebo.

Criteria of treatment effectiveness involved determination of the length of successful participation in the project, attrition rates, reasons for dropouts, and the number of deviations from abstinence.

RESULTS

Sample Characteristics

During a 13-month intake period, 119 subjects were accepted for study and randomly assigned to the three treatment groups. Forty-one of the subjects were assigned to the concurrent control, 39 to placebo, and 39 to Naloxone. The descriptive characteristics of the three subgroups and of the total sample are presented in Table 1.

The subjects were, for the most part, single, Black, and in their middle 20s. They had a low average level of intelligence and had dropped out of school during junior high after demonstrating poor to mediocre performance. Most had had multiple arrests, the average age at the time of the first arrest being approximately 18 years. Except for race, there were no differences among the three subgroups on the demographic measures in question. The effect of the race discrepancy on outcome was subsequently found to be inconsequential.

Table 1
Demographic Characteristics of the Three Subgroups and of the Total Sample

Characteristics		Treatment: Concurrent control ($N = 41$)	Placebo ($N = 39$)	Naloxone ($N = 39$)	Total sample ($N = 119$)
Mean age, years		26.2	25.7	24.2	25.4
Race:	Black	39	29	29	97
	White	2	10	10	22
Marital status:	Single	26	22	25	73
	Married	8	7	5	20
	Separated or divorced	7	10	9	26
Education (mean years)		9.0	9.0	9.1	9.0
Mean IQ		95.0	94.7	91.1	93.6
Mean arrests		3.6	3.6	3.8	3.7
Age at first arrest		17.2	18.8	17.4	17.8

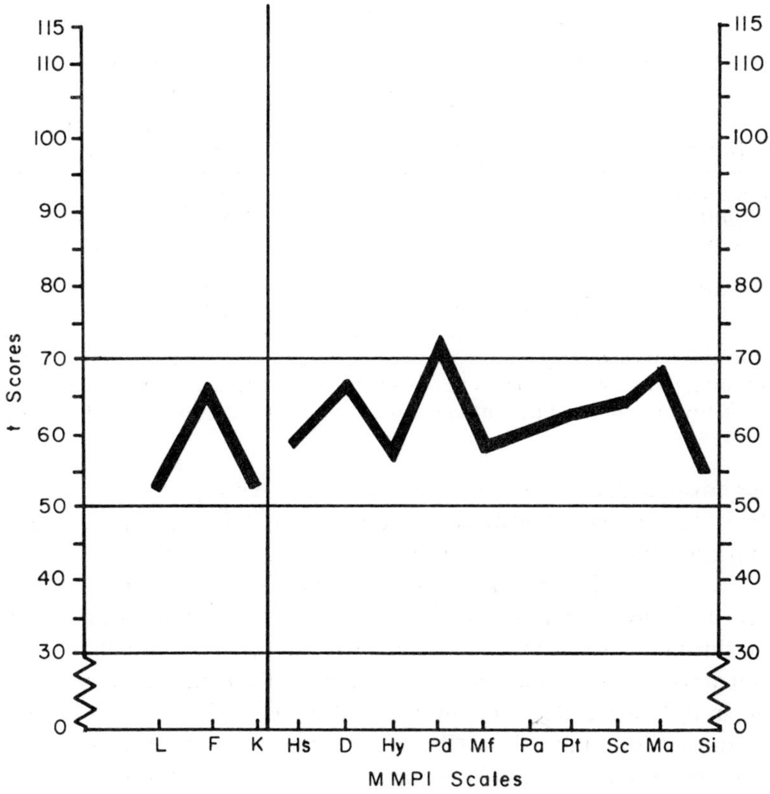

Fig. 1. Composite MMPI profile of total study population ($N = 119$).

The average MMPI profile for the entire sample is presented in Fig. 1. The profile code revealed a "4–9" peak characteristic of acting-out sociopathic individuals. There were no significant differences in the MMPI profiles of the three subgroups involved.

Treatment Outcome

In assessing outcome, two major criteria were employed: completion of the prescribed 9-month treatment course and the maintenance of narcotic drug abstinence. Completed cases were subdivided into the following types: Type I, completed program with abstinent record; Type II, completed program with minimal narcotic drug use; Type III, completed

Table 2
Outcome Data—Nine Months

Group	Completed[a] Type I	Completed[a] Type II	Completed[a] Type III	Uncompleted Ab-sconded	Uncompleted Institution-alized	Total
Concurrent control	6 (15%)	3 (7.5%)	1 (2.5%)	26 (65%)	4 (10.0%)	40[b]
Placebo	10 (25.6%)	5 (12.8%)	5 (12.8%)	17 (43.6%)	2 (5.1%)	39
Naloxone	11 (28.2%)	6 (15.4%)	0 —	19 (48.7%)	3 (7.7%)	39

[a] Type I, Completed program with abstinent record; Type II, Completed program with some drug use; Type III, other, e.g., completed after hospitalization or arrest.
[b] Excluding one nontreatment related terminator (hospitalization due to foot injury).

after hospitalization or arrest. Uncompleted cases were categorized as either absconded or institutionalized. Results for the three treatment groups in terms of these various classifications are presented in Table 2.

Type I and II completions indicate successful program participation since these involved subjects who were neither hospitalized nor incarcerated during their involvement in the program. Correspondingly, the clinic attendance of these subjects was exceptionally high and their narcotic drug usage nonexistent to minimal. Although still participating in the program at 9 months, Type III cases, besides having been briefly hospitalized or incarcerated, had poor attendance and abstinence records. Five of the six Type III cases became readdicted to narcotic drugs during the course of treatment and the remaining case, a placebo subject, required hospitalization for detoxification from alcohol. Those institutionalized, i.e., declared parole violators and returned to their original institutions, were obvious treatment failures. Although less obvious, absconders were also considered treatment failures. The discontinuance of one concurrent control case early in the teatment course was due to a hospitalization for a nontreatment-related injury. This case was not used in determining disposition percentages for the remaining concurrent control cases.

The data in Table 2 reveal that Naloxone fared no better than placebo in terms of final disposition at 9 months. Except for the five interrupted completers (i.e., Type III cases) receiving placebo, the results of active and inactive medications in terms of disposition were remarkably similar.

Although failing to reach the .05 level of significance, outcomes for concurrent control subjects were generally less favorable than those for subjects taking oral medication, whether active or inactive. Only one out of six controls compared to one out of four "pill-takers" managed to remain abstinent for the entire 9-month treatment course. Considering an uninterrupted, completed treatment course with either none or minimal narcotic drug use (i.e., Type I and Type II completions) as indication of successful program participation, the respective "success" rates for controls and "pill-takers" were 9 of 40 vs 32 of 78, a difference significant of a trend in favor of the "pill-takers" ($\chi^2 = 2.89$, $p < .10$).

Most of the subjects who deviated from abstinence did so early in the treatment course. Narcotic positive specimens were obtained on 58% of the "pill-takers" and 73% of the controls during the first 3 months of project involvement. Comparative abstinence results at 6 months were essentially the same as those at 9, i.e., yielding slightly more favorable results for those subjects on oral medication.

Although obviously accompanied by the consumption of a variety of illicitly obtained drugs, there was no evidence to indicate that in the dosage range utilized, the administration of Naloxone resulted in increased hazards or complications for the subjects involved.

DISCUSSION

Regarding the double-blind aspect of the study, the above results reveal little differential effect between placebo and Naloxone, at least as far as retention rates and the maintenance of complete abstinence are concerned. Although retention rate can be considered an appropriate criterion in the present instance, the maintenance of complete abstinence on the part of the addict actually precludes the testing of the real worth of a narcotic antagonist.

The only initial deterrent to narcotic drug-seeking behavior operating in an antagonist approach is the expectation on the part of the addict that he is unlikely to experience the same familiar reaction when he resorts to narcotic drug use. In a double-blind study, this expectation is associated with the administration of both placebo and the antagonist prior to the resumption of narcotic drug usage. The above differential abstinence results favoring "pill-takers" over concurrent controls, however meager, is evidence of this type of nonspecific deterrence.

As with other antagonists, there is no pharmacological reason to expect that Naloxone will insure complete abstinence since it does not reduce the urge to take narcotics. Its specific usefulness lies in its deterrent action once narcotic drugs are again taken. Rather than the insurance of

Table 3
Mean Narcotics Usage and Clinic Participation Data Following Deviation from Abstinence

Group	Days after 1st positive	Days absent after 1st positive	Days not providing adequate speci-mens	No. of specimens provided after 1st positive	No. of narcotic positive speci-mens	Percen-tage of positive specimens
Placebo ($N = 29$)	117.8	20.4	2.3	95.1	28.7	30.2
Naloxone ($N = 26$)	105.3	15.4	0.8	90.2	9.8	10.9

complete abstinence, the question at issue as far as Naloxone is concerned is whether it has any effect on subsequent narcotic drug-taking behavior once narcotics are resumed.

Table 3 presents narcotics usage and clinic participation data for 29 placebo and 26 Naloxone subjects following determination of their first narcotic drug-positive urine specimen in the present program.

Although placebo subjects tended to remain in the program longer after their first deviation, they were also absent or failed to provide an analyzable specimen on more occasions. Also, the number of specimens positive for narcotics among those analyzed yielded respective percentages of 30.2 and 10.9 for placebo and Naloxone, indicating significantly more narcotic drug usage in the placebo sample (difference between proportion corrected for continuity, $p < .01$). Total deviance, an overall measure of uncooperativeness including narcotics usage, absence, and failure to provide an adequate specimen, was found to be 43.6% for placebo vs 24.6% for Naloxone, a difference significant at the .01 level.

To determine whether these results reflected extreme deviance on the part of only one or two placebo cases, the mean narcotics usage percentage (positive specimens over total specimens analyzed), was determined for each double-blind subject remaining in the project for at least 60 days after his first deviation. The resulting percentages ranged from 0.4 to 90.9 for placebo subjects ($n = 21$) and from 0.4 to 33.8 for those administered Naloxone ($n = 16$). Twelve of the 21 placebo subjects had narcotics usage percentages above the percentage range for the Naloxone group. Total deviance data revealed essentially the same results in favor of Naloxone.

While they remain in the program, at least, Naloxone subjects appear to fare better than those on placebo. The fact that a slight difference between the two groups in terms of dropouts actually favors placebo possibly reflects a negative relationship between effectiveness and satisfaction in the less motivated subject. Conceivably, the less motivated placebo subject soon realizes that he can experience his customary "high" and still remain marginally involved in the program, while the less motivated Naloxone subject leaves the program when he no longer obtains gratification from narcotic drug-taking behavior.

Now that the limitations of partial blockade with lower dosage Naloxone are clear as far as outcome is concerned, the question now remains whether a higher dosage approach will be of greater benefit in this respect. A study of the administration of 500 to 2,000 mg of Naloxone contingent upon narcotic drug intake is currently underway at the same clinic and will hopefully provide further direction regarding the most effective use of this agent. For the present it appears that motivation is the key determinant in the success of the antagonist approach. In the properly motivated addict, the use of this approach can provide an important buffer to the process of readdiction.

SUMMARY

Within the framework of an ongoing urine monitoring program, 119 paroled narcotic addicts were randomly assigned to either urine monitoring alone (concurrent control) or to double-blind treatment with either placebo or Naloxone at a partial blockade dosage level (200 to 800 mg daily). Outcome assessments at 6 and 9 months tended to favor "pill-takers" over concurrent controls. Although there were no significant differences between placebo and Naloxone in terms of retention rates and the maintenance of complete abstinence, there was considerably less narcotic drug use by Naloxone-treated subjects. Side effects were judged to be minimal and of little consequence. The importance of motivation on the part of the addict in the narcotic antagonist approach is stressed.

ACKNOWLEDGMENTS

Appreciation is extended to Ralph Jacobsen, M. D., Deputy Medical Director of the Endo Laboratories, Inc., Subsidiary of E. I. du Pont de Nemours and Co., Inc., for providing the Naloxone utilized in this study. Financial support was provided by National Institute of Mental Health Grant ROI-DA-00079, and administrative support and provision of facilities by Friends Medical Science Research Center, Inc., Baltimore, Maryland. Appreciation is also due to the staffs of the Aftercare Narcotic Clinic and the Maryland Department of Parole and Probation, particularly

Mr. Fred Geelhaar of the latter agency, without whose collaboration the study could not have been implemented.

REFERENCES

BLUMBERG, H., DAYTON, H.B., GEORGE, M., and RAPPAPORT, D.N. *N*-Allynoroxymorphine: A potent narcotic antagonist. *Fed. Proc.* 20: 311, 1961.

FINK, M., ZAKS, A., SHAROFF, R., MORA, A., BRUNER, A., LEVIT, S., and FREEDMAN, A.M. Naloxone in heroin dependence. *Clin. Pharmacol. Therap.* 2: 568–577, 1968.

FRASER, H.F., and ROSENBERG, D.E. Comparative effects of (I) chronic administration of cyclazocine, (II) substitution of nalorphine for cyclazocine, and (III) chronic administration of morphine: Pilot crossover study. *Intern. J. Addictions* 1: 86–98, 1966.

FREEDMAN, A.M., FINK, M., SHAROFF, R., and ZAKS, A. Clinical studies of cyclazocine in the treatment of narcotic addiction. *Amer. J. Psychiat.* 24: 1499–1504, 1968.

JAFFE, J.H., and BRILL, L. Cyclazocine, a long-acting narcotic antagonist: Its voluntary acceptance as a treatment modality in narcotic abusers. *Intern. J. Addictions* 1: 99–123, 1966.

JASINSKI, D.R., MARTIN, W.R., and HAERTZEN, C.A. The human pharmacology and abuse potential of *N*-allylnoroxymorphine (Naloxone). *J. Pharmacol. Exp. Therap.* 157: 420–426, 1967.

MARTIN, W.R., GRODETSKY, C.W., and McLANE, T.K. An experimental study in the treatment of narcotic addicts with cyclazocine. *Clin. Pharmacol. Therap.* 7: 455–465, 1966.

SADOVE, M.S., BALAGOT, R.C., HATANO, S., and JOBGEN, E.A. Study of *N*-allylnoroxymorphine—A narcotic antagonist. *J. Amer. Med. Assoc.* 180: 771, 1962.

ZAKS, A., JONES, T., FINK, M., and FREEDMAN, A.M. Naloxone treatment of opiate dependence: A progress report. *J. Amer. Med. Assoc.* 215: 2108–2110, 1971.

The International Journal of the Addictions, 9(5), 673–699, 1974

Evaluation of a 6-Day Course in Alcoholism Education and Orientation

James H. Williams, Ph.D.

Alan VanLewen, M.A.

Tessa Breen

Florida Alcoholism Treatment and Research Center
Avon Park, Florida

This paper reports on a study of the Seventh Annual Florida School of Alcohol Studies, a 6-day course in alcoholism education and orientation.

The short-term instructional course is a tool frequently used for imparting knowledge and attempting to change attitudes. In the field of alcoholism, these efforts generally consist of institutes and seminars similar to the summer institute offered annually by the Rutgers' Center of Alcohol Studies. The alcoholism training programs offered by some states and communities seem to be abbreviated versions of the Rutgers' program, containing lectures, discussions, seminars, and workshops.

Even though the institute approach has enjoyed a growth, some authorities have questioned that participation in these ventures produces significant long-term improvement in services for alcoholics (Chafetz et al., 1970). Nevertheless, the impact of short-term institute training upon students can only be answered by appropriate evaluation studies. This investigation was undertaken with the objective of evaluating the Florida School of Alcohol Studies.

Recent investigations suggest that short courses on alcoholism can bring about attitude, knowledge, and behavioral changes (Mackey, 1969; Williams et al., 1962; Williams et al., 1968; and Mellen et al., 1969). Even though attitudes, knowledge, and behavior can not necessarily be assumed to change together, the school had as its broad purpose the presentation of materials that would effect changes in the student's attitudes, knowledge, and behavior. The study was conducted so that the outcome of the course could be assessed and recommendations made to assist persons in charge of subsequent schools.

Specifically, the major variable under investigation was the Florida School of Alcohol Studies and the impact it had upon the individuals who attended. The actual influence of the school could not be measured directly. However, the objectives of the course were explicit—to bring about a shift in the attitudes, knowledge, and behavior of its students. Therefore, measures were developed to assess indirectly changes the school was attempting to motivate, and an analysis of the results was used to draw conclusions relative to the course's objectives.

The goals of the school were to: motivate attitude changes in students in accordance with specified concepts of alcoholism; enable subjects to gain general information about and an understanding of alcoholism, including the recognition of symptoms in an individual or family unit, referral practices, and treatment methods; encourage students to seek continuing alcoholism education; motivate its subjects to experience alcoholism related activities; and involve students in community services.

METHOD AND PROCEDURE

Subjects

The sample contained 172 students attending the Seventh Annual Florida School of Alcohol Studies and 144 persons not attending. Student and comparison group members were matched on sex, county of residence, and occupation.

Questionnaires

Schedules were constructed to obtain information on the respondents' background characteristics and alcoholism attitudes, general knowledge, information, and activities. The questionnaires were administered to student and comparison group persons on the day the school began (*before*), the day that it ended (*after*), and at 6 months following the school (*follow-up*).

The schedule contained items on attitudes concerning alcoholism. These questions were scaled utilizing an item analysis technique (Likert, 1967). The attitude scales derived were: alcoholism as an illness or a moral weakness (7 items), social responsibility (7 questions), and rehabilitation of alcoholics (7 items).

Eleven knowledge of alcoholism subscales were used (Pennington and McGlammery, n.d.). The tests measured the individual's general knowledge of alcoholism and contained 4 items each. They were: etiology of alcoholism, physiological action of alcohol, treatment procedures for alcoholism, effectiveness of treatment, symptoms of alcoholism, prevalence of alcoholism, state treatment facilities in Florida, effect of alcohol on overt behavior, legal control of alcohol, manufacture of alcoholic beverages, and drinking customs.

The third category of items, information about alcoholism, from which eight scales were developed, was based upon the specific subject matter of the curriculum. The sources of questions were school instructors, research personnel, and others (Pennington and McGlammery, n.d.; Passey and Pennington, 1960). Included then, were general information about alcoholism (14 questions), based upon general sessions of the school, and the following workshop scales: alcoholism and other public health problems (6 questions), alcoholism and industrial problems (7 items), therapy for the alcoholic and his family (15 questions), alcoholism and Halfway Houses (3 items), alcoholism and the law (5 questions), alcoholism and community action (4 items), and alcoholism and health education (14 questions).

A separate schedule containing 33 questions relating to alcoholism activity was administered to the subjects 6 months after the school. The questions were classified as continuing education (5 items), experience with alcoholism (21 items), and community services (7 questions).

The Seventh Annual Florida School of Alcohol Studies

This course offered 6 days of intensive instruction on alcoholism including general and workshop sessions. The general sessions contained daily series of lectures, panel discussions, question and answer periods, and demonstrations–a total of $14\frac{1}{4}$ hr of instruction. They were of general relevance and were scheduled so that all students could attend. On the

Table 1

Topics Given in the General Workshop Sessions at the Seventh Annual Florida School of Alcohol Studies

General and workshop sessions	Name of topics by day given					
	Sunday	Monday	Tuesday	Wednesday	Thursday	Friday
General sessions	Where the action is	Introduction	Approaches to treatment	Teenage use of alcoholic beverages	Educational resources	Wrap up
		The disease concept	A community approach	Approaches to prevention	Current trends	
Workshops						
Public health		Overview	Identifying the alcoholic	Treatment philosophy	Treatment model	Summary and conclusions
		The addiction process	Emergency situations	Family involvement	Referral	
Therapy for the alcoholic and his family		Etiology of alcoholism	Nature of alcoholism. Part II	Inpatient care	Family therapy	Summary and conclusions
		Nature of alcoholism. Part I	Treatment modalities	Outpatient care	Referral	
Industrial problems and approaches		Nature of problem	Early detection. Part II	Supervisory personnel training in confrontation	The workers' return to job	Summary and conclusions
		Early detection. Part I	Management decisions	Supervisory personnel training in referral to	General company program	

			treatment and community resources		
Law as a factor in rehabilitation and prevention	Law oriented rehabilitation	Detoxification	Court programs. Part II	Adult programs	Summary and conclusions
	Medical problems at time of arrest	Court programs. Part I	Community resources	Juvenile programs	
Health teachers	Review of alcohol education	Current alcohol education	Basic principles for teaching	Review of study guide. Part II	Summary and conclusions
	Role of the teacher	Goals	Review of study guide. Part I	Health teachers resources	
Community action	First steps	Local resources	Government action program supervision	Financing. Part II	Summary and conclusions
	Information and referral	Professional education	Financing. Part I	Public relations	
Halfway houses	Desocialization process	Continuance of care	Halfway house staffing	Halfway house organization. Parts I and II	Summary and conclusions
	Rehabilitation process	Starting a halfway house	Halfway house procedures		

other hand, workshop sessions offered instruction on specific topics or situations: public health, health education, community action, the law, industry, Halfway Houses, and treatment. They took place at the same time each day, making it necessary for a student to choose among them. Table 1 contains an outline of the program.

Faculty for the school was recruited from the professional staff members of the Florida Bureau of Alcoholic Rehabilitation, instructors at Florida Technological University, and treatment experts including physicians, psychiatrists, social workers, and psychologists.

Study Design and Procedure

The primary purpose of the study was to investigate what influence the school, the major intervening variable, had upon the persons who attended. The instrument for measuring the course's impact was the questionnaire.

The students' before and after scores were compared with those of the comparison group. However, the administrative structure of the school was such that any qualified applicant was admitted, thus prohibiting a random assignment of subjects to groups as required by the classical experimental design.

The questionnaires were completed by the students at the school immediately preceding its beginning and end, while the comparison group subjects filled out theirs by mail. All respondents completed the follow-up survey through the mail.

RESULTS

Characteristics of Student and Comparison Groups

Most of the background characteristics did not differentiate the students from the comparison group (Table 2). The student group was composed of: 54% males; 96% Caucasians; persons averaging 40 years of age; 61% married individuals; 76% Protestants; persons who averaged 15 years of school completed; 40% of subjects with an undergraduate major in social science; 30% of its individuals with a graduate major ($N = 46$) in social work, criminology, or psychology; and 43% of its subjects with professional school majors in nursing. Students were Florida residents (97%), but they had lived in the state fewer years than comparison

Table 2
Background Characteristics of Students Attending the Seventh Annual Florida School of Alcohol Studies and Controls

Background characteristics	Total ($N = 316$)	Student group ($N = 172$)	Comparison group ($N = 144$)	Significance
Sex	($N = 310$)		($N = 138$)	
Male, %	56	54	62	[a]
Color	($N = 296$)	($N = 162$)	($N = 134$)	
White, %	97	96	98	[a]
Age	($N = 303$)	($N = 165$)	($N = 138$)	
Mean	41	40	42	[b]
Marital status	($N = 301$)	($N = 164$)	($N = 137$)	
Married and living with spouse, %	67	61	74	
Widowed, %	5	7	3	
Single, never married, %	16	17	15	[a]
Divorced or separated, %	12	15	9	
Church preference	($N = 284$)	($N = 149$)	($N = 135$)	
Protestant, %	77	76	77	
Catholic, Roman or Orthodox, %	13	13	13	[a]
Jewish, %	3	3	3	
None, %	7	8	7	
Years resided in Florida	($N = 305$)	($N = 167$)	($N = 138$)	
Mean	20	17	22	[d]
Size of place of residence	($N = 305$)	($N = 167$)	($N = 138$)	
Large city (100,000 or over), %	32	36	26	
City (25,000 to 100,000), %	32	28	38	
Town (2,500 to 25,000), %	29	28	30	[a]
Small town or under, %	8	8	6	
Years of school completed	($N = 304$)	($N = 165$)	($N = 139$)	
Mean	15	15	16	[b]
Highest academic or professional degree	($N = 202$)	($N = 105$)	($N = 97$)	
Doctorate Ph.D., M.D., D.D., Th.D., L.L.D., Litt. D., %	8	6	11	
Master, %	33	31	35	
Bachelor, %	46	49	42	[a]
R.N., %	13	14	11	
Undergraduate major	($N = 196$)	($N = 107$)	($N = 89$)	
Social science, %	36	40	30	
Education, %	17	15	19	
Nursing, %	6	6	6	

(*continued*)

Table 2 (continued)

Background characteristics	Total (*N* = 316)	Student group (*N* = 172)	Comparison group (*N* = 144)	Significance
Liberal arts, %	22	21	24	[a]
Business, %	9	9	9	
Science, %	11	9	12	
Graduate major	(*N* = 103)	(*N* = 46)	(*N* = 57)	
Counseling, rehabilitation counseling, %	18	17	19	
Social work, criminology, psychology, clinical psychology, %	25	30	21	
Public health, %	4	4	4	
Education, health education, school administration, %	18	26	10	
Theology, philosophy, %	13	13	12	[a]
Law, %	5	2	7	
Medicine, %	14	4	21	
Liberal arts, %	3	0	5	
Business, %	1	2	0	
Professional school major	(*N* = 71)	(*N* = 35)	(*N* = 36)	
Nursing, %	48	43	53	
Theology, %	16	14	17	
Medicine, %	7	9	6	
Law, %	8	9	8	[a]
Social work, %	1	3	0	
Other, %	20	23	17	
Number years employed *on* present job	(*N* = 280)	(*N* = 147)	(*N* = 138)	
Mean	5	4	7	[d]
Occupational level of present job	(*N* = 305)	(*N* = 167)	(*N* = 138)	
Professional, technical, and kindred workers, %	70	73	68	
Managers, officials, and proprietors, %	11	7	16	
Clerical and kindred workers, %	6	4	7	
Sales workers, %	2	2	1	[c]
Craftsmen, foremen, and kindred workers, %	1	0	1	
Service workers, %	6	6	6	
Other occupations, %	4	7	0	
Name of company, business organization, unit of govern-				

(*continued*)

Table 2 (continued)

Background characteristics	Total (N = 316)	Student group (N = 172)	Comparison group (N = 144)	Significance
ment, self or others for whom respondent works on present job	(N = 289)	(N = 152)	(N = 137)	
Professional and related services, %	62	55	69	
Public administration, %	30	36	23	c
All other businesses, %	8	9	8	
Training in any aspect of alcoholism				
Attended another school of alcohol studies, %	10	13	6	c
Attended orientation at Avon Park Center, %	11	12	9	a
Attended other training directly involving alcohol, %	5	8	3	a
Other training not mentioning alcoholism or mentioned in connection with other studies, %	22	21	23	a
Informal training, %	8	9	6	a
Very little or none, %	36	31	41	a
Experience in any aspect of alcoholism				
Worked with or treated alcoholics in psychiatric or medical center for alcoholics, %	5	5	4	a
Worked with or treated alcoholics in other treatment settings, %	17	17	17	a
Contact or work with alcoholics; Vocational rehabilitation, pardon and parole, law enforcement agencies, %	13	14	12	a
Contact or work with alcoholics; social or welfare, clergymen, or industry, %	16	17	15	a
In alcoholism organization, %	10	12	6	a

(*continued*)

Table 2 (continued)

Background characteristics	Total ($N = 316$)	Student group ($N = 172$)	Comparison group ($N = 144$)	Significance
Halfway or A.A. house for alcoholics, %	7	10	4	[c]
A.A. related, %	12	17	6	[c]
Personal experience with alcoholics, %	18	19	17	[a]
"Have you had a problem drinker (or alcoholic) as a client during past year?"	($N = 272$)	($N = 143$)	($N = 129$)	
Yes, %	66	77	54	[c]
"To what extent did this person change regarding drinking?"	($N = 144$)	($N = 93$)	($N = 51$)	
Doesn't drink at all now, %	34	42	24	
Still drinks but rarely, %	18	22	12	[c]
Not at all or became worse, %	46	37	65	

[a] Not statistically significant at .05 level based upon the chi-square test.
[b] Not statistically significant at .05 level based upon analysis of variance and the *F* distribution.
[c] Statistically significant at .05 level or beyond using the chi-square test.
[d] Statistically significant at .05 level or beyond using analysis of variance and the *F* distribution.

group subjects, an average of 17 years for the former and 22 years for the latter.

Students had held their last job less time (mean of 4 years) than comparison group persons (mean of 7), while 73% of students were professional, technical, and kindred workers compared with the control group's 68%. A majority of the respondents were employed by agencies engaged in professional and related services (55% among students and 69% in the comparison group).

As to previous alcoholism training, 13% of the students and 6% of the comparison group had attended another such school. Student subjects training included: 12% receiving orientation at the Florida Alcoholism Treatment and Research Center in Avon Park, Florida; 8% who had received other training directly involving alcohol; 21% who reported unspecified alcoholism training; 9% listed informal; and 31% reported very little or none.

Previous alcoholism experience in Halfway Houses was claimed by

10% of students and 4% of the comparison group. Further, 17% of students and 6% of comparison group individuals had some A.A. related experience. On a different question nearly 77% of the students and 54% of the comparison group stated that they had a problem drinker as a client during the past year. Sixty-three percent of the student subjects, but only 35% of comparison group ones, claimed that their client had become abstinent or nearly so after treatment.

Othr types of prior alcoholism experience showed students with 19% of their number reporting personal experience; 17% listed work with or treated alcoholics in treatment settings; 17% gave contacts or work with alcoholics in a social or welfare, industrial, or church settings; 14% reported contact or work with alcoholics in conjunction with vocational rehabilitation, pardon and parole, or law activities; 12% of students had experience with alcoholics in an organization not previously mentioned; and 5% had worked or treated alcoholics in a psychiatric or medical center for alcoholics.

School of Alcohol Studies Attendance Record

Eighty-eight percent of school enrollees attended some activity every day, while 7% missed only 1 day. Workshop participation was assessed for each day of the course. However, the *first* workshop attended by a student was considered indicative of this person's primary area of interest, or perhaps need. Thus instruction most often sought after was therapy for the alcoholic and his family, attended on the first day by 27% of the course participants; law as a factor in rehabilitation and prevention came next with 18%; and then community action, attended by 16%. The industrial problems and approaches workshop was attended by 13% of the student members, and the public health workshop by 12%. The two workshops with the lowest first session sttendance were Halfway Houses (8%) and health teachers (6%).

Attitudes toward Alcoholics

Attitudes concerning alcoholics were measured by three scales. A cutoff point was established for each scale based upon the median for the total sampled distribution of scores *before* the school. The attitude scores ranged from 0 to 5 with high values considered favorable and low ones unfavorable.

Responses that defined "alcoholism as an illness" were rated favorable while the ones that depicted it as "a moral weakness" were unfavorable. Before the school, the two study groups were not statistically different on this attitude scale. However, after the course, 63% of the student subjects and 35% of the comparison group members reached high scores. This time the groups did differ significantly. The change (difference) between the before and after frequencies was statistically significant only for the student responses (Table 3).

Answers indicative of the acceptance of "social responsibility for alcoholism" were considered favorable while the denial of responsibility was unfavorable. Before the school, the student group did not differ from the comparison group on the proportion of persons with a high score on the social responsibility scale; but on the after scores the groups did differ significantly (59% of persons attending the course had a high score while for individuals not attending, the comparable figure was 33%). The difference between the before–after scores for each study group was

Table 3
Attitudes toward Alcoholism Before and After the Seventh Annual Florida School of Alcohol Studies of Student and Comparison Group Members

Attitude scales	Student group	Comparison group	Significance
Alcoholism as an illness or a moral weakness. Score: 4.00 high	(N = 150)	(N = 89)	
After, %	63	35	[c]
Before, %	53	43	[a]
Difference, %	+10	−8	
Significance	[d]	[b]	
Social responsibility. Score: 3.50 high	(N = 149)	(N = 89)	
After, %	59	33	[c]
Before, %	46	43	[a]
Difference, %	+13	−10	
Significance	[d]	[d]	
Rehabilitation of alcoholics. Score: 3.00 high	(N = 149)	(N = 89)	
After, %	60	51	[a]
Before, %	62	53	[a]
Difference, %	−2	−2	
Significance	[b]	[b]	

[a] Not statistically significant at .05 level using the chi-square test.
[b] Not statistically significant at .05 level using the McNemar (1955) test.
[c] Statistically significant at .05 level or beyond using the chi-square test.
[d] Statistically significant at .05 level or beyond using the McNemar (1955) test.

statistically significant. However, the students showed an increase in the percentage of their after scores favorable while the comparison group decreased.

There were no statistically significant differences between the groups before or after the school, or in the before–after differences within each group on the attitude toward rehabilitation of alcoholics. The school did not appear to have an impact on the students' feelings about alcoholism prognosis.

Knowledge of Alcoholism

An assessment of the respondents' level and change in knowledge of alcoholism was a concern of the evaluation study. The general knowledge of alcoholism test consisted of a total score and 11 subtest scores adapted from the Alabama Alcoholism scales. The study groups were not significantly different on the before values of the total score. However, on the after test the proportions reaching a high score came to 91% among students and 71% for comparison group members; the group difference was statistically significant. Student subjects went from 71% high before the school to 91% after; the difference was significant. For the comparison group respondents, no significant before–after difference was found (Table 4).

The student group exhibited after knowledge scores significantly different from before ones on 6 of 11 subscales: etiology of alcoholism,

Table 4

Total General Knowledge of Alcoholism Before and After the Seventh Annual Florida School of Alcohol Studies of Student and Comparison Group Members

General knowledge scale	Student group	Comparison group	Significance
Total general knowledge of alcoholism. Score: .70 high	(N = 150)	(N = 89)	
After, %	91	71	[c]
Before, %	71	61	[a]
Difference, %	+20	+10	
Significance	[d]	[b]	

[a] Not statistically significant at .05 level using the chi-square test.
[b] Not statistically significant at .05 level using the McNemar (1955) test.
[c] Statistically significant at .05 level or beyond using the chi-square test.
[d] Statistically significant at .05 level or beyond using the McNemar (1955) test.

treatment procedures for alcoholism, effectiveness of treatment, state treatment facilities in Florida, effects of alcohol on overt behavior, and manufacture of alcoholic beverages. Student differences were not significant on symptoms of alcoholism, prevalence of alcoholism, legal control of alcohol, and drinking customs. This group did produce one negative change that was statistically significant, physiological action of alcohol. Finally, the comparison group was observed to have one significant before–after favorable change, on the manufacture of alcoholic beverages.

When subscale scores between student and comparison group members were considered, no significant differences were found on any of the general knowledge tests before the course. However, on the after values, the two groups differed significantly on 4 out of the 11 subscales: state treatment facilities in Florida, effects of alcohol on overt behavior, manufacture of Alcoholic beverages, and drinking customs.

Information on Alcoholism

The information about alcoholism tests covered the content of the school's general sessions and workshops. Only students had a significant before–after difference of persons with high scores on general information about alcoholism (general sessions test). This group had 73% with an after proportion high which produced an increase of +32% over the before percentage (41%). Furthermore, a significant difference appeared between the after, but not the before, scores of student and comparison group members (Table 5).

Table 5

General Information about Alcoholism Before and After the Seventh Annual Florida School of Alcohol Studies of Student and Comparison Group Members

General information scale	Student group	Comparison group	Significance
General information about alcoholism.			
Score: .80 high	(N = 150)	(N = 89)	
After, %	73	36	[c]
Before, %	41	29	[a]
Difference, %	+32	+7	
Significance	[d]	[b]	

[a] Not statistically significant at .05 level using the chi-square test.
[b] Not statistically significant at .05 level using the McNemar (1955) test.
[c] Statistically significant at .05 level or beyond using the chi-square test.
[d] Statistically significant at .05 level or beyond using the McNemar (1955) test.

Student respondents exhibited after percentages high that were significantly different from their before proportions on every workshop information about alcoholism test except alcoholism and community action. In the comparison group none of the workshop scale changes reached significance. Before workshop scores of student and comparison group members significantly differed only on one scale, alcoholism and Halfway Houses. After the school, however, 4 out of 7 workshop values showed that student subjects differed significantly from the comparison group (Table 6).

Table 6

Information about Alcoholism Before and After the Seventh Annual Florida School of Alcohol Studies of Student and Comparison Group Members

Information scales	Student group	Comparison group	Significance
Alcoholism and other public health problems. Score: .70 high	(N = 146)	(N = 86)	
After, %	62	41	c
Before, %	43	35	a
Difference, %	+19	+6	
Significance	d	b	
Alcoholism and industrial problems. Score: .60 high	(N = 147)	(N = 88)	
After, %	59	38	c
Before, %	42	42	a
Difference, %	+17	−4	
Significance	d	b	
Therapy for the alcoholic and his family. Score: .80 high	(N = 149)	(N = 87)	
After, %	77	59	c
Before, %	60	55	a
Difference, %	+17	+4	
Significance	d	b	
Alcoholism and Halfway Houses. Score: .60 high	(N = 147)	(N = 83)	
After, %	54	33	c
Before, %	48	33	c
Difference, %	+6	0	
Significance	b	b	
Alcoholism and the law. Score: .80 high	(N = 150)	(N = 88)	
After, %	71	63	a
Before, %	53	61	a
Difference, %	+18	+2	
Significance	d	b	

(*continued*)

Table 6 (continued)

Information scales	Student group	Comparison group	Significance
Alcoholism and community action.			
Score: .60 high	(N = 149)	(N = 87)	
After, %	69	62	[a]
Before, %	63	66	[a]
Difference, %	+6	−4	
Significance	[b]	[b]	
Alcoholism and health education.			
Score: .80 high	(N = 147)	(N = 87)	
After, %	49	43	[a]
Before, %	38	33	[a]
Difference, %	+11	+10	
Significance	[d]	[d]	

[a] Not statistically significant at .05 level using the chi-square test.
[b] Not statistically significant at .05 level using the McNemar (1955) test.
[c] Statistically significant at .05 level using the chi-square test.
[d] Statistically significant at .05 level using the McNemar (1955) test.

Participation in Follow-up Alcoholism Related Activities

Alcoholism activities of the subjects following the course were assessed in the areas of continuing education, experience with alcoholism, and community services. Table 7 presents data from the follow-up survey on the 25 out of 33 items that differentiated student from comparison group members. The student group proportions "yes" were larger on every item than the comparison group's. Continuing education alcoholism activity differentiated students from comparison group members on 3 questions, experience with alcoholism 18, and community services 4.

Follow-up Alcohol-Related Activities Correlated with Previously Held Attitudes about, Knowledge of, and Information on Alcoholism

This part of the findings examines what relationship, if any, exists between the subjects' follow-up alcoholism activities and their previously held attitudes, knowledge, and information concerning alcoholism. The respondents' test scores obtained before and after the school were used. Also, "difference" scores were calculated by subtracting the before value from the after one and adding a constant. Arbitrary scores were assigned follow-up responses to facilitate the use of product moment correlation

Table 7

Alcohol Related Activity Reported by Student and Comparison Group Members 6 Months after Completion of Course[a]

Type of activity	Student group (N = 112), %	Comparison group (N = 70), %
Continuing education		
Have you read books related to alcoholism? "Yes"	81	67
Have you pursued further education in alcoholism workshop seminars? "Yes"	47	24
Have you pursued further education in alcoholism from college courses related to alcoholism? "Yes"	21	6
Experience with alcoholism		
Have you referred alcoholics to helping		0
professions, such as psychiatrists, physicians, social workers, etc.? "Yes"	84	71
Have you counseled alcoholics? "Yes"	80	56
Have you referred alcoholics' families to helping professions, such as psychiatrists, physicians social workers, etc.? "Yes"	80	54
Have you referred alcoholics to A.A.? "Yes"	78	52
Have you referred alcoholics to treatment facilities for alcoholism excluding state mental hospitals? "Yes"	76	53
Have you counseled alcoholics' families? "Yes"	74	49
Have you referred alcoholics' families to Al-Anon or A.A.? "Yes"	72	44
Have you referred alcoholics to other agencies? "Yes"	70	48
Have you referred alcoholics' families to other agencies? "Yes"	66	36
Have you referred alcoholics' families to facilities for alcoholism, excluding state mental hospitals? "Yes"	62	30
Have you participated in study groups dealing with alcoholism? "Yes"	47	26
Have you participated in counseling groups dealing with alcoholism for individuals who are alcoholic? "Yes"	47	26
Have you participated in ongoing functioning of A.A. groups? "Yes"	40	13

(*continued*)

Table 7 (continued)

Type of activity	Student group ($N = 112$), %	Comparison group ($N = 70$), %
Have you participated in counseling groups dealing with alcoholism for individuals who are *not* alcoholic? "Yes"	33	19
Have you organized or helped organize A.A. groups? "Yes"	26	7
Have you organized counseling groups dealing with alcoholism for individuals who *are* alcoholic? "Yes"	25	6
Have you organized counseling groups dealing with alcoholism for individuals who are *not* alcoholic? "Yes"	21	4
Have you organized study groups dealing with alcoholism? "Yes"	27	9
Community services		
Have you distributed educational materials, such as pamphlets, dealing with alcoholism? "Yes"	77	44
Have you given lectures or talks on alcoholism? "Yes"	58	25
Have you participated in community and school alcohol education activities? "Yes"	50	31
Have you served as a member of a planning or advisory group attempting to cope with the problem of alcoholism? "Yes"	41	19

[a]All values are statistically significant at .05 level using the chi-square test.

analysis. Coefficients of correlation were computed between each attitude, knowledge, and information scale scores and the response to the alcoholism activity questions. [Space restrictions prohibit the inclusion of the tables. The author will furnish copies of the correlation tables (1,800 coefficients of correlations) to interested persons upon request].

Continuing Alcoholism Education Correlated with Attitudes, Knowledge, and Information about Alcoholism. Alcoholism as an illness or moral weakness was the only attitude scale which produced statistically significant correlations with the follow-up continuing education questions. Students with a favorable before school attitude score tended to pursue further education in alcoholism workshop seminars ($r = .23$), while those with favorable after school attitudes pursued further education in alcoholism from college courses related to alcoholism ($r = .33$). The comparison group, however, had a significant negative correlation ($r = -.24$) between this before school attitude scale value and the latter follow-up item.

No significant correlations resulted in either study group when continuing education activities were correlated with test scores on the total general knowledge or general information scales.

When the information scores on the seven separate workshop tests were correlated with continuing education responses, the student group had only two significant correlations. Students who increased their scores on the therapy for the alcoholic and his family scale during the school tended to read books related to alcoholism ($r = .22$) and to pursue further education in alcoholism workshop seminars ($r = .21$). Two significant correlations were found in the comparison group. One was between the law workshop scores (after) and further education in alcoholism from other continuing education related to alcoholism ($r = .26$) and the other was between the scores on the community action test (difference) and reading professional journal articles related to alcoholism ($r = .39$).

Alcoholism Experience Correlated with Attitudes, Knowledge, and Information about Alcoholism. Students who scored favorable on alcoholism as an illness or a moral weakness scale (before) tended subsequently: to refer alcoholics' families to helping professions ($r = .26$); to refer alcoholics to treatment facilities for alcoholism ($r = .24$); to refer alcoholics' families to facilities for alcoholism ($r = .28$); to organize study groups dealing with alcoholism ($r = .25$ before and $r = .20$ after); and to organize or help organize A.A. groups ($r = .19$). The comparison group exhibited no comparable significant correlations.

When scores on the other attitude scales were correlated with experience responses, only a few significant correlations resulted. Students scoring favorable on social responsibility (before) referred alcoholics' families to other agencies ($r = .21$). However, comparison group members with favorable scores on this scale had organized study groups dealing with alcoholism ($r = .29$ difference) and had organized counseling groups dealing with alcoholism for individuals who are not alcoholic ($r = .30$ after).

The remaining attitude test, rehabilitation of alcoholics, when correlated with experience, indicated that students with favorable scores both before and after the school tended subsequently to have organized study groups dealing with alcoholism ($r = .24$). Finally, favorable scoring comparison group persons had referred alcoholics' families to Al-Anon or A.A. ($r = .27$ before).

Alcoholism experience questions, when correlated with the total general knowledge scale, indicated that students with high knowledge scores tended to participate in counseling groups dealing with alcoholism for individuals who are alcoholic ($r = .26$ after) but not to participate in study groups dealing with alcoholism ($r = -.26$ difference). No comparison group correlations were statistically significant.

Students with high scores on the general information about alcoholism test (after) tended to: refer alcoholics to A.A. ($r = .24$); refer alcoholics to other agencies ($r = .40$); refer alcoholics' families to other agencies ($r = .20$); refer alcoholics' families to facilities for alcoholism ($r = .26$); participate in study groups dealing with alcoholism ($r = .22$); participate in counseling groups dealing with alcoholism for individuals who are alcoholic ($r = .34$) and who are not alcoholic ($r = .21$); organize study groups dealing with alcoholism ($r = .22$); organize counseling groups dealing with alcoholism for individuals who are alcoholic ($r = .20$); and participate in and organize A.A. groups ($r = .21$ after and $r = .21$ before). The comparison group had no significant correlations.

It can be seen from the preceding paragraph that students' scores on the general information scale outlined a broad connection between information concerning alcoholism taught at the school and alcoholism experience following it.

Significant coefficients of correlation were found when the 7 workshop information scale scores were correlated with the 18 experience items. The therapy workshop test showed that students with high scores had: organized counseling groups dealing with alcoholism for individuals who are not alcoholics ($r = .21$ difference); participated in counseling groups dealing with alcoholism for individuals who are not alcoholics ($r = .20$ difference); not referred alcoholics' families to other agencies ($r = -.24$ after); and not participated in study groups dealing with alcoholism ($r = -.24$ before). Of interest here were the comparison group's correlations. These persons went from a $-.33$ correlation before the school to a $+.27$ after it on their participation in counseling groups dealing with alcoholism for individuals who are alcoholics. Favorable scoring members had referred alcoholics to state mental hospitals ($r = .25$ after and $r = .24$ difference); did not refer alcoholics' families to other agencies ($r = -.29$ difference); did not participate in study groups dealing with alcoholism ($r = -.24$ after); did not counsel alcoholics' families ($r = -.26$ after);

and did not refer alcoholics' families to helping professions ($r = -.24$ before and $r = -.34$ after).

When considering the workshop test on alcoholism and health education, students who were high on the difference score tended to counsel alcoholics ($r = .22$), and to refer both alcoholics ($r = .30$) and their families ($r = .21$) to other agencies. In addition, high-scoring students organized or helped organize A.A. groups ($r = .23$ after), and tended not to refer alcoholics to helping professions ($r = -.21$ before). Definite patterns appeared when the comparison group was noted. Thus high-scoring members participated in counseling groups dealing with alcoholism for individuals who are not alcoholics ($r = .28$ after and $r = .25$ difference), referred alcoholics to A.A. ($r = .28$ after and $r = .25$ difference), referred alcoholics to other agencies ($r = .23$ after), and counseled alcoholics' families ($r = .68$ after).

When the alcoholism and the law workshop scores were correlated with alcoholism experience, significant coefficients were evident only in the comparison group. The questions that produced a significant coefficient of correlation with these workshop scores were: Have you referred alcoholics to A.A.? ($r = .27$ after), Have you participated in study groups dealing with alcoholism? ($r = .31$ difference), Have you organized or helped organize A.A. groups? ($r = .27$ before and $r = .29$ difference), and Does the organization you work for have a stated policy concerning alcoholic employees? ($r = .30$ difference).

No clear pattern was evident in the relationships between the remaining workshops test scores and alcoholism experience.

Follow-up Community Services Correlated with Attitudes, Knowledge, and Information about Alcoholism. When responses to community services follow-up questions were correlated with the three attitude scale scores, only four significant relationships were found. Students with favorable attitudes on the illness concept scale tended subsequently to participate in community and school alcohol education activities ($r = .23$ before) and to serve as a member of a planning or advisory group attempting to cope with the problem of alcoholism ($r = .28$ before). Futhermore, school participants with favorable feelings of social responsibility tended to distribute educational materials, such as pamphlets, dealing with alcoholism ($r = .26$ after). Finally, comparison group members with favorable attitudes concerning the rehabilitation of the alcoholic reported giving lectures or talks on alcoholism ($r = .30$ before).

Students with high total general knowledge of alcoholism scores had a positive correlation ($r = .24$ after) with the question, Have you served as a member of a planning or advisory group attempting to cope with the problem of alcohol? Further, those persons who had high general information about alcoholism scores tended to: give lectures or talks on alcoholism ($r = .27$ after) and participate in community and school alcohol education activities ($r = .25$ after). The comparison group had no significant correlations.

Community services questions were significantly correlated with only four workshop scales; health education, Halfway Houses, community action, and industrial problems. High-scoring students on the health education workshop test had given lectures or talks on alcoholism ($r = .22$ after) and had participated in community and school alcohol education activities ($r = .26$ after). However, the comparison group members scoring high on this workshop scale tended to have: distributed educational materials, such as pamphlets, dealing with alcoholism ($r = .32$ after); given lectures or talks on alcoholism ($r = .26$ after); participated in community and school alcohol education activities ($r = .48$ after and $r = .35$ difference); and served as a member of a planning or advisory group attempting to cope with the problem of alcoholism ($r = .25$ before). In addition, students who were high scorers on the alcoholism and Halfway House scale had given lectures or talks on alcoholism ($r = .24$ before).

The remaining five workshop scales had no significant correlations with community service activities among student participants. However, comparison group members with high scores on the community action scale had given lectures or talks on alcoholism ($r = .28$ difference) and on the industrial problems scale, tended *not* to have distributed educational materials, such as pamphlets, dealing with alcoholism ($r = -.26$ after).

DISCUSSION

Many professional persons are reluctant to provide services to alcoholics. This may be due to mistaken ideas that are held about the nature of alcoholism. The Florida School of Alcohol Studies promotes and reinforces positive attitudes in relation to alcoholism. It furthers the idea that alcoholism is a treatable illness; that the responsibility for coping with the problems of alcoholism lies not *only* with the patient and his family, but is shared by the health care institutions of the community and the larger society; and that alcoholics can recover from alcoholism when they receive appropriate treatment. In addition, the school supports the concept that if misconceptions concerning alcoholism can be replaced with appropriate knowledge and favorable attitudes, then students will increase their treatment skills, look for ways to cope with the alcoholism problem, and be better able to establish rapport with their alcoholic clients. The desirable situation would be that knowledge, attitudes, and behavior of the students change in a concurrent manner.

The study used three scales to assess the respondents' attitudes; alcoholism as an illness or a moral weakness, social responsibility for alcoholism, and rehabilitation of alcoholics. The first attitude concerned the illness concept which poses contrasting viewpoints regarding alcoholism. On the one hand, alcoholics are seen as ill persons in need of treatment, while on the other, only they are blamed for all their difficulties and thus are labeled weak-willed persons who lack the will power or the moral character to control their drinking. The second attitude, social responsibility for alcoholism, makes the family, club, employer, community, and the larger society also accountable for the alcoholics' condition. The last attitude concerns the alcoholics' potential for recovery. The favorable viewpoint is that alcoholics can recover when appropriately treated.

When attitudes of alcoholism as an illness or moral weakness and social responsibility were assessed after the school, students made favorable gains. This school, then, appeared to exercise at least a short-term influence on the students' attitudes. However, they did not make appreciable changes in their views on the alcoholics' potential for lasting recovery. This expressed pessimism of the students is of considerable concern since the majority of the students work with alcoholics.

The study findings suggest that scores on the illness conception of alcoholism, when correlated with the subjects follow-up behavior, were more closely related to their level of belief about the illness concept before the school rather than to any positive influence the school may have had on them. This indicated that a short-term school may not be sufficient to modify both the illness conception attitude and concomitant behavioral effects.

The attitude scores of social responsibility for alcoholism, when correlated with the subjects' follow-up alcoholism activities, produced very little connection (only 4 significant coefficients of correlation on 33 items). No clear pattern was established between attitudes of social responsibility or the rehabilitation of alcoholics subsequent alcoholism-related behavior.

Although the school influenced attitude shifts in its students, it seems evident that there was little relationship between the attitude changes and alcohol related behavior following the course.

The respondents' knowledge and information on alcoholism were assessed by a wide range of test questions. The general knowledge and information scale scores showed that students made significant changes while the comparison group did not. The information about alcoholism workshop test scores showed significant student before–after gains in five out of seven scales, while comparison group members had none. Considering all tests—attitude, knowledge, and information—15 out of the 23 tests indicated that school participants made positive gains after the course over their before figures.

The follow-up alcohol-related activities demonstrated that students were significantly different from comparison group members on 25 out of 33 items. The types of activities included continuing education, experience with alcoholism, and community services.

The total general knowledge of alcoholism student scores, when correlated with these follow-up activities, produced only three significant coefficients of correlation. However, the comparison group had none.

When general information about alcoholism scores were correlated with alcoholism activities, students had 12 or almost one-half of the after or difference values to reach the level of statistical significance. None of the continuing education items were among those yielding significant correlations. However, experience questions, when correlated with student scores on general information, yielded 10 significant coefficients. Under community services activities, the student group produced only two significant ones.

The pervasive relationship between student general sessions scores and follow-up activities, and the student test score changes relative to the comparison group, indicated that the content of the general sessions constitute a meaningful part of the school's curriculum.

The seven workshop tests when correlated with follow-up responses showed students with significant coefficients; nevertheless, the comparison group came up with more of them. In general, then, the workshop content, unlike the general sessions, did not seem to be consistently related to follow-up responses.

It is the opinion of the authors that the Florida School of Alcohol Studies needs to be reviewed critically in light of the tremendous changes that have occurred in the alcoholism field during the last 5 years. The considerable effort and resources put into the Annual Florida School should be weighed against its less tangible benefits. The following specific changes would seem in order: Add two workshops, one for clergymen and another for public school teachers. These two professional groups are intergal parts of their communities and any alcoholism training effort can scarcely afford to overlook these professionals. Offer an advanced course that would take up where the previous one ended. Ways should be explored to offer a practicum especially in connection with treatment and therapy workshops. Curriculum materials such as books, outlines, notes, proceedings, or syllabi should be made available to students during the course so that they may take them home for reference purposes when the school is over. Arrange for an exhibit area and encourage a wide range of participants. Exhibits, for example, could include new books, pamphlets, programs, and audiovisual aids.

The roles of treatment and the general community in the training program are viewed as follows. Alcoholism treatment personnel tend to be utilized to the extent of their specialty but little beyond this. The general community eventually is the recipient of training services provided students. It would seem to be in the community's interest to foster efforts to train persons to work with alcoholics, assuming that the community does not have its own school.

CONCLUSIONS AND RECOMMENDATIONS

It is concluded that the Florida School of Alcohol Studies contributed to: changing student test scores and, therefore, attitudes on the concept of alcoholism as an illness and social responsibility for alcoholism; changing student knowledge and information about alcoholism in a broad range of areas; and motivating students to use their acquired information in at least the 6-month period after the school ended.

Moreover, the school revealed a broad relationship between knowledge and information test scores and follow-up behavior. Thus before–after tests as an evaluation of the impact of general lecture sessions seem pertinent; a weak relationship between attitudes and follow-up behavior indicated that attitude score shifts alone probably are insufficient for an assessment of impact; and an inconsistent pattern of relationships between workshop test scores and follow-up behavior indicated that workshops may need their impact assessed by means dissimilar to those used for lecture and discussion content areas.

Since the Florida School is similar to others, and since it seemed to have a considerable impact, it is recommended that a well-structured short-term alcoholism instructional format be used where appropriate, and supported by concerned persons. It seems clear at this point that this type of school does not meet the state's needs for professional training that requires an intern-like relationship. Within its objectives of education and orientation, the school succeeded. In evaluating subsequent schools, it is recommended that attitude score changes as a measurement tool be supplemented by other means of assessment. Futhermore, in evaluating school workshops, special measures must be developed and employed.

SUMMARY

This study evaluated Florida's School of Alcohol Studies. Students' attitudes, knowledge, and follow-up behavior were assessed to determine the course's impact. The sample contained 172 students attending the school and 144 matched subjects not attending. Results showed that students made favorable after over before gains in attitudes and knowledge as well as alcoholism activities. Correlations on general information about alcoholism with follow-up experience and community services were significant. Short-term training was recommended but it needs to be viewed in the context of the state's alcoholism effort.

ACKNOWLEDGMENT

The study was supported, in part, by funds provided for evaluation under Traineeship Grant for Short-Term Training, Number STT-1151, from the Bureau of Health Professions Education and Manpower Training of the U.S. Department of Health, Education, and Welfare, National Institutes of Health.

REFERENCES

CHAFETZ, M.E., BLANE, H.T., and FEINHANDLER, S.J. On the training of leaders. In *Recent Advances in Studies on Alcoholism, An Interdisciplinary Symposium* (Washington, D.C., June 25–27, 1970. Rockville, Maryland: National Institute of Mental Health, National Institute on Alcohol Abuse and Alcoholism, 1970, pp. 845–862.

FERNEAU, E.W., JR. What students think about alcoholic patients. *Quart. J. Studies Alc.* 28: 1056, 1967.

LIKERT, R. The method of constructing an attitude scale. In M. Fishbein (ed.), *Readings in Attitude Theory and Measurement.* New York: Wiley, 1967, pp. 90–95.

MACKEY, R.A. Views of caregiving and mental health groups about alcoholics. *Quart. J. Studies Alc.* 30: 655–671, 1969.

MCNEMAR, Q. *Psychological Statistics*, 2nd ed. New York: Wiley, 1955, pp. 228–231.

MELLEN, S.W., FOX, V., DRUCKER, M.B., and LOWE, G. *Introduction to the Attitudes and Techniques Useful in the Rehabilitation of the Chronic Alcoholic.* Atlanta, Georgia: Georgian Clinic Division, Georgia Mental Health Institute, August 1969.

PASSEY, G.E., and PENNINGTON, D.F., JR. *Techniques for the Assessment of Se-*

lected Attitudes toward Alcohol and Its Use. Montgomery, Alabama: Alabama Commission on Alcohol, 1960.

PENNINGTON, D.F., JR., and MCGLAMMERY, C.D. *Surveys of Attitudes and Knowledge Concerning Alcohol and Its Use. II. Decatur, Alabama.* Montgomery, Alabama: Alabama Commission on Alcohol, n.d.

WILLIAMS, A.F., DICICCO, L.M., and UNTERBERGER, H. Philosophy and evaluation of an alcohol education program. *Quart. J. Studies Alc.* 29: 685–702, 1968.

WILLIAMS, J.H., WILLIAMS, H.M., GAVIN, J., and GRIGG, C.M. *Attitudes toward the Mentally Ill of a Sample of College Students and Professional Nurses* (Institute for Social Research, No. 5). Tallahassee, Florida: The Florida State University, 1962.

The International Journal of the Addictions, 9(5), 701–717, 1974

Rehabilitating the Ex-Offender, Ex-Addict

George S. Snyderman, Ph.D.

Philadelphia Public Offender Program
Pennsylvania State Employment Service
Philadelphia, Pennslvania

INTRODUCTION

This paper is based on a year's study, June 1971 to June 30, 1972, conducted by the Special Placement Service Staff of the Public Offender Program. Funds for this Research and Demonstration Program were allocated to the Pennsylvania State Employment Service by the United States Department of Labor—Manpower Division. The program was conducted in cooperation with the staff of the Philadelphia House of Correction, the Philadelphia County Prison, and the Pennsylvania Correctional Institution at Graterford for those offenders who were to be released in the near future and wished to avail themselves of special vocational services. Inmates released from other institutions were accepted into the program in the local office units. As the program progressed, it was established that a great percentage of the ex-offenders accepted into the rehabilitation program were ex-addicts.

The paper, therefore, is devoted to an intensive examination of the characteristics and problems of these ex-addicts and the methods used to help them rehabilitate themselves. The facts which emerged during the study are placed in simple tables to give the reader a quantitative picture of the problem, the successes, and the failures. Sixty-two percent of the total number served were found to be ex-addicts. Although the sociological literature was researched, we have omitted most of it from our references since it had no relevance to the population studied.

GENERAL BACKGROUND

From time immemorial, man has sought escape from frustration and pain. The literature of behavioral sciences contain an almost endless list of drugs used to induce euphoria and relieve physical and emotional stresses. In present-day society, people who seek this type of release include the "hard drug users." They comprise the major portion of the inmates of our penal institutions who have been adjudicated guilty of possession of drugs, breaking and entering, purse snatching, and other similar crimes against property. Concomitant with the growth in the number of these hard drug users, there has been a significant increase in crimes committed since the 1950s. Prior to this era, crimes consisted mainly of such offenses as burglary, second-story robbery, and bootlegging. Today, the pattern of criminality has changed, violence against persons has become far greater and more vicious. Popular opinion and law enforcement agencies have attributed this significant increase to the users of hard drugs.

Surprisingly enough, the user of hard drugs has, most often, not resorted to violence of this type (Nurco and Lerner, 1972). As a matter of fact, only 2.0% of the crimes committed by hard drug users in New York City in 1966 were felonies against persons. The remainder of the crimes committed by these addicts were crimes against property (Newman, 1971). A review of the literature fails to unearth any hard data regarding crimes committed by users of the so-called "soft drugs." We must therefore assume that the crimes of violence against persons are being committed by other social deviants and that addictive drugs, if used by these deviants, play a secondary role in the causation of these crimes.

The relationship of specific drugs to crime is confused by the fact that arresting and convicting institutions fail to differentiate the drug used by the offender and tend to lump all drug users in one category. It is clear, however, that the heroin users, arrested and convicted, are numerically in excess of the users of soft drugs (Mandel, 1971; Eldridge, 1967).

Americans are seriously concerned with the increase in violence against persons, i.e., rape, murder, and a variety of other physical assaults. Community pressures, even though distorted by misinformation regarding the relationship between hard drugs and violent crimes, have stimulated the federal government to invest sizeable sums of money to develop a variety of treatment modalities aimed at rehabilitating the addict. Many of these treatments are still in their experimental stages. One approach to rehabilitating the ex-offender drug addict is incorporated in the Public Offender Program.

THE POPULATION

The hard drug or heroin user remains an outcast from the American mainstream, and he in turn rejects its norms. The recent ex-offender, ex-addict finds it easy to regress and obtain a fix in the drug subculture when he is confronted with stresses and pain brought on by our overly mechanized, impersonal, and unfeeling way of life. It is obvious that these hard drug users are alienated from society.

The rich and the poor, the college graduate and the high-school dropouts, the urban dweller and the rural resident—all are affected regardless of previous criminal records, educational levels, or social status. While in the drug subculture, the ex-offender, ex-addict rubs shoulders with the more affluent addict who visits the ghetto or the "scene" to secure a fix. When such a range of persons reject society's goals, they substitute other norms and goals which are at variance with middle-class standards. The fact is, there is a "drug scene" and we are living in or on the fringe of a drug culture which is, as one applicant put it, "all around us." And violence is used in this drug culture as a last resort of those who are desperate for a fix. Violence is minimal because the real addict is "strung out."

The "drug culture," as any other culture, is learned. It includes ways and means of securing and using drugs, avoiding arrest, conviction, and incarceration. Individuals living in the drug culture share certain traits. That is why there are relatively few "loners" who are addicts—users tend to concentrate in specific geographic areas to secure mutual support. These areas are not necessarily in slums; there are similar sites in or near the "silk stocking" neighborhoods and affluent suburbia. Ex-addict, ex-offenders, the man on the street, and the legal authorities know where these sites are, and periodic police raids and arrests are made there for the illegal possession, sale, and use of these drugs.

Since the ex-addict, ex-offender population represents attitudinal and behavior patterns which are so different from middle-class society norms, special treatment programs must be aimed at helping the ex-addict, ex-offender change his lifeways and take his place in the world of work and the community at large.

OBJECTIVES

One of the aims of this paper is to describe the behavior characteristics of the ex-addict, ex-offender and to demonstrate that many of them can be rehabilitated and that the Public Offender Program can play a decisive role in their rehabilitation. Data provided to the staff of the program by the ex-addict, ex-offender during the period of counseling, placement, and follow-up services must be evaluated and interpreted. No single procedure must be short changed if maximum help is to be given.

By now it has been established that the rehabilitation of drug offenders in the "total" sense involves no single step, but rather a configuration of treatments tailored to meet the needs of each offender. The Special Placement Services approach, or POP as it is commonly known, offers the ex-addict, ex-offender a variety of services. These services include counseling, job development, referral to other agencies, and continuing follow-up to help him adjust and sever his reliance on drugs. The program is aimed at helping him accept and use the services he needs.

A major problem which faces any rehabilitation staff is its inability to obtain accurate information from the person seeking services. The ex-addict and the addict alike are suspicious, fearful, and seldom willing to admit that they are users or have used hard drugs. This deficiency contributes to inaccurate official records and conflicting estimates which in turn makes definition and solution of the problem difficult. Our aim, here, was to secure as detailed and accurate data as possible.

POP STAFF

Aside from supervision and management, the services are delivered by a team which includes a counselor, an interviewer, and a human-service aide. The team is supplemented by an employer relations representative. The teams are flexible and may, on occasion, change roles. For example, the interviewer or the human-service aide may actually perform all or many of the tasks of the counselors. All members of the team are expected to devote time discussing vocational plans and performing job development and follow-up for specific applicants. Flexibility also extends to shifting team members from the local employment office to prisons and community agencies serving ex-offenders, as needed.

Staff is selected on the basis of their interest and desire to help ex-offenders and ex-addict, ex-offenders. Counselors are required to have graduate training in psychology or the behavioral sciences; interviewers may or may not be college graduates, but are expected to have knowledge about ghetto lifestyle; human-service aides are not required to have any specific educational backgrounds, but must be able to read and write at approximately 7th grade levels. These aides are selected from the indigenous community and several of them are ex-addict, ex-offenders. In-service training is conducted by the manager and his assistant as well as other state personnel who are technicians and specialists in specific areas of knowledge, i.e., counseling techniques, interviewing techniques, etc. Where indicated and feasible, the Employment Service enrolled staff members in relevant courses at several local colleges and universities.

EXTENT OF DRUG ADDICTION

There is reason to question the reliability of published data regarding incidence. For example, talks with penal authorities yielded estimates that from 50 to 80% of the prison population were users or ex-addicts. Discussions with the inmates, however, lead us to believe that these estimates are too low. Dr. Stanley Yolles (1969), as Director of the National Institute of Mental Health, stated that there were between 80,000 and 90,000 drug users in the United States. In the same paper, however, he acknowledged that his data were not valid and said the drug problem was growing and by 1979 it would increase one-hundredfold (April 26, 1969). It can be argued that even this is a gross understatement. In 1971, Senator Hatfield introduced a bill to authorize treatment for "certain narcotic addicts." The senator noted that there are between 150,000 and 400,000 addicts in our country. Despite this sharp increase of estimates, various sources have informed us there were more than a quarter of a million users in New York City *alone*.

Before abandoning this somewhat fruitless battle of the estimators, we cite the recent statement of Wade (1972) that between six-and-a-half and ten tons of pure heroin are imported into the United States each year. This tonnage, Wade believes, supports the habits of 56,000 addicts. He does not state to what extent the heroin is cut before it is peddled. This information, if available, would reveal an alarming increase in the number of user addicts.

Content of Rehabilitation

Many ex-offenders are also ex-addicts or resume their addiction upon release from the penal institution. If our communities are to survive, ways which are constructive, humane, and intelligent must be found to deal with the problems of the individual ex-addict, ex-offender. The techniques and resources of other agencies, particularly the community mental health centers, should be reoriented and beefed up so that they are better able and more willing to serve the ex-addict, ex-offender. These agencies, working in concert with the Special Placement Service teams of the United States Employment Service, can help many more ex-addict, ex-offenders resolve personal problems associated with drug use. Similarly, public and private agencies must exhibit a greater willingness to help the addicts handle family, child care, housing, and a host of other problems before and after the POP teams begin to cope with the employment problem.

Total rehabilitation means more than psychotherapy, family counseling, methadone programs, etc. It includes an on-going counseling and job placement service geared to the needs and aspirations of the individual ex-addict, ex-offender. Our view that medical, social, and vocational services, including job placement, vocational training, and follow-up, are the best way to rehabilitate addicts and prevent ex-addicts from resuming their "habits," is supported by Raskin (1964).

Rehabilitation, thus defined, is somewhat different than the recommendation of Police Lt. Cathcart (1972) of Linden, New Jersey, who plugs for clinics where addicts can get free shots of heroin from a qualified physician. This, Cathcart feels, will remove the profit motive from the sales of heroin thus forcing the pushers and their bosses out of business. Many experts express doubt that this method would rehabilitate a single ex-addict, ex-offender or put any pushers out of business.

ATTITUDES OF THE EX-ADDICT, EX-OFFENDER

Ex-offenders are not a homogeneous group (Podnes, 1972; Hartke, 1972; Mirabel, 1972; Nurco and Lerner, 1972). They are individuals and differ widely in interests, aptitudes, and behavior patterns. But when an ex-offender is also an ex-addict, the rehabilitation problem is compounded and a much wider spectrum of behavior patterns emerges. While this means that all ex-addict, ex-offenders are not the same, and do not share all the same behavior patterns, the fact is that they had shared the drug habit and behavior patterns this usage necessitated. They had to support the habit—and this was often the cause for arrest and conviction.

The addict in treatment frustrates easily. During interviews with team members, many were uncooperative because they feared the frustrations found in the world of work. Accordingly, some became uncontrollable; some deliberately exaggerated previous work experiences by building up skill variables required to do the work involved; others denigrated themselves and either denied a previous work record or downgraded the skill content of the jobs they had held. When referred to a job their negativism "gets in their way"—and some deliberately "blow the employer interview"; some do not report for the interview; some sell themselves and are hired, but never report for work. Slovenly and inappropriate dress often compounds the problem presented by the ex-addict, ex-offenders.

This is a generalized picture of the applicants who refused service or dropped out. The team members feel that most of this group resume the "habit." Some commit another crime and are caught; some take an overdose and suffer the consequences. In any event, if this type of applicant resumes his addiction, he becomes locked into the "drug scene" and is apt to leave it only after reinstitutionalization or death.

A small percentage of the ex-addict, ex-offenders react toward rehabilitation services in much the same manner as the normal "handicapped applicants." They use counseling, coaching, job placement, and ancillary services positively. They are not secretive, or hostile, and ask for help whenever they need it.

The above statements are interpretations of interviews by Special Service team members with the applicant. Some of the most meaningful interpretations were those of the human-service aides who are equal partners with the counselors and interviewers in this program. The reason for their realistic reactions is that several are ex-addit, ex-offenders and all are products of the ghetto.

The meaningful point stressed by all staff members is that most ex-addicts and even some addicts, who are in constructive and helpful treatment programs, can work successfully in a variety of jobs. However, since few of those served have saleable skills and knowledge, they have to begin in less demanding jobs and progress slowly. This tends to be frustrating and several ex-addicts "slipped back—lost their jobs and dropped out of sight." None of these was ever located and there is no way to determine the extent of their recidivism.

An obvious question is, "How do we recognize that an ex-addict, ex-offender is slipping back into the drug culture?" There is no single answer or even a group of symptoms. The following behavior patterns are signals to the team members that the individual *may* be beginning to use drugs: nodding off to sleep during the interview; excessive slowness of speech; enlarged pupils; a tendency to be overly elusive or secretive; excessively hostile or abusive; a tendency to talk at great length about subjects unrelated to the problem of "staying clean, and finding and holding a job."

Perhaps these symptoms are more exaggerated with the ex-addict, ex-offender seen by our teams than the "normal ex-addict" who is usually middle-class and White, and therefore does not have the same life experiences. Our applicants, in the main, are products of poverty-ridden ghettos. Their environment has not been conducive to good adjustment and does not foster White, middle-class attitudes.

As expected and already noted, some of the applicants served returned to their old habit. A few reconsidered and returned for further services. They tended to express a series of rationalizations such as "It was just too tough out on the street"; "I was not able to cut it"; "I could not make it on the money"; "A friend started me back on it"; "I needed a kick so bad I went out and bought a 'nickle bag' ($5 worth)"; and "God knows I tried to stay clean but just could not."

If one leafs through the literature relating to addiction, it would appear that the backsliders use the same rationalization as persons who are confirmed addicts. Our experience has unveiled *no* new evidence to the contrary. Why these men returned to the drug culture remains a subject for study which is beyond the purview of this paper. However, we can say some did return to the teams for help. This is a positive factor and perhaps the team is a kind of Court of Last Resort! Team members say "If we do not listen who will?" and "If we don't let the applicant talk it out he will never come back and we will lose him forever. This way there is some hope." To paraphrase it differently, and perhaps in a lighter vein, the team serves as the backslider's Father Confessor.

It must be noted that a number of men in the program effected a cure by their own efforts with assistance from groups in the Black community. Their Black brothers and sisters taught them that they, the ex-addict, ex-offenders, had roles to play in their own community, i.e., helping their "brothers and sisters" stay clean and driving the pushers out. Unquestionably, the "rap sessions" in the Black community helped some of our applicants build or restore their self-image. This help was instrumental in giving them the courage to desert the "drug culture." The White community may profit from the Black experience in the years ahead.

THE SPECIAL PLACEMENT SERVICES PROGRAM

Initially, the program was designed to handle ex-offenders per se. No special thought was given to the changing populations in the various penal institutions. Today, for example, there are virtually no safe-crackers, second-story men, or highwaymen. Many of the men involved in crime today were convicted and/or confined "for drug-related offenses." The latter caption does not appear in the records though many penal officials are aware of the underlying cause for the conviction.

Methods and Procedure

Accordingly, we have and shall continue to develop new and restructure present procedures and policies so that maximum rehabilitative services can be delivered to all ex-offenders including ex-addicts. The brief summation of present policies should suffice to give most readers a picture of the direction the Employment Service is taking. It includes the belief that the staff of the Special Placement Service Units must begin with the lifestyle of the ex-offender and learn how he is attempting to resolve his problems. If the staff learned or suspected that the applicant was using drugs, it had to find ways and means of dealing constructively with this problem before tackling the vocational problem. Thus the staff dealt with the here and now so that proper remedial measures would eventually lead to the development and implementation of vocational goals.

The ex-addict, ex-offender was personally involved by the staff from the outset in all the planning. Any actions taken were understood and accepted by him. The treatments, just as the vocational goals, differed and depended on the lifestyle of the applicant, his personality, aptitudes, interests, physical, and emotional capacities as well as the nature and cause of his addiction. How he arrived at a vocational goal and how he implemented his decision was, for the most part, his own choice.

The nature of the ex-addict, ex-offender population made counseling a necessity for each of these applicants. Individual counseling was the modus operandi, but group rap sessions were tried with varying degrees of success. Individual rap sessions, which were not considered counseling interviews but really are, were extremely useful when conducted by the human-service aide.

Testing was used sparingly and selectively. Most ex-addicts were burdened with a variety of educational, vocational, and psychosocial failures. They resented or feared tests. One man claimed "Its just another con to prove I'm nothing." But, as in all human situations, there are occasional exceptions. For these, aptitude tests were scheduled.

Counseling, testing, and even ancillary services alone were viewed as hoaxes by the ex-offender when these services did not result in a suitable job placement. Accordingly, it was imperative that the teams contact many employers as often as possible in the presence of the applicant in order to find the one who would be willing to give the applicant a chance to prove that he was a good worker. Jobs paying less than $2 an hour were deemed unacceptable except for weekend work or if they had an on-the-job training ladder built in.

If the plan of service included use of ancillary help such as medical, dental, psychiatric, and drug treatment, the counselor or interviewer might ask the human-service aide to accompany the applicant to the helping agency. The aide visited the applicant's home and neighborhood periodically to determine whether the applicant was making an adjustment and was "drug free." Follow-up was not discontinued until the applicant was in a permanent job and was adjusting in the community.

Since the program's ultimate aim was suitable placement for the applicant, it cannot be overemphasized that the employer service representative, who was the link between the team and the employer, played an important role. It was his responsibility to educate employers that this category of ex-offenders could learn to be good producers. Telephone job development calls by all the other team members supported his efforts.

ANALYSIS OF DATA

Demographic data were collected at intake, recorded on forms, and placed in folders. To this team assessment, social, medical, and psychiatric evaluations made by the institution or other agencies were added. The summary tables included here show successes as well as failures. The obvious inference is that the program was, to a degree, attempting to cope with a problem far beyond its capacities. Less obvious, however, is the fact that the teams were helping many ex-addict, ex-offenders stay clean and achieve maximum rehabilitation. This information filtered into the total community as well as to the "drug scene." More and more addicts and ex-addicts called on local office teams because, as one applicant put it, "they listen, we talk and don't get chewed out or get jive talk." This statement alone could underscore the need for drug treatment, mental health centers, and other community agencies to get closer to the kind of applicants we are attempting to rehabilitate.

Let us clarify certain aspects about "failure cases." While some rejected service, others found employment without help and did not communicate this information; some disappeared; some died; and 99 were reincarcerated for parole violation or new convictions. This situation creates a "mixed bag" which defies real study. Of the 99 who were reincarcerated, 61 were never seen more than one time and could not be induced to complete their vocational development plans. None were working at the time of arrest and only 3 of the remaining 38 had been employed when rearrested. It is safe to assume that working in a suitable job is related to keeping recidivism at a minimum. This is a bold assumption and should be tested out on a larger and similar population in Philadelphia and other cities.

The data summarized in the tables encompasses services rendered between June 30, 1971 and June 30, 1972. During this period the Special Service Placement Units registered 2,192 persons. These are shown in Table 1.

The population was obviously youthful since 1,546 or 70.6% of the individuals were younger than 35.

Table 2 lists the ex-offenders who were known to be addicts when sentenced together with those whom we learned had had a habit or were still addicted.

If one combines Tables 1 and 2, it is clear that 62% of 2,192 persons served had at one time or other been addicted. More than 20% of the 1,376 in the age group 18–24 and almost 65% of the age group 25–34 were known as addicts or ex-addicts to the institution or told team members about their habit after release. Thus more than 85% of the group were under 35

Table 1

Total Ex-Offenders Served by Age

18–24	%	25–34	%	35–44	%	45–54	%	55 and over	%	Total	%
379	17.3	1167	53.3	571	26.0	44	2.0	31	1.4	2192	100

Table 2

Total Ex-Addicts Receiving a Service by Age and Offense

	18–24	%	25–34	%	35–44	%	45–54	%	55 and over	%	Total	%
Known	189	17.4	795	73.2	92	8.5	9	0.8	1	0.09	1086	99.9
Told team	92	31.7	99	34.1	83	28.6	16	5.5	0	0.0	290	99.9
	281	20.4	894	64.9	175	12.7	25	1.8	1	0.1	1376	99.9

years of age. The surprising fact that emerges from Table 2 is that 290 or 21% of the ex-offender addicts were convicted and sentenced, and the authorities did not recognize the fact that these persons had a history of drug use.

Table 3 shows the number of ex-addicts and addicts who dropped out of the Special Service Placement Program. The reader will note that 2,192 men were registered initially (Table 1). Of this number, 346 failed to complete their rehabilitation. Note, too, that 211 of the 346 (61%) were addicts or suspected addicts. It is significant that only 3 of the 346 were able to find jobs. This does not mean that more did not "make it" in the world of work. The teams could not locate them to verify this fact.

Table 3 also indicates that 82.9% of the ex-addict, ex-offenders who did not complete the program were under 35 years of age. This raises a host of questions regarding the community's failure to recognize its responsibility to prevent and treat the younger addict's problems. It suggests that innovative rehabilitation programs must be introduced while these men are still in prison or made mandatory for probation. It also suggests programs for preventing drug addiction and crime must begin with very young populations who are apt to become addicts and/or offenders.

Table 4 is a listing of the ex-addicts placed in jobs by age grouping. Note that the total number of persons placed in the program by the teams was 441; 277 or 62.8% of the total were ex-addicts or addicts in treatment programs.

The younger addict appeared easier to place—219 or 79% of the total were younger than 35. Although we know that American culture has been labeled a youth-enamored culture by behavioral scientists, and that growing older is almost akin to being sinful, many employers have mixed

Table 3
Ex-Addicts and Addict Dropouts

18–24	%	25–34	%	35–44	%	45–54	%	55 and over	%	Total	%
34	16.1	141	66.8	30	14.2	6	2.8	0	0.0	211	99.9

Table 4
Ex-Addicts Placed

18–24	%	25–34	%	35–44	%	45–54	%	55 and over	%	Total	%
79	28.5	140	50.5	39	14.1	12	4.3	7	2.5	277	99.9

feelings about hiring younger persons. Many seek maturity, skills, and experience which take considerable time to develop. However, it cannot be denied that some employers wish to develop young people because they "do not have to unlearn bad work habits," etc. So, generally, despite stated equal opportunities, young persons are usually easier to place than persons 45 or over, especially if they do not demand too high wage rates and are "willing to learn and are motivated."

This appears to be the reason for the higher success placement rate for the younger ex-addict, ex-offender. It follows, then, that if ways and supports can be devised to hold the younger applicant in a rehabilitation program, many more will be placed in suitable jobs. With respect to the older applicant served, there is tentative narrative data in the records that some employers fear not only the individual's age but also his lengthy record of arrests and rearrests. Further study of this discriminatory fear is contemplated.

Table 5 details the type of jobs found for the ex-addict, ex-offender.

The type of occupation in which the ex-addict, ex-offender was placed underscores his lack of skills and knowledge. Thus 71.8% were placed in unskilled or service occupations while less than 4% were placed in occupations commonly known as "white collar."

Regardless of the occupational level in which the ex-addict, ex-offender found work, placement was difficult not only because of the individual's lack of skills and knowledges but because of employer attitudes. Some employers feared the man would resume his habit "and steal me blind." Employer fears were allayed by the fact that there was continuing follow-up with the applicant and his family and that the Employment Service could pay for skills training and, when necessary, bond the applicant.

Table 5

Ex-Offender, Ex-Addicts Placed Initially by Occupaticn and Age

Age	Profes-ional	%	Cleri-cal	%	Service	%	Skilled and trainees	%	Semiskilled	%	Unskilled	%	Totals	%
18–24	0		2		32		8		11		26		79	
25–34	0		6		47		10		15		62		140	
34–44	0		1		6		11		9		12		39	
45–54	1		0		3		0		1		7		12	
55 and over	1		0		2		1		1		2		7	
	2	0.7	9	3.2	90	32.5	30	10.8	37	13.4	109	39.4	277	100

Table 6
Ex-Addict, Ex-Offender Placed Moren Than One Time by Age

Age	Placed 2 times	%	Placed 3 times	%	Placed more than 3 times	%	Total	%
18–24	2		6		20		28	48.3
25–34	4		8		3		15	25.9
35–44	6		2		1		9	15.5
45–54	2		2		0		4	6.8
55 and over	2		0		0		2	3.4
	16	27.6	18	31.0	24	41.3	58	99.9

Sixty-five of the persons placed lost their jobs and had to be placed again. None were fired or discharged for creating disturbances but seven lost their jobs because of excessive absence. Five of the seven could not be located and it is possible that they may have resumed the habit. The other two have been placed in other jobs and appear to be adjusting. Since verification of these two placements was not received until this paper was completed, they are not included in Table 6.

The older ex-addict, ex-offender did not need to be placed as often as the younger. He tended to get a job and stay put. Thus more than 74% of the multiple placements were made in the age groups 18–24 and 25–34. These were persons who were "job ready" but had neither experience nor skills. Any downturn in the labor market was apt to cause the employer to lay them off because they did not have seniority. But, it must be noted that several of the men were not ready psychologically to "stay put" in a regular job. They needed to explore several jobs before they could "settle down."

It is interesting that the youthful ex-addict, ex-offender, once placed, tended to return to the team for additional help. There is subjective data in individual case records that indicates that motivation sometimes increased with each job change. Obviously increasing motivation made it easier to place such men a second or third time. Some had letters of reference from their employers. Such letters tended to eliminate some barriers to placement.

RECIDIVISM

In the annual progress report of the POP Program (Snyderman, 1972), we detailed difficulties in determining the rate of recidivism. It was pointed out that in the total population which included persons never addicted, there was a recidivism rate of 3.9%. This is far below national averages but we could not verify arrests and convictions in other states and even in counties within the Commonwealth of Pennsylvania. The 3.9% figure, therefore, is likely to be incorrect.

Ninety-nine recidivists were known to us. Fifty-nine of them were known as addicts or ex-addicts. Forty of these 59 men were parole violators and 19 had been committed for new offenses. The following comments summarize the characteristics of these recidivists: Only 1 was working at the time of his recommitment; only 1 completed high school—the average educational level was 7.8 years and the lowest 4 years; the oldest man was 39 and the youngest 19 years old; 10 of the 59 were veterans—3 of whom were Vietnam vets.

The statement which follows is quoted from the progress report because it applies equally to ex-addicts, addicts, and nonaddict, ex-offenders: "The recidivists were young, relatively uneducated and untrained with fewer prior incarcerations recorded than we suspect. . . . " We hazard a guess that the data and the conclusions noted above would apply equally to a more accurate listing of ex-addict, ex-offender recidivists.

The lack of skill and work orientation of the recidivist ex-addict and addict is detailed in Table 7.

The data tabulated in Table 7 throws some light on the low socioeconomic class of the men as well as their lack of education and skills which could give them access to better jobs. Comparisons with the placements made by team as indicated in Table 5 show some slight differences. There are, however, greater differences between the recidivists and the population served as noted in Table 2. No firm conclusions are possible, and it is hoped that several additional years of study will enable us to point out some of the factors causing these differences.

Table 7

Recidivists by Occupational Level and Age

Age	Clerical	%	Service	%	Skilled and trainee	%	Semiskilled	%	Unskilled	%	Total	%
18–24	1		7		0		2		5		15	25.4
25–34	2		8		1		3		12		26	44.1
35–44	0		3		1		2		4		10	16.9
45–54	1		2		0		1		3		7	11.8
55 and over	0		0		0		1		0		1	1.7
	4	6.7	20	33.9	2	3.3	9	15.3	24	40.7	59	99.9

Finally, there has been considerable discussion in Philadelphia and other communities regarding the need to curb recidivism. Suggestions have been made which were never implemented fully. It appears that the solution lies in total community commitment. There must be more tolerance for involvement and new approaches. Jobs are not the complete answer to problems of addiction or crime. There is no one way to treat addicts or criminals. Public and private agencies must pool their resources, knowledges, and skills. Such cooperation will help the Employment Service deliver better vocational services to the ex-addict, ex-offender.

SUMMARY

A federally funded research and demonstration program was conducted in Philadelphia from June 30, 1971 to June 30, 1972. The team concept was utilized to deliver services to ex-offenders. More than 62% of the 2,192 persons served were ex-addicts or addicts needing treatment. Greatest successes as well as failures were achieved with applicants younger than 35 years of age. Job placements were most apt to be in unskilled or service occupations. Recidivism as known to the team is noticeably lower than the national figure. Use of a configuration of community services in conjunction with vocational services is indicated and strongly recommended.

ACKNOWLEDGMENTS

This paper results from the work performed by the staff of the Special Placement Services Office. I wish to thank Frank DeFlavia for helping me gather and evaluate the data. I am indebted to the POP teams for descriptions of ex-addict and addict behavior patterns. The encouragement of Charles P. Connolly, Philadelphia District Manager, Pennsylvania State Employment Service, and Eugene Harrow, Assistant District Manager, is appreciated. The support of Edward J. Finnegan, State Director of the Pennsylvania State Employment Service, and John M. Clark, Executive Director of the Bureau of Employment Security, was constant.

REFERENCES

CATHCART, A.J. A policeman advocates free heroin clinics. Cited by Congressman Don Edwards, *Congessional Rec.*, Extension of remarks E 3091–3092, 1972.

ELDRIDGE, W.B. *Narcotics and the Law*, 2nd ed. Chicago: Univ. Chicago Press, 1967.

HARTKE, V. The narcotics problem. *J. Drug Issues* 2: 29–31, 1972.

HATFIELD, M.A. Speech in the U.S. Senate. *Congressional Rec.* 3214–3215, September 17, 1971.

MANDEL, J. Problems with official drug statistics. *Drug Abuse Rev.* 1: 606–681, 1971.

MIRABLE, C.C. Psychologic aspects of the drug problem. *Curr. Med. Dialogue* 33: 255–262, 1972.

NEWMAN, K.E. Heroin, marijuana and crime: A socio-logical analysis. *Drug Abuse Rev.* 1: 354–387, 1971.

NURCO, D.N., and LERNER, M. Characteristics of drug abusers in a correctional system. *J. Drug Issues* 2: 49–56, 1972.

PODNES, B. Stages of community response to the drug problem. *J. Drug Issues* 2: 1–5, 1972.

RASKIN, H. Rehabilitation of the narcotic addict. *J. Amer. Med. Assoc.* 189: 956–958, 1964.

SNYDERMAN, G.S. *Progress Report Special Placement Services Program.* Philadelphia: Bureau of Employment Security, 1972.

WADE, N. Heroin: Role and technology in curtailing supply. *Science* 177: 1083–1085, 1972.

YOLLES, S.F. Drugs and human behavior. In *Symposium: Manipulating and Controlling Human Behavior by Drugs.* Ellicott City, Maryland: Taylor Memorial Hospital, 1969.

The International Journal of the Addictions, 9(5), 719–730, 1974

The Hippie Turns Junkie: The Emergence of a Type

Richard S. Campbell, Ph.D.

Jeffrey B. Freeland, M.A.

NIMH Clinical Research Center
Lexington, Kentucky

The past decade has seen the emergence of new and different patterns of drug abuse in the United States. Previous to the "psychedelic revolution," abuse of drugs (other than alcohol) was largely limited to urban minorities and a Bohemian fringe. Beginning in the early 1960s, however, the use and abuse of new and nonconventional psychoactive substances became increasingly common among young people of many socioeconomic strata—most notably among the middle class. During its formative stages, the use of such drugs (primarily marijuana and LSD) was associated with what has commonly been termed a youth movement oriented toward the creation of a new consciousness. Psychedelic drugs were viewed in the esoteric sense as sacraments, and in the most mundane sense as pleasant and harmless means of enhancing one's sense of well-being. In any event, the prevalent rationalizations underlying the use of such substances were couched in philosophical terms. Psychotogens (especially LSD) were seen by many as liberating agents, aids in engendering new and better qualities of being in those who used them.

Within a short span of time, the signs and symbols of this "hipness" were being adopted by youth across the nation. A sense of identity and esprit de corps was enhanced both by the in-group feeling of shared knowledge and by the rejection of the hip ethic and style by the "establishment." By accepting the philosophy and etchics of "hipness," alienated or disenchanted young people could associate themselves with a positive and viable social group. A "hippie" subculture emerged as an intermediate result of this process.

The very attractiveness of the subculture, however, proved overwhelming to its early philosophy and goals. The ranks of youth swelled more quickly than the ability of the proponents of hipness to influence them. From the early emphasis on the essential goodness of drugs in an esoteric sense grew a hedonistic emphasis on the goodness of drugs in a mundane sense. The "core" hippies, the genuine mystics, slowly withdrew from the scene and were replaced largely by representatives of the new wave.

This change in the character of the hippie scene was reflected behaviorally in changing patterns of substance abuse. In keeping with the emerging emphasis on the hedonistic correlates of drug use, a variety of different drugs came into use. In addition to the "traditional" use of marijuana and LSD, there was an increasing use of amphetamines as well as a variety of barbiturates and new psychotogens coupled with a growing experimentation with heroin and other opiates. Despite this polydrug use, even as late as 1969, Hamburger observed that hippies were averse to the use of narcotics. Even at this time, however, the Haight-Ashbury clinic staff was noting the growing use of narcotics in San Francisco. By 1970, Sheppard et al. were reporting the emergence of the "middle-class junkie." As some observers had cautioned, the hip aversion to addictive drugs had begun to break down, and opiate addiction had moved into the middle class.

The present research grew out of the authors' study of drug abuse sequences or patterns among narcotic addicts. In comparing the social characteristics of addicts with differing patterns of substance abuse in their drug histories, the psychotogen abuser emerged as a distinctive social and demographic type. Psychotogen abusers tended to be young, White, and of middle-class background, with a drug abuse pattern characterized by the abuse of marijuana followed by abuse of psychotogens and/or stimulants in turn followed by narcotic abuse. The critical variable in the drug abuse pattern which differentiated this type of addict from all others was the abuse of psychotogens. The present study, therefore, focuses on narcotic addicts who have (1) abused psychotogens, (2) tried psychotogens, and (3) never used psychotogens. The major theme of this study is that increasing numbers of addicts are being drawn from the ranks of "freaks," and that such addicts are culturally distinct from the traditional "street addicts." As such, these people constitute a distinctive type and may require different kinds of therapeutic approaches if they are to readapt successfully to the larger society.

In order to establish the parameters and characteristics of the "hippie" type of narcotic addict, we will describe the social and demographic characteristics of psychotogen abusers admitted to the Clinical Research Center (CRC), Lexington, Kentucky, and compare these characteristics with those of samples analyzed by other researchers. The sample is drawn from 3,772 narcotic addicts admitted to the CRC under the Narcotic Addict Rehabilitation Act (NARA) during the period from May 20, 1969 to December 31, 1971. Following withdrawal from narcotics, each subject was interviewed using the Lexington Social Data Form, which contains items regarding social, demographic, drug history, and attitudinal information.

Of the 3,772 subjects, 508 reported having abused psychotogens,* 933 had tried them at least once, and 2,331 had never used them. (Abuse is defined for purposes of this study as regular use, frequent use, or use for sprees).

For intrasample comparison, the subjects were divided into three categories: (1) abusers, (2) users, and (3) nonusers. For almost every variable where a difference was found between abusers and nonusers, the users were intermediate in their responses. Apparently even willingness to try psychotogens differentiates between drug users, while the tendency to abuse psychotogens differentiates even further.

TEMPORAL TRENDS IN PSYCHOTOGEN ABUSE

Admissions to the CRC over the past 4 years reflect observations by other authors that increasing numbers of young opiate abusers are becoming involved in psychotogen abuse (Table 1).

While some part of the increase may be due to the operation of NARA commitment procedures, it seems clear that the strength of this trend reflects the growing use of opiate drugs among middle-class, White youth. As the following discussion will show, these are people who are socially

* Psychotogens, as defined for this study, include LSD, DET, DMT, DOM-STP, mescaline, peyote, psilocybin-psilocin, belladonna alkaloid, scopolamine, and atropine.

Table 1
Temporal Trends in Psychotogen Abuse as Reflected in CRC Admissions

Year of discharge	Abusers, %	Users, %	Nonusers, %
1969 (after May 20)	6.9	17.4	75.7
1970	13.2	24.1	62.7
1971	17.3	30.1	52.6
1972 (through April 30)	21.6	32.4	46.1
Not yet discharged	32.0	30.0	38.0

and demographically distinct from the street addict of the urban ghetto. They are presenting themselves for treatment in sufficient numbers to warrant serious investigation.

CHARACTERISTICS OF THE SAMPLE

Subjects classified as psychotogen abusers and users comprise 38.2% of the sample. The most notable demographic characteristic of this subgroup is its racial composition. Ninety-one percent of the abusers and 54.7% of the users of psychotogens are White, whereas Whites comprise only 38.2% of the total sample. In this respect the sample is comparable to those of other studies. Shick et al. report that 86.2% of their sample of Haight-Ashbury drug users were White, and Sheppard et al. found that 81.2% of their group of "new junkies" in the same area were White. Thus there seems to be a breakdown in the aversion psychotogen users feel toward narcotics but no significant tendency for street addicts to engage in psychotogen use (cf. Hamburger, 1969).

Other demographic characteristics of the sample support these racial distinctions. The abuser category contains a disproportionately large number of females (24.4%) in relation to the sample as a whole. Sixty-four percent of all White females in the sample fell into the abuser or user categories as compared with only 16.8% of Black females. In comparison, Shick et al. (1968) report 46.2% of their sample as female, and Sheppard et al. (1972) show 33.0% of their "new junkies" as female.

There are large social class differences between categories, with psychotogen abusers consistently having higher social class backgrounds than users or nonusers (Table 2). The largest percentage of abusers (36.9%) come from families of middle- and upper-range occupations, while families from semiskilled and unskilled occupations contributed the largest percentage of users and nonusers (39.0 and 51.6%, respectively). Table 2 shows a clear relationship between occupational background and tendency to use or abuse psychotogens. The same trend is supported by other SES measures. Abusers' heads of household tend consistently to have higher educational levels than those of users and nonusers (see Table 3). Thirty-seven percent of the abusers' heads of household in our sample had at least some college, as compared with 44.3% in the Shick et al. study. Although the figure for our sample is somewhat smaller, it differentiates well within the sample, contrasting with 18.2% for the users and 10.2% for the nonusers.

The abusers in our sample show a remarkably lower level of educational achievement than those studied by Shick et al. (15.5% with at least some college as compared to 51.8%). This may reflect sampling bias, or

Table 2
Occupational Level of Subjects' Families

Occupational level	Abusers		Users		Nonusers	
	N	%	*N*	%	*N*	%
Executives, managers, administrators	181	36.9	145	16.1	220	9.8
Clerical, sales	90	18.4	122	13.5	151	6.7
Skilled manual	102	20.8	205	22.7	448	19.9
Semiskilled, unskilled	93	19.0	353	39.2	1161	51.6
Entertainment, sports	2	0.4	2	0.2	11	0.5
Unemployed, other	22	4.5	74	8.2	257	11.4

Table 3
Educational Levels of Subjects and Their Heads of Household

Educational level	Abusers		Users		Nonusers	
	Own, %	H of H, %	Own, %	H of H, %	Own, %	H of H, %
0–8	6.3	17.5	8.9	33.6	13.6	45.7
Some high school	46.9	17.9	49.5	23.0	54.9	25.0
High school graduate	31.3	27.2	29.4	25.1	23.1	19.1
Some college	14.8	14.7	11.4	11.4	6.9	6.0
College graduate	0.8	22.7	0.9	6.8	1.5	4.2

it may indicate a greater susceptibility to heroin abuse among youth with lower educational aspirations.

It is particularly interesting to compare the educational backgrounds of the subjects with those of their heads of household. As a group, there appear to be many more educational dropouts among the abusers than in the other categories. Thirty-seven percent of the abusers' heads of household had at least some college as compared with 15.5% of the abusers themselves. Conversely, 45.7% of the nonusers' heads of household had a grade school or less education, while only 13.6% of the nonusers had not progressed beyond that level. Overall, the abuser is downwardly mobile educationally while the nonuser is upwardly mobile in relation to his household head. Despite these contravening trends, the abusers remain at considerably higher educational levels than the nonusers.

Distinctive differences appear in the marital histories of the three categories. Users and abusers are less apt to have been married than nonusers (possibly a function of their generally lower age). Thirty-seven percent of the abusers have never married, as compared with 32.5% of the users and 25.6% of the nonusers. Among those abusers and users who have been married, however, there is a slight tendency for the mean number of marriages (including common law) to be higher than that of the nonuser; 2.1, 1.9, and 1.8 marriages, respectively. In addition, 27.8% of the abusers are currently married as compared with 10.7% of the Shick et al. sample. Overall, the abuser or user of psychotogens is less likely to form a stable and lasting relationship with someone of the opposite sex than is the nonuser.

DRUG USE

Patterns of drug use are clearly differentiated among the three categories. In general, heroin and cocaine are more apt to be the drugs of preference for the nonuser of psychotogens, while amphetamines, psychotogens, and marijuana are more commonly favored by the abuser (Table 4). The differences are particularly interesting considering that the sample consists entirely of narcotic addicts. This fact probably accounts for the generally lower level of preference among our sample for psychotogens and marijuana (10.8 and 12.2% repectively) than among the Shick et al. sample (46.8 and 25.5%, respectively), which contained only 2% heroin abusers.

The most common source of narcotics for the sample as a whole was a pusher or peddler (76.1%). Interestingly, the abusers are more often in-

Table 4
Most Common Preferred Drugs[a]

Drug or drug class	Abusers		Users		Nonusers	
	N	%	*N*	%	*N*	%
Psychotogens	55	10.8	20	2.1	0	0
Cocaine	24	4.7	118	12.6	384	16.5
Other stimulants	32	6.3	29	3.1	34	1.5
Marijuana	62	12.2	88	9.4	128	5.5
Heroin	242	47.6	514	55.1	1346	57.7

[a] Percentages do not total 100 because only the five most common drugs/drug classes are included in this table.

volved in drug sales than the nonusers. Of the abusers, 20.3% reported that their most common source of drugs was a supply bought for resale, as compared with 12.7% of the users and 10.3% of the nonusers.

There were no differences between the three categories regarding usual route of administration of narcotics. Approximately 90% of the subjects used the intravenous injection route.

Abusers and users show a stronger propensity to experiment with a variety of drugs than do the nonusers (Table 5). In contrast to street addicts who tend to use few drugs and move rather quickly to nearly exclusive heroin use, the psychotogen abuser apparently maintains a curiosity about drugs and a willingness to sample their variety. In general, the style of involvement of the psychotogen abuser in a drug culture seems to center on the use of drugs, while the involvement of the street addict is multidimensional, including a variety of factors other than just drugs.

Table 5
Mean Number of Drugs Used and Abused by Drug Class

Drug class	Abusers		Users		Nonusers	
	Used	Abused	Used	Abused	Used	Abused
Narcotics	8.6	2.3	6.9	2.0	4.2	1.6
Sedatives	6.3	2.0	4.5	2.0	3.0	1.8
Tranquilizers	1.7	1.4	1.5	1.3	1.5	1.4
Stimulants	4.9	2.1	3.4	1.6	1.9	1.3
Antidepressants	1.5	1.2	1.2	1.1	1.1	1.0
Psychotogens	5.0	1.8	2.2	NA	NA	NA
Antihistamines	1.0	1.1	1.0	1.0	1.0	1.0

VARIATION WITHIN THE ABUSER CATEGORY

A comparison of the 25 most common drug abuse sequences of the abuser category on the basis of a variety of social, demographic, and criminality variables exposed some variation within the category. In general, the differences were most clearly related to racial differences within the category. Differences related to race were, in turn, signaled by the relative positions of the psychotogens and narcotics in the drug string. Those patterns in which the psychotogen preceded the narcotic were essentially those of Whites, while those in which the narcotic preceded the psychotogen were more strongly those of Blacks. This finding implies that Black psychotogen users initially follow the abuse patterns of street addicts in general, but are then attracted to the abuse patterns of psychotogen abusers. In fact, Black psychotogen abusers do show some differences from other Blacks who do not abuse or use this drug class. In general, they have achieved higher educational levels than the nonusers and are upwardly mobile in relation to their heads of household in terms of education (in contrast to the White abusers who are downwardly mobile in the same situation). On the basis of the variables measured in the present study, the Black abusers appear to be marginal persons who are oriented toward a shift in their group affiliations. It may be that their marginality acts to influence them toward participation in a more middle-class pattern of drug abuse. Overall, the abuser category is composed of Whites who are generally downwardly mobile in relation to their families and of Blacks who are upwardly mobile in relation to theirs.

CRIME

Criminality variables indicate further differences between the abusers, users, and nonusers of psychotogens. Abusers and users apparently become involved in criminal activities at an earlier age, as reflected in the age at first arrest figures which show 16.5, 16.9, and 17.7 years, respectively. This pattern is probably an artifact of the generally lower age of the abusers and users.

Data on number of arrests and bookings and on the amount of time served illuminates the wider experience of the nonusers with the criminal justice system. Abusers have been arrested and booked on an average of 6.2 times, as compared with 9.3 times for the users and nonusers. Mean time served is 23.6 months for abusers, 33.6 months for users, and 45.8 months

Table 6
Types of Criminal Activity

Criminal Activity	Abusers		Users		Nonusers	
	N	%	*N*	%	*N*	%
Drug sales	452	89.0	706	75.9	1327	57.1
Prostitution or pimping	128	25.2	349	37.5	930	40.0
Numbers or gambling	57	11.2	194	20.9	515	22.2
Burglary or theft	432	85.0	801	86.1	1808	77.7
Armed robbery	108	21.3	247	26.6	520	22.4
Con games	270	53.1	501	53.9	1087	46.8

for nonusers. Further, although the majority of subjects in all categories were first arrested after first drug use, the nonusers show a stronger tendency to become involved in criminal activities prior to drug use than those in the other two categories. While 53.4% of the nonusers were first arrested after first drug use, 62.9% of the users and 65.1% of the abusers were not arrested until after involvement with drugs.

Differences in types of criminal activity emerged between the three categories (Table 6). There is a tendency for abusers and users to engage more in drug sale and burglary, while nonusers are more strongly represented in vice-related activities. Such patterns of criminality indicate that abusers are more deeply involved in such typically drug-related crimes as drug sale, burglary, robbery, and con games, while nonusers are relatively more involved in criminal activities which are more "organized," at least on a community or neighborhood level, such as numbers, gambling, and prostitution. This implies that the nonusers are more highly integrated into criminal subcultures than are abusers, an implication which is in line with the quite different socioeconomic backgrounds of the subjects in the two categories.

ATTITUDE VARIABLES

Subjects in all three categories showed a strong tendency to conceptualize themselves as addicts, although the abusers were more willing to see their whole future in terms of being an addict (Table 7). The largest differences between the categories were on the items relating to the role of drugs and drug use in the lives of the subjects. Abusers strongly felt

Table 7
Attitude Variables (percentage agreement)

Attitude variable	Abusers	Users	Nonusers
Most of my close friends use narcotics	70.2	56.9	46.5
I consider myself an addict	83.5	83.5	79.7
Drug use is one of the most important things in my life	79.0	64.4	51.4
I like to try drugs others say they have enjoyed	71.1	46.3	19.9
I will be an addict the rest of my life	16.9	10.2	8.4

that drug use was one of the most important things in their lives, and evinced an interest in trying drugs that others have said that they enjoyed. Additionally, in contrast to the nonusers, abusers report that the majority of their friends are narcotics users.

Abusers appear to have a more focused involvement in activities, ideas, and relationships relating specifically to drugs and drug use than do nonusers. The abusers appear to be primarily involved in and concerned with a world of drugs, in contrast with the street addict whose drug use is only one part of a larger, more complex subcultural milieu (cf. Preble and Casey, 1969; Feldman, 1968; Finestone, 1964).

TREATMENT PERFORMANCE

The data indicate differential responses to treatment among the three categories. Abusers show a higher mean number of days stay in treatment (80.4) than do the users (69.5) and nonusers (59.2). This measure is misleading, however, because abusers show a more erratic response to treatment than do the others. Abusers are more likely to leave the program against medical advice (elope), but those who stay, tend to stay longer. Table 8 summarizes the general treatment performance of the three categories. The treatment response of the abusers is clearly less predictable than that of the nonusers. Interestingly, while the abusers are consistently evaluated as being more suitable for treatment than nonusers, they show a more negative reaction to the treatment process as indicated by their higher elopement rate. Conversely, those who do choose to remain in treatment tend to show more success, at least insofar as program goals are concerned, than do the users or nonusers.

Table 8
Treatment Performance at the CRC

Status	Abusers, %	Users, %	Nonusers, %
Left against medical advice	18.1	13.8	9.4
Not suitable for treatment	42.3	49.3	60.4
Released to aftercare	28.5	24.3	20.5
Not suitable for aftercare	10.0	11.8	9.2
Other	1.2	0.8	0.4

CONCLUSIONS

Working from a sample of narcotic addicts, it is clear that a variety of significant differences emerge when the abuse, use, or nonuse of psychotogens is used as a controlling variable. The psychotogen abuser is more similar to the "hippie" or "freak" reported in the literature than he is to the archtypical street addict of the urban ghetto.

In contrast to the street addict whose drug use can be viewed within a larger cultural context of "institutionalized deviance," the psychotogen abuser appears in some respects to be a casualty of the psychedelic revolution. The abuser shows evidence of being more highly committed to drug use as an end in itself than does the nonuser, and of being more likely to see himself as an addict for the rest of his life. The abuser is more likely to make his money by selling drugs than is the nonuser, and generally appears to be less involved than the nonuser in established or organized types of criminal activity.

Coming from a distinctive sociocultural background, experiencing a different natural history of involvement in drug use, and manifesting a distinctive kind of addictive life style, the psychotogen abuser, and to some extent the user, constitutes a definable type of narcotic addict. As such, treatment and rehabilitation personnel should be sensitive to differential needs on his part within the treatment situation. Both intervention and educational efforts aimed at such a population should take their distinctiveness into account.

REFERENCES

FELDMAN, H.W. Ideological supports to becoming and remaining a heroin addict. *J. Health Social Behavior* 9: 131–139, 1968.

FINESTONE, H. Cats, kicks and color. In H.S. Becker (ed.), *The Other Side*. New York: Free Press, 1964.

HAMBURGER, E. Contrasting the hippie and junkie. *Intern. J. Addictions* 4: 121–135, March 1969.

PREBLE, E., and CASEY, J. Taking care of business—The heroin user's life in the streets. *Intern. J. Addictions* 4: 1–24, March 1969.

SHEPPARD, C.W., SMITH, D.E., and GAY G.R. The changing face of heroin addiction in the Haight-Ashbury. *Intern. J. Addictions* 7: 109–122, 1972.

SHICK, J., SMITH, D.E., and MEYERS, F. Use of marijuana in the Haight-Ashbury subculture. *J. Psychedelic Drugs* 2: 49–66, Fall 1968.

The International Journal of the Addictions, 9(5), 731–740, 1974

A Study of Methadone Failures in an Abstinence Program

O. Lee McCabe, Ph.D.

Albert A. Kurland, M.D.

Dorothy Sullivan, B.S.

Maryland Psychiatric Research Center
Maryland Department of Health and Mental Hygiene
Baltimore, Maryland

The methadone maintenance approach to the treatment of chronic heroin addiction has become exceedingly popular. Evaluations of such programs, however, have been generally inadequate and are particularly remiss in delineating the profile and fate of the methadone dropout. The present report focuses on a group of chronic heroin abusers who: (1) previously had failed on a methadone program (2) subsequently were institutionalized in a correctional facility, and (3) were paroled to a community-based abstinence program. The study addresses itself to the following questions: What are some of the experiences (expectations, fears, drug effects, disappointments, etc) that ex-methadone patients retrospectively associate with their methadone participation? Do methadone dropouts differ on social-demographic and criminal history variables from addict-parolees who never participated in a methadone maintenance program? What will be the adjustment course in an abstinence program of ex-methadone patients compared to a cohort of methadone-naive addicts?

The outpatient abstinence clinic to which both addict groups were admitted was established in 1964. The program requires patients to report to the clinic for daily urinalysis and weekly group psychotherapy sessions. The above procedures complement parole supervision, which includes employment assistance and constant monitoring of social adjustment. Relapse to regular narcotics use occasions hospitalization or reincarceration for parole violation. A series of reports have been published describing the program in which the present study was conducted (Kurland et al., 1966, 1969a, 1969b, 1969c, 1969d).

METHOD

Beginning in March 1971, all inmates in the Maryland correctional system who had previously failed on methadone maintenance programs were interviewed prior to their parole release to the aforementioned abstinence program. The data to be reported are based on the first 50 such inmates interviewed and a concurrent group of 50 inmates applying for admission to the same program who had not participated in a methadone program. Members of the prerelease methadone group were questioned about their methadone experiences, using a modified version of Connor and Kremen's (1971) inventory. The following inquiries were made: (1) What were the motivations, expectations, fears, etc. immediately prior to participation in the methadone program(s)? (2) How many applicants had to wait before being placed on methadone maintenance? (3) What occurred (drug use, arrests, etc.) during that waiting period? (4) Once placed on methadone, what was the typical length of participation? (5) What were the effects of methadone? (6) Did methadone make the patients feel "high," "less uptight," etc.? (7) Did the patients consistently ingest the methadone during the official period of participation? (8) What were the perceived benefits from and disappointments in the program? (9) To what extent did the patients engage in simultaneous illicit drug use while being maintained on methadone? (10) How prevalent was alcohol use? (11) Did patients "hustle" while on the program? (12) What was the incidence of employment and arrests during program participation? (13) What were the addicts' reasons for leaving the methadone program?

In addition to the above questions, assessments were made of each subject's pre-methadone criminal history, encompassing ages of first narcotics use, criminal offense, and penal institutionalization. Also, data on age, marital status, race, and education were collected on all subjects. Program retention rates and abstinence data were calculated for both the methadone and non-methadone cohorts during their participation in the clinic from March 1971 to August 1972.

RESULTS

Background Information

Table 1 summarizes the demographic characteristics of methadone failures contrasted with the non-methadone cohort. No significant differences existed between the two groups. The typical subject in both groups was a ghetto-raised, single Black male in his late twenties who dropped out of high school before completing the second year.

Table 1

Background Characteristics of Ex-Methadone vs Regular Patients in an Outpatient Abstinence Program (N = 100)

	Ex-methadone ($N = 50$)	Regular ($N = 50$)
Age		
Mean years	26.8	28.0
Race		
Black	44 (88%)	41 (82%)
White	6 (12%)	9 (18%)
Marital status		
Single	30 (60%)	31 (62%)
Married	10 (20%)	10 (20%)
Separated	6 (12%)	9 (18%)
Other	4 (8%)	0
Education		
Mean years	9.1	9.7

Table 2

Ages at Which Selected Deviant Behavior First Occurred as Reported by Ex-Methadone and Regular Patients in an Outpatient Abstinence Program (N = 100)

	Type of patient	
	Ex-methadone	Regular
Age first use of narcotic drugs	19.0	18.8
Age first criminal offense	19.1	18.9
Age first penal institutionalization	20.7	21.5

Temporally correlated with the subjects' termination in formal education was the initial use of illicit narcotics (Table 2) and the first arrest, the average of both being age 19. The first penal institutionalization tended to occur at approximately age 21.

The Methadone Program

Program-Related Items. Table 3 summarizes the responses that ex-methadone patients gave to general questions directed toward the methadone program in which they had participated. The salient findings regarding program variables are as follows: the majority (72%) of patients were not required to wait before being placed on methadone maintenance; however, approximately one out of five were delayed 1 week or more

Table 3
Response of Methadone Failures to Overall Program Related Questions

Item[a] and response	*N*	%
* Pre-methadone waiting period		
None	28	72
1–7 days	4	10
8–28 days	4	10
1 month or more	3	8
* Therapeutic expectations from program		
To "kick" the habit for good	6	15
Detoxification	1	2
To return to normal life-style	2	5
No reported therapeutic expectations	30	77
Length of time on program		
Less than 1 month	17	34
1–6 months	18	36
7–12 months	9	18
Over 1 year	6	12
* Greatest benefit from methadone program		
Stayed off other drugs	10	26
Functioned normally	3	8
Remained out of jail	1	2
Therapy	1	2
None	24	62
* Most helpful element in methadone program		
Group counseling	9	26
Individual counseling	4	10
Drug	2	5
None	24	62

(*continued*)

Table 3 (continued)

Item[a] and response	*N*	%
* Biggest disappointment from program		
No counseling	5	13
Dosage lowered too quickly	4	10
Still had a habit	4	10
Problems with staff	2	5
None	24	62
Employed while on program		
Entire period	25	50
Partial period	10	20
Not at all	15	30
Reason for leaving		
Arrest	26	52
"Fed up"	10	20
Disliked methadone	6	12
Wish to participate in another methadone program		
Yes	5	10
No	45	90

[a] Eleven of the 50 patients in the methadone dropout group were administered an abbreviated form of the methadone questionnaire; items with an asterisk were available only in the longer version.

before admission to the program. Interestingly, most (77%) patients reported no specific therapeutic expectations from the program; however, the most frequently reported hope was "to kick the habit for good." The majority of failures dropped out of the program during the first 6 months, with only 12% lasting longer than 1 year.

When questioned about the "greatest benefits" and "helpful elements" in the methadone program, 62% reported "none"; 26% reported that the program enabled them to stay off other drugs and that group counseling contributed most to this. Although most subjects chose not to specify their disappointments while on the methadone program, either "no counseling available," "premature lowering of dosage," or "persistance of the narcotic habit" were mentioned by one-third of all subjects.

Regarding employment during methadone maintenance, 50% reported working during the entire period of participation, 20% for only part of the period, and 30% during none of the period. The most popular reasons given for leaving the methadone program were: arrest, being "fed up," and disliking methadone. When asked if they wished to participate in another methadone program, 90% responded "No."

Table 4
Frequency of Selected Deviant Behaviors During Previously Unsuccessful Methadone Maintenance Participation

	Yes		No	
Item	*N*	%	*N*	%
Illicit narcotics use (during waiting period)[a]	11	100	0	0
Illicit narcotics use	20	40	30	60
Frequent alcohol consumption	22	44	28	56
"Hustling"	18	36	32	64
Arrested	25	64	14	36

[a] Only 11 patients were required to wait before placement on methadone program.

Deviant Behavior Items. Table 4 summarizes the frequency of reported deviant behaviors occurring during methadone maintenance. Every subject who had to wait before being stabilized on methadone reported using illicit narcotics during that waiting period. Nearly half of all patients indicated use of illicit narcotics concurrently with methadone maintenance.

The frequent use of alcohol during program participation was reported by 44% of the population. Although only one-third admitted to "hustling" during their program participation, 64% reported having been arrested while on the program.

Drug-Related-Items. Table 5 indicates responses to drug-specific questions. Only one out of five patients reported any preprogram apprehension about the effects of methadone on their bodies or about long-term addiction. Half of the patients reported feeling "normal" while on methadone, the most common complaints were feeling "slow and sluggish" or "sick." Constipation, which traditionally is reported to be a major side effect of methadone, was mentioned by only one patient. Sixty percent of the subjects reported obtaining a "high" on methadone which lasted up to 12 hours or more. The majority of the patients expressed a distinct feeling of being less "uptight" while they were receiving methadone.

The Abstinence Program

Comparative Adjustment. When former methadone patients were accepted into the clinic, the prevailing question was: How will their participation compare with patients who have not previously participated in a methadone program? One line of reasoning indicated that previous fail-

Table 5
Responses of Methadone Failures to Drug-Related Questions

Item[a] and response	N	%
*Worries or fears about methadone		
Effects on body	4	10
Long-term addiction	3	8
None	13	33
No answer	19	49
*Effects of methadone		
Slow or sluggish	8	20
Sick	5	13
Insomnia	1	2
Constipation	1	2
Lost drug craving	3	8
Felt normal	21	54
Obtained "high" from methadone		
Yes	30	60
No	20	40
Length of "high" from methadone		
1–2 hours	8	27
3–6 hours	8	27
7–11 hours	3	10
12 hours or more	8	27
Not specified	3	10
Felt less "uptight" with methadone		
Yes	35	70
No	15	30

[a] Eleven of the 50 patients in the methadone dropout group were administered an abbreviated form of the methadone questionnaire; items with an asterisk were available only in the longer version.

ure on a program usually viewed as less demanding signified poor prognosis for an abstinence program. To test this hypothesis, the adjustment course of the former methadone patients ($N = 50$) was compared with that of the group of patients ($N = 50$) who previously had never participated in a methadone program. Previously cited background data indicated that the two groups were initially equivalent except for previous methadone experience. Table 6 summarizes the dispositions of both groups. There is a distinct trend indicative of a poorer prognosis of methadone failures. Despite their simultaneous admission to the program, 42% of the non-methadone cohort group were still active in the clinic 18 months after initiation of the study, compared to 26% of the methadone group (21 of 50 vs 13 of 50, $\chi^2 = 2.68$, $p \leq .20$). In terms of abstinence, more than

Table 6
Adjustment Course (Disposition) of Ex-Methadone vs Regular Patients in an Outpatient Abstinence Clinic (N = 100)

	Disposition					
	Active			Discharged		
Type of patient	Abstinent	Nonabstinent	Total	Absconded	Institutionalized	Total
Ex-Methadone ($N = 50$)	5 (10%)	8 (16%)	13 (26%)	26 (52%)	11 (22%)	37 (74%)
Reqular ($N = 50$)	11 (22%)	10 (20%)	21 (42%)	19 (38%)	10 (20%)	29 (58%)

twice as many regular patients than ex-methadone patients (11 vs 5) remained completely free of narcotics use during their participation in the program ($\chi^2 = 2.85$, $p \leq .15$).

CONCLUSIONS

The results of the present study suggest that the criminal histories and social-demographic backgrounds of addicts who have failed on methadone maintenance are virtually indistinguishable from those of addicts who have never participated in such programs. Despite similarity in backgrounds, ex-methadone failures tend to have a relatively poorer prognosis in a community-based, verified abstinence program than non-methadone patients. The data indicate an 80 to 85% probability of methadone failures adjusting significantly poorer on such criteria as abstinence and length of program participation.

Although most methadone failures did not do well on the abstinence program, this observation should not obscure the fact that 25% of these patients satisfactorily participated in the program and that 10% had complete abstinence records for their entire period of participation. For these 10% (five patients), a completely drug-free existence was made possible, an accomplishment impossible to achieve in a methadone program.

Regarding the methadone treatment questionnaire, the authors wish to emphasize that the subjects' responses were not evaluated against an absolute standard of validity. The assumption is that viewpoints expressed by the subjects, despite being liable to various distortions, conscious and otherwise, are valuable data for comprehending the phenomenology of the addict. Moreover, items of the questionnaire were specifically designed in an open-ended fashion, as opposed to a forced-choice or structured alternatives approach, so as to minimize the "programming" phenomenon which a priori categorizations frequently produce.

Despite the limitations of the approach, the addicts' responses raised some significant issues. For example, a "self-fulfilling prophecy" phenomenon is suggested by the finding that the majority of methadone failures did not really expect to be helped by the methadone program. One, therefore, wonders about specific motivations that led them to such programs. Some intriguing hypotheses are the following: (1) Certain addicts may seek admission to methadone programs in the hope that if arrested during the course of their criminal activities, the courts will deal with them less severely because of their apparent motivation to seek help for their problem. Data from Dole and Nyswander's methadone program indicate that this reasoning is sound since approximately half of the charges were dropped in those cases involving patients on their program who were arrested (Joseph and Dole, 1970). (2) Some addicts may use methadone programs as an "insurance policy" to guarantee a "minimum narcotic income." Not only does methadone cost less than street heroin, it insures against discomforting withdrawal symptoms and frantic "hustling" during panic (heroin storage) periods. (3) Some addicts may associate themselves with methadone programs to facilitate the procurement of heroin because of the obvious accessability of a large, concentrated number of other addicts who are continuing to use illicit drugs along with their methadone. (One patient in the present study admitted to having made such "copping" behavior easier for a large number of fellow methadone patients by running a "shooting gallery" in his home during his year-long "successful" participation in a methadone program). (4) Some addicts may attach themselves to such programs to gratify vague anaclitic needs, not consciously specificable.

An important question is whether or not methadone "successes" respond differently to "therapeutic expectation" questions than do methadone "failures." Assuming a differential response tendency would consistently obtain, the utilization of these questions for their screening and prognostic value is indicated. Support for such an assumption exists in Connor and Kremen's (1971) study of *successful* methadone patients, 94% of whom had program contacts lasting 1 to 4 or more years. Reportedly, "... most of these former drug abusers *hoped that methadone would produce very substantial changes in their lives*" (emphasis added).

Other impressions derived from the methadone drop-outs' questonnaire responses: Inasmuch as reports of unemployment were found to be positively correlated with program failure, greater emphasis on job counseling, training, and placement on methadone programs would seem appropriate. Moreover, augmentation of group therapy resources seems warranted, and special treatment for alcoholism should be considered.

The reports that most patients obtained a "high" from methadone contradict the oft-heard repudiations (Dole and Nyswander, 1968) of the "euphorigenic" potential of methadone and suggests that dosages administered on many programs may be too great. Recent findings, such as those of Garbutt and Goldstein (1972), that low dose maintenance is equally efficacious as high dose maintenance, may provide a rationale for the utilization lower, less euphorigenic dosages of methadone.

Finally, patients' reports of feeling less "uptight" on methadone support Wurmser's (1972) thesis that methadone (and other narcotics) have distinct tranquilizing effects on the profound, dysphoric feelings of the addict and emphasize the need for rigorous and comprehensive investigation of the pharmacodynamics of addiction.

REFERENCES

CONNER, T., and KREMEN, E. Methadone maintenance—Is it enough? *Intern. J. Addictions* 6: 279–298, 1971.

DOLE, V.P., and NYSWANDER, M.E. The use of methadone for narcotic blockade. *Brit. J. Addictions* 63: 55–57, 1968.

GARBUTT, G.D., and GOLDSTEIN, A. *Blind Comparison of Three Methadone Maintenance Dosages in 180 Patients.* Presented at the Fourth National Methadone Conference, San Francisco, January 8–10, 1972.

JOSEPH, H., and DOLE, V.P. Methadone patients on probation and parole. *Fed. Prob.* June 1970.

KURLAND, A.A. *The Deceptive Communication and the Narcotic Abuser. Rutgers Symposium on Communication and Drug Abuse,* Rutgers University, The State University of New Jersey, New Brunswick, New Jersey, September 3–5, 1969a.

KURLAND, A.A. Outpatient management of the narcotic addict. In P. Black (ed.) *Drugs and the Brain,* Baltimore, Johns Hopkins Press, 1969b, pp. 363–370.

KURLAND, A.A., KERMAN, F., and BASS, G.A. Laboratory control as a deterrent to narcotic usage—A case study. In J. R. Wittenborn, H. Brill, G. P. Smith, and S.A. Wittenborn (eds.) *Drugs and Youth—Proceedings of the Rutgers Symposium on Drug Abuse,* Springfield, Illinois: Thomas, 1969c, pp. 372–384.

KURLAND, A.A., KERMAN, F., WURMSER, L., and KOKOSKI, R. Intermittent patterns of narcotic usage. In J. O. Cole and J. R. Wittenborn (eds.) *Drug Abuse, Social and Psychopharmacological Aspects,* Springfield, Illinois: Thomas, 1969d, pp. 129–145.

KURLAND, A.A., WURMSER, L., and KERMAN, F. Urine detection tests in the management of the narcotic addict. *Amer. J. Psychiat.* 122: 737–742, 1966.

WURMSER, L. *Methadone and the Craving for Narcotics: Observations of Patients on Methadone Maintenance in Psychotherapy.* Presented at the Fourth National Methadone Conference, San Francisco, January 8–10, 1972.

The International Journal of the Addictions, 9(5), 741–748, 1974

Emotional Openness and Mood Change in Marathon Group Psychotherapy

Henry S. G. Cutter, Ph.D.

Albert B. Samaraweera, M.D., D.P.M.

Richard A. Fish, Ph.D.

Louis Morris, M.A.

Repton Merritt, B.D.

Boston State Hospital
Boston, Massachusetts

Group psychotherapy with drug-dependent persons is usually conducted on the assumption that openness in the expression of feelings is associated with favorable results. The behavioral implications of this assumption have not been adequately studied because of an apparent lack of suitable methodology. The present study attempted to develop a technique that would permit the investigation of the relationship between openness and mood change without undue interference with the ongoing group process.

The conceptual model underlying the treatment program of the Drug

Addiction Rehabilitation Center of Boston State Hospital states that drug-dependent people often use drugs to avoid unpleasant feelings. According to this paradigm, drugs make unpleasant feelings go away temporarily and prevent the drug user from learning to cope constructively with the deteriorating life situation from which the bad feelings originate. Emotional openness is encouraged in therapy partly because it leads to emotional relief, helping the person learn that he need not flee strong feelings, but more importantly is encouraged because emotional relief and mood change may function as positive reinforcers of the undrugged verbal responses occurring in group therapy. Mowrer (1964) in particular emphasizes the necessity to bring out bad feelings about oneself and one's actions—to make a clean breast of it—in order to obtain relief and eventually resolve personal problems.

It was hypothesized consequently that emotionally open people are likely to report greater reductions in unpleasant feelings and increases in pleasant feelings (positive mood change) than emotionally closed people.

The treatment program at the Boston State Hospital Drug Addiction and Rehabilitation Center where this study was conducted is organized as a therapeutic community (Jones, 1968). Staff and drug-dependent patients confront each other with various problems, avoidance of and failures to take responsibility for unpleasant feelings, distortions of reality and inability to make hard decisions that, among patients, were coped with by the prolonged heavy use of drugs. The emphasis on the meaning of one's existence (drug free) and the element of choice are aptly described by Frankl (1959).

The program, by preference, is strongly group oriented. Daily inpatient "feelings meetings" for staff and patients, both together and separately, and monthly 10-hour marathon groups are regularly employed in addition to special purpose problem-solving and decision-making group sessions. The same rules of conduct apply to both staff and patients in the various therapeutic groups. Marathon groups were selected for study because they offer sufficient opportunity for all group participants to openly say what they feel.

SUBJECTS

The 12 marathon participants in the first study included seven professional staff: the chief inpatient psychiatrist, two psychologists (three males), and a nurse, social worker, and two student nurses (four females).

The four staff involved in the second study were the head nurse (female), head social worker, a minister (trainee), and an ex-addict attendant (three males). The 18 patients in the two studies were predominantly Catholic (15), White (16), and male (15). The average age (mean) was 25.16 with a range of 18 to 46, their mean years of education was 11.25, varying from seventh grade to 3 years of college.

METHOD

The Psychiatric Outpatient Mood Scale (POMS) (McNair and Lorr, 1964) was administered at the beginning and end of the 10-hour group session in order to evaluate changes in mood. The POMS contain 52 adjectives that describe various moods or feelings. Factor analyses of these adjectival self-ratings by psychiatric patients have produced seven stable mood factors that have been labeled: depression-dejection, anger-hostility, fatigue-inertia, vigor-activity, tension-anxiety, friendliness, and confusion (McNair and Lorr, 1964).

In using the POMS, *S*s are instructed to rate each adjective on a four-point scale as to whether it describes not at all (0), a little (1), quite a bit (2), or extremely (3) their feelings at that precise moment.

After completing the second postgroup POMS, group members were asked to rate each other and themselves on the degree to which they were: (1) open or honest; "came out straight" in the expression of their feelings; (2) benefited from the group experience; (3) warmth; expressed closeness, warmth, and supportiveness of others; and (4) power; the degree of influence, power, or force exerted in the group. The same type of four-point scale used to obtain self-ratings of mood with the POMS was used with the behavior ratings. The openness, warmth, power, and benefit scores for each person were the sum of his ratings by himself and others. An assessment of the reliability of these group ratings indicated that there was a high degree of concensus among the group members as raters which led the investigators to have a fairly high degree of confidence in assessing the relationship of the openness ratings to changes in mood from pre- to post-group. Correlation ratios, computed to obtain the indices of reliability for the several ratings of the group members, varied from .88 to .92 (Winer, 1962).

The twelve *S*s were divided into high, medium, and low groups of four members each on the warmth, openness, power, and benefit ratings. The beginning and the end POMS mood measures constituted the second variable in a 3×2 analysis of variance.

RESULTS

Because the openness, warmth, power, and benefit ratings were highly intercorrelated, only the results for the openness dimension are presented. The data tends to support the hypothesis that openness with feelings is related to decreases in unpleasant moods; a lack of openness is associated with opposite mood changes. An exception to the hypothesis was the lack of significance in the tension-anxiety factor. Significant results are reported in Tables 1 and 2.

The significant interactions of openness with anger-hostility and with depression-dejection are attributable to decreases in depressive and hostile mood levels among the high and medium openness groups, and to increases in the levels of these moods in the least open group. The patterning of the friendliness mood data indicates that the two more open groups increased in friendliness while the least open group decreased in friendliness.

Table 1

Mood Level Means for Openness Groups Before and After Marathon

Openness groups	Before	After	*F* Ratio
	Depression-Dejection		
High	8.50	2.25	4.78*
Medium	12.25	7.75	
Low	6.75	15.00	
	Anger-Hostility		
High	4.00	2.25	5.38*
Medium	9.50	3.75	
Low	0.25	6.00	
	Friendliness		
High	9.25	11.00	4.87*
Medium	8.50	10.00	
Low	8.00	4.50	

* $F = 4.26$, $p < .05$, $df = 2/9$, $N = 12$.

Table 2

Mood Level Means for Openness Groups

Mood	High	Medium	Low	*F* Ratio
Vigor-activity	8.62	7.37	3.25	4.86*

* $p < .05$, $df = 1/9$

One-way analyses of variance were computed among the high, medium, and low openness groups in order to assess the simple effects of the significant interactions. The results of this analysis indicated that the three groups varying in openness were significantly different from each other on anger-hostility when measured after the group session ($p = .05$). Subtests among adjacent cells were not significant.

DISCUSSION

The initial difference in levels of mood found among the groups differentiated by the openness behavior ratings was felt to merit further investigation. Differences in occupational status, involvement in the operation of the unit, and experience with group therapy may explain some of the "good group member effect" reflected in the ratings of openness of the staff. The chief inpatient psychiatrist and head nurse, both full-time professional staff, were rated members of the high openness, warmth, and power groups. Three part-time workers, a social worker, a clinical psychology graduate student, and a social psychologist, somewhat peripherally related to the day-to-day activities of the treatment program, were placed in the medium openness, power, and warmth groups. Two student nurses, visitors to the unit, were rated members of the low openness warmth and power groups.

The difference in the staff's openness ratings are interpretable in terms either of formal status, experience in encounter groups, and/or involvement in the work of the center. Although there were no such obvious status, work involvement, or encounter experience differences among the patients in the marathon, the high degree of agreement among both staff and patient ratings of each other suggests that similar criteria were employed for both subgroups.

In order to firm up confidence in the stability of the results of this initial study, a second study was undertaken on another marathon group with the same basic methodology. There were four staff and 12 (different) patient participants. Postmarathon ratings of openness were used to divide the group into high and low openness subgroups.

The POMS (McNair and Lorr, 1964) was again used to obtain self-ratings of mood immediately before and after the marathon. A 2×2 analysis of variance was used to analyze the data. Means and significant F ratios are reported in Table 3.

The results of the second study are different from those of the first in that a different mood was implicated—tension-anxiety rather than

Table 3
Significant Mood Levels for High and Low Openness Groups and Overall Mood Levels Before and After the Second Marathon

Openness group	Before	After	F Ratio
	Tension-Anxiety		
High	19.75	8.75	10.70*
Low	14.125	12.125	
Overall means	16.9375	10.4375	22.32*
	Fatigue-Inertia		
Overall means	4.5625	12.250	55.53*
	Vigor-Activity		
Overall means	7.500	3.125	30.68*

* $F = 8.86$, $p = .01$, $df = 1/14$, $N = 16$.

depression-dejection, anger-hostility, and friendliness—in, however, a similiar relationship of openness to initial mood levels and pattern of mood shift. The significant interaction of openness and before and after marathon mood change in tension-anxiety is attributable to the more open participants feeling more anxious before the marathon and less anxious after than the less open participants. The results clearly imply additional and independent support for the hypothesis that emotionally open people have more marked decreases of negative moods than the emotionally closed.

Overall, the other significant results indicate that all participants, regardless of their degree of openness, felt significantly less anxious, more fatigued, and less vigorous after the marathon than they did before it. The results for fatigue, inertia, and vigor-activity were not replicated from one study to the other.

Inspection of the staff openness ratings suggested that the degree of involvement in the day-to-day operation of the center and encounter experience rather than formal status determined the order of the openness ratings. The head nurse, an attendant (ex-addict), and the chief social worker in that order were considered most open. A (professional) trainee was just above the group mean for this variable.

Although the particular mood changes in the two studies differed, the basic pattern of emotional relief associated with openness is consistent. The openness ratings and the before and after mood measures appear to be validly sensitive to individual differences among members and to the effects of the group process on emotional states relevant to a specific group. The methodology used in these studies appears to be useful in studying changes in feelings during group encounters. The insights gained from this procedure suggest replication, because of the necessarily small number of subjects involved, and extension to other types of group therapy and subject populations.

Positive mood change, as per hypothesis, is associated with openness and possibly the reinforcement of openness. Negative mood change, sometimes graphically described by patients as being "jammed," is associated with being closed and has been observed to lead to avoidance responses up to and including "splitting" from the unit prematurely and precipitously. (Data from an additional marathon, for example, was incomplete and unusable because three of the more closed patients "split" from the marathon and the unit before the postmarathon mood adjective check list could be collected.)

Length of stay on the unit studied with a larger sample is strongly correlated with treatment success as measured by degree of drug abstinence and steadiness of employment (beta weights = .238 and .261, respectively, study in progress). It follows that if openness can be increased, negative mood change and "splitting" may be decreased for a net gain in treatment success.

In order to help new patients and others who have poor access to feelings succeed in their stay on the unit introductory feelings meetings, human relations exercises and relaxation-meditation training have been introduced as a part of the regular program during the detoxification (early) phase of treatment. Experimental studies of these and other treatment procedures are suggested in terms of their impact on mood change. Some pilot work by two of the authors (Merritt and Cutter) suggests that it is possible to study marathons experimentally (pre- and posttest design with random assignment to treatment). It is hoped that such studies will specify the conditions and people for whom various treatments are most effective.

Therapeutic communities can perform a valuable public service if they serve as behavior change laboratories continuously exploring and assessing procedures for the treatment of drug-related problems.

REFERENCES

FRANKL, V.E. *Man's Search for Meaning: An Introduction to Logotherapy*. New York, Pocketbooks, 1959.

JONES, M. *Social Psychiatry in Practise: The Idea of a Treatment Community*. Baltimore, Penguin, 1968.

MCNAIR, D.M., and LORR, M. An analysis of mood in neurotics. *J. Abnormal Social Psychol.* 69: 620–627, 1964.

MOWRER, O.H. *The New Group Therapy*. New York: Van Nostrand-Reinhold, 1964.
WINER, B.J. *Statistical Principles in Experimental Design*. New York: McGraw-Hill, 1962.

The International Journal of the Addictions, 9(5), 749–755, 1974

Differences among Youthful Users and Nonusers of Drugs Based on Their Perceptions of Parental Behavior

Fred Streit, Ed.D.

Fred Streit Associates
Highland Park, New Jersey

Donald L. Halsted, Ed.D.

Graduate School of Education
Rutgers—The State University of New Jersey
New Brunswick, New Jersey

Pietro J. Pascale, Ed.D.

Youngstown State University
Youngstown, Ohio

The interactions within the family are recognized as important influences on a child's psychological development, and considerable empirical evidence has been generated examining these interactions. Two major directions in the research are clear.

1. Relating objectively described parental behaviors and attitudes to child response.
2. Studying the child's perception of parents from a phenomenological point of view.

Most of the empirical research has focused on objectively described parental behaviors and indicates a significant influence of parental factors on child behavior (Becker and Krug, 1965; Frankiel, 1959; Schaefer and Bell, 1958; Sears et al., 1957).

In the area of the child's perception of parents and its relationship to delinquency or deviancy, delinquents perceive parents as rejecting. Hayward (1935) found that delinquents report their families as maladjusted; Jackson (1950) disclosed that parents are seen as rejecting; Medinnus (1965) found that delinquents have a less favorable picture of parents; Williams (1958) reported a lower percentage of both parents are seen as high in love; and Zucker (1943) found less attachment to parents.

Delinquents do not see parents as setting limits for responsible social behavior and failing to enforce limits if they are not set. Johnson (1952) and Williams (1958) recorded that delinquents perceive parents as lower in authority than do normal children. They further see parents as controlling through guilt and as being excessively severe (Jackson, 1950; Schaefer, 1965).

Schaefer (1965) reported an hypothesized relationship to develop reliable scales for measuring the concepts of a child's perception of autonomy, autonomy with love, love, love with control, control, control with hostility, hostility, and hostility with autonomy.

Schaefer then developed a 10-item scale for each of the 26 dimensions comprising the 8 concepts above. After administration to a sample population, the conclusion reached was,

> The analyses of differences between groups justify the analysis of specific components of parental behavior . . . and demonstrate the discriminative power of these scales. Both the reliability data and the analyses of group differences suggest that this inventory provides a sensitive method of investigating children's perceptions of parental behavior (p. 420).

STATEMENT OF THE PROBLEM

A recent study (Streit and Oliver, 1972) indicated a strong relationship between a negative perception of family and drug abuse. The study compared the child's response to a question about whether he perceived his family to be close or distant to the various forms of drug abuse or alienated behavior.

The study reported here compares the perceptions of their parents held by drug users and nonusers and compares males versus females as well, using an adaptation of Schaefer's scales.

DATA COLLECTION

Three school districts in the middle Atlantic region participated in the study. The districts selected represented:

1. A suburban, middle, and upper socioeconomic class community with religious and ethnic diversity.
2. An urban community with a high proportion (30%) of Blacks and generally containing a lower and upper-lower socioeconomic population.
3. A suburban-rural community with limited heterogeneity in races, socioeconomic status, or religions.

In each secondary school in the three districts, class selections were made at all levels—grades seven through twelve. In total, 1,050 children completed the instrument. Choices for each statement describing a possible parental behavior included both parents, mother only, father only, and neither parent.

In addition, a lie scale was included to verify the accuracy of responses to questions asking about use or nonuse of drugs.

The content of the questions covering facts about drug use were developed at meetings held with former heavy users and abusers of the listed drugs. The rationale employed in scoring the responses was that if a child responded that he had used a specific drug extensively but could not correctly answer the factual question, his response as using the drug was not accepted.

ANALYSIS

The four forms of drug abuse studied were: marijuana, LSD, barbiturates, and amphetamines. The definitions of a drug user based on self-report data were:

Marijuana	Seven or more times used
LSD	Seven or more times used

Barbiturates	Eleven or more times used
Amphetamines	Eleven or more times used

One-way analysis of variance computations were made comparing male users to male nonusers and female users to female nonusers. The comparisons were made for each of Schaefer's eight dimensions for each drug, and whether it was both parents, mother only, or father only whose behavior was perceived in the manner indicated. Whenever a significance level at $p < .05$ was obtained, Scheffe (1953) post hoc procedures were employed to find the significant contrast.

FINDINGS

Table 1 presents the summary of the analysis of variance procedures. The analysis of the post hoc procedures and conclusions are presented below.

Marijuana

1. Male users perceive significantly more hostility from both parents than do male nonusers, female users, or female nonusers.
2. Both male and female users perceive significantly more hostility with autonomy from both parents than do nonusers.
3. Both male and female users perceive significantly more hostility with autonomy from their fathers than do nonusers.
4. Both male and female nonusers perceive significantly more love from both parents than do users.

LSD

1. Male users perceive significantly more hostility from both parents than do male nonusers, female users, or female nonusers.
2. Male users perceive significantly more autonomy from both parents than do female users.
3. Female users perceive significantly more love with autonomy from their mothers than do female nonusers, male users, or male nonusers.
4. Users, both male and female, perceive significantly more hostility with autonomy from both parents than do nonusers of either sex.
5. Nonusers, both male and female, perceive significantly more love from both parents than do users.

Table 1
Analysis of Variance F *Ratios*
Comparison of Perception of Parental Behavior Among Male and Female, Users and Nonusers

Perception	Marijuana	LSD	Amphetamines	Barbiturates
Autonomy				
Both parents	1.97	2.80*	2.28	3.63*
Mother	.35	.63	.91	.54
Father	.66	.40	.21	.36
Love with autonomy				
Both parents	.85	1.56	2.08	3.76*
Mother	2.45	6.38*	4.46*	5.93*
Father	.70	.48	.66	.53
Love				
Both parents	3.01*	5.46*	5.96*	9.15*
Mother	.24	1.00	.66	1.38
Father	.11	.11	.18	.36
Love with control				
Both parents	1.41	1.95	1.47	2.88*
Mother	.58	.45	.96	1.77
Father	1.67	.36	.56	.44
Control				
Both parents	.96	.53	.54	.58
Mother	1.56	1.02	1.83	1.89
Father	1.42	.79	.23	.12
Control with hostility				
Both parents	1.05	.36	.96	.49
Mother	2.35	1.59	1.38	1.39
Father	.41	.63	2.74*	1.41
Hostility				
Both parents	7.09*	4.33*	2.52	3.56*
Mother	.88	.92	.76	.70
Father	1.57	.71	.72	.93
Hostility with autonomy				
Both parents	5.05*	3.08*	4.62*	3.29*
Mother	.33	.31	.10	.49
Father	3.45*	1.62	4.42*	.74

* Significant at $p < .05$.

Amphetamines

1. Users, both male and female, perceive significantly more hostility with autonomy from both parents than do nonusers.
2. Nonusers, both male and female, perceive significantly more love from both parents than do users.
3. Users, both male and female, perceive significantly more hostility with autonomy from their fathers than do nonusers.
4. Female users perceive significantly more love with autonomy from their mothers than do female nonusers, male users, or male nonusers.

Barbituates

1. Nonusers, both male and female, perceive significantly more love from their parents than do users.
2. Male users perceive significantly more autonomy from their parents than do male nonusers, female users, or female nonusers.
3. Nonusers of both sexes perceive significantly more love with autonomy from both parents than do users of either sex.
4. Users of both sexes perceive significantly more hostility from both parents than do nonusers of either sex.
5. Users of both sexes perceive significantly more hostility with autonomy from both parents than do nonusers.
6. Female users perceive significantly more love with autonomy from their mothers than do female nonusers, male users, or nonusers.

CONCLUSIONS

Examination of the comparisons found to be significant indicates that:

1. The perception of love from both parents is consistently present among male and female nonusers of the four drugs studied.
2. Users of all the drugs except amphetamines perceive hostility from both parents.
3. The granting of autonomy by parents when coupled with hostility is present in the perceptions of parents by drug users.

SUMMARY

There continues to be a need to develop predictive scaling models to predict future drug abuse among a currently nonusing population. Recent efforts have been devoted to identifying personological characteristics to make the prediction. This study provides evidence that the indicators of potential drug abuse within the population lie in the province of a child's perception rather than in demographic or sociological classification.

REFERENCES

BECKER, W.C., and KRUG, R.S. The parent attitude research instrument—A research review. *Child Develop.* 36: 329–365, 1965.

FRANKIEL, R.V. *A Review of Research on Parent Influence on Child Personality.* New York: Family Service Association of America, 1959.

HAYWARD, R.S. The child's report of psychological factors in the family. *Arch. Psychol., New York,* No. 189: 1935.

JACKSON, L. Emotional attitudes towards the family of normal, neurotic, and delinquent children, Part I. *Brit. J. Psychol.* 41: 35–51, 1950.

JOHNSON, T.F. Conceptions of parents held by adolescents. *J. Abnormal and Social Psychol.* 47: 783–789, 1952.

MEDINNUS, C. Delinquent's perceptions of their parents. *J. Consult. Psychol.* 29: 592–593, 1965.

SCHAEFER, E.S. Children's reports of parental behavior: An inventory. *Child Develop.* 36: 413–424, 1965.

SCHAEFER, E.S., and BELL R.Q. Development of a parental attitude research instrument. *Child Develop.* 29: 339–361, 1958.

SCHEFFE, H. A method for judging all contracts in the analysis of variance. *Biometrika* 40: 87–104, 1953.

STREIT, F., and OLIVER, H.G. The child's perception of his family and its relationship to drug use. *Drug Forum* 3: 283–289, 1972.

WILLIAMS, W.C. The PALS tests: A technique for children to evaluate both parents. *J. Consult. Psychol.* 22: 487–495, 1958.

ZUCKER, H. The emotional attachment of children to their parents as related to standards of behavior and delinquency. *J. Psychol.* 15: 31–40, 1943.

The International Journal of the Addictions, 9(5), 757–760, 1974

General and Specific Perceived Locus of Control in Heroin Addicts

Frederick W. Obitz, Ph.D.*

Veterans Administration Hospital
Phoenix, Arizona

Kimberly Cooper, M.A.

Arizona State University
Tempe, Arizona

Donald C. Madeiros, Ph.D.

United States Army
Fort Bliss, Texas

Persons labeled "internals" on the I-E scale (Rotter et al., 1961) perceive themselves as being in control of their own behavior, while persons labeled "externals" perceive fate, chance, or others as being in control of their own behavior. Individuals addicted to alcohol or drugs might logically be predicted to be persons who do not perceive themselves in control of their own behavior. In this regard, Goss and Morosko (1970)

* To whom requests for reprints should be addressed at Veterans Administration Hospital, Phoenix, Arizona, 85012.

were surprised to find that alcoholics scored as internals on the I-E scale. Further, Oziel et al. (1972) found that alcoholics perceive themselves in control of their behavior in general and in control of their drinking behavior in particular. Obitz et al. (1972) were further surprised to find that a sample of delinquent drug users scored as extreme externals with regard to their behavior in general and as neither externals nor internals with regard to their drug taking behavior in particular. Although the sample of delinquent drug users was heterogeneous in that the subjects were multiple drugusers, the sample was characterized by marijuana as the drug of choice and little use of the so-called hard drugs, i.e., heroin (Obitz et al., 1972). The purpose of this study was to ascertain whether heroin addicts are perceivers of internal or external control of their behavior in general, and perceivers of internal or external control of their drug-taking behavior in particular.

PROCEDURE

Fifty heroin addicts in a heroin detoxification program at Fort Bliss, Texas constituted the sample of subjects. The sample had the following characteristics: all were male, all were Caucasian, all were in a heroin detoxification program at the time they were tested. The mean age of the sample was 20.6 years, with a range of 18 to 26 years of age. Subjects were recruited on a voluntary basis, were informed they were participating in research, and were not asked to identify themselves on any of the testing materials. Table 1 characterizes the (multiple) drug usage of the sample.

All *S*s were administered two tests. The first was the I-E scale (Rotter et al., 1961). The second was a scale specifically designed to measure perceived locus of control of drug-taking behavior. This scale was patterned after the I-E scale with regard to number of items, forced choice

Table 1
Percent of Sample Using Drugs

	Two to ten times in last 12 months	More than ten times in last 12 months
Alcohol	26	60
Amphetamines	32	38
Hashish	34	36
Heroin	00	100
LSD	30	36
Marijuana	12	74

format, and scoring each item in either an internal or external direction. In essence the scale translated generalized perceived locus of control into specific perceived locus of control with regard to drug-taking behavior. A sample item:

a. There is no such thing as an irrestistable temptation to take drugs.
b. Many times there are circumstances that force you to take drugs.

RESULTS

The mean I-E score for the sample was 10.84 with a range of 1 to 18 and a standard deviation of 4.1. Using Rotter's (1966) general norms for comparison, *S*s in the present study were significantly more external ($t = 4.40$, $df = 1{,}258$, $p < .001$). The sample mean score of 10.84 converts to approximately the 78th percentile in terms of a normative description. *S*s in the present study were also significantly more external than the following groups reported by Rotter (1966): (1) a national stratified sample of 10th, 11th, and 12th graders ($t = 4.03$, $df = 1{,}048$, $p < .001$), (2) prisoners age 18 to 26 ($t = 5.38$, $df = 128$, $p < .001$), and (3) 18-year olds from the Boston area ($t = 2.21$, $df = 105$, $p < .05$).

*S*s did not endorse items keyed "external" on the perceived locus of drug-taking control scale significantly more frequently than they endorsed items keyed "internal" ($\chi^2 = .08$, $df = 1$, N.S.). The mean score on this measure was 8.44 with a range of 1 to 23 and a standard deviation of 5.5. The correlation between the I-E scale and the drug locus of control measure was .26. This relationship was not statistically significant.

DISCUSSION

Clearly the results of this study parallel those reported earlier for soft-core drug users (Obitz et al., 1972). Both heroin addicts and drug users not classified as heroin addicts perceive themselves as not in control of their behavior in general. Further, heroin addicts perceive no relationship between control over their behavior in general and control over their drug-taking behavior in particular. In fact, the scores of the general and drug-specific I-E scales were not significantly related. Why heroin addicts should perceive themselves as not having control over their behavior in general but as having relatively more control over their drug-taking behavior (i.e., they are neither external nor internal) is paradoxical.

The results of this study reaffirm the conclusion that alcoholics and drug users do not have similar beliefs regarding their respective roles in causing whatever difficulties they experience in life. It does not appear, then, that individuals addicted to different drugs can be treated homogeneously under a unitary rubric that "addiction is addiction."

SUMMARY

A group of 50 heroin addicts was administered the I-E scale and a scale specifically designed to measure perceived locus of control of drug-taking behavior. The group scored as externals on the I-E scale and did not score as either internals or externals on the perceived locus of control of drug-taking behavior scale. The scores on the two scales were not significantly related. Results for heroin addicts were similar to those reported earlier for so-called "soft" drug abusers.

REFERENCES

GOSS, A., and MOROSKO, T. Relation between a dimension of internal-external control and the MMPI with an alcoholic population. *J. Consult. Clin. Psychol.* 34: 189–192, 1970.

OBITZ, F., OZIEL, L., and UNMACHT, J. General and specific perceived locus of control in delinquent drug users. *Intern. J. Addictions.* 8 (4): 723–727, 1973.

OZIEL, L., OBITZ, F., and KEYSON, M. General and specific perceived locus of control in alcoholics. *Psychol. Rep.* 30: 957–958, 1972.

ROTTER, J. Generalized expectancies for internal versus external control of reinforcement. *Psychol. Monographs* 80: (*1*, Whole No. 609), 1966.

ROTTER, J., LIVERANT, S., and CROWNE, D. The growth and extinction of expectancies in chance, controlled and skilled tasks. *J. Psychol.* 52: 161–177, 1961.

A Statement of Purpose

INSTITUTE FOR THE STUDY OF DRUG MISUSE, Inc.

The Institute for the Study of Drug Misuse, Inc. (formerly the Institute for the Study of Drug Addiction) was established in 1965 as an international organization to develop clear channels of communication and to encourage research in the field of drug abuse. To fulfill its goals, the Institute participates in research, professional training, and education. In addition, it serves as a consulting agency in the establishment of treatment programs in the United States and abroad. As professional, government, and lay concern increases in the field of drug abuse, the Institute has been called upon to serve as a resource agency for the dissemination of scientific materials through the press, television, radio, and other media.

In order to achieve its purposes, the Institute for the Study of Drug Misuse:

Sponsors the INTERNATIONAL JOURNAL OF THE ADDICTIONS, published by Marcel Dekker, Inc.

Sponsors national and international conferences and workshops in cooperation with universities, medical teaching centers, governmental agencies, and private industry.

Sponsors a lecture series "The Use and Misuse of Drugs and Alcohol," for professionals and interested lay people.

Sponsors international awards for significant research reports focusing upon various aspects of drug abuse.

The expanding programs of the Institute have been dictated by the present crisis in drug abuse. It is apparent that in the United States and in the world at large, certain social forces are at work which have magnified the scope of the problem. In order to insure that the Institute reaches the broadest group of interested individuals, it has become necessary to establish several categories of membership.

Membership in the Institute for the Study of Drug Misuse is tax exempt.

For membership information, write:

Institute for the Study of Drug Misuse, Inc.
111 Fifth Avenue
New York, N.Y. 10003

INFORMATION FOR AUTHORS SUBMITTING MANUSCRIPTS

Send a clear double-spaced typewritten original and two duplicate copies to the Editor, *International Journal of the Addictions*, Institute for the Study of Drug Misuse, Inc., 111 Fifth Avenue, New York, N.Y. 10003. DOUBLE-SPACE the entire manuscript; do not use single spacing anywhere.

Include authors' academic degrees and present affiliation. If applicable, cite auspices under which work being reported was done. Specify address to which requests for reprints should be sent.

Begin your TITLE with a word useful in indexing. Put news of your finding or a statement of the problem first. Major and minor headings may be used in the text; indicate major headings by typing in capitals. Provide a 100-word SUMMARY at the end.

Use METRIC UNITS of measure. If measurements were made in English units, give metric equivalents.

Cite all TABLES and FIGURES in the text. Tables should have titles, and figures should have brief legends. In tables, give each column a heading. Indicate units of measure in parentheses in the heading for each column. Do not use vertical rules. Do not use horizontal rules other than those in the heading and at the bottom. Submit PHOTOGRAPHS as glossy prints, untrimmed and unmounted; identify each with pencil lightly on the back and indicate top.

ARTWORK will not be returned unless specifically requested, and will be disposed of three months after publication.

REFERENCES in the text should be enclosed in parentheses and include the author's surname and the date of the item cited. Keep footnotes to a minimum.

The BIBLIOGRAPHY (double-spaced) should be given at the end of the article in alphabetical order. Journal references should include authors, title, name of journal abbreviated according to *Chemical Abstracts List of Periodicals,* inclusive page numbers, and date. Book references should include authors, title, place of publication, publisher, and date.

CLINICAL TOXICOLOGY

Volume 7 Number 3 1974

CONTENTS OF THIS ISSUE

RICHARD T. RAPPOLT, SR.: Drug Abuse 231

RAMESH C. GUPTA, SALLIE H. MONTGOMERY, AND GEORGE D. LUNDBERG: Quantitative Determinations of Street Drugs in the Los Angeles Area 241

MALCOLM D. SOLOMON: A Study of Codeine Metabolism . . 255

TOD H. MIKURIYA: Synthetic Heroin-Like Drugs 259

ABSTRACTS: Second International Symposium-Drug Addiction 261

WHERE WE STAND ON DRUG ABUSE: California Medical Association Committee on Alcoholism and the Committee on Dangerous Drugs 321

EDITORIAL
HONORABLE FRANCIS MC CARTY: A Case for Heroin Maintenance 337

RICHARD T. RAPPOLT, SR.: Narcotic Antagonists Administered Sublingually in Heroin Overdoses 343

CHARLES E. BECKER: Changing Medical Complications of Illicit Drug Use 347

NEWS ITEMS 351

A complimentary copy will be sent on request

Contributions to This Journal Are Published Free of Charge

MARCEL DEKKER, INC., New York

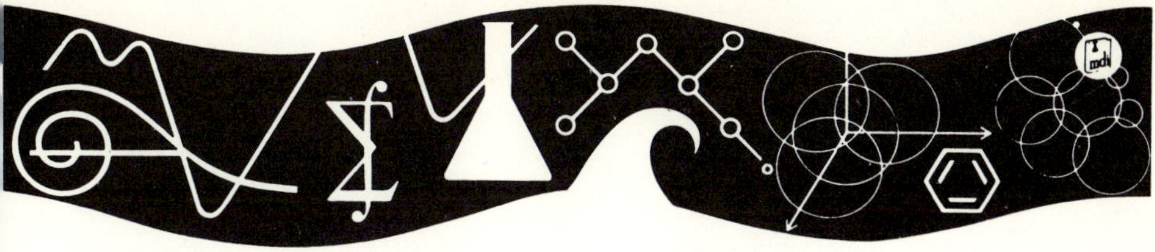

STATEMENT OF OWNERSHIP, MANAGEMENT, AND CIRCULATION. Title of Publication: The International Journal of the Addictions. Frequency of Issue: Bimonthly. Location of Known Office of Publication: 270 Madison Avenue, New York, New York 10016; Names and addresses of Publisher, Editor, and Managing Editor: publisher: Marcel Dekker, Inc., 270 Madison Avenue, New York, New York 10016; editor: Stanley Einstein, 111 Fifth Avenue, New York, New York 10003; managing editor: none. Owners: Marcel Dekker, 146 Cat Rock Road, Cos Cob, Connecticut 06807; Maurits Dekker, 60 Heights Road, Plandome, New York 11030; Rozetta Dekker, 60 Heights Road, Plandome, New York 11030. Extent and Nature of Circulation (Average No. Copies each Issue during Preceding 12 Months): A. Total No. Copies Printed (Net Press Run): 2000: Actual Number of Copies of Single Issue Published Nearest to Filing Date: 2000. B. Paid Circulation: 1. Sales Through Dealers and Carriers, Street Vendors, and Counter Sales: 0; 2. Mail Subscriptions: 1257. C. Total Paid Circulation: 1257. D. Free Distribution (including samples) by Mail, Carrier, or Other Means: 117. E. Total Distribution (sum of C and D): 1374. F. Office Use, Left-Over, Unaccounted, Spoiled After Printing: 626 (mail house). G. Total: 2000. I certify that the statements made by me above are correct and complete.

Marcel Dekker

THE INTERNATIONAL JOURNAL OF THE ADDICTIONS

Published by Marcel Dekker, Inc., New York
Sponsored by The Institute for the Study of Drug Misuse, Inc., New York

THE INTERNATIONAL JOURNAL OF THE ADDICTIONS

Volume 9 Number 5 1974

CONTENTS

Short- and Long-Term Therapeutic Communities: A Follow-up and Cost Effectiveness Comparison: William S. Aron and Douglas Daily ... 619

Value Change in Drug Education: The Role of Encounter Groups: Michael Peretz and Frederick B. Glaser ... 637

Amphetamines in the District of Columbia. III. Stimulant Abuse in Narcotics Addicts in Treatment, with an Emphasis on Phenmetrazine: Mark H. Greene, Napoleon Turner, Jr. and Robert L. DuPont ... 653

Naloxone and the Narcotic Abuser: A Controlled Study of Partial Blockade: Albert A. Kurland, Thomas E. Hanlon, and O. Lee McCabe ... 663

Evaluation of a 6-Day Course in Alcoholism Education and Orientation: James H. Williams, Alan VanLewen, and Tessa Breen ... 673

Rehabilitating the Ex-Offender, Ex-Addict: George S. Snyderman ... 701

The Hippie Turns Junkie: The Emergence of a Type: Richard S. Campbell and Jeffrey B. Freeland ... 719

A Study of Methadone Failures in an Abstinence Program: O. Lee McCabe, Albert A. Kurland, and Dorothy Sullivan ... 731

Emotional Openness and Mood Change in Marathon Group Psychotherapy: Henry S. G. Cutter, Albert B. Samaraweera, Richard A. Fish, Louis Morris, and Repton Merritt ... 741

Differences among Youthful Users and Nonusers of Drugs Based on Their Perceptions of Parental Behavior: Fred Streit, Donald L. Halsted, and Pietro J. Pascale ... 749

General and Specific Perceived Locus of Control in Heroin Addicts: Frederick W. Obitz, Kimberly Cooper, and Donald C. Madeiros ... 757

Cover illustration: "Your sign has tumbled down."
From the National Temperance Society and Publishing House (1877).
Courtesy of the Picture Collection, The Branch Libraries, New York Public Library.

MARCEL DEKKER, INC., New York

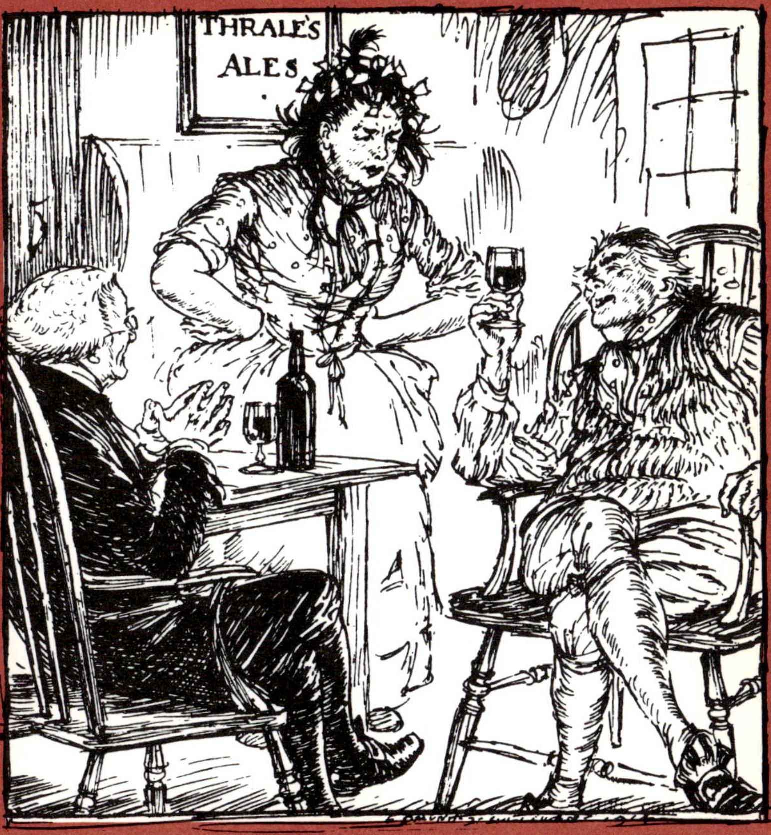

THE INTERNATIONAL JOURNAL OF THE Addictions

INDEX TO VOLUME 9 INCLUDED

Volume 9 Number 6 1974

THE INTERNATIONAL JOURNAL OF THE ADDICTIONS

See inside back cover

The International Journal of the Addictions, December 1974

Published six times annually—February, April, June, August, October, December—by Marcel Dekker, Inc., 270 Madison Avenue, New York, N. Y. 10016. The subscription rate for Volume 9 (1974), containing 6 issues is $40.00 (prepaid). Postage outside the United States is $5.10 per volume for all subscriptions. The special discounted rate for individual professionals and students is $20.00. Back volume prices will be sent on request. Please *mail payment with order* to the following address: Marcel Dekker Journals, P. O. Box 11305, Church Street Station, New York, New York 10249.

Second-class postage paid at New York, N. Y., and at additional mailing offices.

Contributions to This Journal Are Published Free of Charge

The International Journal of the Addictions, 9(6), pp. 761–773, 1974

Drinking, Drugs, and Death*

Paul W. Haberman, M.B.A.

Division of Sociomedical Sciences
Columbia University School of Public Health
New York, New York

Michael M. Baden, M.D.

Office of Chief Medical Examiner
and
New York University School of Medicine
New York, New York

This paper deals specifically with alcoholism and narcotism among decedents at the Office of Chief Medical Examiner in New York City. The emphasis is, first, on the extent to which alcoholism and narcotism are underreported by relatives or other persons identifying decedents, or are not evident in post-mortem medical findings; and, second, on the similarities and differences among deceased alcoholics, narcotic addicts, and those with both conditions. Data are also presented on toxicological evidence of alcohol ingestion just prior to death in these medical examiner cases.

BACKGROUND

A search of the literature reveals no data on the use of narcotics and few publications dealing with the use or misuse of other drugs by decedents

* Presented at 28th Annual Conference of the American Association for Public Opinion Research, Asheville, North Carolina, May 1973.

classified primarily as alcoholics. There are, however, a number of references on the misuse of nonnarcotic drugs, principally barbiturates and tranquilizers, by alcoholic clinic or hospital patients (Devenyi and Wilson, 1971a, 1971b; *Maryland State Medical Journal*, 1967). There are also considerable data on alcoholism and alcohol ingestion just prior to death by decedents classified as narcotic addicts.

Narcotism in conjunction with alcoholism was reported to be the cause of death for one-tenth of the narcotic addicts in New York City from 1950 to 1961 by Helpern and Rho (1967). Baden (1972) has reported that more than one-fifth of the heroin addicts who die in New York City have evidence from medical histories or autopsy findings of concomitant chronic alcoholism; and cirrhosis of the liver in narcotic addicts is much more likely to be the result of alcoholism than of prior hepatitis.

In a group of decedents at the Chief Medical Examiner's Office who had used narcotics, more than two-fifths of those tested for blood or brain alcohol were positive (Cherubin et al., 1972). One-half of such decedents with detectable alcohol had blood or brain levels of 0.10 g% or over (Thalinger, 1970), the critical point in New York State equivalent to operating a motor vehicle while intoxicated (*McKinney's*, 1972–73). These post-mortem medical findings on the occurrence of alcoholism and alcohol ingestion just before death by narcotic addicts at the Chief Medical Examiner's Office have also been confirmed in several reports to the Health Research Training Program of the New York City Department of Health (Austerlitz and Sattler, 1969; Cybuch and Shaw, 1971; Cybuch and Thaller, 1972).

The role of alcohol in "narcotism" deaths has been suggested by the high proportion of narcotic addicts who had detectable post-mortem alcohol levels (Cherubin et al., 1972). The only factor differentiating a group of dead narcotic addicts from a control group, both of which had been previously hospitalized, was heavy alcohol use (Jackson and Richman, 1971). The implication of alcohol as a contributing factor to mortality among narcotic addicts has been attributed to liver damage caused by alcohol, greater risk of violent death among alcohol users, and the synergistic effect of these two depressant drugs, with their relative contribution not yet determined. In any event, narcotic addicts who use alcohol excessively are undoubtedly overrepresented among those who are medical examiners' cases.

It should also be noted that chronic alcohol abuse has been a major reason for discharge from the Methadone Maintenance Treatment Program in New York City (Gearing, 1970), and that alcohol abuse was an immediate precursor to heroin addiction in almost one-fifth of a group of patients at the Public Health Service Hospital in Lexington, Kentucky (Weppner and Agar, 1971).

METHODOLOGY

The collaborative arrangement between the Columbia University School of Public Health and the Office of Chief Medical Examiner, New York City, made it possible to investigate narcotism and alcoholism in the same population of decedents. This cooperative study provided a unique opportunity to present new data on the understimation of mortality from narcotic and alcoholic disorders and their distribution among demographic subgroups.

The total sample consisted of 1,000 decedents 18 years of age or older, recorded consecutively and identified by a relative or other person at the Office of Chief Medical Examiner from February to April 1972. Those decedents who were not identified by an informant during the interviewing period and a few who were identified when neither of the two interviewers was in the Medical Examiner's office are excluded from the sample.

Any sudden, medically unattended, traumatic or potentially unnatural deaths, including all those from homicide, suicide, accident, drug addiction, and acute (but not necessarily chronic) alcoholism in New York City are investigated by the Office of Chief Medical Examiner. All such deaths which occur anywhere in the city—except in Brooklyn—are investigated at the Medical Examiner's Office in Manhattan. The questioning of persons identifying decedents about drug addiction and alcoholism or problem drinking is completely within the routine course of the official investigation by the Office of Chief Medical Examiner into the circumstances of death and of prior medical history.

The data used in this study include the results of post-mortem medical findings and answers to questions which informants were uniformly asked at the time of identification of decedents about their demographic characteristics and about any problems due to drinking and drug use. Questions about such problems are usually asked, but not in this consistent manner.

Informant identification of the decedent as an alcoholic or narcotic addict was made primarily on the basis of affirmative answers to the following questions:

> Did the decedent *ever* have any health problems because of drinking (alcoholic beverages)?
>
> Did the decedent *ever* have any family, money, job, or other problems because of drinking?

Did the decedent *ever* have any problems because of drug use? *If yes*: What drug(s) did the decedent take?

Those decedents reported to be "heavy drinkers" without any resulting problems were not considered to be alcoholics.

Information related to the case of death routinely obtained at the Office of Chief Medical Examiner or from prior investigation of the scene of death by a medical examiner is: nature of the place and circumstances of death; evidence of drinking or drug use at the scene, if available; cause-of-death certification; and, depending on the type of examination, autopsy and toxicology findings. The autopsy findings of most interest are those indicative of alcoholism, particularly liver abnormalities. The toxicological data relevant to this investigation are evidence of drug use and blood or brain alcohol concentration.

Medical examiner identification of the decedent as an alcoholic or narcotic addict was made either on the basis of official cause-of-death certification (when death was directly attributed to alcoholism or narcotism), on prior medical history—or for the alcoholics, on autopsy findings, and for the narcotic addicts, on toxicological test results. Thus decedents whose autopsies revealed moderate or severe fatty change in the liver, cirrhosis of the liver, pancreatitis, or ruptured esophageal varices, not attributable to some other disease or condition, were classified as alcoholics, and those with positive toxicological tests for narcotics or methadone were classified as narcotic addicts.

It should be noted that complete autopsies were performed on three-fifths of the 1,000 cases (58.5%) and on the same proportion of alcoholics (58%), but on more than nine-tenths of the narcotic addicts (93%). An additional 5.0% of the total sample, one-eighth (13%) of the alcoholics, and 3% of the narcotic addicts underwent partial autopsies, which may only encompass an abdominal incision.

It must also be emphasized, before presenting the findings, that not all deaths of persons 18 years of age and over in New York City, but only those investigated by the Office of Chief Medical Examiner—those which are sudden, medically unattended, traumatic, or in some way suspicious—are included in this analysis. Moreover, there is undoubtedly some seasonal bias in a sample of such decedents obtained during a 3 month period—February, March, and April—rather than over the entire year.

FINDINGS

Of the total sample of 1,000 decedents, three-tenths (29.7%) were classified as alcoholics and one-sixth (15.9%) as narcotic addicts (Haberman and Baden, 1974). Included in these two proportions were 4.7% classified as both alcoholics and narcotic addicts.* Thus 30% ($N = 159$) of the narcotic addicts were also alcoholics and 16% ($N = 297$) of the alcoholics were also narcotic addicts.

As shown in Table 1, almost three-fifths (58%) of the alcoholics and three-quarters (72%) of the narcotic addicts were identified as such by informants, with or without corroborating post-mortem medical evidence. Three-quarters (76%) of the alcoholics and four-fifths (80%) of the narcotic addicts had medical examiner identification, with or without confirmation by informants. These proportions indicate that a substantial minority of

Table 1

Method of Identification of Decedents as Alcoholics and Narcotic Addicts[a]

	Alcoholics[b] $N = 297$		Narcotic addicts[b] $N = 159$	
Method of identification	Totals %	Subtotals %	Totals %	Subtotals %
Informant only	24		20	
Autopsy (alcoholics) or toxicologic tests (narcotic addicts)		14		12
No autopsy or toxicologic tests		10		8
Office of Chief Medical Examiner only	42		28	
Cause-of-death certification		16		20
Autopsy[c] or toxicologic findings[d]		26		8
Both informant and Office of Chief Medical Examiner	34		52	
Cause-of-death certification		27		39
Autopsy[c] or toxicologic findings[d]		7		13
Total	100	100	100	100

[a] $\chi^2 = 15.1$, $df = 2$, $P < .01$; $\chi^2 = 28.5$, $df = 4$, $P < .01$.

[b] Both alcoholics and narcotic addicts, $N = 47$, included in both groups.

[c] Autopsy findings for classification as alcoholic: moderate or severe (bright yellow) fatty change in the liver, liver cirrhosis, pancreatitis, or ruptured esophageal varices, not attributable to other disease or condition.

[d] Toxicologic findings for classification as narcotic addict: narcotics or methadone.

* Barbiturates were the only drugs other than narcotics or methadone to be implicated with sufficient frequency in this sample for analysis. However, only one-half of those decedents with abuse of barbiturates indicated ($N = 68$) were *not* classified as alcoholics or narcotic addicts. The cause of death for nine-tenths (91%) of these other 34 cases, moreover, was certified as suicide, three-quarters (77%) by ingestion of pills. An examination of nonnarcotic drugs, therefore, is not included in this particular report.

alcoholics and narcotic addicts would not have been classified as such without both informant and medical examiner identification—ranging from one-fifth (20%) of the narcotic addicts with informant identification only and no supporting post-mortem medical findings to two-fifths (42%) of the alcoholics with only Medical Examiner identification and no confirmation by informants.

The medical examiner identification for one-third (33%) of all alcoholics and one-fifth (21%) of all narcotic addicts, moreover, was based only on autopsy or toxicological test findings which would not be included on the death certificate as presently constituted. Under the present system of death certification in the United States, evidence of alcoholism or narcotic addiction is recorded only when it is the immediate cause of death. Furthermore, violent deaths involving alcohol or drugs usually do not implicate the substance taken, and deaths resulting from a combination of drugs and alcohol are usually attributed to drugs alone.

For more than two-fifths (43%) of the alcoholics and three-fifths (59%) of the narcotic addicts, death was directly attributed to alcoholism or narcotism and recorded as such on the death certificate. One-third (33%) of the alcoholics were identified by the medical examiner on the basis of complete or partial autopsies when liver damage or other abnormalities due to alcoholism were observed, and one-fifth (21%) of the narcotic addicts were identified by the medical examiner on the basis of toxicological findings of narcotics and/or methadone. Of those decedents with just informant identification, it should be noted that two-fifths of the alcoholics (40%, $N = 73$) did not have autopsies and the same proportion of such narcotic addicts (41%, $N = 32$) had no toxicological tests.

Comparable data on the method of identification for those 47 decedents classified as both alcoholics and narcotic addicts are presented in Table 2. The major difference in identification of the two conditions for this subgroup is that informants were more likely to report that decedents had problems with narcotics than with alcohol. Three-quarters (74%) were identified by informants as narcotic addicts, compared to about one-half (53%) identified as alcoholics—with or without concurrent medical examiner identification.

The characteristics of decedents classified as alcoholics, narcotic addicts, or those with both conditions, and the significance level of subgroup differences in characteristics are shown in Table 3 and 4, respectively.

The alcoholic decedents differed markedly from the narcotic addicts in demographic characteristics—notably in respect to age, marital status, education, principal activity in the past year, and place of birth. The nar-

Table 2

Evidence of Alcoholism and Narcotism for Decedents Classified as Both Alcoholics and Narcotic Addicts[a]

Method of identification as alcoholic	Method of identification as narcotic addict: Informant, %	Medical Examiners,[b] %	Informant and Medical Examiner, %	Totals $N = 47$ %
Informant	4	7	19	30
Medical Examiner	13	17	17	47
Informant and Medical Examiner	13	2	8	23
Totals	30	26	44	100

[a] $\chi^2 = 7.4$, $df = 4$, NS.
[b] Toxicologic findings for classification as narcotic addict: narcotics or methadone.
[c] Autopsy findings for classification as alcoholic: moderate or severe (bright yellow) fatty change in the liver, liver cirrhosis, pancreatitis, or ruptured esophageal varices, not attributable to other disease or condition.

Table 3

Characteristics of Decedents Classified as Alcoholics and Narcotic Addicts

Characteristics	Decedents: Alcoholics, $N = 250$, %	Narcotic addicts, $N = 112$, %	Both alcoholics and narcotic addicts, $N = 47$, %
Sex			
Percentage male	74	79	89
Color			
Percentage white	54	48	38
Age at last birthday			
Under 30 years	8	68	43
30 to 59 years	66	30	57
60 years or older	26	2	—
Total	100	100	100
Median age	50 yr	26 yr	32 yr
Marital status			
Never married	29	63	51
Married[a]	34	24	30
Previously married	36	13	17
Unknown	1	—	2
Total	100	100	100

(*continued*)

Table 3 (continued)

Characteristics	Decedents: Alcoholics, $N = 250$, %	Narcotic addicts, $N = 112$, %	Both alcoholics and narcotic addicts, $N = 47$, %
Usual occupation			
White-collar	23	25	23
Blue-collar	61	54	47
Other	8	7	9
None, unknown	8	14	21
Total	100	100	100
Birthplace			
New York City	27	47	51
Southern states[b]	34	17	17
Other continental United States	17	13	13
Puerto Rico	10	15	13
Foreign country	11	5	2
Unknown	1	3	4
Total	100	100	100
Principal activity in past year			
Working	30	34	32
Sick	25	17	26
Doing nothing, drinking, taking drugs	17	14	17
Retired	11	—	—
Jail	1	12	4
Other, unknown	16	23	21
Total	100	100	100
Religion (at time of death)			
Catholic	45	47	36
Protestant	44	39	49
Jewish	2	5	2
Other, none, unknown	9	9	13
Total	100	100	100
Education			
Grade school or none	30	11	15
Some high school	18	50	49
High school graduate or more	37	32	30
Unknown	15	7	6
Total	100	100	100
Cause-of-death classification			
Natural (cardiovascular disease or other)	23	3	4

(*continued*)

Table 3 (continued)

Characteristics	Decedents: Alcoholics, $N = 250$, %	Narcotic addicts, $N = 112$, %	Both alcoholics and narcotic addicts, $N = 47$, %
Accident (motor vehicle or other)	16	5	2
Suicide	3	7	2
Homicide	11	22	19
Narcotism	—	63	51
Alcoholism: chronic	30	—	11
acute and chronic, or acute	17	—	11
Total	100	100	100
Hospitalization for liver trouble, ulcer, or jaundice			
Liver trouble, irrespective of other conditions	16	5	17
Ulcer or jaundice	5	4	6
No such hospitalization	64	84	66
Unknown	15	7	11
Total	100	100	100
Blood or brain alcohol concentration			
Alcohol absent	19	50	36
.01 to .09	3	15	15
.10 or higher	16	22	32
Not obtained	62	13	17
Total	100	100	100

[a] Includes small percentages in common-law marriages.
[b] Southern states are Alabama, Arkansas, Delaware, District of Columbia, Florida, Georgia, Kentucky, Louisiana, Maryland, Mississippi, Oklahoma, North Carolina, South Carolina, Tennessee, Texas, Virginia, and West Virginia.

cotic addicts were much younger; more apt to be single, rather than previously married; and to have some high school, rather than only grade school education. The main differences in principal activity are that more narcotic addicts than alcoholics had been in jail during the past year; and reflecting their age, no narcotic addicts were retired. The alcoholics were more frequently born in Southern States, whereas the narcotic addicts most often were born in New York City.

Those decedents with both conditions resembled the narcotic addicts

Table 4

Significance Level of Differences in Characteristics among Decedents Classified as Alcoholics and/or Narcotic Addicts[a]

Characteristics	df	Alcoholics (A) cf. narcotic addicts (NA) χ^2	P	A cf. both A & NA χ^2	P	NA cf. both A & NA χ^2	P
Sex	1	0.8	NS	5.2	.05	2.6	NS
Color	1	1.2	NS	4.1	.05	1.3	NS
Age at last birthday	2	146.8	.01	47.6	.01	10.7	.01
Marital status	2	38.1	.01	10.4	.01	2.4	NS
Usual occupation	1	0.7	NS	0.5	NS	0.0	NS
Birthplace	4	23.0	.01	15.2	.01	1.0	NS
Principal activity in past year	4	45.5	.01	16.4	.01	3.3	NS
Religion (at time of death)	2	1.2	NS	1.6	NS	1.7	NS
Education	2	37.9	.01	18.1	.01	0.6	NS
Cause-of-death classification	3	38.4	.01	16.6	.01	2.0	NS
Hospitalization for liver trouble	1	10.1	.01	0.0	NS	6.1	.05
Blood or brain alcohol concentration	2	8.2	.05	2.5	NS	2.9	NS

[a] A = Alcoholics; $N = 250$. NA = Narcotic addicts; $N = 112$. A & NA = Both alcoholics and narcotic addicts; $N = 47$.

much more than the alcoholics in these characteristics, differing from the simple addicts only in that they were older and somewhat more likely to be male and Black.

The decedents with both conditions, however, were similar to the alcoholics in respect to more reported hospitalizations for liver trouble and illness during the past year than for the narcotic addicts. The alcoholics were more likely to have died from natural causes or accidents, while more of the narcotic addicts and those with both conditions were homicide victims. Alcohol was present in a large proportion of those decedents in all three subgroups for whom post-mortem blood or brain concentrations were obtained. Most cases with detectable alcohol, particularly the alcoholics and those with both conditions, had levels of 0.10 or higher, indicating impairment or intoxication by ingestion just prior to death (*McKinney's*, 1972–73).

CONCLUSION

Narcotic addicts, in conclusion, were more likely to be labeled by relatives or other persons identifying decedents than were alcoholics, because narcotics are illegal, and perhaps also due to the more rapid onset of narcotic addiction and problems resulting from the daily struggle to support this habit. Likewise, narcotism more than alcoholism was apt to be recorded as the immediate cause of death in this medical examiner population.

The findings indicate that those decedents with both conditions were in almost all cases primarily narcotic addicts rather than alcoholics, differing from the simple addicts mainly in that they were older. Alcohol abuse by narcotic addicts probably occurs most frequently during periods when heroin is more difficult to obtain and when they are trying to take drugs less often or not at all. The relevant literature supports the classification of decedents with evidence of both alcoholism and narcotism as narcotic addicts primarily; there are no references to the use of narcotics by alcoholics, but considerable data on alcohol abuse by narcotic addicts.

It might be useful to close with profiles of a typical alcoholic and narcotic addict in this sample of medical examiner cases. The typical alcoholic decedent was likely to be a male blue-collar worker in his 40s or 50s who had a grade school education or graduated high school. He migrated from the South if he was Black, and if White, was born in New York City. The typical dead narcotic addict, with or without concomitant alcoholism, was likely to be a single Black male blue-collar worker near 30 years of age, with some high school education, and born in New York City.

SUMMARY

In a sample of 1,000 consecutive adult decedents at the Office of Chief Medical Examiner, New York City, in 1972, three-tenths were classified as alcoholics and one-sixth as narcotic addicts, including 5% classified as both. A substantial minority of alcoholics and narcotic addicts would not have been so classified without both post-mortem medical findings and information from respondents when identifying decedents. Narcotic addicts were much younger, more often born in New York City, single, and likely to be homicide instead of accident victims than were alcoholics. Decedents with both conditions were similar to the narcotic addicts in these characteristics.

ACKNOWLEDGMENT

This study has been supported by the National Institute on Alcohol Abuse and Alcoholism, Grant R01-MH20997, for the project, "Alcoholism among Decedents in New York City," from the Columbia University School of Public Health, with the cooperation of the Office of Chief Medical Examiner, New York City.

The assistance of David H. Rosenthal and Loretta Hervey are very much appreciated.

REFERENCES

AUSTERLITZ, M., and SATTLER, S. *Analysis of heroin addict deaths in Manhattan—1968* (Baden, M.M., preceptor). Unpublished report, Health Research Training Program, New York City Department of Health, 1969.

BADEN, M.M. Homicide, suicide and accidental death among narcotic addicts. *Human Pathol.* 3: 91–95, 1972.

CHERUBIN, C., et al. The epidemiology of death in narcotic addicts. *Amer. J. Epid.* 96: 11–22, 1972.

CYBUCH, W., and SHAW, L. *A study of deaths of narcotic users in New York City—1970* (Baden, M.M., preceptor). Unpublished report, Health Research Training Program, New York City Department of Health, 1971.

CYBUCH, W., and THALLER, S. *Deaths of narcotic abusers in New York City—1971* (Baden, M.M., preceptor). Unpublished report, Health Research Training Program, New York City Department of Health, 1972.

DEVENYI, P., and WILSON, M. Barbiturate abuse and addiction and their relationship to alcohol and alcoholism. *Can. Med. Assoc. J.* 104: 215–218, 1971a.

DEVENYI, P., and WILSON, M. Abuse of barbiturates in an alcoholic population. *Can. Med. Assoc. J.* 104: 219–221, 1971b.

GEARING, F.R. *Successes and failures in methadone maintenance treatment of heroin addiction in New York City.* In *Proceedings of 3rd National Conference on Methadone Treatment, New York City, 1970.* Washington, D.C.: NIMH, Public Health Service Publication No. 2172, 1971.

HABERMAN, P.W., and BADEN, M.M. Alcoholism and violent death. *Quart. J. Studies Alc.* 35: 221–231, 1974.

HELPERN, M., and RHO, Y. Deaths from narcotism in New York City. *Intern. J. Addictions* 2: 53–84, 1967.

JACKSON, G.W., and RICHMAN, A. *Risk factors in mortality of narcotic addicts.* Paper presented at 99th annual meeting of American Public Health Association, Minneapolis, 1971.

Maryland State Medical Journal, Pennsylvania Department of Health Notes Dangers of Conjunctive Use of Alcohol and Drugs, 16: 134–139, May 1967.

McKinney's Consolidated Laws of New York. Vehicle and traffic law. 62A: section 1192, as amended in 1972. St. Paul, Minnesota: West Publishing Co., supplement 1972–73.

THALINGER, A. *A study of deaths of narcotic users in New York City—1969* (Baden, M.M., preceptor). Unpublished research report, Office of Chief Medical Examiner, 1970.

WEPPNER, R.S., and AGAR, M.H. Immediate precursors of heroin addiction. *J. Health Social Behavior* 12: 10–18, 1971.

The International Journal of the Addictions, 9(6), pp. 775–784, 1974

Addiction to Propoxyphene (Darvon): A Second Look

Barry M. Maletzky, M.D.

Department of Neuropsychiatry
Lyster Army Hospital
Ft. Rucker, Alabama

Abstract

Addiction to propoxyphene hydrochloride has been reported in the literature previously, although usually in patients afflicted with a variety of psychiatric ills or those already prone to drug and alcohol abuse. The author first reviews previous case reports of propoxyphene addiction, and then discusses basic experimental data which indicate that the potential of propoxyphene addiction is greater than previously suspected. Seven additional cases of propoxyphene addiction are described in patients with no prior history of psychiatric difficulties or other drug abuse. The physician's role in unknowingly abetting propoxyphene abuse is stressed and suggestions for further definitive research offered.

Although abuse of propoxyphene is a well-known entity, the belief still strongly exists that only those somehow psychologically deficient can become addicted. Thus literature (Lilly Research Laboratories, 1972) from the manufacturer boldly states:

> It should be noted that *all* patients involved in . . . case reports had a history of previous drug abuse or psychiatric disability prior to their misuse of Darvon.

Indeed, several case reports seem to verify the manufacturer's claim. Elson and Domino (1963), Claghorn and Schoolar (1966), and Collins and Mathis (1967) report a total of five cases of propoxyphene abuse in narcotic addicts who used the drug as an erstwhile, albeit largely unsatisfactory, substitute. Moreover, Claghorn and Schoolar (1966), Wolfe et al. (1969), and Kane and Norton (1969) report a total of three patients previously diagnosed as "disturbed" or "psychopathic" who appeared to be addicted to propoxyphene.

Various broadly available publications now seem to lend a quasi-official sanction to the notion that propoxyphene can only be abused by the addiction-prone individual. Salter (1970), writing in the "Drug Information Digest" Section of the *American Journal of Hospital Pharmacy* claims that "propoxyphene dependence does not appear to be a great problem," while the widely-distributed *Medical Letter on Drugs and Therapeutics* states, "most cases involved had a prior history of abuse of other drugs" (Anonymous, 1970). As a seemingly final statement, the World Health Organization, reviewing the abuse potential of propoxyphene in 1963 and again in 1969, concluded that the potential for abuse was so low as to not warrant any type of narcotic control.

In the face of such complacency, one can only be disturbed by the occasional report of propoxyphene's addiction potential in patients without apparent prior psychiatric difficulty. Salguero and his colleagues (1969), for example, describe a 20-year old man who had undergone numerous surgical procedures with concomitant abdominal distress. After an initial period of relief while not abusing propoxyphene, he steadily increased his use of the drug until addiction was apparent. Barrow and Souder (1971) describe a 35-year old woman who manifested signs of addiction while taking up to 2,000 mg of propoxyphene per day. Again, there was no psychiatric history.

A more recent report is especially intriguing. Chambers and Taylor (1971) have delineated, from their reservoir of experience with narcotic addiction, six patterns of propoxyphene abuse among a total of 120 subjects. Unfortunately, just five of these cases can be isolated technically as *addicttion* to propoxyphene; these cases manifested dependency and tolerance *without a past psychiatric or drug history*. It is equally unfortunate that the authors could not attempt withdrawal in these cases. Among many of the remaining cases, propoxyphene was abused for its immediate effects of euphoria and drunkenness, but not depended upon. In several cases, propoxyphene, as previously reported (Anonymous, 1970), was dissolved in water and intravenously injected.* However, of primary importance was the use of propoxyphene either as a drug of narcotic substitution or a drug of self-detoxification. Chambers and Taylor have discovered 15 opiate addicts who used propoxyphene to temporarily maintain their habit until the desired narcotic could be obtained. Although propoxyphene could only be successfully used for this purpose for 3 to 4 days, the fact that it substitutes for a narcotic increases the suspicion of addiction potential. Adding to this suspicion, Chambers and Taylor further describe 7 opiate addicts who routinely used propoxyphene to withdraw from narcotics. Most distressing was the fact that, in virtually all of Chambers and Taylor's subjects, propoxyphene had been obtained through perfectly legal channels: physicians' prescriptions.

Because of the present uncertainty surrounding the addiction potential of propoxyphene, and because of the enormous amount of propoxyphene daily prescribed, the following seven case reports of clear addiction to propoxyphene in nonpsychiatric patients are offered in an effort to justify inincreasing clinical caution and stimulate more definitive experimental research.

Case 1

A 20-year-old man had been given propoxyphene by his physician for pain secondary to injuries sustained in an automobile accident. Over a 2-year period the patient continued to complain of intermittent pain, receiving additional prescriptions. His physician began to grow suspicious and discontinued all propoxyphene, resulting in complaints of tremor and diaphoresis. Blood pressure measurements were elevated at that time. Upon admission to the hospital, pulse and blood pressure were again elevated and the patient was noted to be disoriented and tremulous, and to manifest "goosefleshing" and dilated pupils. Subsequent history revealed he had been obtaining propoxyphene from several different physicians for "pain" when, in fact, he took the drug to prevent the symptoms of withdrawal mentioned above. He was taking, prior to abrupt discontinuance, up to 1,560 mg daily in six divided doses. In hospital he was gradually withdrawn

* The manufacturer now produces propoxyphene in a form which discourages dissolving and injecting the drug.

from propoxyphene, beginning with 1,560 mg daily in four divided doses and decreasing by 130 mg every other day. On this regime he experienced no withdrawal symptoms except on the 10th hospital day when placebo was abruptly substituted. Such substitution resulted in a rise in blood pressure and pulse, agitation, and diaphoresis. Follow-up over the succeeding 2 years of close medical supervision revealed no drug abuse and no craving for propoxyphene. There was no prior history of psychiatric consultation or other drug abuse.

Case 2

A 45-year-old veteran, injured in a farming accident at the age of 38, was given propoxyphene by his physician. He steadily increased his own dose, first noticing he enjoyed the relief of pain and the "slight high" produced, then discovering he could not do without the drug. He experienced craving for the drug and agitation, tremor, insomnia, nausea, and muscle cramps without it. Beginning to purchase the drug illegally from a narcotics "pusher," he was soon spending several hundred dollars monthly to support his habit. He came voluntarily for treatment, plagued by his deteriorating financial condition and by the necessity to camouflage his complicity in the illicit drug trade. Upon hospitalization, he admitted to taking up to 35 Darvon compounds with ASA per day. It is of interest that he had been treated for severe gastric ulceration the year before. He was given 2,080 mg of plain Darvon daily in 4 doses and immediately noticed an improvement in the chronic epigastric pain associated with his ulcer. Tapering occurred at the rate of 130 mg of Darvon every other day without evidence of withdrawal. He has been followed by a Mental Health Service since hospitalization (6 months) with evidence of slight craving but with no return to propoxyphene. There was no prior history of psychiatric consultation or drug abuse.

Case 3

A 35-year-old housewife was treated for headaches of unknown origin over a period of 3 years with propoxyphene. She began to request increasing supplies of the drug and was usually accommodated. Suddenly hospitalized for acute lower abdominal pain secondary to ureteral lithiasis, she became disoriented and tremulous on the third hospital day. Although she had passed her "stones," she began to complain of abdominal and leg cramping and was noted to have elevations in pulse, temperature, and blood pressure, dilated pupils, and "goosefleshing" on the anterior chest. Her husband then volunteered her past history of propoxyphene abuse at this point, and because of the uncertainty of how much she had been taking, she was given 260 mg every 4 hr until symptoms of withdrawal ceased. Over a 24 hr period, most symptoms remitted at this dosage, thus withdrawal proceeded from this point at the rate of 130 mg every other day without further incident. A 2-year follow-up revealed absence of craving or drug abuse. There was no prior history of psychiatric consultation or other drug abuse.

Case 4

A 19-year-old man had been given propoxyphene by his physician the previous year for a severe toothache. Although dental work alleviated the original problem, he claimed that when he stopped propoxyphene he experienced recurrence of dental pain, as well as generalized tremor and agitation. He was taking, at this point, 520 mg daily. He subsequently increased his dosage by visiting different physicians in various cities until, at the time of voluntary admission to hospital, he was taking 1,625 mg of propoxyphene (Darvon compound) daily. Because his treating physicians expressed doubt about the addicting potential of propoxyphene, this medication was abruptly discontinued. By the second hospital day he was noted to have increases in pulse, blood pressure, temperature, dilated pupils, and to complain of agitation and nausea. He could not sleep that night and was observed to have a grand mal convulsion the next morning. An EEG revealed generalized fast activity and diffuse spiking. Propoxyphene was begun at 1,625 mg daily in four divided doses and reduced by 130 mg every other day. This schedule resulted in no recurrence of withdrawal symptoms. An EEG on the 12th hospital day (9th propoxyphene day) was normal. Mental Health Clinic follow-up revealed persistent craving with suspected return to propoxyphene abuse over 1 year. There was no prior history of psychiatric consultation or other drug abuse.

Case 5

A 52-year-old man began to take propoxyphene, originally prescribed for his wife, when he experienced pain secondary to a back sprain. Over the succeeding 2 years he used the drug more and more often for minor pains before he began to notice that he needed it almost daily. Frightened, he abruptly stopped the medication, only to experience nausea, tremors, and agitation. For 2 more years he tried sporadically to decrease propoxyphene without success. At the time of self-referral, he had stopped the drug for 18 hr and was extremely agitated and diaphoretic. He had been taking 2,600 mg daily. He was hospitalized and withdrawn at the rate of 130 mg every other day without incident. An EEG on admission revealed some diffuse spiking and exceedingly fast activity; on the 12th withdrawal day the EEG was normal. This patient has been without propoxyphene for 1½ years to date and still experiences craving. There was no prior history of psychiatric consultation or other drug abuse.

Case 6

A 23-year-old woman complained to her physician of lower abdominal cramping associated with menses and received large supplies of propoxyphene compound. She began to enjoy the slight euphoria high doses produced and soon found she could not receive enough through legal channels. Contacting a local drug "pusher," she began to satisfy her habit through illegal sources of supply, only to discover the cost was too much to bear. Abruptly discontinuing the drug, she soon experienced insomnia and agitation, for which she was seen in the emergency room and admitted. She had been taking up to 1,950 mg/day for a period of 6 months. Withdrawal of 130 mg every other day was begun without deleterious effect except for a 2-day placebo period on days 10 and 11. During this time symptoms of insomnia and agitation returned, along with a rise in temperature and blood pressure, dilated pupils, and "goosefleshing" of the anterior chest and upper arms. Follow-up over a 6-month period has been uncomplicated by drug craving. There was no prior history of psychiatric consultation or other drug abuse.

Case 7

A 32-year-old man was hospitalized in 1968 following an automobile accident and given propoxyphene compound for pain secondary to a fracture of the femur. He was discharged with a large supply of the drug and found that when he decreased the dose of four per day his pain recurred. Over a period of several months he was surprised to discover that even at that dose, pain began to recur. He increased his dose over the next several years, always finding an obliging physician to cater to his demands for more. Finally, unable to fill his needs from local physicians, he began to visit various emergency rooms complaining of bizarre pain syndromes, and literally pleading for propoxyphene. Suspected of heroin abuse, he was hospitalized and treated for 2 days with methadone, 10 mg every 6 hr, until he finally divulged his true history. Methadone was tapered gradually and on 1 year follow-up, while slight craving for propoxyphene existed, no return to the drug had occurred. There was no prior history of psychiatric consultation or other drug abuse.

DISCUSSION

The cases described above clearly indicate the need to regard propoxyphene as a potentially addicting substance. They underscore the following points relating to propoxyphene abuse.

1. Addiction to propoxyphene can occur in patients not previously regarded as psychiatrically ill or as "addiction-prone." To assert that development of the addiction by itself signifies a defect seems both scientifically unsound and, in these cases, clinically unverifiable. The present cases, added to several already described (Salguero et al., 1969; Barrow and Souder, 1971; Chambers and Taylor, 1971) in which addiction occurred without prior psychiatric impairment, emphasize the need to closely monitor propoxyphene prescriptions in the general population.
2. Addiction can occur under the usual circumstances of medical prescribing. Cases 1, 3, 4, 5, and 7 amply demonstrate the ease with which physicians will unknowingly initiate and maintain a propoxyphene addiction. Cases described were not suffering overwhelming pain; indeed, retrospectively it seemed impossible to delineate which factors contributed to addiction in these cases. In the face of such ignorance, increasing caution must be urged.
3. Clear evidence of addiction in these cases exists. Cases 2, 3, 4, and 7 demonstrated unmistakable tolerance. All cases manifested at least three of the following signs of withdrawal: tremor; insomnia; agitation; diaphoresis; elevated blood pressure, pulse and temperature; recurrence of original pains; abdominal and other muscular cramping; hyperactive deep tendon reflexes; dizziness; nausea and vomiting; and seizures.
4. Addiction can occur without intravenous use; the usual oral route appears sufficient. None of our cases injected the drug.
5. Addiction can occur without the initial experience of euphoria. Cases 1, 3, 4, 5, and 7 did not describe any initial "high" from the drug nor did any of our cases claim to experience any immediately noticeable effect after addiction was truly established. Rather, almost all admitted to need-

ing the drug to prevent the dreaded appearance of withdrawal. It is of interest that, occasionally, upon abrupt (but not gradual) withdrawal, the original pain for which the patient first received propoxyphene recurred despite the absence of the original lesion.

Propoxyphene is now the most widely prescribed analgesic in the United States (Salter, 1970). A major thrust in the advertising for this drug has been that it is equivalent to codeine in intensity of analgesic action without codeine's potential for abuse and addiction. The above cases not only contribute to a growing caution against such a sanguine view, but also draw attention to some similarity between addiction to propoxyphene and addiction to narcotic substances, including pentazocine. In both cases, substances were initially touted as major advances in analgesia, only subsequently discovered to be potentially addicting; in both cases, substances occasionally produce a "high" or "rush" yet do not rely upon this effect to produce addiction; and in both cases, symptoms upon withdrawal are strikingly similar: dilated pupils, elevations of vital signs, abdominal and skeletal muscle cramping, extreme agitation, insomnia, and chest "goose-fleshing." Even more convincing is apparent cross tolerance with narcotics (Chambers and Taylor, 1971). Indeed, in Case 7, methadone was unknowingly used to withdraw the patient from propoxyphene without difficulty. The major differences between propoxyphene and narcotics may be quantitative (although no rhinorrhea on withdrawal may be another difference): propoxyphene is undeniably less dangerous than most narcotics in terms of percentage taking these drugs who will subsequently become addicted; moreover, propoxyphene is less expensive and more available, thus sparing its addicts the social turmoil consequent upon most narcotic abuse.

Nonetheless, there is sufficient evidence for an addiction potential to warrant increasing caution in prescribing propoxyphene and careful follow-up for those patients already taking the drug. A heavy burden for the cases reported rests with the physicians who prescribed more analgesic than absolutely necessary or who allowed refills without apparent purpose. Caution here may exert a preventive effect: it has already become clear that among those families where unnecessary analgesic and minor tranquilizer abuse exists, children carry a heightened probability of experimenting with potentially addicting drugs (Smart and Fejer, 1972).

While conservatism is thus urged in propoxyphene's clinical use, it is also apparent that more research of a basic nature is necessary. The first controlled experiments detailing propoxyphene's ability to produce dependence were reported by Fraser and Isbell (1960). Shemano and Wendel

(1964) produced a definitive method of rank ordering propoxyphene's addictive liability in 1964. However, animal self-infusion procedures (Schuster and Thompson, 1963), so helpful in clarifying relationships among narcotic, alcohol, amphetamine, and diazepoxide addictions (Schuster and Thompson, 1963; Findley, Robinson, and Peregrino, 1972) have as yet not been applied to propoxyphene. It is hoped this logical next step will soon be forthcoming, along with a greater recognition of the need for caution in propoxyphene use.

SUMMARY

Case examples are provided which demonstrate the following points relative to propoxyphene addiction.

1. Addiction to propoxyphene can occur in individuals neither psychiatrically ill or "addiction-prone."
2. Addiction can occur under the usual circumstances of medical prescribing.
3. Tolerance and withdrawal can be clearly demonstrated.
4. Addiction can occur without initial euphoria.

A review of pertinant literature, combined with these case reports, provides sufficient evidence of addiction potential to warrant not only caution in prescribing propoxyphene, but the institution of careful follow-up measures as well.

REFERENCES

ANONYMOUS. Propoxyphene hydrochloride (Darvon) and Darvon compounds. *Med. Letter on Drugs and Therap.* 12: 5–6, 1970.

BARROW, M.V., and SOUDER, D.E. Propoxyphene and congenital malformations. *J. Amer. Med. Assoc.* 217: 1551, 1971.

CHAMBERS, C.D., and TAYLOR, W.J.R. Patterns of propoxyphene abuse. *Intern. J. Clin. Pharmacol.* 4: 240–250, 1971.

CLAGHORN, J.L., and SCHOOLAR, J.C. Propoxyphene hydrochloride, a drug of abuse. *J. Amer. Med. Assoc.* 196: 1089, 1966.

COLLINS, M.S., and MATHIS, J.L. Addiction to intravenous Darvon, case report. *J. Oklahoma State Med. Assoc.* 60: 609, 1967.

ELSON, A., and DOMINO, E.P. Dextro-propoxyphene addiction: observations of a case. *J. Amer. Med. Assoc.* 183: 482, 1963.

FINDLEY, J.D., ROBINSON, W.W., and PEREGRINO, L. Addiction to secobarbital and chlordiazepoxide in the Rhesus monkey by means of a self-infusion preference procedure. *Psychopharmacologia* (Berl) 26: 93–114, 1972.

FRASER, H.F., and ISBELL, H. Pharmacology and addiction liability of *dl*- or *d*-propoxyphene. *Bull Narcotics* 12: 9, 1960.

KANE, F.J., and NORTON, J.T. Addiction to propoxyphene. *J. Amer. Med. Assoc.* 211: 300, 1969.

LILLY RESEARCH LABORATORIES, Letter, August 9, 1972. Personal communication.

SALGUERO, C.H., VILLAREAL, J.E., HUG, C., Jr., and DOMINO, E.F. Propoxyphene dependence. *J. Amer. Med. Assoc.* 210: 135, 1969.

SALTER, F.J. Propoxyphene: dependence, abuse and treatment of overdosage. *Amer. J. Hosp. Pharmacol.* 28: 208–210, 1970.

SCHUSTER, C.R., and THOMPSON, T. A technique for studying self-administration of opiates in Rhesus monkeys. *Commun. Drug Addiction and Narcotics, NRC-NAS.* Ann Arbor, Michigan, 1963.

SCHUSTER, C.R., and THOMPSON, T. Self-administration of and behavioral dependence on drugs. *Ann. Rev. Pharmacol.* 9: 483–502, 1969.

SHEMANO, I., and WENDEL, H. A rapid screening test for potential addiction liability of new analgesic agents. *Toxicol. Appl. Pharmacol.* 6: 334, 1964.

SMART, R.G., and FEJER, D. Drug use among adolescents and their parents: closing the generation gap in mood modification. *J. Abnormal Psychol.* 79: 153–160, 1972.

WOLFE, R.C., RUDENBERG, M., and VISPO, R.H. Propoxyphene (Darvon) addiction and withdrawal syndrome. *Ann. Int. Med.* 10: 773, 1969.

The International Journal of the Addictions, 9(6), pp. 785–804, 1974

The Indexing and Analysis of Drug Indulgence

K. H. Lu, Ph.D.

University of Oregon Health Sciences Center
Portland, Oregon

Abstract

An index of drug indulgence is constructed by deriving sets of appropriate index weights for each state of use of each drug from the data distribution. A user thus has one weight from each drug scale according to his involvement, and his drug-use index is defined as the average of these weights. The index inherently places more weight on drugs less commonly used than the more commonly used ones. Data from 38 males and 35 female users are analyzed, and it is found that males are 11 points higher than the females and that there are no significant correlations between drug uses.

It is a well-known fact that drug indulgence by young people has assumed epidemic proportions in recent years. Unfortunately, the drug use data as collected by the police or by the free clinics reflect only a very special segment of the population of the drug culture; namely, those who were arrested or in need of clinics. The majority of the volitional users who never skirmished with the law and had no need of clinics have thus far eluded systematic evaluation in their pristine states (Zili et al., 1971). The difficulty in gathering drug use information lies in the fact that the possession of drugs is illegal. Most users are reluctant to give such personal information to an inquirer, especially when the inquirer is a nonuser and not of their generation. The inquirer is usually viewed with suspicion, contempt, and sometimes open hostility. The author, through his reading of poetry and knowledge of Bhuddism, was fortunate to have a friendly relationship with and ready acceptance by the drug colony. In time they knew that he was not a "lark," nor did he wish to judge or condemn. Finally, they realized that he was trustworthy enough to "rap" with and friendly enough to listen. They became open and eager to talk.

In order to study the drug scene objectively, it appears desirable to have an index of drug use which measures the user's total involvement with the entire spectrum of drugs (Sadava, 1972; Feinstein, 1967). The data thus collected should lend themselves to statistical analysis for epidemiological purposes. The purposes of this paper are as follows:

1. To develop a procedure of obtaining index weights which are relevant to the different stages of use for each drug.
2. To compute an overall index value for each user such that it is relevant of his total involvement with the entire spectrum of drugs.
3. To derive statistical characterizations of the users in different percentiles of the drug-using population according to their respective involvements with each drug.
4. To assess the relative importance of each drug on their influence upon the overall index.

The sample of study is admittedly small, but the heuristics thus developed may be of interest to those who are concerned with this problem.

HEURISTICAL CONSIDERATIONS

In addition to the difficulties associated with data collection, another handicap is that young drug users as a rule are quite unprecise in assessing their own drug using habits. The unpreciseness, though not deliberately intended, is an unpleasant defect of the basic data. Consequently, they can only be classified into broad categories arranged in ordinal sequence according to the extent of use. Thus, in actual handling of the data, we face further theoretical difficulties.

1. The insummability between qualitatively different drugs. The dif-

ferences between different drugs are not only in substance but in effects as well. We cannot say two users are "alike" because they each use two drugs, nor can we say a three-drug user is a more "involved" user than a two-drug user. It depends very much on what drugs they are using and how much. A user of marijuana and barbiturates is qualitatively different from a user of amphetamines and narcotics (heroine and opiates), etc.

2. The insummability of categories bearing the same names or ranks. The ordinal categories of drug use are (1) nonuser, (2) experimental, (3) occasional, (4) regular, and (5) heavy for all drugs. However, the same ordinal names or labels may denote quite different extents of use in different drugs. For example, a person who "drops acid" once every 2 or 3 weeks is a regular user of LSD, but a person who smokes marijuana that often is an experimental user as generally considered by the groups.

3. The insummability of ordinal ranks within a drug. The sequence of ordinal categories in each drug denotes an ordered set of degrees of drug use. The ranks, however, do not themselves denote the quantitative difference between the degrees they represent. In other words, though we may say Rank 2 is more involved than Rank 1, but we cannot say exactly by how much. The underlying true difference between Rank 1 and Rank 2 may or may not be equal to that between Rank 3 and Rank 4. The insummability of ranks is due to (1) the unequal true differences between adjacent ranks, and (2) the obvious fact that a first plus a second does not equal a third.

It is now clear than in order to measure drug use, we must first construct a metric such that it is (1) capable of measuring the involvement of all drugs, and interdrug currency of exchange, so to speak, and (2) capable of regular mathematical operations.

THE DEVELOPMENT OF THE INDEX OF DRUG INVOLVEMENT

Let C_{ij} be the ith category of use of the jth drug, and y_{ijk} be the status of user, S_k, with respect to C_{ij} such that

$$y_{ijk} = 1 \quad \text{if } S_k \in C_{ij}$$

or

$$= 0 \quad \text{if } S_k \notin C_{ij}$$

where $i = 1, 2 \ldots, t$; $j = 1, 2, \ldots, m$, and $k = 1, 2, \ldots, n$. Let the following array represent the observed data on a sample of n users:

Categories	Drugs 1	2	. . . j . . .	m	Σ
1	n_{11}	n_{12}	n_{1j}	n_{1m}	n
2	n_{21}	n_{22}	n_{2j}	n_{2m}	n
⋮					
i	n_{i1}	n_{i2}	n_{ij}	n_{im}	n
⋮					
t	n_{t1}	n_{t2}	n_{tj}	n_{tm}	n

where n_{ij} = number of users belong to C_{ij}

$$= \sum_{k=1}^{n} y_{ijk}$$

We shall utilize the observed n_{ij}'s to derive index weights for the C_{ij}'s so that each subject $S_k \in C_{ij}$ will be given the derived index weight, w_{ij}.

Let x_j = the usage of the jth drug, and x_j is conceptually a continuous random variable with frequency function $f(x)$ and finite first two moments. In practice we have to use ordinal categories to represent the continuum because of our inability to gather precise data. Note that since C_{ij} covers a segment of the continuum, then

$$P_r\{S_k \in C_{ij}\} = \int_{C_{ij}} f(x)\,dx$$

It is a well-known fact that if we let w be the distribution function of x,

$$w = F(x) = \int_{-\infty}^{x} f(u)\,du$$

then the frequency function of w,

$$f(w) = f(x)\left|\frac{dx}{dw}\right| dw = \frac{f(x)}{f(x)}\,dw = dw$$

We see that w is always uniformly distributed with mean $\frac{1}{2}$ and variance 1/12, regardless what form $f(x)$ may have been.

We now compute the set of index weights appropriate for the C_{ij}'s as follows. Let

$$w_{ij} = \text{the weight of } C_{ij}$$
$$= \sum_{r=1}^{i-1} P_{rj} + \tfrac{1}{2}P_{ij}$$

where $P_{ij} = n_{ij}/n$. Note that w_{ij} denotes the proportion of subjects who are less than or equally as involved as category i in drug j. Thus we have assigned index weights to the categories of the jth drug with a probabilistic meaning (Lu, 1971).

The observed data in terms of the transformed probabilistic scale are therefore as follows:

	Drugs						
Categories	1	2	. . .	j	. . .	t
1	$n_{11}w_{11}$	$n_{12}w_{12}$		$n_{1j}w_{1j}$		$n_{1t}w_{1t}$
2	$n_{21}w_{21}$	$n_{22}w_{22}$		$n_{2j}w_{2j}$		$n_{2t}w_{2t}$
⋮						
i	$n_{i1}w_{i1}$	$n_{i2}w_{i2}$		$n_{ij}w_{ij}$		$n_{it}w_{it}$
⋮						
m	$n_{m1}w_{m1}$	$n_{m2}w_{m2}$		$n_{mj}w_{mj}$		$n_{mt}w_{mt}$

Each subject S_k shall have one w_{ij} value from each drug scale, the total value of S_k is therefore the sum of the t values.

We define the overall involvement index of S_k as the average of the w_{ij}'s of each subject, i.e.,

$$z_k = \frac{1}{t}\left(\sum_{i=1}^{t} \sum_{j=1}^{m} y_{ijk}w_{ij}\right)$$

By virtue of being the average of the distribution functions of t drugs, the index value, say, z_k, is therefore an average percentile denoting S_k's position of drug use in relation to his peers. Since each w_{ij} is uniformly distributed with mean $\frac{1}{2}$, we know that an index value of .5000 is the average.

In other words, an average user is expected to have an index value of .5000. Users with indices less or greater than .5000 are consequently considered to have less or greater involvements than the average user.

A word on the distribution property of z_k seems appropriate here. Since z_k is a mean of t uniform variables, thus when t is large, z_k becomes a normal variable in virtue of the central limit theorem. When t is small ($t = 2, 3, 4$), the exact distributions of z_k are known (Kendall and Stuart, 1958). These distributions, though not normal, can nontheless be approximated by a normal distribution (Bell, 1970; Hoyt, 1968). For practical and computational purposes, z_k may be considered as approximately normal.

THE INDEXING AND THE ANALYSIS

Seventy-three users, 35 females and 38 males, self-rated themselves according to their involvements with five types of drugs. The five types of drugs are (1) marijuana, (2) LSD, (3) amphetamines, (4) barbiturates, and (5) narcotics. The ranks of involvements are (1) nonuser, (2) experimental,

Table 1
Definitions of States of Use of Five Drugs

	Marijuana	LSD	Amphetamines	Barbiturates	Narcotics[a]
Nonuser	0	0	0	0	0
Experimental	Less than 2 joints in a month	Tried once	Tried once	Use when depressed	Tried once
Occasional	1 to 2 joints per week	Tried 3 or 4 times in 6 months	About 1 to 2 times a month	Use whenever available	Tried more than 2 times and will try again
Regular	3 to 6 joints per week	1 to 2 times a month	About once per week	Keep a supply once a week	Must have a fix sometimes
Heavy	More than 1 joint a day	3 or more times per month	More than once a week	More than once a week	Must have a fix at least once a week

[a] Heroine and opiates.

(3) occasional, (4) regular, and (5) heavy. The definitions of the ranks of involvement for each type of drug are summarized in Table 1.

The frequencies of users classified by sex and drug-use are given in Table 2.

The Computation of Index Weights for Each Drug and Overall Indices

The stepwise computation of categorical weights for marijuana is shown in Table 3 as an example.

The category weights for all drugs are given in Table 4.

One inherent property of the index weights is that it places less weight on drugs which are commonly used. For instance, since marijuana is the most frequently used drug, its index weights are considerably lower than

Table 2
Distribution of 73 Subjects' Involvement in Drug Use According to Drugs, Sex, and States of Use

States of use		Types of drugs[a]				
		D_1	D_2	D_3	D_4	D_5
Female	Nonuser	4	12	13	10	12
	Experimental	6	15	18	8	19
	Occasional	8	5	3	15	2
	Regular	10	2	1	1	1
	Heavy	7	1	0	1	1
	Σ	35	35	35	35	35
Male	Nonuser	0	2	10	14	13
	Experimental	4	14	19	4	19
	Occasional	5	13	5	9	3
	Regular	17	5	3	5	1
	Heavy	12	4	1	6	2
	Σ	38	38	38	38	38
Both sexes	Nonuser	4	14	23	24	25
	Experimental	10	29	37	12	38
	Occasional	13	18	8	24	5
	Regular	27	7	4	6	2
	Heavy	19	5	1	7	3
	Σ	73	73	73	73	73

[a] D_1 = marijuana. D_2 = LSD. D_3 = amphetamines. D_4 = barbiturates. D_5 = narcotics (cocaine, morphine, heroin, etc.).

Table 3
Stepwise Computation of w_{ij} for Marijuana

Categories	(1) Observed frequency f_i	(2) (1)/2	(3) $\sum_{r=1}^{i-1} f_r$	(4) (2) + (3)	(5) w_{ij}
Nonuser	4	2	0	2	.0274
Experimental	10	5	4	9	.1233
Occasional	13	6.5	14	20.5	.2808
Regular	27	13.5	27	40.5	.5548
Heavy	19	9.5	54	63.5	.8699

Table 4
Index Weights of Drugs According to States of Use

	Types of drugs[a]				
State of use	D_1	D_2	D_3	D_4	D_5
Nonuser	.0274	.0959	.1575	.1644	.1712
Experimental	.1233	.3904	.5685	.4110	.6027
Occasional	.2808	.7123	.8767	.6575	.8973
Regular	.5548	.8836	.9589	.8630	.9452
Heavy	.8699	.9658	.9932	.9521	.9795

[a] D_1 = marijuana. D_2 = LSD. D_3 = amphetamines. D_4 = barbiturates. D_5 = narcotics.

those of other drugs in every category. On the other hand, since narcotics is the least used drug in the drug culture, it has higher values in every category than do all the others. For example, a regular user of marijuana shall be given an index value of .5548, and be considered less involved than an occasional user of LSD, amphetamines, and barbiturates. Narcotic being the most advanced drug, an experimental user of it has an index value of .6027, and is therefore considered as being more involved than a regular marijuana user.

Substituting the category ranks of each user with the appropriate weights, each user thus has five weights, one from each type of drugs according to the user's own involvement. The average of the five weights of each user is taken as the index value of the user in question.

The Analysis

The Reflectiveness of the Indices. We are now in the position to see how well the indices represent the total drug involvements of the users.

Let us examine the indices for some users who are at the two extremes. For example, female users F-2 and F-6 have indices of .22876 and .22466, respectively. We see that F-2 is a regular marijuana user and a nonuser of all others, and F-6 is an experimental user of amphetamines and a nonuser of all others. The index thus considers a regular marijuana user and an experimental user of amphetamines as approximately equally involved in drug indulgence. This seems to agree with the drug culture's own consensus that "speed kills" whereas to "roll a roach" (to smoke marijuana) is harmless. Male user M-9 is a regular user of marijuana; a heavy user of LSD, amphetamines, and barbiturates; and an occasional user of narcotics. He has an index value of .86578, far above the average indeed.

The Classification of Users. The mean and standard deviation of the 73 indices are .5000 and .2238, respectively. It appears that .5000 $\pm$ .0500 would be a reasonable center class for classification purposes, i.e., the class width is approximately one-half the size of the standard deviation. The 73 indices are thus classified into seven classes. The results are summarized in Table 5.

From Table 5 we observe the following points of interest:

1. The indices enable us to classify the users according to their index values without trying beforehand to define the range of involvement in each drug for each class. For example, anyone with index value $.4500 \leq x \leq .5500$ is classified in the "average" class with the center at .5000. The actual ranges of involvement in each drug of each class can be obtained from the data after the classification has been made. In other words, instead of subjectively "defining" the boundaries of the classes, we let the data suggest the boundaries themselves.

The advantage of this type of classification is that the class boundaries are always relevant to the population, whereas if the boundaries were suggested by an "authority," his "authoritative" pontification may or may not be relevant to the population in question.

2. The concept of the "average users." Since w_{ij}'s are by definition to have a mean equal to .5000, theoretically, an "average" user can be one who is "average" all the way, i.e., he has all $w_{ij} = .5000$. In reality, however, such a user does not exist because none of the $w_{ij} = .5000$. In practice, while the w_{ij}'s of the users may vary from user to user, as long as their average indexes are between .4500 and .5500, they are considered as members of the "average" class, therefore, they are "average users."

Translating the average index values of each type of drugs of the average

Table 5
Mean Drug Involvement of 73 Users Classified According to Overall Index Value and Sex

		Type of drugs[a]					
		D_1	D_2	D_3	D_4	D_5	$\Sigma/5$
15–25	Female	.3391	.0959	.3630	.1644	.1712	.22671
	Male	0	0	0	0	0	0
	All	.3391	.0959	.3630	.1644	.1712	.22671
25–35	Female	.1861	.2432	.2260	.3699	.4826	.30154
	Male	0	0	0	0	0	0
	All	.1861	.2432	.2260	.3699	.4826	.30154
35–45	Female	.2957	.3670	.4983	.4110	.4720	.40879
	Male	.4635	.5289	.4749	.2466	.3959	.42192
	All	.3676	.4364	.4883	.3405	.4393	.41441
45–55	Female	.6439	.5206	.3630	.7089	.2791	.50307
	Male	.5675	.5047	.4341	.5638	.4947	.51296
	All	.5854	.5085	.4174	.5979	.4440	.51063
55–65	Female	.6196	.4695	.5778	.5722	.6370	.57521
	Male	.5665	.6448	.7730	.4178	.4802	.57647
	All	.5989	.5377	.6537	.5122	.5760	.57570
65–75	Female	0	0	0	0	0	0
	Male	.7124	.7997	.5428	.8082	.6027	.69315
	All	.7124	.7997	.5428	.8082	.6027	.69315
85–95	Female	0	0	0	0	0	0
	Male	.5548	.9658	.9589	.9521	.8973	.86578
	All	.5548	.9658	.9589	.9521	.8973	.86578

[a] D_1 = marijuana. D_2 = LSD. D_3 = amphetamines. D_4 = barbiturates. D_5 = narcotics.

class into the descriptive language of Table 3, we see that the average user is (1) a regular-to-heavy user of marijuana, (2) an experimental-to-occasional user of LSD and barbiturates, and (3) a non-to-experimental user of amphetamines and narcotics.

The females of the average class are more involved in marijuana and barbiturates than males, and the males are more involved in amphetamines and narcotics. The involvement in LSD of both sexes appeared to be equal.

The Differences between Sexes. Note that there are no males in the two lower classes and no females in the two uppermost classes, clearly indicating the males are more involved in drug use than the females. An

Table 6
Mean Index Values between Sexes

	♂	♀	♂ − ♀	P_r(♂ > ♀)[a]
Marijuana	.5728	.4209	.1519*	.6519*
LSD	.6105	.3800	.2305*	.7305*
Amphetamines	.5429	.4534	.0895	.5895
Barbiturates	.5234	.4746	.0488	.5488
Narcotics	.5019	.4878	.0141	.5141
Index	.5503	.4431	.1072*	.6072*

[a] Where P_r(♂ > ♀) = P_r(a randomly chosen male has greater involvement than a randomly chosen female).

analysis of variance showed that the differences between sexes and drug-sex interaction are significant. We shall interpret these findings in terms of the table of means as in Table 6.

The meaning of the differences between sexes, .5503 − .4431 = .1072, means that the probability of a randomly chosen male be more involved in drugs than a randomly chosen female is .5000 + .1072 = .6072, or roughly at six to four odds. The differences between sexes within each drug may be interpreted in the same way. Note that only the cases of marijuana and LSD are significant.

It might be of interest to see the extent of involvement of the average male and female users in terms of individual drugs. By regrouping the data from Table 6, we define the average male user class as $.50 \leq z_k \leq .60$ and the average female user class as $.40 \leq z_k \leq .50$. The results are summarized in Table 7.

We see that the average male user is a regular-to-heavy user of marijuana and an experimental-to-occasional user of all other drugs. The

Table 7
The mean Index Values of "Average" Male Users ($.50 \leq z_k \leq .60$) and "Average" Female Users ($.40 \leq z_k \leq .50$)

	♂	♀
D_1(marijuana)	.6199	.2983
D_2(LSD)	.5088	.3470
D_3(amphetamines)	.6120	.4749
D_4(barbiturates)	.5090	.5434
D_5(narcotics)	.4926	.5395
Index	.5485	.4406

average female user is an occasional-to-regular user of marijuana, an experimental-to-occasional user of barbiturates, and a non-to-experimental user of others.

The Correlation Analysis. The correlation matrices of the individual and overall indices of males and females are given in Table 8.

We observe the following salient points.

1. The only significant correlation is the correlation between marijuana and amphetamines, −.3470 in the males. The correlations between drugs in most cases are negative and of low magnitude. The negative correlations may be explained by the fact that the various drugs must compete with one another for the limited funds at the disposal of the users, thus the increase in the use of one must be at the expense of the others. The low magnitudes may be due to the fact that as funds become more available, there may be general increases in the use of all drugs, but the increases may not be proportional to one another.

2. The relative importance of the component drug indices to the overall index. All correlations between the individual index weights of each drug and the overall indices are significant except for the case with mari-

Table 8

Correlation Matrices of Drug Indices According to Sex

Females

	Type of drugs[a]					
	D_1	D_2	D_3	D_4	D_5	Index
			Females			
D_1	1.0000	–.0334	–.0966	.1900	.0149	.5315*
D_2		1.0000	–.0026	–.0307	–.1068	.3809*
D_3			1.0000	.1553	–.0397	.4334*
D_4				1.0000	–.0520	.5341*
D_5					1.0000	.3500*
			Males			
D_1	1.0000	–.1632	–.3470*	.2318	–.1019	.2900
D_2		1.0000	.1507	.0941	–.0259	.4850*
D_3			1.0000	–.1872	.0623	.3283*
D_4				1.0000	–.1480	.5535*
D_5					1.0000	.3678*

[a] D_1 = marijuana. D_2 = LSD. D_3 = amphetamines. D_4 = barbiturates. D_5 = narcotics.

juana in the male group. The overall index is the arithmatic mean of the five individual indices, thus the multiple correlation between the overall index and its components is, by definition, unity, i.e.,

$$R^2_{\mathrm{I}\cdot 12345} = 1$$

A partition of $R^2_{\mathrm{I}\cdot 12345}$ in terms of the contribution from each component drug is useful in assessing their relative importance in terms of the determination of the amount of variation in the overall index. The partition of R^2 for the males and the females is given in Table 9.

The values in Table 9 indicate the amount of variation in the overall index that can be accounted for by the variation in the component index weights. For instance, the barbiturates is the most important component for the males, and it alone accounts for 31.6% of the variations in the overall index; LSD is second, accounting for about 21.47%, etc. For the females, the indices of marijuana and barbiturates account for 26.87 and 21.71%, respectively.

The relatively larger determination of R^2 by barbiturates in the males and marijuana in the females is due, in addition to the larger correlations, to the fact that they also have wider variation as compared to other drugs, as evidenced by the large coefficient of variation C.V.(D_4) = .6038 for the males and C.V.(D_1) = .6936 for the females.

3. A discussion in the correlation results in conjunction with the generally held "truism" that "marijuana smoking leads to the use of narcotics."

The paralogical arguments. A rather startling phenomenon from the correlation matrices is the lack of strong correlations among the component drug indices (w_{ij}). In order to discuss this matter in sharp focus, let

Table 9

Amount of Determination of Five Drugs in the Variation of the Overall Index

	Amount of determination of $R^2_{\mathrm{I}\cdot 12345}$			
	Males		Females	
D_1(marijuana)	.1306	5	.2687	1
D_2(LSD)	.2147	2	.1742	4
D_3(amphetamines)	.1625	4	.1895	3
D_4(barbiturates)	.3161	1	.2171	2
D_5(narcotics)	.1761	3	.1505	5
$R^2_{\mathrm{I}\cdot 12345}$	1.0000		1.0000	

us bear in mind that a strong correlation between two variables simply implies a linear association between them, but in no way implies it is a cause-and-effect relationship. On the other hand, if a strong linear cause-and-effect association is known to exist between two variables, then a strong correlation necessarily exists. Thus the lack of significant correlation among the drug suggests two alternatives:

1. Drug use habits are independent of each other, i.e., there is no cause and effect relationship between drug use.
2. The association between drug use habits may be caused by other common factors in a nonlinear manner.

Neither one of the alternatives supports the "truism" that the use of marijuana leads to the use of narcotics. In the passages to follow, we shall attempt a probable explanation.

The existence of a drug-prone subpopulation: It is safe to say that not all young people exposed to the lure of drugs become users. It is also safe to say that not all marijuana users open to the temptation of narcotics become narcotic addicts; after all, there are narcotic addicts who never used marijuana at all. Consequently, it appears reasonable to say that there exists a subpopulation of youth who are more prone to drug use than others, and there is a subset of marijuana users who are more prone to become narcotic users than others. According to the young users, the reasons most frequently given for turning to drugs are boredom, noncommunication with parents, and feelings of being unwanted, unloved, and useless. Some of them take drugs to enter a "better world," some to spite their parents, and some just to get "kicks." The above observation seems to agree with other studies (Robbins et al., 1971; Braucht and Berry, 1973).

There are dilligent research works probing into the social, economical, and psychological forces responsible for the evolvement of a drug-prone subpopulation. It is important to realize that as long as there are "alien-nated" youth, there will be young drug users. If they have no drugs to use, they probably will turn to something else.

An explanation on why most addicts started with marijuana: To be sure, there is a general stepwise pattern of drug use. Most drug users did indeed start with marijuana,and moved on to other drugs. The pertinent points of this phenomenon is that marijuana is the cheapest and the most available, and the knowledge that it is relatively harmless and nonaddictive. The most potent restraining force preventing the young from trying narcotics first was that they know narcotics are expensive as well as addictive. It is possible that many zealous compaigns against marijuana may have actually encouraged experiments with narcotics. As far as we know to date, there has been no definite proof that smoking marijuana is harmful, except for its mild euphoric effect. It is no worse than and not as addictive as alcohol (Gorodetzky, 1970). Yet a great number of the "educational" materials overstated the "harmful" effects of marijuana, hoping to "scare" the youth away from it. Unfortunately, most of them have at one time or another been exposed to it, and they know from their own experience that all the "scare facts" are not facts at all.

Once they realized that a "straightman's lie" has been dealt to them as the "straight goods," they tend to distrust and dismiss most if not all the utterances of the "straight" world, including scientific and medical facts about other drugs.

CONCLUSIONS AND SUMMARY

1. A uniform transformation of the distribution function is used as the basic indexing device. The index system is used to index 73 drug users (35 females and 38 males), with respect to five drugs: marijuana, LSD, amphetamines, barbiturates, and narcotics. The computed indices have a mean of .5000 and a standard deviation of .2238.

2. The above indexing system allows the investigator to rate the users on a probabilistic scale. It weighs users' involvements with drugs in terms of their standing with their peers, without a priori definition of involvement with each drug. The statistical characteristic of each class may be ascertained after the classification is completed. It lets the data themselves suggest the range of involvement with each drug. Therefore, it is always relevant to the population under observation.

3. A user of the average class is a regular-to-heavy user of marijuana, experimental-to-occasional user of LSD and barbiturates, and none-to-experimental user of amphetamines and narcotics. The females in this group are more involved in marijuana and barbiturates than the males; the males of the class are more involved in amphetamines and narcotics than the females.

4. There are significant differences between sexes with respect to the overall index as well as in the individual drugs. The males' average index is .55 and the females' .44.

5. The correlations among the five drugs are mostly negative and of low magnitude. The only significant correlation is between marijuana and

amphetamines in the males ($r = -.3470$). The above finding does not support the general belief that "the use of marijuana leads to the use of narcotics."

6. There exists a subpopulation of youth which is more susceptible to the lure of drugs than other groups. The reasons most frequently given for turning to drugs are boredom, noncommunication, and alienation. If this subpopulation has no drugs to turn to it will turn to something else.

ACKNOWLEDGMENT

The author wishes to express his appreciation to those young persons who, in spite of their personal plight, freely gave the drug use information used in this study. It is hoped that this paper may in some way help to bring some understanding to a group of human beings who are so mercilessly condemned, so hopelessly trapped, and so helplessly young!

REFERENCES

BELL, S. Approximating the normal distribution with the triangular, *Continuous Univariate Distributions,* Volume 1. New York: Houghton Mifflin, 1970, p. 55.

BRAUCHT, G.N., and BERRY, K.L. Deviant drug use in adolescence: a review of psycho social correlates, *Psychol. Bull.* 79(2): 92–106, 1973.

FEINSTEIN, A.R. *Clinical Judgment.* Baltimore: William and Wilkins, 1967, pp. 247–263.

GORODETZKY, C.W., Marijuana, LSD, and amphetamines. *Drug Dependence* 5: 18–23, 1970.

HOYT, J.P. A simple approximation to the standard normal probability density function, *Amer. Statistician* 22(2): 25–26, 1968.

KENDALL, M.G., and STUART, A. *The Advanced Theory of Statistics,* Volume 1. New York: Hafner, 1958, pp. 257–259.

LU, K.H. A measure of agreement among subjective judgments. *Educ. Psychol. Measurement,* 31 (1): 75–84, 1971.

ROBBINS, L., ROBBINS, E.S., and STERN, M. Psychological and environmental factors associated with drug abuse. *Drug Dependence* 5: 1–6, 1971.

SADAVA, S.W. Stage of college student drug use. A methodological contribution to cross-section study. *J. Consult. Clin. Psychol.* 38(2): 298, 1972.

ZILI, A., et al. The use of the narcotic register for follow-up of a cohort of adolescent addicts. *Intern. J. Addictions* 6(2): 225–239, 1971.

APPENDIX I

Female Users

	*D_1	D_2	D_3	D_4	D_5
F–1	1	3	2	2	1
F–2	4	1	1	1	1
F–3	3	1	1	2	2
F–4	4	2	2	3	2
F–5	5	3	1	3	1
F–6	2	1	2	1	1
F–7	2	2	1	1	2
F–8	1	2	2	3	2
F–9	3	2	4	2	1
F–10	4	1	1	3	2
F–11	1	2	2	2	2
F–12	3	4	1	4	1
F–13	2	5	2	1	1
F–14	2	2	2	2	2
F–15	3	2	2	1	1
F–16	2	1	1	3	2
F–17	4	2	2	3	2
F–18	5	3	1	2	2
F–19	3	1	1	3	1
F–20	4	2	2	1	1
F–21	3	1	2	3	2
F–22	4	3	2	2	2
F–23	5	1	3	2	2
F–24	3	2	3	5	2
F–25	4	2	2	3	2
F–26	5	3	1	1	5
F–27	4	1	2	3	2
F–28	2	1	2	1	3
F–29	4	2	3	3	2
F–30	1	2	1	1	4
F–31	3	4	2	3	2
F–32	4	2	1	1	3
F–33	5	1	2	3	2
F–34	5	1	1	3	1
F–35	5	2	2	3	1

*D_1 = marijuana
D_2 = LSD
D_3 = amphetamines
D_4 = barbiturates
D_5 = narcotics

APPENDIX I (Cont.)

Male Users

	D_1	D_2	D_3	D_4	D_5
M–1	4	2	1	2	2
M–2	4	4	2	4	2
M–3	2	4	2	1	5
M–4	4	2	2	5	1
M–5	5	2	2	3	1
M–6	4	2	2	1	5
M–7	5	2	2	1	3
M–8	5	2	1	3	2
M–9	4	5	4	5	3
M–10	4	4	3	3	2
M–11	3	3	5	1	2
M–12	5	2	1	2	1
M–13	4	3	1	2	1
M–14	5	4	3	1	1
M–15	5	5	2	3	2
M–16	4	5	2	4	2
M–17	2	3	4	1	1
M–18	4	3	2	1	1
M–19	3	5	2	1	1
M–20	4	3	3	1	4
M–21	5	3	1	2	1
M–22	5	4	1	4	2
M–23	4	2	2	3	2
M–24	2	3	1	4	2
M–25	5	3	1	5	2
M–26	4	3	2	5	1
M–27	4	1	3	5	1
M–28	4	2	2	1	2
M–29	4	3	1	4	1
M–30	3	3	4	3	1
M–31	3	2	2	3	2
M–32	3	3	2	1	2
M–33	4	1	2	1	2
M–34	5	2	1	3	2
M–35	4	3	3	3	2
M–36	5	2	2	1	2
M–37	5	2	2	5	2
M–38	2	2	2	1	3

APPENDIX II

Female Users

	*D_1	D_2	D_3	D_4	D_5	Index
F–1	.0274	.7123	.5685	.4110	.1712	.37808
F–2	.5548	.0959	.1575	.1644	.1712	.22876
F–3	.2808	.0959	.1575	.4110	.6027	.30958
F–4	.5548	.3904	.5685	.6575	.6027	.55478
F–5	.8699	.7123	.1575	.6575	.1712	.51368
F–6	.1233	.0959	.5685	.1644	.1712	.22466
F–7	.1233	.3904	.1575	.1644	.6027	.28766
F–8	.0274	.3904	.5685	.6575	.6027	.44930
F–9	.2808	.3904	.9589	.4110	.1712	.44246
F–10	.5548	.0959	.1575	.6575	.6027	.41368
F–11	.0274	.3904	.5685	.4110	.6027	.40000
F–12	.2808	.8836	.1575	.8630	.1712	.47122
F–13	.1233	.9658	.5685	.1644	.1712	.39864
F–14	.1233	.3904	.5685	.4110	.6027	.41918
F–15	.2808	.3904	.5685	.1644	.1712	.31506
F–16	.1233	.0959	.1575	.6575	.6027	.32738
F–17	.5548	.3904	.5685	.6575	.6027	.55478
F–18	.8699	.7123	.1575	.4110	.6027	.55068
F–19	.2808	.0959	.1575	.6575	.1712	.27258
F–20	.5548	.3904	.5685	.1644	.1712	.36986
F–21	.2808	.0959	.5685	.6575	.6027	.44108
F–22	.5548	.7123	.5685	.4110	.6027	.56986
F–23	.8699	.0959	.8767	.4110	.6027	.57124
F–24	.2808	.3904	.8767	.9521	.6027	.62054
F–25	.5548	.3904	.5685	.6575	.6027	.55478
F–26	.8699	.7123	.1575	.1644	.9795	.57672
F–27	.5548	.0959	.5685	.6575	.6027	.49588
F–28	.1233	.0959	.5685	.1644	.8973	.36988
F–29	.5548	.3904	.8767	.6575	.6027	.61642
F–30	.0274	.3904	.1575	.1644	.7452	.29698
F–31	.2808	.8836	.5685	.6575	.6027	.59862
F–32	.5548	.3904	.1575	.1644	.8973	.43288
F–33	.8699	.0959	.5685	.6575	.6027	.55890
F–34	.8699	.0959	.1575	.6575	.1712	.39040
F–35	.8699	.3904	.5685	.6575	.1712	.53150

*D_1 = marijuana
D_2 = LSD
D_3 = amphetamines
D_4 = barbiturates
D_5 = narcotics

APPENDIX II (Cont.)

Male Users

	D_1	D_2	D_3	D_4	D_5	Index
M–1	.5548	.3904	.1575	.4110	.6027	.42328
M–2	.5548	.8836	.5685	.8630	.6027	.69452
M–3	.1233	.8836	.5685	.1644	.9795	.54386
M–4	.5548	.3904	.5685	.9521	.1712	.52740
M–5	.8699	.3904	.5685	.6575	.1712	.53150
M–6	.5548	.3904	.5685	.1644	.9795	.53152
M–7	.8699	.3904	.5685	.1644	.8973	.57810
M–8	.8699	.3904	.1575	.6575	.6027	.53560
M–9	.5548	.9658	.9589	.9521	.8973	.86578
M–10	.5548	.8836	.8767	.6575	.6027	.71506
M–11	.2808	.7123	.9932	.1644	.6027	.55068
M–12	.8699	.3904	.1575	.4110	.1712	.40000
M–13	.5548	.7123	.1575	.4110	.1712	.40136
M–14	.8699	.8836	.8767	.1644	.1712	.59316
M–15	.8699	.9658	.5685	.6575	.6027	.73288
M–16	.5548	.9658	.5685	.8630	.6027	.71096
M–17	.1233	.7123	.9589	.1644	.1712	.42602
M–18	.5548	.7123	.5685	.1644	.1712	.43424
M–19	.2808	.9658	.5685	.1644	.1712	.43014
M–20	.5548	.7123	.8767	.1644	.7452	.61068
M–21	.8699	.7123	.1575	.4110	.1712	.46438
M–22	.8699	.8836	.1575	.8630	.6027	.67534
M–23	.5548	.3904	.5685	.6575	.6027	.55478
M–24	.1233	.7123	.1575	.8630	.6027	.49176
M–25	.8699	.7123	.1575	.9521	.6027	.65890
M–26	.5548	.7123	.5685	.9521	.1712	.59178
M–27	.5548	.0959	.8767	.9521	.1712	.53014
M–28	.5548	.3904	.5685	.1644	.6027	.45616
M–29	.5548	.7123	.1575	.8630	.1712	.49176
M–30	.2808	.7123	.9589	.6575	.1712	.55614
M–31	.2808	.3904	.5685	.6575	.6027	.49998
M–32	.2808	.7123	.5685	.1644	.6027	.46574
M–33	.5548	.0959	.5685	.1644	.6027	.39726
M–34	.8699	.3904	.1575	.6575	.6027	.53560
M–35	.5548	.7123	.8767	.6575	.6027	.68080
M–36	.8699	.3904	.5685	.1644	.6027	.51918
M–37	.8699	.3904	.5685	.9521	.6027	.67672
M–38	.1233	.3904	.5685	.1644	.8973	.42878

The International Journal of the Addictions, 9(6), pp. 805–826, 1974

A Follow-up Study of Former Residents of a Therapeutic Community

Walter V. Collier, M.A.

Yasser A. Hijazi, M.A.

Research Division
Daytop Village, Inc.
New York, New York

INTRODUCTION

In a recent review article, Vaillant (1970) discusses at great length the point that the long-term approach to doing follow-ups on individuals once in treatment for drug dependency is far superior to that of the short-term approach. In defining these two approaches, the long-term one would, for example, involve an elapse of 5 or more years before attempting follow-up; and with the sort-term approach, the time lapse would be anywhere from less than 1 to about 2 years. Vaillant bases his argument on some of his own research (1966a, 1966b, 1966c) as well as on that of O'Donnell (1969), and concludes that final remission of drug dependency probably occurs only after a long elapse of time during which the individual goes through a relatively drawn out process of trial and error in re-adjusting to a drug-free existence. Given this, Vaillant is, therefore, of the opinion that short-term follow-up studies are inappropriate—for short periods following treatment involvement are not sufficiently adequate to be able to discern if or to what extent prior treatment of the individual has been ultimately successful.

The present authors are in agreement with Vaillant's argument. However, there are some practical realities involved in outcome evaluation of drug rehabilitation programs which Vaillant apparently does not consider. Within recent years, pressure has been put on the rehabilitation programs—particularly those financed through public funding—to show how many drug abusers in and/or following treatment have ceased to use drugs and commit illegal acts. Such pressure has not only emanated from governmental agencies in assessing the cost/benefit status of the programs, but also from other civic quarters which are concerned with how and for what tax monies are being spent. This situation has led drug treatment programs to produce outcome data and statistics within relatively short periods of time. Consequently, most of the programs are forced to do short-term follow-up evaluation studies or else run the risk of violating contractual requirements of their funding agencies and possibly jeopardizing continued financial support. One solution to this problem could be to educate funding administrators and the public as to the need for extended time periods to adequately evaluate treatment outcome. Unfortunately, such an idea would probably fall on ears that are selectively deaf to anything that does not, at least, give the appearance of quick and easy answers to the drug problem.

There does, of course, remain a middle-ground alternative. That is, a longitudinal type follow-up approach wherein follow-up data are obtained and reported periodically over an extended time span. Utilizing this approach would not only satisfy public informational demands, but also would be in accord with adequate evaluation methodology: any early follow-up feedback reported would be explicitly qualified on the basis that the data reflect posttreatment activities of an individual at a given point in time, and should not be taken as conclusive until further feedback can be obtained. The present paper gives an interim report of results obtained from a longitudinal follow-up on former residents of Daytop Village from April 1971 to December 1972. The study specifically focused on terminees from Daytop's drug-free residential therapeutic community. (Included in the 1972 Annual Report of Daytop is a follow-up report on former participants within the program's drug-free ambulatory modality.)

Finally, it has been the experience of the present authors that follow-up studies usually proceed on the sole basis of determining posttreatment behavior of drug abusers, with little or no concern given to assessing how these individuals perceive the program they were once in. Information bearing on such subjects could be of value for any therapeutic program in evaluating its operations. As part of the present study, an attempt was therefore made to obtain feedback data from the resident sample as to their personal assessments of the way Daytop is run and the problems they encountered while in the program.

METHODOLOGY

Sample and Time Criteria

The present sample of terminees from the residential program consisted of individuals who had completed the full treatment cycle, i.e., 20 months, and those who left treatment prior to completion. Both sample groups were drawn from larger populations in terms of the following criteria. Individuals in the first group (graduates) were selected for their initial follow-up interview on the basis of having been out of the program for a minimum of 6 months. Individuals in the second group (dropouts) were selected on the basis of having been in the program for at least 6 months and out of the program for the same amount of time. In view of the full length of the treatment cycle, the criterion of 6 months in treatment was considered to be a reasonable minimum base from which effects of treatment could be safely judged for the dropouts. Following the initial follow-up, each individual in the present sample was scheduled for a subsequent 18-, 30-, and 48-month follow-up. Moreover, since the study was designed as an ongoing part of Daytop's basic evaluation activities, the sample size would, of course, increase over time.

Initial follow-ups were scheduled for *272* graduates who had entered the the program in 1969 or before, and *280* resident dropouts who had entered during the same period. All individuals (graduates and dropouts) had left the program by June 1972. Specific data pertaining to the overall termination populations of Daytop, along with time spent in treatment, are given in the results section of the report.

Procedure

An initial contact letter was sent to all individuals, explaining the nature of the study and requesting that they contact a specific office within Daytop's administrative headquarters to set up an interview appointment. Each individual was given the assurance that his interview would remain in the strictest of confidence, and would not be revealed under his name to any staff member or resident of Daytop or to outside agencies without his expressed permission.

Six interviewers were assigned to the study, three of whom were former addicts employed in paraprofessional positions within Daytop and an outside program; the remaining three interviewers were professional staff members of Daytop's research division. All six were experienced in doing field investigation work and were given orientation training as to protocols. Wherever possible, the interviewee and interviewer were matched in terms of sex, ethnicity, and age as a means of facilitating rapport and degree of conversational openness.

The interviews were conducted either at the home of the resident or his place of employment, depending on which was more convenient. No limit was imposed on how long the interviews would last. The information obtained during the sessions was guided by an interview schedule. The schedule was an eight-page questionnaire which focused on several areas of readjustment to the outside community and post-Daytop involvement with drugs, alcohol, and criminal activities. Specific items included in the schedule were:

1. What kinds of problems (if any) have you had in readjusting to the outside since leaving Daytop?
2. Has your social life changed from what it was prior to entering Daytop?
3. Current employment: place and type of work, salary, and length of employment.
4. If unemployed, source of financial support.
5. Current and planned involvement in school: school, program, and length of involvement.
6. Current marital status.
7. Current household (with whom do you live?).
8. Post-Daytop drug usage: types of drugs, how long since leaving Daytop, frequency and recency of drug use, and in what context, i.e., alone or with others.
9. Alcohol usage: frequency and context.
10. Post-Daytop arrests: nature of charge, convictions, and length of incarceration.
11. Current legal status, i.e., probation, parole.
12. Reinvolvement in drug treatment or psychiatric program since leaving Daytop.

13. Main reasons for dropouts leaving Daytop.
14. In what ways was Daytop helpful and not helpful to you.
15. During stay in Daytop, did you feel there were serious sexual and racial problems among residents?
16. What are your opinions about the following:
    (a) "The atmosphere in Daytop is too strict and rigid."
    (b) "More individual therapy should be included in the program."
    (c) "The amount of time involved in completing the program is too long."
17. What services do you feel should be added to the program?

Those questionnaire items which were subject to change analysis on a pre- and post-Daytop basis were compared with resident record information, e.g., drug usage, marital status, criminal offenses.

The usual sources for directly obtaining information to corroborate the response data received from the residents, e.g., police and hospital records, proved unusable. Instead, what is called the "grapevine" among using addicts and their nonusing associates was employed. The grapevine is an informal communication network existing within the so-called drug subculture through which information flows on the whereabouts and activities of addicts and former addicts. Much like the communication network of the criminal underground, which is effectively employed in police and intelligence work, the addict grapevine showed a high degree of informational reliability. Further discussion on this point is presented below under Methodological Issue.

Follow-Up Evaluation Criteria

The major items used in evaluating the out-of-program status of the sample included: (1) current drug use; (2) alcohol use; (3) involvement in illegal activities, i.e., arrests; and (4) prosocial involvement, e.g., employment or school.

General Analysis of Data

Analysis of the data preceded along the lines of determining (1) the proportion of terminees who were found leading productive vs nonproductive lives, post-Daytop; (2) a profile description of these individuals in terms of background (e.g., sex, age, ethnicity, time in and out of the program). Specific analytic work included the use of percentage distributions and the chi-square (χ^2) technique for comparison tests.

A Methodological Issue

It was originally planned that information corroborating the interview response data would be sought from central social and legal information banks, such as the New York City Narcotics Register. However, the investigators were subsequently confronted with a reality that only "authorized" agencies could gain access to police and hospital records on former residents of Daytop. Several attempts were made to secure such information indirectly (i.e., in anonymous aggregrate data forms) from local governmental narcotics service agencies, but to no avail.

The general issue of confidentiality of information regarding service or correctional involvement of addicts and the nonreciprocity in information exchange between agencies has become increasingly problematic within the last few years. While it is recognized that individual agencies do have a civil obligation to protect file information on their clients from potential misuse, some type of legal arrangement should be, nevertheless, reached among agencies so that legitimately needed client information can be exchanged without risk of transgression of confidentiality. If not, this issue of "classified information" will continue to frustrate research efforts in documenting the effectiveness of addict treatment programs, as well as to foster noncooperation and noncoordination among the various agencies that deal with addicts or addict-related information.

As an alternative to use of central information sources, the "communication grapevine" method was utilized in obtaining corroborative follow-up data. This approach involved using information obtained from abusers, former abusers (not included in this study), and nonabusers. Information which was fed to the research unit of Daytop narrowed down the possibilities of the whereabouts and activities of the former residents. Once obtained, the information was then followed through on by direct contact made with specific penal institutions or hospitals, whenever possible, to validate the data originating from the street network.

The grapevine network has thus far been able to generate certain information that would otherwise remain unknown through using agency sources alone. For instance, data on whether a person was using drugs but had not been rearrested or rehospitalized could be obtained from the street sources, whereas agencies like the Narcotics Register are forced to depend on police and hospital records for tracking information, and consequently data pertaining to such an individual could not be picked up by an agency system. While some may argue that street networks may not be "scientifically valid" in the traditional sense and that information derived from such sources should be dismissed as mere hearsay, the utilization of such information sources is probably better in situations where nothing else exists—and given nothing else, they certainly can serve as "leads" to other sources.

The Program

The treatment modality in which the sample had been involved was Daytop's drug-free residential therapeutic community. Since the program has been exhaustively described elsewhere (Calof, 1967; Collier, 1970; Casriel, 1971), it is not profiled here.

RESULTS

The overall resident termination statisfics are given in Table 1.

Resident Terminees Satisfying Initial Follow-Up Time Criteria

Of the total number of graduates as of the June 1972 cut-off date, 85% ($N = 272$) met the time-out-of-program criterion for initial follow-up. Of the total number of drop-outs, 45% ($N = 327$) satisfied the time-in-and-out-of-program cirteria. Table 2 gives the statistics on rate of follow-up contacts actually made.

Table 1

Overall Resident Termination Statistics

	No.	%
Entries to program (1971 and prior)	1,367[a]	100.0
Net dropouts from entries (as of June 1972)	729	63.3
Graduates (as of June 1972)	318	23.3
Resident deaths	3	0.2
Medical, legal discharges	28	2.0
Resident entries remaining in program as of June 1972	289	21.2

[a] This figure represents only the total number of actual resident entries. The total for number of preadmission interviews could not be verified by the investigators, particularly for the period prior to 1971.

Table 2
Number of Resident Terminations Who Met Time In-and-Out-of-Program Critieria For Follow-up as of December 31, 1972

Groups	Total number of persons scheduled for follow-up	Total number of interviews completed by December 31, 1972	Contact letters returned: Address unknown or no response to letter as of December 31, 1972
Graduates	272 (100%)	173[a] (64%)	99 (36%)
Dropouts	280 (100%)	78 (39%)	202 (61%)
Totals	552 (100%)	251 (46%)	301 (54%)

[a] Included in this figure are 47 long-term graduates who have been out of Daytop for 5 years or more. A special follow-up investigation on these 47 will be published separately. From this point on, these individuals are excluded from the present sample.

As indicated in Table 2, the dropout group proved to be more difficult in finding than graduates from the program. Several attempts at contacting the dropouts were made, but as of the closing date of this report, these attempts have been unsuccessful. As for the nonrespondent graduates, while they had yet to contact the program, their whereabouts were at least ascertained.

Although one could generally assume current drug reusage or criminal recidivism as reasons for one-third of the graduate sample not responding to follow-up contacts, the investigators were of the opinion that some of these individuals probably refused follow-up interviews because of possible negative feelings they held toward certain program staff or because of a perceived threat to the privacy of their lives (e.g., fear that employer might become aware of former addiction involvement).

Sample Profile

Below are profile descriptions of the initial (respondent and nonrespondent) graduate and dropout groups. The social background descriptors analyzed were selected on the basis of a resident profile study in which determination was made as to what background variables were associated with stay vs nonstay in treatment (Collier, 1973).

Graduates ($N = 225$)

The median age of graduates (upon entry to Daytop) was 22.3; 84% were males; 12.3% were Black, 12.8% were Puerto Rican, and 74.9% were White; and two-thirds were from middle economic class background, with the remainder from the lower classes. The average length of prior drug use for this group was 6 years, with a majority (88%) having used heroin as a main drug. Finally, the average amount of time the graduate group spent in Daytop was 22 months, and the average time spent outside before initial followup was 11.8 months.

Dropouts ($N = 280$)

The median age for dropouts was 22.1; 81% were males; 25.3% were Black, 12.2% were Puerto Rican, and 62.5% were White; and half were from middle class backgrounds, with the remainder from the lower classes. The average length of drug use for the dropouts was 5 years, with a majority (91%) having used heroin as a primary drug. Lastly, the average time the dropout group stayed in Daytop was 13 months, and the average time out prior to follow-up was 11.6 months.

Respondents Versus Nonrespondents

On the basis of the above and other background variables, comparisons were made between those individuals who received a follow-up interview and those who did not (see Table 3). The results were that age was the only variable which significantly differentiated between the two groups. Within

Table 3
Profile of Follow-up Respondents

	Graduates ($N = 126$)	Dropouts ($N = 78$)
Average age	21.3 years	20.0 years
Male	83%	78%
Female	17%	22%
Black	10%	22%
Puerto Rican	11%	6%
White	79%	72%
Catholic	68%	69%
Protestant	10%	16%
Jewish	16%	9%
Other	6%	6%
Upper middle class	13%	16%
Middle class	46%	36%
Lower class	41%	48%
Primary drug used	Heroin	Heroin
Average length of drug use	6 years	5 years

the graduate sample, those who responded to follow-up contact tended to be older (25 and above) than those who did not respond ($\chi^2 = 12.0$, $p < .01$). A reversed trend was found among the dropouts: respondents tended to be younger (under 25) than the nonrespondent dropouts ($\chi^2 = 11.2$, $p < .01$). The significance of this age differential between respondents and nonrespondents was not exactly clear to the investigators. However, the investigators did attempt to discern possible sample self-selection biases, i.e., whether there were any unique characteristics or motivations shared by those residents who responded to a follow-up interview and those who did not. Such artifacts would, of course, have implications for how the interview data should be interpreted. At first we thought we had come across something when during the first batch of interviews we found that some of the dropouts indicated their willingness to be interviewed was related to their wanting to obtain "good standing" or a job with the program. Subsequently, however, this ulterior motive did not bear out with most of the remaining dropouts nor with any of the graduates. Without totally dismissing the possibilities of other sample biases, the investigators were led to assume the nonexistence of such biases that would greatly alter the present findings—at least until further research could be done on this issue.

FOLLOW-UP FINDINGS

Reliability of Interview Response Data

In all cases where a subject received a follow-up interview, the following major response items were either corroborated or disconfirmed by information obtained from street sources and/or social/legal agencies: (1) current drug usage, (2) arrests, and (3) current employment or school involvement. While these results were impressive, the investigators, nevertheless, felt that cross-checking of the interview data on an ongoing basis would be required as a means of testing any fluctuations in reliability. As such, any feedback obtained subsequent to this report that points to respondent untruthfulness within the present and later samples will be reported in future Daytop reports on follow-ups.

Interview Responses

Item 1. Problems in Readjustment to Community. Of the total graduate sample ($N = 126$), 21% indicated that they had not experienced any major problems in readjusting to the outside community. Of the dropout sample ($N = 78$), 8% said they had not experienced any problems.

Among those graduates who experienced adjustment difficulties, the specific problem areas were ranked as follows from the most problematic to the least: (1) socializing and being able to deal with outside social realities (e.g., social/racial prejudices, interpersonal game-playing, dishonesty) which were felt to be in conflict with the teachings of the program; (2) not being able to make enough money from current employment; (3) readjusting to family setting; and (4) being able to relate intimately to opposite sex in a mutually satisfying way. Profile-wise, young (under 25) males experienced these four problems more so than any other profile group. Also, those who remained the longest in treatment (22 + months) showed greater readjustment problems.

Among the dropouts who experienced adjustment difficulties, the specific problem areas were ranked identically to those of the graduates. The profile of the dropouts who experienced these problems was also the same as for graduates, with the one exception that Blacks and Puerto Ricans seemed to have a slightly higher rate of adjustment problems than White dropouts.

Item 2. Changes in Social Life. Three percent of the graduates reported that they had made no real changes in their social life at present as compared with the time prior to entering Daytop. Nine percent of the dropouts said they had made no changes.

Both graduates and dropouts who had made changes in their social life gave the following specific changes which are ranked in order: (1) socialize more with nondrug users; (2) socialize more with opposite sex; and (3) socialize both with drug and nondrug users. In analyzing these data on the basis of profiles, nothing significant became evident.

Item 3. Current Employment Status. Eighty-eight percent of the graduates were employed, with 4% unemployed but who were full-time students (Table 4). Seventy-seven percent of the dropouts were employed, with 11.5% as full-time students (Table 5). Of those graduates who were unemployed and not full-time students, two were receiving unemployment insurance, one was on welfare, and nine were being supported by their families. Among the dropouts, three were receiving unemployment insurance, one was on welfare, and five were receiving family support.

In comparing the sample's pre- and post-Daytop employment status, the employed graduates ($N = 114$) had increased their average annual

Table 4

Pre- and Post-Daytop Employment Level for Graduates

Pre-Daytop employment levels (annual income)	Original N	Post-daytop changes in income				
		Upward	Downward	No change	Student[a]	Not working
$7,500–15,000	45	3	20	14	2	6
Less than $6,000–7,000	70	50	—	14	3	3
Unemployed	11	11	—	—	—	—
Totals	126	64	20	28	5	9

[a] Full-time student.

Table 5

Pre- and Post-Daytop Employment Level for Dropouts

Pre-Daytop employment levels (annual income)	Original N	Post-daytop changes in income				
		Upward	Downward	No change	Student	Not working
$7,500–15,000	28	2	11	9	3	3
Less than $6,000–7,000	40	22	1	7	4	6
Unemployed	10	8	—	—	2	—
Totals	78	32	12	16	9	9

earnings by approximately $2,500. A little less than half of these individuals ($N = 50$) were working as staff within drug rehabilitation and prevention programs. The remaining employed graduates were working in various other fields. Employed dropouts ($N = 60$) showed a similar upward trend in income, but their average salary increase was about $1,000 less than that for the graduates. Almost three-quarters of the dropout group were working in areas other than the drug field. And of those remaining ($N = 17$) dropouts, all were employed in drug rehbilitation programs—representing 28% of the dropouts as compared with almost 50% of the graduates who were employed within the drug field.

Item 4. Current Educational Involvement. Almost one-third of the graduates (31%) were involved in a school program: 32 were in a liberal arts college and eight in a technical school. Among dropouts, 31% were also involved in a school program. Unlike graduates, however, most of the dropouts (14) were enrolled in a technical vocational program, and the remainder (11) in a college program.

Item 5. Changes in Marital Status. Of the graduates who were single prior to entering the program ($N = 95$), 42% had gotten married after leaving Daytop; and of those who were initially married ($N = 14$), 50% had either become separated or divorced. Such striking changes in marital status were not observed among the dropout sample.

One interesting observation made with respect to residents who married after treatment was that a very small minority ($N = 2$) of the graduates had married other graduate residents. No within-dropout marriages had occurred. The significance of this is that a kind of "inbreeding" is assumed to exist among participants of a therapeutic community. While the present data are numerically insufficient to support or reject this assumption, preliminary information on Daytop's total graduate sample does suggest that about 5% of the graduates married among themselves and that this percentage predominantly includes females. Why female graduates tend to marry other graduates more than male graduates was unknown to the investigators, but was planned for future research.

Item 6. Changes in Household. Thirty percent of the graduates had initially lived alone, and since Daytop, only 5% lived alone. Fifty-seven percent had initially lived with their parents, and after leaving Daytop, 12% remained with their parents. In contrast to this, 72% of the dropouts had initially lived with their parents; and since leaving Daytop, 42% remained with their parents. Eleven percent of the dropouts lived alone pre-Daytop, and 5% remained alone after the program.

Item 7. Post-Daytop Drug Use. Ninety-four percent of the graduates have remained drug-free since leaving the program. Those who returned to using drugs ($N = 7$) used marijuana primarily on a weekly or less periodic basis. In contrast to the graduates, 53% of the dropouts remained drug free. Of the 38 who returned to drugs, most used a variety of drugs, including methadone. Thirteen used drugs daily, 10 weekly, and the remaining 15 less than weekly.

In analyzing the duration of drug use for both reusing graduates and dropouts, most started using drugs during the first 6 months of being out of Daytop.

Item 8. Alcohol Use. While a majority of both graduates and dropouts used alcohol, none used it in excess.

Item 9. Criminal Involvement. Both graduates and dropouts exhibited a marked decline in legal violations. Before entering Daytop, 67% of the graduates had been arrested for criminal activities involving, e.g., assault and theft; and after leaving the program, only 7% were rearrested. The charges involved for these recidivists were all of a minor nature, with no convictions received. Among the dropouts, 72% had been arrested before entering Daytop, and after leaving, only 15% were rearrested. Unlike the graduates, however, most of these recidivists were convicted for major violations of drug selling and theft.

Item 10. Reinvolvement in Treatment. Nine percent of the graduates had become reinvolved in a treatment program. Of these, five had reentered a drug-free residential program and six had become involved in individual psychotherapy. Four of the graduates were still involved in treatment, and the remaining seven had remained for an average of about 6 months. Thirty-three percent of the dropouts had returned to some form of treatment: 11 entered a methadone maintenance program, 10 entered a drug-free residential program, four entered a drug-free day-care setting, and one entered individual psychotherapy. Eight of the dropouts were still involved in treatment, and the other 18 had remained for an average of 6 months.

In asking whether an individual felt he needed further rehabilitation service at this point, 12% of the graduates currently uninvolved in a program indicated *yes*. Most indicated that what they specifically needed was individual psychotherapy. As for the dropouts, 18% of those uninvolved in a program said they needed additional treatment, viz., individual psychotherapy.

Item 11. Main Reason for Dropouts Leaving Daytop. In ranked order, the following reasons were given by dropouts for leaving the program:

1. Felt staff treatment was unjust by playing favoritism with some residents and ignoring individual needs of others.
2. Pressures of the therapeutic process of the therapeutic community became too great, i.e., staff demands placed on residents.
3. Felt that therapy was no longer needed.
4. Had sexual difficulties, i.e., were either homosexual or felt restrictions on heterosexual relationships while in-residence were unjust.
5. Used drugs while socializing outside of the therapeutic community.
6. Older dropouts felt an age-identification problem in a setting of younger residents.

SUMMARY ANALYSIS AND OVERALL FOLLOW-UP STATUS

Based on the foregone data, it appeared that the Daytop program had a distinct influence in altering the life styles of most of the sample's graduates and residents who did not stay to complete treatment. A majority of the sample were no longer abusing drugs or committing crimes, and were regularly employed and/or in school. In terms of more personal areas, the sample showed a significant change in their interpersonal lives: many of them who had been loners or marginal socializers had either become married or socialized with others more than before. Those who had been married during their previous drug-use had decided to separate themselves from what was apparently a negative marital situation.

More specifically, on the basis of the four major evaluation criteria, 84% of the graduates were no longer using drugs or abusing alcohol, were not arrested for criminal violations, and were employed and/or involved in furthering their formal education (Table 6).

Whether all of the remaining 16% ($N = 20$) should realistically be evaluated unfavorably is quite frankly debatable, and would actually depend on one's personal perspective. For instance, those graduates who used drugs after leaving Daytop primarily used marijuana on an infrequent basis. Taking into account other factors, some of these individuals were unemployed at the time of interview but none had been arrested for serious criminal offenses. If nothing else, the post-Daytop behavior of these individuals was at least seen as an improvement over their initial behavioral patterns. In any event, the present investigators have attempted to refrain

Table 6
Follow-up Status of Graduates[a]

	Number	%
Infrequent drug use	2	2
Not employed or in school and infrequent drug use	4	3
Not employed or in school	6	5
Arrested	7	6
Arrested and infrequent drug use	1	1
Employed/school, not arrested, and no drug use	106	84
Total	126	100

[a] Alcohol-use is excluded on the basis that none of the graduates abused alcohol.

from what might be taken as a personal bias; instead, presented below for the reader's own consideration and evaluation are specific follow-up status data on the graduate sample.

In terms of background profiles, those graduates evaluated most favorably upon initial follow-up tended to be mainly older (25–30) and of both sexes (although females slightly outnumbered males proportionately). While Whites numerically outnumbered both Black and Puerto Rican graduates, percentage-wise, ethnicity did not prove to have any significant relationship to which ethnic group was evaluated more favorably. The long-term drug abusers (6+ years) of heroin, barbituates, and amphetamines were evaluated more favorably upon follow-up than any other drug-using group. Finally, the amount of time spent in and out of Daytop as of this initial follow-up had no significance.

Forty-six percent of the dropout sample were no longer using drugs or abusing alcohol, were not arrested for illegal actions, and were employed and/or involved in school (Table 7). Although there was, again, some equivocalness in evaluating the remaining dropouts, the degree of uncertainty was less than that of the graduate situation. Of the remaing dropouts ($N = 42$), 15 of them were clearly recidivists to frequent drug abuse, serious criminal involvement, and unemployment; the other 27 were evaluated only as using marijuana on an infrequent basis.

Those drop-outs who were evaluated most favorably upon follow-up were characteristically similar to their graduate counterparts: age 25–30, of both sexes, and long-term users of heroin, barbituates, and marijuana. Again, ethnicity played no significant part. As for time spent in Daytop, those who stayed in treatment from 12 to 18 months showed a favorable

Table 7
Follow-up Status of Dropouts[a]

	Number	%
Infrequent drug use	23	29
Not employed or in school and frequent drug use	5	6
Not employed or in school	2	3
Arrested	2	3
Arrested and frequent drug use	8	10
Arrested, unemployed, and frequent drug use	2	3
Employed/school, not arrested, and no drug use	36	46
Total	78	100

[a] Alcohol-use is excluded on basis that none of the dropouts abused alcohol.

follow-up. Nothing significant was generated from the data on time spent out of treatment upon initial follow-up.

Results of Resident Feedback

During the follow-up interviews, the former residents were asked several questions as to what they thought about the Daytop program. The responses, ranked in order from the most frequent to the least are given below. *Question 1. In What Ways Did Daytop Help You?*

Graduate Response:

1. Instilling a new set of values and life style.
2. In getting off drugs.
3. Building self-confidence.
4. Furthering self-knowledge.
5. Solving sexual problems.

Dropout Response:

1. Furthering self-knowledge.
2. Instilling a new set of values and life style.
3. Building self-confidence.
4. In getting off drugs.
5. Solving sexual problems.

Question 2. In What Ways Did Daytop Not Help You?

Graduate Response:

1. None.
2. Insufficient preparation for outside readjustment (i.e., in coping with general outside stress).
3. No help in solving individual psychological problems.
4. Inadequate educational/vocational services.
5. Not enough individual attention from staff.

Dropout Response:

1. None.
2. No help in solving individual psychological problems.
3. Insufficient preparation for outside readjustment.
4. Not enough individual freedom within program.
5. Staff failure to deal with ethnic/cultural identity problems.

While most of both the graduates and dropouts felt they had been helped psychologically, many of them, nevertheless, felt that additional psychological help—on an individual basis—should have been provided. Moreover, most individuals among graduates and dropouts felt the program should have provided them with better coping behaviors in dealing with outside environmental stress, as was further evidenced by the responses to the earlier question, "What problems have you had in readjusting to the outside?"

Question 3. During Your Stay in the Program, Did You Feel There Were Any Major Problems Because Residents of Different Ages Were Mixed (in One Setting)?

Graduate and Dropout Response:

1. No.
2. Yes. Older residents had problems in relating and identifying with younger ones.
3. Yes. Younger residents had problems in relating and identifying with older ones.

Question 4. Did You Feel There Were Any Major Racial Conflicts Among Residents and Staff?

Graduate and Dropout Response:

1. No.
2. Yes. Between Black residents and White staff.
3. Yes. Between Puerto Rican and White residents.
4. Yes. Between Puerto Rican residents and White staff.
5. Yes. Between White residents and Black staff.
6. Yes. Between Black and White residents.

In looking at the foregoing response data in terms of ethnic breakdown of the sample, it turned out that Black, Puerto Rican, and White residents particularly concurred that racial conflict existed, mainly between the predominant White staff vs Black and Puerto Rican residents. Also, the longer the stay within the program, the more evident these racial conflicts became evident to the residents. It should be pointed out that, at the writing of this report, the ethnic composition of the program's staff and residents included more Blacks and Puerto Ricans. As to whether this shift has produced any changes in racial conflict is, however, uncertain at this point.

Question 5. What About Problems Relating to Males and Females Living Together Within the Same Center?

While most of the sample indicated no real problem in the coed situation, some did feel that both sexes living together in a setting which prohibited sexual intercourse among the residents did cause undue frustration and sexual deviance, e.g., casual homosexual encounters.

The next three items relate to resident opinions about some statements on the program.

Question 6. "The Atmosphere in Daytop Is too Strict and Rigid."

Response	Graduates, %	Dropouts, %
Strongly agree	8	22
Agree	35	42
Disagree	48	24
Strongly disagree	6	1
No opinion	3	11
Total	100	100

Question 7. "Individual Therapy Should Be as Available as Group Therapy."

Response	Graduates, %	Dropouts, %
Strongly agree	27	24
Agree	61	51
Disagree	9	13
Strongly disagree	1	—
No opinion	2	12
Total	100	100

Question 8. "The Amount of Time Involved in Completing the Program Is too Long."

Response	Graduates, %	Dropouts, %
Strongly agree	12	31
Agree	41	45
Disagree	38	15
Strongly disagree	3	1
No opinion	6	8
Total	100	100

Finally, in response to the question, "What services do you feel Daytop could provide that it does not provide now?", most of the sample of graduates and drop-outs indicated a need for more (1) vocational counseling and training, and (2) individual psychological help.

CONCLUDING COMMENTS

While the overall results of this follow-up study indicated significant behavioral improvement among graduates of the Daytop residential program and a fair degree of improvement among dropouts who remained in the program for at least a year, the findings should be viewed within the context of "early feedback." Those of us who may tend to perceive the preliminary as conclusive, should bear a reality in mind: individuals who have manifested behavioral problems for any extensive period of time should not be expected to extinguish those behaviors in a puff of smoke. Changing bad habits takes time, recognizing, of course, that some individuals may require less time than others. This point cannot be emphasized enough. For the public as well as people in the drug field, in their enthusiasm to be rid of the abuse problem, tend to set themselves up for disappointment when possibly prematured optimism over certain research findings becomes thwarted by subsequent reports of relapse rates among treated abusers. If the tone of all this sounds pessimistic, that is not our intent. Our posture is merely one of cautiousness in communicating the present findings on initial follow-ups.

In closing, some remarks on resident feedback on the Daytop program are in order. A majority of the sample followed-up on were in accord that that the program is not flexible enough in its use of the group approach. They felt that more attention should be paid to the psychological needs of the individual on an individual basis. In the opinion of the investigators, this point probably has at least some validity. For all the economic and clinical benefits derived from using a group dynamic, there is always the risks involved of obliterating the individual. For those readers who may be unfamiliar with the Daytop process, individual therapy does go on within the program. The point being made here is, however, that perhaps the program ought to consider striking a more balanced situation involving both the individual and group treatment approaches.

The sample also expressed the opinion that the program's reentry process may be deficient in that not enough preparation is given to residents for their return to the outside community. While this subject entails a need for more vocational preparation, which is clearly needed and is presently being tackled by Daytop's staff, there is an even more crucial issue involved here. That is, how to better prepare residents to cope with the stresses of the outside world which are probably reexperienced by the residents as a kind of culture shock. Essentially, what takes place in the early treatment phases of the program is a stripping away of a resident's self-defeating and antisocial behaviors, which are then replaced by a more personally positive and socially acceptable life-style. The values that are imparted to the resident relate to honesty with self and others, and communal concern and responsibility as opposed to preoccupation with self. The later phases, reentry, serve as a testing ground, a point at which the resident must then learn to apply in his day-to-day living on the outside that which he has been taught within the therapeutic community. In so doing, however, the resident may find it difficult to behave in ways that are not practiced by the outside community. He may find it difficult to be honest about himself with others, for fear that his honesty may be turned against him. Or he may come to realize that his concern for others may go unrequited. What the resident needs at this point is some additional coping assistance in realizing that what he has learned in the therapeutic community must now be modified so he is able to deal with the world as it is without having to totally unlearn or greatly compromise his Daytop experience. A rather delicate situation, but one that must be worked through.

Within the last year or so the program staff of Daytop has been working toward improving the reentry process. Certain structural modifications have been effected in terms of earlier resident reexposure to the outside community, in actuality as well as through techniques such as environmental structuring wherein residents act out anticipated readjustment problems in a setting which simulates the outside social milieu. The outcome of such changes in the reentry process will, of course, have to await future evaluation.

SUMMARY

In an attempt to measure the outcome of the Daytop drug abuse program, a longitudinal follow-up study was initiated on former residents of the program. Interim findings indicated that most of the "graduates" and drop-outs who remained in treatment for about one year had remained drug-free and were pursuing productive life styles. In discussing some methodological problems encountered, it was pointed out that the issue of confidentiality of agency's files on former residents of Daytop led the investigators to use street sources in obtaining corroborative followup data.

Finally, in commenting on the overall findings of the resident re-adjustment problems, some issues surrounding the therapeutic community re-entry process were discussed.

ACKNOWLEDGMENTS

This Project was supported in part by a grant from NIMH, MH 21080–01 and by the new York City Addiction Services Agency.

REFERENCES

CALOF, J. *A Study of Four Voluntary Treatment and Rehabilitation Programs for New York City's Narcotic Addicts,* Part I. New York: Community Service Soc., 1967.

CASRIEL, D., and AMEN, G. *Daytop.* New York: Hill and Wang, 1971.

COLLIER, W. *An Evaluation Study on the Therapeutic Program of Daytop Village.* New York: Daytop Press, 1970.

COLLIER, W. A profile study on the residents of Daytop Village. *J. Drug Issues* 3(1): 10–21, 1973.

O'DONNELL, J. *Narcotic Addicts in Kentucky* (Public Health Service Publication #1881). Washington, D.C.: U.S. Government Printing Office, 1969.

VAILLANT, G. A 12-year follow-up of New York narcotic addicts: I. The relationship of treatment to outcome. *Amer. J. Psychiat.* 122: 727–737, 1966a.

VAILLANT, G. A 12-year follow-up of NewYork narcotic addicts: II. The natural history of a chronic disease. *New England J. Med.* 275: 1282–1288, 1966b.

VAILLANT, G. A 12-year follow-up of New York narcotic addicts: III. Some social and psychiatric characteristics. *Arch. Gen. Psychiat.* 15: 599–609, 1966c.

VAILLANT, G. The natural history of narcotic drug addiction. *Seminars Psychiat.* 2(4): 486–498, 1970.

The International Journal of the Addictions, 9(6), pp. 827–839, 1974

Family Characteristics Associated with Marijuana Use among Adolescents

Thomas J. Prendergast, Jr., M.D.

Community Health Sciences
University of Missouri—Columbia
Columbia, Missouri

In the broadest sense, human behaviors can be thought of as occurring in response to stresses. Furthermore, while almost any behavior may have health implication (Stewart, 1969), it is clear that certain behaviors in our society are critical influences of health. Suchman distinguished such obvious examples as alcohol use, cigarette smoking, the use of illicit drugs, and risk-taking behaviors (Suchman, 1970). The methodology and conceptual framework described in this study of marijuana use has been applied to alcohol use and cigarette smoking as well and is equally applicable to other forms of behavior of less critical health relevance.

The use of marijuana and other illicit drugs is an activity acquired during adolescence (Gossett, 1972; Surgeon General's Report, 1971). This applies equally well to other important health-related behaviors such as patterns of alcohol consumption and cigarette smoking (Gossett, 1972; Prendergast, 1973; Surgeon General's Report, 1964; Weitman, 1972).

A study was conducted to determine whether marijuana use by adolescents was related to certain characteristics of the adolescent's family. Three categories of mechanisms were considered as possible influences on the adolescent's behavior. The three categories were modeling, parental attitude toward marijuana use, and the general parent–child relationship.

In order to be able to assess the importance of factors already known to be associated with different patterns and frequency of drug use, selective demographic information on the age, sex, and race of respondents as well as parental educational achievement was collected. These variables have been previously discussed in relationship to drug use among young people (Blackford, 1969; Surgeon General's Report, 1971; Prendergast, 1973).

METHODS AND MATERIALS

Subjects and Statistical Analysis

A detailed description of the population sampled, reasons for nonparticipation, results for other variables, and statistical methods of analysis have been previously presented (Prendergast, 1973).

Survey Instrument

The survey questionnaire utilized included two principal parts. The first part ascertained each respondent's own experience with regard to marijuana use as well as the use of othet illicit drugs. Each repondent also gave information regarding his perception of the use by each of his parents of over-the-counter and prescription drugs (parents as models); and the attitude of each of his parents about possible or actual marijuana use by the respondent (parents as educators). These were analyzed as indices with values from 1 ("never" and "strongly approve," respectively) to 5 ("almost daily" and "strongly disapprove," respectively). Standard demographic variables including age, race, sex, grade, and maximum level of educational achievement of each of the parents were also obtained.

Part two of the questionnaire utilized consisted of a modified version of Schaefer's "Child's Report of Parent Behavior Index" (CR-PBI). This instrument and the modifications employed have been previously reported (Schaefer, 1971; Schludermann, 1970). The following scales of behavior index were included: (1) Rejection; (2) Control; (3) Enforcement; (4) Positive Involvement; (5) Control Through Guilt; (6) Inconsistent Discipline; (7) Nonenforcement; (8) Acceptance of Individuation; (9) Control Through Withdrawal of Relations; (10) Control Through Instilling Persistent Anxiety; (11) Hostile Detachment; and (12) Extreme Autonomy.

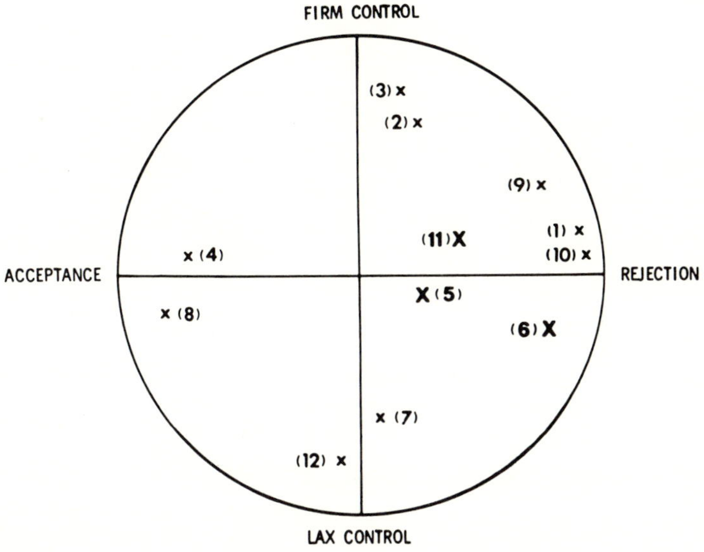

1. REJECTION (-.05)
2. CONTROL (+.22)
3. ENFORCEMENT (+.25)
4. POSITIVE INVOLVEMENT (-.09)
5. CONTROL THROUGH GUILT (+.02)
6. INCONSISTENT DISCIPLINE (-.17)
7. NONENFORCEMENT (-.25)
8. ACCEPTANCE OF INDIVIDUATION (-.12)
9. CONTROL THROUGH PERSISTENT ANXIETY (-.11)
10. CONTROL WITH HOSTILE DETACHMENT (-.08)
11. CONTROL THROUGH WITHDRAWAL OF RELATIONS (-.17)
12. EXTREME AUTONOMY (-.11)

X HIGH PSYCHOLOGICAL TENSION
x AVERAGE PSYCHOLOGICAL TENSION
x LOW PSYCHOLOGICAL TENSION

Fig. 1. Child's report of mother's behavior index showing the relationship between individual scales of the index. The linear correlation coefficient between each scale and the respondents marijuana use index is given after the name of each scale. The diagonals of the circle represent the factors of the parent–child relationship; the third factor (psychological tension) being on an axis in and out of the plane of the paper.

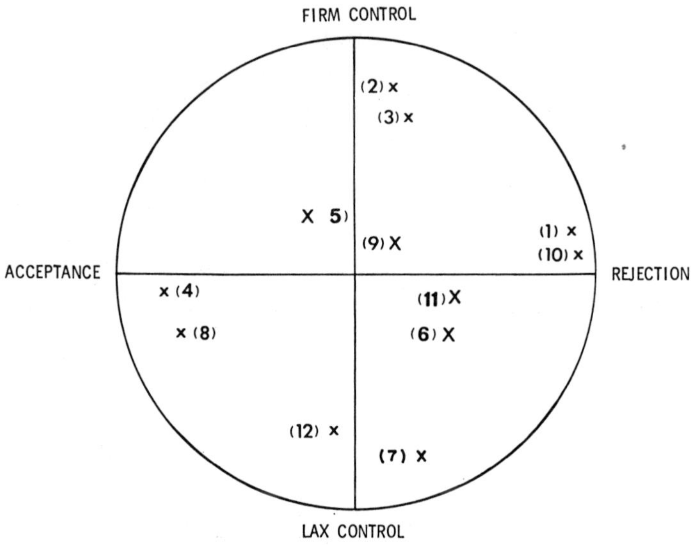

X HIGH PSYCHOLOGICAL TENSION
x AVERAGE PSYCHOLOGICAL TENSION
x LOW PSYCHOLOGICAL TENSION

1. REJECTION (-.13)
2. CONTROL (-.03)
3. ENFORCEMENT (-.08)
4. POSITIVE INVOLVEMENT (-.06)
5. CONTROL THROUGH GUILT (-.14)
6. INCONSISTENT DESCIPLINE (+.08)
7. NONENFORCEMENT (-.07)
8. ACCEPTANCE OF INDIVIDUATION (+.13)
9. CONTROL THROUGH PERSISTENT ANXIETY (-.36)
10. CONTROL WITH HOSTILE DETACHMENT (-.25)
11. CONTROL THROUGH WITHDRAWAL OF RELATIONS (-.25)
12. EXTREME AUTONOMY (-.10)

Fig. 2. Child's report of father's behavior index showing the relationships between individual scales of the index. The linear correlation coefficient between each scale and respondent's marijuana use index is given after the name of each scale. The diagonals of the circle represent the factors of the parent–child relationship; the third factor (psychological tension) being on an axis in and out of plane of the paper.

Figures 1 and 2 demonstrate graphically the statistical relationship between scales, between the scales and the major factors, and among the scales and the respondent's marijuana use index.

Obtaining Parent–Child Relationship Factors

In agreement with previous researchers who have utilized the CR-PBI, we found that three major parent–child relationship factors can be derived from these 12 scales (using the PA-1 option of subprogram FACTOR in SPSS). The derivation of these three factors has been previously described. The three factors have been designated: "Acceptance–Rejection," "Firm Control–Lax Control," and "Psychological Control" (Schaefer, 1971; Schludermann, 1970). The last of these is labeled "Control Involving Psychological Tension" or "Psychological Tension" in this report, since the scales which load highly on this factor assess the use of psychological techniques in the control of the child which result in a tense relationship with the parent. These three factor scores for each parent were utilized in data analysis. The relationship between the scores on each of the scales can be displayed in the form of a "map" in which the principal "factors" are the major axes of a sphere.

RESULTS

Child's Report of Parent Behavior Index

The "Firm Control–Lax Control" factor from the mother–child relationship was found to be significantly correlated with respondents' marijuana use index values ($r = .28, p \doteq .05$). The direction of the correlation was such that increasing perception of control was associated with decreasing marijuana use. Neither the "Acceptance–Rejection" factor or the "Psychological Tension" factor in the mother–child relationship inventory significantly correlated with respondents' marijuana use (see Fig. 1).

From the respondents' reports of perceived relationships with their fathers, the factor "Control Involving Psychological Tension" was significantly correlated with respondents' marijuana use index ($r = .35, p \doteq .01$). The direction of the association was such that increasing perception of the use of psychological tension mechanisms in control by the father was associated with increasing marijuana use by the respondent. Neither the father's "Acceptance–Rejection" factor nor the "Firm Control–Lax Control" factor was significantly correlated with repondent's marijuana use index. Figures 1 and 2 present the "maps" of the scales of the parent–child relationships. The location on the map of each scale is determined by its correlation coefficient with each of the other scales. The correlation coefficients written in represent the correlation between each scale of the mother or father–child relationship index and the dependent variable, the marijuana use frequency index (see Fig. 2).

The similarity in sign and numerical value for the correlation coefficients of closely related scales with the dependent variable provides a measure of the reliability of the relationship.

The relationship of the maternal "Firm Control–Lax Control" factor is illustrated by the positive correlations of both the "Control" and "Enforcement" scales with the marijuana use index, while "Lax Control" and "Extreme Autonomy" have negative correlations (Fig. 1).

The relationship of the paternal "Psychological Tension" factor is illustrated by the relatively high negative correlations of scales near the center in Fig. 2 since the third factor lies on an axis in front of and behind the plane of the circle. These scales include "Control through Guilt," "Control Through Withdrawal of Relations," and "Control Through Persistent Anxiety."

Parental Use of Prescription and Over-the-Counter Drugs (Parents as Models)

The use of over-the-counter drugs by parents was not associated with marijuana use by their adolescent children. Nor was there any indication that the use of prescription drugs by the mother was related to marijuana use by the students ($r = -.06$). The use of prescription drugs by the father, however, did significantly correlate with respondent's marijuana use index ($r = .30$, $p < .05$).

Parental Attitudes toward Marijuana Use (Parents as Educators)

There was a significant positive correlation between marijuana use and the attitudes of the father ($r = .41$, $p \doteq .001$) and of the mother ($r = .41$, $p \doteq .001$) toward possible or actual use of marijuana by the child. Most parents agreed about marijuana use ($r = .86$) and most "strongly disapproved" of its use. An increase in marijuana use by respondents was thus associated with less disapproval by parents.

DEMOGRAPHIC AND "CONTROL" VARIABLES

Race

The correlation between race and the marijuana use index was significant ($r = .35, p \doteq .01$), with the White students reporting more marijuana use.

Age and Sex

There was no evidence to suggest that there were significant differences between boys and girls with regard to marijuana use ($r = .09$). In addition, no systematic variation was found with age ($r = .04$) since essentially only high school seniors were studied.

Parental Education

There was a significant positive relationship found between respondent's ma rijuana use index score and the father's level of educational achievement ($r = .44, p \doteq .001$), as well as with the mother's level of educational achievement ($r = .32, p \doteq .02$). Those reporting greater use of marijuana also reported higher levels of education attained by their parents. The correlation between father's and mother's level of educational achievement was quite strong ($r = .68, p < .001$). Also race and educational achievement by the father and mother were closely associated ($r = .57, p < .001$; and $r = .41, p \doteq .001$, respectively), with White parents having completed more years of formal education.

MULTIPLE CORRELATIONS

Controlling for the Effects of Parental Education

After statistically accounting for the reduction in variance of the marijuana use index due to father's level of educational achievement, the partial correlations of race (partial $r = .14$, $p =$ NS) and of the "Psychological Control" factor from the father–child relationship (partial $r = .22, p \doteq .10$) were no longer significant. However, after controlling for father's education level, the partial correlation with the mother's "Firm Control–Lax Control" factor becomes more impressive (partial $r = .38, p \doteq .005$).

Also, significant partial correlations persist with father's attitude toward marijuana use (partial $r = .34$, $p < .02$), mother's attitude toward marijuana use (partial $r = .34$, $p < .02$), and father's use of prescription drugs (partial $r = .30$, $p > .05$).

Taken together, father's level of educational achievement and the "Firm Control–Lax Control" factor from the mother–child relationship "explain" (multiple R^2) 30% of the variance in respondents' marijuana use index scores. This reduction in variance is highly unlikely to be due to random variation $p(F_{2,51} = 11.18) < .001$.

"Best" Statistical Model for Predicting Marijuana Use

After considering a large number of statistical models for "predicting" marijuana use from this data set, the model in Table 1 was selected. This model provides nearly the maximum reduction of variance attainable with all of the data available, utilizing a minimum number of independent variables each of which contributes significantly to the overall reduction in variance of the dependent variable.

Table 2 demonstrates the efficiency of the "best-predicting" model at categorizing individual responses with regard to marijuana use. Since the index was derived from the same data, this table does not constitute a confirmation of the index, it is simply a demonstration of the meaning of the 43% reduction in variance achieved by the combination of factors in the statistical model for "predicting" marijuana use. In order from lowest to highest quartile of scores derived from this multiple regression model, the rate of regular involvement with marijuana use (monthly or more often) is 8% (1/13), 24% (4/17), 35% (5/14), and 83% (10/12).

Table 1
Best Statistical Model for "Predicting" Marijuana Use by Adolescents[a,b]

Variable	B	β	Partial F	Statistical significance
Father's level of educational achievement	.40	.36	9.97	$p < .005$
Maternal "firm control–lax control" factor	.24	.24	4.51	$p < .05$
Mother's approval of possible or actual marijuana use	.61	.30	6.76	$p < .025$
Father's use of prescription drugs	.34	.27	5.77	$p < .025$
Constant	.26			

[a] Based on survey data from 54 North Carolina high school students, 1972.
[b] Multiple $R^2 = .43$, $p[F_{4,49} - 9.24] \ll .001$.

Table 2
Distribution of Marijuana Use Responses by Quartiles of Marijuana Use Index

Quartiles of marijuana index derived from "best-predicting" model	Marijuana use				
	Never	Less than 5 times	A few times each year	Monthly	Weekly
1st	8	1	3	1	0
2nd	10	3	0	3	1
3rd	5	2	2	3	2
4th	0	0	3	2	7

[a] High school students, North Carolina, 1971.

DISCUSSION

Adolescence is recognized as a period of major stress for individuals in our society (King, 1969). It is also a period during which peer influences on behavior become increasingly strong (Lanese, 1972). However, the most significant representation of the attitudes and behavior of the larger adult society to the adolescent continues to be his parents. Furthermore, firm, supportive parental relationships can be an important source of strength toward the resolution of adolescent stresses. Alternatively tense and unsupportive parental relationships can add to the problem of adolescence, and not be part of the solution (King, 1969).

Parents as Educators

In this study, parental attitudes toward possible or actual use of marijuana were significantly associated with frequency of marijuana use by their adolescent children. This was true despite the fact that there was very strong consensus against marijuana use and agreement between parents. Using cross-sectional data as this study does, it is possible that the attitude of the parents (or the child's perception of it) changed after the use of illicit drugs was acquired rather than preceding the behavior change.

Parents as Models

The significant correlation between father's use of prescription drugs and respondent's use of marijuana is of considerable interest and was somewhat unexpected, particularly since there was no significant correlation observed with the use of over-the-counter drugs. The American Osteopathic Association has sponsored television statements suggesting that physicians have contributed to the creation of a "pill-oriented" society in which illicit drug use by children is presumably "modeled" after the behavior and attitudes of adults. This concern has also appeared in the medical literature (Thompson, 1972). In Canadian adolescents, at least, a strong association was found between the use of prescription drugs by parents, specifically stimulants and barbiturates, and the frequency of use of marijuana by adolescents (Smart, 1972).

Parent–Child Relationship (Parents as Supports vs Parents as Problems)

Two factors from the parent–child relationship were significantly correlated with adolescent drug use. The perception by the child of increasing use by the father of control mechnisms and methods which might result in psychologically tense relationship was correlated with increasing use of marijuana. This may be analogous to the importance placed on intrafamilial tension by others (Wurmser, 1970; Solomon, 1970). This supports the hypothesis that the parent may be one of the problems of adolescence. On the other hand, the network of correlations, in this study, between race, parental education, and the "psychological control" factor make it impossible to select the variable of primary importance.

Individuals who perceived that they were under lax maternal control reported a greater frequency of marijuana use. This suggests two partially divergent interpretations. It is possible that maternal "firm control" might function as an effective barrier to the unlimited freedom necessary to acquire illicit drug use as an "extracurricular" activity. It would seem equally reasonable, however, that the perception of "firm control" is an important part of a supportive relationship with the mother which facilitates the resolution of conflicts in the adolescent's life with fewer adaptive behaviors.

Influence of Demographic and "Control" Variables

In this study, significant correlations were identified between the frequency of reported marijuana use and race (White excess), as well as increasing level of parental education, particularly that of the father. Previous studies have also demonstrated that marijuana use is more frequent in adolescents whose fathers are well educated (Shafer, 1972). Differences between the races observed in this study may well be secondary to differences in socioeconomic status, of which paternal education is a good indicator. On the other hand, previous authors have suggested that the use of illicit drugs is not really limited by socioeconomic factors, but the motivations may differ for the advantaged youth as opposed to the relatively disadvantaged (Keniston, 1969). In any case, no entirely satisfactory explanation for the relationships between drug use and socioeconomic status or race is available.

Family Typology

The "best" statistical model for "predicting" adolescent marijuana use consisted of four factors, each of which made a significant contribution to the overall reduction of variance. Such a model permits the proposal of a typology of the family in which marijuana use is most likely to occur. Such a family would be headed by a well-educated father. The children perceive relatively lax control on the part of the mother. The father uses prescription drugs frequently. The mother does not strongly disapprove of marijuana use.

This combination of factors, if confirmed on other groups, may separate otherwise unselected students into subgroups with a likelihood of regular drug use varying from as little as 8 % to as much as 83 %. This demonstration of the meaning of the statistical results quoted emphasizes the potential value of such an approach.

This study suggests that we must understand the influence of a variety of mechanisms in order to explain the undeniable influences of parents on the use of illicit drugs by their adolescent children. Since all of the data presented is based on the child's report of his perceptions, it should be recognized that it is possible that the child's perception of his parents was altered after he became a drug user. Only a longitudinal study design can resolve this issue (Jessor, in press).

SUMMARY AND CONCLUSIONS

Marijuana use among 54 North Carolina high school students was evaluated as a function of family characteristics reported by the students. Particular attention was directed toward the evaluation of the child's perception of his relationship with each of his parents, using Schaefer's Child's Report of Parent Behavior Index.

Significant linear correlations were found between respondent's increasing reported use of marijuana and each of the following variables: race

(White), increasing use of prescription drugs by the father, increasing level of parental (particularly father's) level of educational attainment, less disapproval of either parent about possible or actual marijuana use, "lax control" in the mother–child relationship, and "psychological tension" in the father–child relationship.

The "best" statistical model for "predicting" adolescent marijuana use from this sample suggests that marijuana use is more likely to occur among young people from families in which the father is well educated, the parents do not strongly disapprove of marijuana use, the father uses prescription drugs, and the relationship with the mother as perceived by the child includes relatively lax control. These results suggest that multiple causation of adolescent drug use is conceptually accurate.

ACKNOWLEDGMENT

Research conducted in the Department of Epidemiology, School of Public Health, University of North Carolina, Chapel Hill, supported in part by Department of Health, Education and Welfare, Public Health Service Training Grant Environmental Epidemiology Research 5 to 1 E 500134–02 ESTC.

REFERENCES

BLACKFORD, L. Trends in student drug use in San Mateo County. *California's Health* 27: 3–11, 1969.

GOSSETT, J.T., LEWIS, J.M., and PHILLIPS, V.A. Extent and prevalence of illicit drug use as reported by 56,745 students. *J. Amer. Med. Assoc.* 216(9): 1464–1470, 1972.

JESSOR, R., JESSOR, S., and FINNEY, J. A social psychology of marijuana use: Longitudinal studies of high school and college youth. *J. Personality Social Psychol.* In press.

KENISTON, K. Search and rebellion among the advantaged. In *Drug Dependence: A Guide for Physicians.* Chicago: American Medical Assoc., 42–52, 1969.

KING, S.H. Youth in rebellion: An historical perspective. In *Drug Dependence: A Guide for Physicians.* Chicago: American Medical Assoc., pp. 30–41, 1969.

LANESE, R.R., BANKS, F.R., and KELLER, M.D. Smoking behavior in a teenage population: A multivariate conceptual approach. *Amer. J. Public Health.* 62: 807–813, 1972.

NIE, N., BENT, D.H., and HALL, C.H. *Statistical Package for the Social Sciences.* New York: McGraw-Hill, 1970.

PRENDERGAST, T.J., Jr. Parent-child relationships associated with important health related behaviors in adolescents. Presented at the Social Epidemiology Seminar, University of North Carolina, April 20, 1973. Proceedings in press.

PRENDERGAST, T.J., Jr., TENNANT, F.S., Jr., and PREBEL, M.R., Jr. Drug use and its relations to alcohol and cigarette consumption in the U.S. military community of West Germany. *Intern. J. Addictions* 8(5): 791, 1973.

SCHAEFER, E.S. Development of hierarchical, configurational models for parent behavior and child behavior. In *Minnesota Symposium on Child Psychology,* Vol. 1. Minneapolis: Univ. Minnesota Press, 1971.

SCHLUDERMANN, E., and SCHLUDERMANN, S. Replicability of factors in children's report of parent behavior (CRPBI). *J. Psychol.* 76: 239–479, 1970.

SHAFER, R.P. (Chairman). *Marijuana: A Signal of Misunderstanding.* (Report of the National Commission of Marijuana and Drug Abuse). Washington, D.C.: U.S. Govt. Printing Office, March 1972, pp. 294–295.

SMART, R.G., and FEJER. D. Drug use among adolescents and their parents: Closing the generation gap in mood modification. *J. Abnormal Psychol.* 79(2): 153–160, 1972.

SOLOMON, N. The communication gap and the drug problem. *Maryland State Med.* J. 19: 78–81, November 1970.

STEWART, G.W. Promotion of health and behavioral change. Presented to the International Conference of Health and Health Education, Buenos Aires, 1969.

SUCHMAN, E.A. Health attitudes and behavior. *Arch. Environmental Health.* 20: 105–110, 1970.

SURGEON GENERAL'S REPORT. *Smoking and Health, Report of the Advisory Committee to the Suregon General of the Public Health Service.* Washington, D.C.: U.S. Govt. Printing Office, 1964.

SURGEON GENERAL'S REPORT. *Marijuana and Health, A Report to the Congress from the Secretary, Department of Health, Education and Welfare.* Washington, D.C.: U.S. Govt. Printing Office, 1971.

THOMPSON, R.F. Too much use of drugs (Letter to the Editor). *Ann. Int. Med.* 77(1): 150, July 1972.

WEITMAN, M., SCHUBLE, R., JOHNSON, K.C., and ABBEY, H. Survey of adolescent drug use. III. Correlations among use of drugs. *Amer. J. Public Health.* 62: 166–170, 1972.

WURMSER, L. Why people take drugs: Escape and search. *Maryland State Med. J.* 19: 62–64, November 1970.

The International Journal of the Addictions, 9(6), pp. 841–849, 1974

Counseling Utilization Related to Dose Reduction in Methadone Maintenance

S. Creel, M.D.

R. Berkson, M.D.

J. Reilly, A.B.

P. Butler, M.Ed.

B. Walker, M.S.W.

L. Carrozza, R.N.

J. Morrison, R.N.

R. O'Connell

V. Patch, M.D.

Brighton Clinic
City of Boston Drug Treatment Program
Boston, Massachusetts

INTRODUCTION

Counseling is an effective adjunct to methadone maintenance in the treatment of heroin addiction (Connor et al., 1971). This study attempts to demonstrate a relationship between increased counseling activity and dose reduction in 79 patients at the Brighton "Turnoff" Clinic in Boston, Massachusetts.

METHODS

The clinic, a unit of the Boston City "Turnoff" Program, is located in a partitioned 400 ft^2 room staffed by one full-time psychiatrist, one half-time psychiatrist, two professionally trained counselors, a psychiatric social worker, two nurses, and a secretary, all of whom share to some extent the counseling load.

The average census is 100 patients. All receive methadone on a daily basis and are allowed to determine their own dosage levels within limits of the Federal Guidelines. Limited counseling is available on request. Patients frequently present in crisis and feel most comfortable in an atmosphere of informality, openness, and empathy. Emphasis is placed on eventual drug abstinence and employment as treatment goals. Family members are often involved, and there are three evening groups: one for patients and family members, one for patients alone, and a third for patients who are in the process of detoxification.

The study population was made up of 79 patients (67 male, 12 female), 90% caucasion with an age range of 18 to 42 and a median age of 23. Average estimated length of addiction prior to treatment was $2\frac{1}{2}$ to 3 years. They entered the Brighton Clinic in late 1971 and early 1972 and were on continuous maintenance from 6 months to 1 year.

Without anticipating any specific results, each staff member provided a wide range of raw data concerning their patients on a standard questionnaire for both the first and second 6-month periods of treatment. Dosage behavior was analyzed by calculating the individual mean dose for each treatment period.

A 0–4 rating scale for utilization of counseling by patients was employed as follows:

0 no contact with counselor.
1 minimal contact, crisis oriented, approximately 1 hr/month.

2 sporadic contact, crisis oriented, approximately 2 hr/month.
3 frequent contact, nonscheduled, often crisis oriented but with relationship building, 3 hr/month.
4 regular scheduled interviews, 4 or more hours per month with specific treatment goals.

A rating of 2 was considered average for the clinic.

The patients were divided into two groups: those who showed an increase in counseling activity between the first and second 6 months of treatment ($N = 41$, mean counseling change $+1.4$) and those who showed no increase ($N = 38$, mean counseling change -0.4) (Fig. 1).

A statistical comparison was then made of the individual mean dose changes between the two groups for the first and second 6 months of treatment using the Two-Sample Ranks Test ($p < .01$) (Mainland, 1964).

As seen from Fig. 1, the group that increased its counseling is distributed in a bimodal curve at the two extremes of mean dose change, with dose raises to the right and dose reductions to the left of zero, or no change.

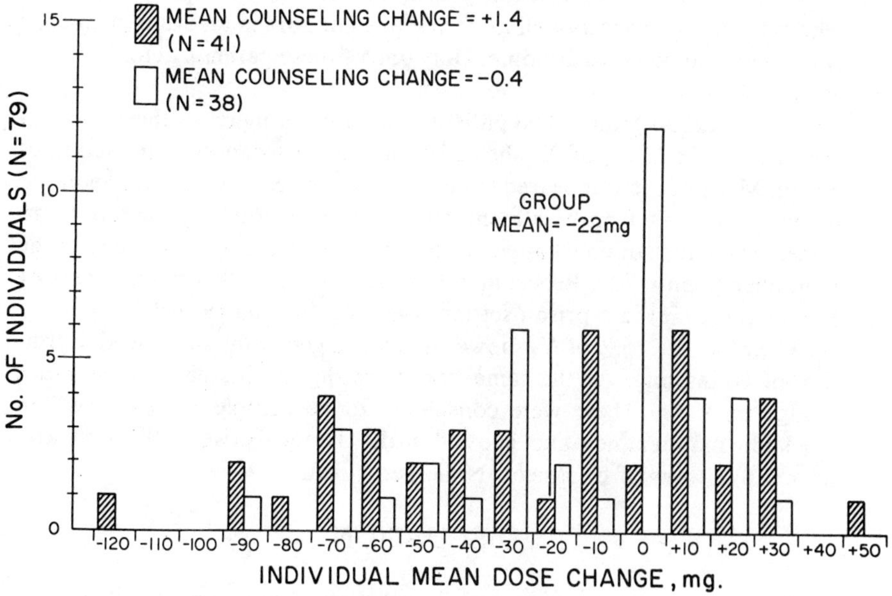

Fig. 1. Relationship between individual mean dose change and utilization of counseling from the first to the second 6-month period of treatment.

The group that did not increase counseling is distriubted closer to the group mean (—22 mg) with one tail extending to the left, toward the dose reduction end of the scale.

OBSERVATIONS AND INTERPRETATIONS

The characteristic patterns of distribution for the two groups were further analyzed and four basic patterns of dose behavior were identified, two for each of the two groups (Table 1).

First, of the 41 patients with increased counseling activity, 26 (33% of *N*) showed a low initial counseling level of 1. As they increased their counseling level to 3 in the second 6-month period of treatment, they reduced their mean dose by 80 mg. These were identified as patients whose primary goal was to reduce dosage slowly, often erratically at first. This in itself constituted a continuing crisis for which they sought more counseling. Eight or 31% of this group detoxified.

The other 15 (23% of *N*) who increased their counseling also increased their mean dose considerably, by 22 mg. These were found to be basically unstable patients, most with dirty urines indicating multiple drug abuse, who were using drugs as well as counseling support in an attempt to cope with a continuing crisis at home. Only one of these patients detoxified successfully.

Of the second group of 38 patients who did not increase their counseling activity, 18 (23% of *N*) showed a significant mean dose reduction of 39 mg. Many of these appeared to be reacting to external crises that required them to withdraw from treatment, such as an ultimatum by the family, an impending arrest, or court appearance. This is referred to as the "end of the road phenomenon" by Bess et al. (1972), and was also described in part by Lipkowitz (1971) in a prison setting. Eight or 44% detoxified.

The other 20 (25% of *N*) showed a low and generally unchanged utilization of counseling. At the same time they slightly increased their mean dosage by 9 mg. These were considered to be completely stabilized on blockade maintenance and showed little change between the first and second 6 months of treatment. None detoxified.

DISCUSSION

Evidence that counseling and dose behavior are significantly related suggests that the two modalities of treatment may be more effective in combination than when offered alone (Connor et al., 1971; Capparell,

Table 1

Four Basic Patterns of Dose Behavior Related to Utilization of Counseling

	Mean dose, mg		Differ-ence M, mg	% Change	Average dose change, mg	r, dose change, mg	Mean counsel-ing (0–4), 0/6–6/12 months	Differ-ence, M	Number/ percent detoxified
	N	0/6–6/12 months							
Increased utilization counseling									
Dose reducers	26	139–59	−80	−58	−47	105	1–3	+2	8/31
Nondose reducers	15	87–111	+22	+25	+18	50	1–2.5	+1.5	1/6
All	41	114–85	−29	−25	−14	165	1–2.7	+1.7	9/22
No increased utilization counseling									
Dose reducers	18	96–57	−39	−41	−39	90	2–2	0	8/44
Nondose reducers	20	98–107	+9	+1	+8	30	1.5–1	−0.5	0/0
All	38	97–82	−15	−16	−16	120	1.7–1.3	−0.4	8/21
All patients	79	105–88	−22	−21	−15	165	1.4–2	+0.6	17/22

1972). Although available counseling services fell short of overall patient need, the drug abstinence rate of 22% in this study compares favorably with similar figures for other programs (Levy, 1972).

The relationship of addiction to disordered personality, as well as to familial and social st ress, has been the subject of continuing study. Merry (1972) found no differences between 63 addicts and nonaddict personality disorders, and noted a marked contrast between 20 female addicts and 20 healthy primipara. Mott (1972) cites MMPI results of addicts showing gross deviation from normals, with high scores in psychopathy and neurosis in that order. They were described as "overactive, drug oriented, incapable of delay or modification of behavior." Yet no clear evidence of a distinct addict personality is said to exist as yet due to biased sampling in studies.

That this population is subject to considerable psychosocial stress leads to the conjecture that heroin, in addition to hedonistic properties, is utilized as a tranquilizer (St. Pierre, 1971). This is recorded in the history of opium in psychiatry (Carlson and Simpson, 1963). The drug was widely used in European medicine by the time of the Renaissance, largely as a result of Arabic influence. Paracelsus perscribed it for a wide range of excited states collectively called "mania," and for hysteria and hypochondriasis.

In the seventeenth century, Sydenham introduced laudanum as a drug of choicc for the treatment of these same conditions, and by the eighteenth century the demand fo r opium in psychiatric illness led to other formulas, such as blackdrop and paregoric. Intense research began to determine its mode of action. Physicians regarded it as a panacea, prescribing it for a wide range of medical and psychiatric problems. With the nineteenth century came the introduction of morphine and use by hypodermic syringe. In America the opiates were highly recommended for the treatment of melancholia hypochondriaca, a form of agitated depression, and their use as a substitute for mechanical restraints was recognized. Woodward, at Worcester Asylum in Massachusetts, used moderate long-term doses of opiates as an effective adjunct to moral treatment.

Popularity of opiates waned in the 1880s after the dangers of habituation became widely recognized with the emergence of a new psychiatric syndrome called morphinomania or morphinism. Hope that new preparations would be addiction-free led to the use of cocaine in 1885 in the treatment of morphinism and to enthusiastic statements about heroin after it became available in 1898. Around this time many psychiatrists still did not recognize addiction as a disease, and addicts were frequently turned away from overcrowded mental hospitals in favor of patients with other types of disorders.

The data from this and other studies, plus historical information, suggest that we are dealing with a disturbed, self-medicated population which tends to become more anxious during drug withdrawal, due in part to the symbolic loss of the drug itself, to the physical reaction, as well as to the emergence of psychopathology with preexisting unresolved conflicts of sexual identity (Connor et al., 1971). This is supported by Lipkowitz (1971) who states that the principle responses to abrupt heroin withdrawal are subjective, yet not by Goldstein (1972) who states that slow, blind decreases of methadone from high doses down to 40 mg are without significant side effects.

Improved interpersonal relations and support from families and treatment programs is vital for continued drug abstinence, whereas relapses to drug use are associated with deteriorating intrapsychic and interpersonal situations (Stephens and Cottrell, 1972). Likewise, successful narcotics renunciation has been correlated with more intact families and with fathers who provide suitable role-models (Bess et al., 1972). Important is the "rose-colored-glasses syndrome," described by Bess et al., which is pervasive in successful ex-addicts. They see themselves as popular, attractive, secure, and superior, a self-image which is thought to be a personalized combination of hope and reality that provides a new gratification and a source of strength for renunciation of drug use.

Finally, the importance of staff attitudes toward treatment must be mentioned. In this study the emphasis on drug abstinence, with maintenance as a means to this end, provided consistent motivation for outpatients. St. Pierre (1971) observes that addicts are often initially unmotivated to discontinue drug use and employ the defenses of blocking and isolation to sustain their behavior. He stresses the need to confront the patient with his addiction and then to motivate him to struggle against it through the use of will power, a greater awareness of feelings and responses to drug temptation, and a clearer understanding of the disadvantages of drug use. At the same time, our staff suggests substitute goals, such as full employment or education, and that patient interest in this direction should be positively reinforced.

Butler (1973) provides further evidence to support the effectiveness of therapeutic staff attitudes in a study just completed at our clinic, using the Edwards Personal Preference Schedule to measure the manifest needs of patients on methadone. It was observed that patients in the process of detoxification scored significantly higher on "deference" (following instructions, conforming to custom) and "abasement" (feeling guilt, accepting blame) but lower on "affiliation" (participating in groups, making friends) than did patients remaining on long-term maintenance. This latter group scored significantly higher on "succorance" (needing assistance, sympathy, nurturance). Therefore, it would seem that patients with a greater capacity to feel guilt and to follow the advice of the counselor are more likely to respond to motivation and to accept treatment goals.

QUESTIONS FOR FURTHER RESEARCH

Further work needs to be done to define the exact nature of the effect of methadone as it is related to specific intrapsychic and interpersonal variables involved in overall patient management, especially those that influence drug withdrawal and motivate the patient to seek counseling.

SUMMARY

Counseling is an important adjunct to methadone maintenance in the treatment of heroin addiction.

Patients who increase their counseling activity are in a state of change. Most are in the process of reducing their dosage of methadone, whereas a lesser number are unstable, in crisis, show multiple drug abuse, and raise their doses.

Patients with no increased counseling activity are generally stable and are unlikely to change dosage. However, a smaller percentage may be in the process of withdrawing from treatment because compelling outside pressures require them to detoxify.

Addicts are known to employ heroin in part for relief of psychic tension. Successful drug renunciation is correlated with supportive interpersonal relations and staff attitudes, and the development of a positive self-image.

Opiates have a long history of use in psychiatry. From the above it is inferred that methadone may exert a tranquilizing effect with the result that the disturbed, self-medicated addict in the process of dose reduction will seek conseling for support, in order to deal not only with the drug withdrawal syndrome but with emerging psychopathology.

REFERENCES

BESS, B., JANUS, S., and RIFKIN, A. Factors in successful narcotics reunuciation. *Amer. J. Psychol.* 128: 861, 1972.

BUTLER, P. Personality differences between maintenance patients and patients progressing toward detoxification on a methadone treatment program. Unpublished thesis, Boston Univ. School of Education, 1973.

CAPPARELL, H. Drugs versus psychotherapy. *New York State J. Med.* 72: 1830, 1972.

CARLSON, E., SIMPSON, M. Opium as a tranquillizer. *Amer. J. Psychol.* 120: 112, 1963.

CONNOR, P., and KREMEN, E. Methadone maintenance—is it enough? *Brit. J. Addictions* 66: 53, 1971.

GOLDSTEIN, A. Heroin addiction and role of methadone in its treatment. Arch. *Gen. Psychiat.* 26: 291, 1972.

LEVY, B. Five years after: a follow-up of 50 narcotic addicts. *Amer. J. Psychiat.* 128: 7, 1972.

LIPKOWITZ, M., SCHWARTZ, D., and LAZARUS, R. Abrupt withdrawal of maintenance methadone. *J. Amer. Med. Assoc.* 217: 1860, 1971.

MAINLAND, D. *Elementary Medical Statistics.* Philadelphia: Saunders, 1964, p. 284.

MERRY, J. Social characteristics of addiction to heroin. *Brit. J. Addictions* 67: 322, 1972.

MOTT, J. The psychological basis of drug dependence—the intellectual and personality characteristics of opiate users. *Brit. J. Addictions* 67: 89, 1972.

ST. PIERRE, A. Motivating the drug addict in treatment. *Social Work* 16: 80, 1971.

STEPHENS, R., and COTTRELL, E. A follow-up study of 200 narcotic addicts committed under the Narcotic Addiction Rehabilitation Act. *Brit. J. Addictions* 67: 45, 1972.

The International Journal of the Addictions, 9(6), pp. 851–861, 1974

Student Drug Use and the Perceived Peer Drug Environment

Lee H. Bowker, Ph.D.

Washington State University
Pullman, Washington

INTRODUCTION

Though the number of studies dealing with perceived peer drug environments in colleges and universities is small, the pattern of results is consistent. Drug users and nonusers may share the same physical world on the campus, but their perceived social worlds are different.

King (1971, p. 216) found that 88% of nonusers and 100% of marijuana users knew other students who smoked marijuana. Imperi et al. (1968, pp. 1022–1023) found that 76% of Yale nonusers and 80% of Wesleyan nonusers knew students who used illegal drugs, and that student estimates of the extent of student drug use tended to double or triple the figures obtained through the surveys. Brown (1972, p. 461) presents a correlation of .24 between desire to try marijuana (among nonusers) and identification with others who approve of marijuana use, and a correlation of .52 between marijuana use and identification with other drug users.

Goldstein et al. (1970, p. 26) agree that drug users tend to overestimate the amount of drug use, and add that nonusers tend to underestimate it. They found that heavy drug users had had many more drug-using friends of all types (even tobacco) than occasional users, who in turn had more drug-using friends than nonusers (Goldstein et al., 1970, p. 49). Johnson (1971, p. 103) reports that only 16% of students in his sample who had few marijuana-using friends had tried the drug. In comparison, 90% of students who had mostly marijuana-using friends had tried it.

Suchman (1968, p. 148) also found that students perceived more marijuana use occurring among other students than actually existed. He found that more students felt at least some pressure to use alcohol (51%) than to use marijuana (20%), but that as pressure to use marijuana increased, the use of the drug also increased. A similar pattern emerged among users of LSD. Approximately two-thirds of the students who reported that most of the students they knew smoked marijuana did so themselves, while less than one in a hundred of those whose friends did not smoke marijuana had tried it themselves (Suchman, 1968, p. 149).

Campbell (1970, pp. 52–53) found that marijuana users had been offered the drug much more than nonusers, and that they perceived marijuana as easier to obtain. Marijuana users were fairly accurate in their estimate of the extent of marijuana use at Bishop's University, but nonusers underestimated it to a considerable degree (Campbell, 1970, p. 54). There were strong relationships between knowledge of people who used marijuana and both marijuana and LSD use (Campbell, 1970, p. 56). Marijuana users were more likely than nonusers to have a large number of marijuana-smoking friends (Campbell, 1970, p. 57). Forty-three percent of marijuana users felt some degree of social pressure to use the drug, compared to 24% of the nonusers.

METHODOLOGY

A 100% sample of students enrolled on February 1, 1972 at Ivy College, a small liberal arts college located west of the Mississippi River, was asked to complete a lengthy anonymous questionnaire on factors associated with the use of legal and illegal drugs on the campus.

The Ivy College drug survey departs from traditional studies in deviance and symbolic interaction, such as those by Lindesmith (1947) and Becker (1953), by opting for a methodology leaning heavily on standard sample survey techniques rather than participant observation and extended unstructured interviews. However, it remains in the tradition of symbolic interaction because of its approach to the data. Student drug use is not seen as the direct product of stated empirical conditions such as whether the drug users are from broken homes. Instead, it is conceptualized as arising out of definitions of the situation (Thomas and Thomas, 1928, p.

Table 1
Cross-Sectional Surveys Relevant to College Student Drug Use and the Perceived Peer Drug Environment

First author	Date	School	Response rate, %	Sample size
Imperi	1968	Yale, Wesleyan	80, 66	327, 251
Suchman	1968	"West Coast university"	81	497
Blum	1969	Five California schools	66 to 99	201 to 300
Gallup	1969a, 1969b, 1972	National samples	Not given	1,063[a]
Campbell	1970	Bishop's University	62 to 76[b]	609 to 774
Goldstein	1970	Carnegie-Mellon University	72	2,274
Gergen	1971	National sample	Not given	5,050
Johnson	1971	Twenty New York area schools	[c]	3,500
King	1971	Dartmouth	67 to 79[d]	518 to 576
Brown	1972	University of Southern California	81	257

[a] A sample size is given only for the 1972 report. The other reports do not give data on sample sizes.
[b] Campbell selected three samples fıom the Bishop's University student body over a period of 2 years.
[c] Johnson used essentially availability samples from his schools so the concept of a response rate is not applicable.
[d] King selected two samples from Dartmouth in successive years.

575). The only variables treated as causal agents are perceived states of the peer drug environment. Demographic variables are used as controls, but these are seen as predisposing factors within which definitions of the peer drug environment occur.

Approximately 20 students from a methodology class in the Sociology Department at Ivy College were trained to deliver and pick up the questionnaires and to answer all possible questions that could be asked about the study by respondents. The questionnaires were distributed to students in the residence halls and off-campus apartments one evening after supper. Over 75% of the questionnaires were returned within 48 hr, and 95% were returned within 1 week of the initial distribution. A number of students also returned signed cards giving permission for a personal interview with the researcher, which resulted in 53 in-depth interviews lasting up to 4 hr.

The returned questionnaires were coded, punched on computer cards, and summed into tables and indexes by the Ivy College computer center. The composite index of the self's drug use was correlated with other indexes using the gamma measure for ordered data, and these correlations were examined for specification by the variables of sex, parental income, home community size, religion, and religiosity. Relationships between specific types of drug use and a variety of independent variables were tested using the chi-square test of statistical significance.

The reliability and validity of the study for the Ivy College student body were found to be adequate based on (1) the high return rate, (2) consistency of responses demonstrated by internal checks built into the questionnaire, (3) comparison with a student-conducted survey on the same topic that was completed a few months earlier, and (4) comparisons between those completing the questionnaire and the total student body on selected demographic variables. There is no way to establish the degree to which results from the Ivy College study can be generalized to other colleges. Data from several national surveys of student drug use indicate that colleges with similar characteristics tend to experience comparable patterns of drug use, but an examination of studies of drug use at colleges comparable to Ivy College suggests that drug use at Ivy is unusually low.

RESULTS

The relationships among 11 measures of the perceived peer drug environment and five categories of student drug use were examined using chi-square. All six of the relationships between measures of the perceived peer drug environment and the student drug use index (a composite of 10 separate categories of drug use covering the spectrum of legal and illegal drugs) were statistically significant. Seven of eight relationships involving perceived peer drug environment and the use of "soft" hallucinogens (marijuana and hashish) were significant, as were two of three relationships involving "hard" hallucinogens (LSD, mescaline, etc.), two of three dealing with alcohol, and all three involving amphetamines. These are summarized in Table 2.

In addition to the student drug use index, indexes were formed by combining responses in the areas of the perceived opposite sex best friend's drug use, perceived same sex best friend's drug use, perceived drug use of other students, perceived friends' attitudes toward drug use, and perceived attitudes of other students toward drug use. The student drug use index

Table 2

Significance Levels of Relationships[a] between Student Drug Use and the Perceived Peer Drug Environment

Dimensions of perceived peer drug environment	Dimensions of student drug use				
	Drug use index	"Soft" hallucinogens	"Hard" hallucinogens	Amphetamines	Alcohol
Perceived friends' attitude toward drug use	.001	.001	.001	.001	.001
Perceived same sex best friend's drug use	.001	—	—	—	—
Perceived opposite sex best friend's drug use	.001	—	—	—	—
Perceived attitudes of other students	.001	.02	.001	.001	.001
Perceived drug use of other students	.001	.02	NS	.001	NS
Number of pushers known	—	.001	—	—	—
Pressure to use marijuana	—	.001	—	—	—
Pressure not to use marijuana	—	.01	—	—	—
Proportion of social marijuana use	—	.001	—	—	—
Marijuana group size	—	NS	—	—	—
Comparative perception of Ivy College drug use	.02	—	—	—	—

[a] Significance levels are based on the analysis of 2 × 2 and 2 × 3 tables using the chi-square test of statistical significance.

Table 3

The Specification by Sex, Parental Income, Home Community Size, Religion and Religiosity of Relationships[a] *between Measures of the Perceived Peer Drug Environment and Student Drug Use*

Dimensions	Measures of the perceived peer drug environment					
	Perceived opposite sex best friend's drug use	Perceived same sex best friend's drug use	Perceived drug use of other students	Perceived friends' attitudes toward drug use	Perceived attitudes of other students toward drug use	*N*[b]
Total sample	–.04	.06	.26	.61	.18	948
Males	–.34	–.10	.34	.61	.23	529
Females	.30	.22	.18	.60	.14	407
Parental income under $25,000	–.05	.07	.22	.65	.13	614
Parental income $25,000 and up	.00	.09	.33	.55	.34	288
Home town size under 50,000	–.03	.12	.35	.65	.24	471
Home town size 50,000 and up	–.06	.02	.21	.58	.12	468
Protestant	.13	.03	.29	.62	.17	430
Catholic	–.11	.25	.24	.56	.20	99
Other religion or no religion	–.21	.00	.31	.58	.14	399
Religious services attended once per month or less	–.19	.01	.21	.64	.13	503
Religious services attended more than once per month	.13	.11	.37	.55	.22	435

[a] Correlations are gamma correlations, based on the analysis of 2 × 2 and 2 × 3 tables.
[b] Because some respondents did not complete all the demographic items, the *N*'s for each control variable differ slightly from the *N* of 948 on which the correlations were computed for the uncontrolled relationships.

was correlated with the other five indexes using gamma. Correlations varied from .62 to —.04, and these were specified to some degree by the control variables of sex, parental income, home town size, religion, and religiosity. These correlations are presented in Table 3.

All of the five relationships between the perceived attitudes of friends toward drug use and dimensions of student drug use were statistically significant at the .001 level. In every case the more positive the perceived attitudes of friends toward drug use, the higher the level of student drug use. The correlation between the index of attitudes of friends toward drug use and the index of student drug use was .61. Multivariate analysis using the five control variables, one at a time, failed to reveal any appreciable specification.

The relationships between the student drug use index and perceptions of both same and opposite sex best friend's drug use were significant at the .001 level, but the correlations were very small— .06 for same sex best friend and —.04 for opposite sex best friend. Sex, religion, and religiosity specified these two relationships to a considerable degree.

All five of the relationships between the index of student drug use and dimensions of the perceived attitudes of other students toward drug use were found to be statistically significant. In each of these relationships the more positive the perceived attitudes of other students toward drug use, the higher the level of student drug use. The correlation between the student drug use index and the index of the perceived attitudes of other students toward drug use was .18. The degree of specification by the control variables was small, except for parental income.

Only three of the five relationships between the perception of other students' drug use and dimensions of student drug use were statistically significant. In both the significant and the nonsignificant relationships, higher perceived drug use of other students was associated with higher self's drug use. The correlation between the index of student drug use and the index of the perceived drug use of other students was .26. There was some specification of this relationship by the variables of sex, community size, and religiosity.

Six additional factors from the perceived peer drug environment were included in the survey, and each factor was tested with a single measure of student drug use using chi-square. There were significant relationships between the use of marijuana or hashish and the number of dealers known, perceived pressure to use marijuana, proportion of instances of social marijuana usage, and perceived pressure not to use marijuana. The first two relationships were direct and the last two were inverse. Students seeing

Ivy College as having higher than average drug use tended to be low users of drugs, while students seeing Ivy as having equal or lower drug use than other colleges were more likely to be high in drug use.

DISCUSSION

The studies surveyed in the first section of this paper found that drug users were different from nonusers in that they were more likely to overestimate the extent of peer drug use, to feel more social pressure to use drugs, to know more drug users, to have more friends who used drugs, and to be more exposed to the presence of drugs in their social and physical environment. There is nothing in the Ivy College survey that is inconsistent with these findings.

The general tendency of drug users to overestimate the amount of drug use around them was the same at Ivy College as in earlier studies in the literature, but the Ivy College study also asked the question of how drug use on the campus compared with drug use at other colleges with similar characteristics. In this question, high drug users were more likely than low drug users to see Ivy College drug use as equal to or lower than drug use at comparable colleges. This is not inconsistent with other findings, since the comparison of drug use between colleges is a perceptual task of a very different nature from estimating the amount of drug use among friends or fellow students.

In this question it was not the drug users, but rather the nonusers, who distorted the facts. All of the information about raw drug use rates and the variation in rates between colleges of different characteristics that is available in the literature (Gallup, 1969a, 1969b, 1972; Gergen et al., 1971) suggests that drug use at Ivy College is lower than current use levels at comparable colleges. The drug users may have been able to make more accurate statements because they were more aware of the amount of drug use at other colleges through drug culture contacts on these campuses.

The specification of the relationships between student drug use and perceptions of opposite and same sex best friend's drug use as well as the perceived drug use of other students by the control variable of sex produced some interesting results. In all three cases there was a positive relationship for females, but the relationships for males were quite different. Correlations for males were negative for perceptions of opposite and same sex best friend's drug use, but positive and lower for the perceived drug use of other students.

Material from the 53 in-depth interviews that were part of the Ivy

College study indicates that female students are largely turned on to drug use of various kinds by male companions. The correlation between perceived opposite sex best friend's drug use and student drug use for all students was −.04, but this was specified to .30 for females and −.34 for males. In the survey, 91% of the 119 males who were classified as heavy drug users perceived their female best friend as using much less, less, or the same amount of drugs as they did, while only 35% of the 71 females classified as heavy drug users perceived their male best friend in this way. The comparison between correlations for males and females suggests that females are more positively oriented toward their immediate social environment than males. Comparing perceptions of best friend's with other students' drug use, one concludes that sexual differences in orientation toward the social environment decrease as social distance from the self increases.

One possibility to be considered is that sexual differentiation in drug use patterns is due to distorted perceptions arising out of sex role stereotypes (analogous to the sexual double standard discussed by Reiss, 1967) rather than a reflection of true sexual differences. However, bivariate relationships between drug use and sex of respondent showed statistically significant relationships for all ten categories of drug use tested. On the composite index of student drug use, 21% more males than females were rated as high users of drugs.

The pattern of sexual differentiation in drug use was examined by translating differences into ratios of male to female drug use for each category of drugs. When this was done, the drugs fell into three groups. The first group consisted of drugs with serious effects that were fairly often abused and obtained illegally. These were amphetamines, barbiturates, and "hard" hallucinogens. Ratios of ever-use for these drugs ranged from 1.72 to 1.89.

The second group was composed of alcohol and marijuana (including hashish), with ratios of 1.25 for alcohol use once or more per week and 1.48 for marijuana ever used. These were the common drugs of choice for the average Ivy College student. The final group included tobacco, tranquilizers, aspirin, and other legal drugs. The male–female ratios were calculated on the basis of ever-use for tranquilizers and use once per week for the other three categories of drugs. These drugs are legal in American society and their use within reason is normally defined as legitimate. The ratios for this group of drugs varied from .24 to .90.

Cooperstock (1971) has suggested that it is sexual differentiation along an instrumental-expressive continuum that leads to different patterns of drug use between the sexes. This is consistent with reports of higher female use of amphetamines and barbiturates by Goldstein et al. (1970, p. 20) and of sedatives and tranquilizers by Blum and Associates (1969, p. 64). However, the instrumental-expressive continuum of sexual differentiation does not explain why males at Ivy College used barbiturates and amphetamines more than females.

A different model suggested by the Ivy College data is sexual differentiation along the dimension of access to illegal sources of drugs. Males have greater access than females to sources of illegal drugs. Even when females use illegal drugs, they have usually been given to them by male friends in the college peer culture. All of the drugs in the Ivy College study that show higher female use than male use were generally obtained through legal sources of supply. The three drugs showing the largest degree of male over female use were all commonly obtained through illegal sources.

Differentiation by sex in the use of legal and illegal drugs is better explained by the model of differential access to drugs because of their legal status than by Cooperstock's model of an instrumental-expressive continuum, but this does not mean that one model supplants the other. Instead, it may be said that both models have some explanatory power in illuminating the relationship between sex and drugs.

SUMMARY

Data on the use of legal and illegal drugs at Ivy College, a small liberal arts college located west of the Mississippi River, were gathered using questionnaires returned by 95% of the student body and 53 in-depth interviews. Student drug use was found to be related to a number of measures of the perceived peer drug environment. Twenty of the 23 relationships examined were statistically significant at the .05 level or better. Zero-order correlations ranged from −.04 to .61. These correlations were specified by the variables of sex, home community size, parental income, religion, and religiosity. An intriging pattern emerged when the relationships between perceptions of same and opposite sex best friend's drug use and self's drug use were specified by sex.

REFERENCES

BECKER, H.S. Becoming a marihuana user. *Amer. J. Sociology* 49: 235–242, November 1953.

BLUM, R.H., and Associates. *Drugs II: Students and Drugs*. San Francisco: Jossey-Bass, 1969.

BROWN, J.W. A test of a three-stage learning model of drug use. *Criminology* 9: 449–466, February 1972.

CAMPBELL, I.L. *Non-Medical Psychoactive Drug Use at Bishop's University, 1965 to 1970*. Unpublished report. Lennoxville, Canada: Bishop's University, 1970.

COOPERSTOCK, R. Sex differences in the use of mood-modifying drugs: An explanatory model. *J. Health Social Behavior* 12: 238–244, September 1971.

GALLUP OPINION INDEX. *Report Number 48,* June 1969a, pp. 21–31.

GALLUP OPINION INDEX. *Report Number 53,* November 1969b, pp. 7–12.

GALLUP OPINION INDEX. *Report Number 80,* February 1972, pp. 10–30.

GERGEN, M.K., GERGEN, K.J., and MORSE, S.J. *Correlates of Marijuana Use Among College Students*. Unpublished manuscript. Swarthmore, Pennsylvania: Swarthmore College, 1971.

GOLDSTEIN, J.W., KORN, J.H., ABEL, W.H., and MORGAN, R.M. *The Social Psychology and Epidemiology of Student Drug Usage: Report on Phase One* (Report Number 70–18). Pittsburgh: Department of Psychology, Carnegie-Mellon Univ., 1970.

IMPERI, L.L., KLEBER, H.D., and DAVIE, J.S. Use of hallucinogenic drugs on campus. *J. Amer. Med. Assoc.* 204: 1021–1024, June 17, 1968.

JOHNSON, B.D. *Social Determinants of the Use of "Dangerous Drugs" by College Students*. Doctoral dissertation, Columbia Univ., 1971.

KING, F.W. Users and non-users of marijuana: Some attitudinal and behavioral correlates. *J. Amer. College Health Assoc.* 18: 213–217, February 1971.

LINDESMITH, A.R. *Opiate Addiction*. Bloomington, Indiana: Principia Press, 1947.

REISS, I.L. *The Social Context of Premarital Sexual Permissiveness*. New York: Holt, Rinehart and Winston, 1967.

SUCHMAN, E.A. The "hang-loose" ethic and the spirit of drug use. *J. Health Social Behavior* 9: 146–155, June 1968.

THOMAS, W.I., and THOMAS, D.S. *The Child in America*. New York: Knopf, 1928.

The International Journal of the Addictions, 9(6), pp. 863–872, 1974

Methadone on Demand as a Heroin Detoxification Procedure

Roy Stern, M.D.

N. B. Edwards, M.D.

Furey A. Lerro, M.D.

Department of Psychiatry
Temple University Hospital
Philadelphia, Pennsylvania

Abstract

Detoxification procedures for heroin addiction have been, until now, physician-directed. Despite claims that this kind of withdrawal should minimize staff–patient conflicts, our experience has been exactly the opposite. We therefore instituted an addict-controlled detoxification program and tested it on 11 patients. Our findings indicate that addicts do not abuse such a program (they actually use less methadone), staff–patient and staff–staff interactions improve markedly, and the ability to observe the addict as an individual is facilitated.

INTRODUCTION

The process of "detoxification" of the heroin addict tends to be, at best, an unhappy affair. Our experience with this procedure on the inpatient psychiatric unit of the Temple University Health Sciences Center had been, up until a year ago, invariably unpleasant. While an addict was on the floor undergoing detoxification, ward procedures were set topsy-turvy, verbal battles between staff and addict were the rule, problem rounds tended to be dominated by the staff's concern about the addict's "sociophathic" behavior, and thefts tended to increase. The usual impression was that the addict was trying to "con" the staff, i.e., he seemed to be using a combination of charm, withdrawal symptoms, anger, tears, etc. to coerce the physician into increasing his methadone dosage. Generally, as part of the drama, the staff, like a Greek chorus, provided background social commentary composed of an unharmonious blend of optimism, pessimism, overindulgence, hard-nosedness, outright moral indignation, etc.

In trying to decide why this unfortunate state of affairs existed, we came upon the notion that perhaps a crucial variable was the detoxification procedure itself. The addict is taken from one authoritarian system (viz., society), which he continually tries to "beat" in order to get his drug, and is thrown into another equally authoritarian system where dosage of methadone and dosage schedules are determined for him. It seemed to us that the stimulus "authoritarian system" might be sufficient to produce the response consisting of an entire array of sociopathic behaviors that we had consistently observed.

Our detoxification procedure, prior to 1 year ago, most closely approximated that of Blachly (1968) who recommends the use of up to 40 mg on day 1 of withdrawal with 10 mg decrements daily once the addict is stabilized. Other authors have suggested alternative schedules. Wesson et al. (1972) suggest starting all inpatients on 40 mg methadone daily, then withdrawing 5 mg daily after stabilization. It is interesting to note that although Wenson et al. admit that this dosage may be far in excess of the addict's needs, they feel that this standardizing approach will avoid staff–patient conflict over dosage. Another schedule is recommended by the AMA Council on Mental Health and Committee on Alcoholism and Drug Dependence (1972); they suggest up to 40 mg of methadone initially with daily decrements of 20% once stabilization occurs.

More important than these slight differences in dosage regimens, however, is that they all share the quality of being physician–staff controlled. Hence, no matter what schedule is used, they would all tend to reproduce the adversary relationship which we had come to know so well.

A further undesirable phenomenon, which seemed to go along with our previous detoxification procedure, was that we seemed to know little about our addicts as either individuals vis-a-vis their habits or simply as people. On reflection this seemed to be a side effect of the "adversary relationship" described above, i.e., the "conning behavior" was so dramatic as to obscure our vision of other behaviors, while on the addict's part he was so busy reacting to the system that he had little time left for other behaviors. It seemed that our rigidly defined treatment program, by reducing the freedom of the patient to act spontaneously on his environment, was erasing clues about individual differences, including motivation.

The primary purpose of this study was to devise and test a detoxification procedure which might avoid these problems. Therefore, we decided to place the responsibility for withdrawal directly under the control of the addict, thereby relieving him of the need to control by manipulation with the hope that this would reduce many of the difficulties in staff–patient interactions. We further hoped that having removed both the staff and the patient from the adversary relationship, the individual differences in addicts (i.e., motivation and character structure) might be more accurately and consistently observed.

The specific questions which we attempted to answer were:

1. Can the withdrawal schedule be left to the patient without his abusing the privilege?
2. Would such a program change staff–patient and staff–staff interactions?
3. What indicators will such a program yield as far as describing the individual who is addicted?

It should be noted that no "cure" for the heroin addiction was intended. We were aware that the real problems of "kicking the habit" seem to begin only on leaving the hospital.

Patients and Treatment Setting

Patients were drawn from the Temple catchment area, a predominantly Black urban ghetto, and from nearby surburban communities. We applied no selection procedure other than to limit the number of addicts on the floor to one at a time, a restriction we have assiduously followed for several years.

The variety of individuals and problems of addiction encountered in this study are well represented by the following examples.

Patient 1 was a veteran from a suburban community whose girl friend was being withdrawn at another hospital. When she died while being withdrawn, he increased his dosage and signed out AMA.

Patient 2 was a 25 bag/day, 18-year-old city addict with two prior withdrawal attempts.

Patient 3 was also from a suburban community with an 8 bag/day, $1\frac{1}{2}$ year addiction, who had previously been detoxified using up to 60 mg methadone per day.

Patient 4 was a 25 bag/day, 8-year-old city addict from a family where addiction was endemic.

Patient 5 was an 18-year-old, 14 bag/day city addict, in many senses the most professional of the group, who commented that the ease of his withdrawal was a reflection on the street drugs commonly on the market.

Patient 6 was a young woman from a suburban community who used an occasional 3 to 4 bags/day over a $1\frac{1}{2}$-year period. After discharge she managed to get herself into a methadone maintenance program which necessitated a daily trip into the city.

The treatment setting was Temple University Health Sciences Center's inpatient psychiatry unit. This is a 25-bed short stay unit (average of 21 days) specializing in differential diagnosis and the acute treatment of practically all severe behavior disorders (behavior problems of childhood, severe neuroses, functional psychoses, various organic brain disorders ranging from acute metabolic disturbances to Alzheimer's and Pick's Disease, and, of course, drug addictions).

METHOD

Patients seeking detoxification for heroin addiction were informed that methadone would be dispensed to them in 5 mg doses at their request, with no limitations. We asked only that drugs be taken, as is all medication, under observation at the nursing station. We felt this to be necessary for the accurate tabulation of dosage and timing and to reduce the possibility of individual doses being saved and then taken at one time. Nursing staff was instructed to do nothing to discourage patients from taking methadone. To overcome staff trepidations concerning the possibility of overdosage, we decided to maintain some short-run control by requesting that if more than a certain amount of methadone (i.e., 40 mg in 2 hr) was taken, the nursing staff was to contact the physician who then had the option of abandoning the program. Minor tranquilizers were only occasionally used. We also instructed each addict that, should it become obvious after a week to 10 days that he was making no real attempt to withdraw, we would consider discharging him but that this would be open to negotiation.

RESULTS

As can be seen from Table 1, practically all patients reached a dosage level of 0 mg/day for at least 1 day prior to leaving the hospital. Of the two who did not, one left the hospital against medical advice soon after learning his girl friend had died in another hospital.

Tables 2 and 3 compare the present and prior Temple programs on habit strength (bags/day and duration) and detoxification indices (amount of methadone taken and duration of stay).

The information shown in Table 2 regarding size and duration of habit was obtained from a number of sources. A complete history was obtained on each patient on admission. Many items of this history, including size and duration of habit, were reviewed with the patient every 2 or 3 days until the day of discharge. Confirmatory historical data on these variables were also collected from relatives, friends, and referral agencies. When any large discrepancies existed between the patient's history and that obtained from other sources, the resident met with the patient and family member, friend, or agent of the referral source to clear up these differences. In all cases it was possible, using all these sources, to come to a consensus on size and duration of habit.

Table 1
Individual Detoxification Schedules

	Hospital day												
Patient record no.	1	2	3	4	5	6	7	8	9	10	11	12	13
46–20–02 (1)	30	25	20	10	60	50		(Signed out AMA)					
46–43–51 (2)	5	15	10	10	10	0	0	0	15	10	5		
46–41–22 (3)	10	10	10	10	0	0	0	0	0	0	0		
30–69–41 (4)	10	15	5	5	10	5	0						
46–83–56 (5)	10	20	15	15	15	15	10	10	5	0	0	0	0
46–55–74 (6)	10	10	0	0									
47–43–45 (7)	15	10	10	0	0								
47–44–65 (8)	20	20	15	10	0	0	0	0					
44–40–46 (9)	15	15	0	0	0								
47–42–50 (10)	0	0	0										
47–59–31 (11)	20	25	35	25	30	25	5	0	10	10	0		

Table 2
Habit and Detoxification under Present Program

	Habit		Detoxification		
Patient	Bags/day	Years addicted	Days in hospital	Total methadone, mg	Average methadone day, mg
1	5	3	6	185.	30.8
2	25	18	11	80	7.3
3	8	1.5	11	40	3.6
4	25	8	7	50	7.1
5	7	5	13	115	8.8
6	5	1.5	4	20	5.0
7	5	4	5	35	7.0
8	14	18	8	65	8.1
9	12	2	5	30	6.0
10	4	1.5	6	0.	0.
11	45	5	11	185.	16.8
Total:	155	67.5	87	805.	100.5
Average:	14	6.1	7.9	73.1	9.14

Table 3
Habit and Detoxification Prior to Present Procedure

	Habit		Detoxification		
Patient	Bags/day	Years addicted	Days in hospital	Total methadone, mg	Average methadone day, mg
44–08–25	6	2	6	50	8.33
44–54–25	15	2	14	150	10.71
44–32–37	8	11	12	235	19.56
45–14–57	30	3	6	60	10.00
41–18–26	22	2	9	78.5	8.72
43–54–79	5	2	21	175	8.33
39–46–89	2	2	4	50	12.5
X	8	5	11	80	7.27
Total:	96	29	83	878.5	85.44
Average:	12	3.625	10.375	110.	10.65

It is noteworthy that some patients chose practically no methadone at all and, in the case of Patient #10, absolutely none. From our data it is impossible to single out any one variable as critical in this respect. No doubt personality factors, motivation, and habit strength and duration are all relevant. Certainly, in the case of Patient #10, his relatively small size and short duration of habit were important, although he might have simply been in a hurry to get out of the hospital for reasons unknown to us. One patient (Patient #5) reflected on his ease of withdrawal as an indicator of the relatively bad stuff available on the street. However, on a more general level, the ease of withdrawal noted by us may simply be a result of removing the patient from the adversary relationship, i.e., giving him the *responsibility* he has asked for by taking it on his shoulders to get off drugs.

Figure 1 compares length of hospital stay and total methadone required (on the average) of our present program, our previous program, and three other published regimens.

In terms of hospital stay, our present program lies about in the middle, but in terms of total methadone required, our current figures are decidedly smaller. The present group treated at Temple remained an average of 2.4 fewer days in hospital and required, on the average, 3.7 mg less methadone than those detoxified under the physician-controlled program.

CHANGES IN WARD INTERACTION

The most striking results took place in staff–patient and staff–staff interactions. The atmosphere of the adversary relationship was, for all practical purposes, gone. The mood of excitement which had previously been

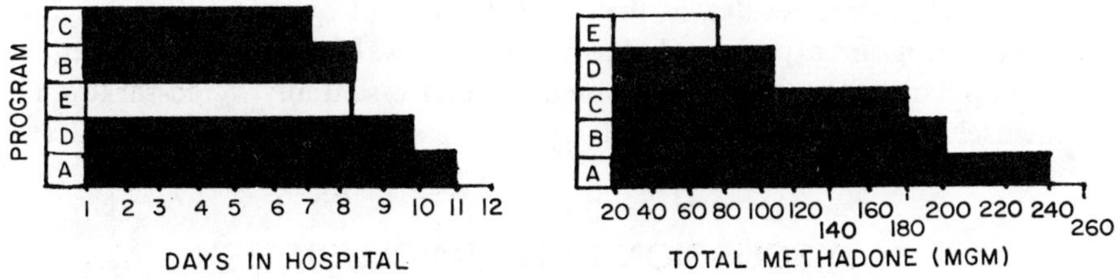

Fig. 1. Comparison of length of stay and total methadone used in five programs, A = University of California (estimated); B = American Medical Association recommended (estimated); C = Lexington (estimated); D = Temple prior to present program; E = Temple during present program. The figures for A, B, and C are estimates based on descriptions of typical withdrawal regimens found in publications from these institutions. We have assumed a "stabilization period" of 3 days for each set of figures.

generated by the question of who was going to outfox whom was no longer present. No longer did the addicts regale staff and other patients with the heroic aspects and sizes of their street habits or the amount of pain they were suffering from withdrawal. The preoccupation on the part of the staff with how much methadone was taken and whether a particular dose was "really necessary" also declined markedly. Gone also were Messianic therapeutic efforts and the traditional disagreements between "knowledgable" senior staff and "naive" residents as to the "motivation" of the particular addict. There was, moreover, a sudden, unexplained decrease in thefts (purses and cash) and consequently in the fear of thefts.

Although we repeatedly instructed the staff that no attempt should be made to convince patients to reduce their dosages, some continued to find it diffcult to entirely inhibit this therapeutic urge. Considering the orientation of "Helping Professionals," it may well be impossible to eliminate this completely. Furthermore, it did not seem to materially interfere with the addict's voluntary withdrawal.

Seemingly as a consequence of these improved ward interactions, it became much easier for us to deal with various problems of the *individual* addict—problems we had previously agonized about. For example, one patient from a middle-class community who had decided to come in, mainly to escape the last of a series of criminal charges for dealing in drugs, was discharged without qualms when marijuana was found in his bed. Another patient who was admitted for addiction and impulsive behavior was also found to have signs of mental retardation and hypomania and was taken off methadone and placed on thorazine. Still a third patient who showed no signs of decreasing his dosage was discharged after he attempted to molest an extremely seductive but psychotic patient.

An interesting result was the fact that none of our patients under the present program experienced objective withdrawal symptoms (piloerection or pupillary dilatation) even though several essentially "cold-turkeyed" themselves. Also G.I. complaints and restlessness were noted only a few times and were invariably mild.

DISCUSSION AND CONCLUSIONS

The answers to the three questions posed previously would now seem to be apparent.

1. The withdrawal schedule *can* be left to the addict without his abusing the privilege.

2. Such a program does change staff–patient and staff–staff interactions.
3. These changes do seem to free us to observe more accurately the individual who is addicted.

The question as to whether some of our patients were actually fully detoxified might easily be raised since only seven of the 11 spent two or more drug-free days in the hospital. The likelihood that some patients merely reduced their requirements for heroin certainly exists. However, as the large overall rate of recidivism would indicate, we doubt that the actual breaking of the habit occurs very often in the hospital. Therefore, insisting on every patient reaching a stable zero level seemed rather pointless and might easily have hampered our obtaining meaningful results in the areas of interactions and individual patient behaviors.

Admittedly, our results in the interactions between staff and patients and staff and staff were nonobjectified, but they were too glaringly obvious to ignore. A typical day on our ward with an addict undergoing withdrawal was almost magically transformed from a practically continuous hassle (previous program) to a rather pleasant routine day in the care of the psychiatrically disturbed (present program).

As to our reactions to the individuals concerned, we found that, having broken the preoccupation with withdrawal and the stereotyped staff–addict relationship, we felt able to act more appropriately to each individual patient, to assess motivation more accurately, and to escape provocations which we had previously accepted passively in order to complete withdrawal.

Since the methadone-on-demand technique seemed to avoid pathological confrontations by placing the major onus of treatment on the addict himself, and since this inclusion of the addict in the treatment planning has the effect of appealing to his maturity rather than to the regressive and childish aspects of his personality, we believe there is reasonable justification for this approach to detoxification. Although some patients showed a somewhat lagging interest in decreasing their dose of methadone, we did not encounter any gross misuse of this program, nor did there seem to be a tendency to escalate the dosage.

Addiction is, after all, the responsibility and predicament of the addict, and it seems somewhat inappropriate for the physician to pretend, act, or feel that either the responsibility or ability for successful withdrawal is in his powers. For the physician to take part in such a charade does harm not only to his capacity to relate to the addict, but to his ability to conceptualize the problem as well. What was striking, after even a brief period of detoxification under these circumstances, was the remission, overtly at least, of the usual patterns of interaction, thus enabling the staff to view the addict as a person.

ACKNOWLEDGMENT

The authors wish to express their appreciation to Dr. John Ball, Professor of Psychiatry, Temple University, for his critical assistance.

REFERENCES

A.M.A. COUNCIL ON MENTAL HEALTH AND COMMITTEE ON ALCOHOLISM AND DRUG DEPENDENCE REPORT. Treatment of morphine-type dependence by withdrawal methods. *J. Amer. Med. Assoc.* 219: 1611–1615, 1972.

BLACHLY, P.H. Management of the opiate abstinence syndrome. *Amer. J. Psychiat.* 122: 742–744, January 1968.

WESSON, D.R., GAY, G.R., and SMITH, D. Managing narcotic and sedative withdrawal, *Hosp. Physician* 8: 52–55, January 1972.

The International Journal of the Addictions, 9(6), pp. 873–878, 1974

Social and Psychological Factors Associated with Length of Stay in a Drug Treatment Facility

Vitali V. Rozynko, Ph.D.

Veterans Administration Hospital
Palo Alto, California

Kenneth B. Stein, Ph.D.

Psychology Department
University of California, Berkeley
Berkeley, California

Recent widespread concern about drug abuse has resulted in the establishment of an increasing number of drug rehabilitation facilities throughout the nation. Certain types of rehabilitation programs, however, seem to have little appeal to drug addicts (O'Malley et al., 1972). While some other programs report high treatment success rates (DeLeon et al., 1972), they are very selective in their admission policy (Cummings and McGarraugh, 1972). Thus it appears that many drug addicts in the population receive little or no treatment.

In the context of another study (Stein and Rozynko, 1973) the authors had the opportunity to interview and administer psychological tests to a large sample of drug addicts who admitted themselves voluntarily to a drug detoxification ward. The drug detoxification ward was located in a California State Hospital which also offered a limited number of possibilities for long-term treatment. The study sought to identify some existing relationships between demographic, social, and psychological variables and whether the addict entered into longer term treatment.

THE SETTING

During the 7-month period of the study, the drug detoxification patients were admitted, for the most part, from an urban area 120 miles from the hospital. Over 95% of these admissions were voluntary and constituted referrals from one of the many city agencies from which the drug addict initially sought assistance. The detoxification program consisted of drug-assisted (methadone and tranquilizers) withdrawal, after which the patient was discharged with referrals to one of the continued treatment agencies. Longer term treatment was available to a minority of patients, namely, those who might be admitted to "The Family," a confrontation-type long-term rehabilitation program; and a 30-day short-term treatment program whose treatment methods were heavily "Family" influenced. In addition, those patients who were observed to be disorganized or to have severe psychiatric symptomatology were admitted to psychiatric wards for the acutely disturbed. The admission rate of drug addicts to the detoxification ward during the study period averaged 210 admissions per month. Although admission to longer term treatment averaged 20%, only 10% of those admitted to the detoxification ward stayed in treatment for 20 days or more.

METHOD

Two-hundred forty-two randomly selected voluntary male admissions to the detoxification ward of a California State Hospital were interviewed. The structured interview extracted information about demographic characteristics, drug use history, and family background. Psychological tests were administred to 201 of the 242 sample. They included the Minnesota Multiphasic Personality Inventory (MMPI) (Hathaway and McKinley, 1951), Tryon-Stein-Chu scales (TSC) (Stein, 1968) derived from the MMPI, the Motoric Ideational Sensory Test (MIST) (Stein and Lenrow, 1970), the Socialization (So) scale of the California Psychological Inventory (CPI) (Gough, 1957), and the Future and Past Time Perspective Tests (Stein and Craik, 1965). In addition, two measures of intellectual level were administered: Extended Range Vocabulary Test -V-3- (Educational Testing

Service, 1962a) and the Hidden Patterns Test -CF-2- (Educational Testing Service, 1962b).

Forty-one fewer patients were tested than interviewed because that number was discharged before they could be tested. The fact that a substantial minority of the patients left before testing could be accomplished (within 2 days) provided an opportunity for a preliminary and exploratory study of social background differences related to very early departures from the detoxification unit.

The interview responses of the 41 patients who left early were compared with the responses of the 201 patients who stayed long enough to be tested. This comparison yielded suggestive results and a more differentiated analysis was therefore undertaken. In the more differentiated analysis, the 201 subjects who completed both interview and testing were divided into four groups according to length of stay—2 days or less, 3 to 6 days, 7 to 19 days, and 20+ days. The number of subjects in each group was 26, 123, 27 and 25 respectively. Since the standard detoxification period was 6 days, the relatively great number of subjects in the second group was expected. Statistical comparisons between groups were calculated, utilizing chi square and t tests. Significance levels were uniformly set at the .05 level or below.

RESULTS

The differentiated analysis showed few significant differences to be present between either the two shorter stay groups (2 days or less and 3 to 6 days) or between the two longer stay groups (7 to 19 days and 20+ days). On the other hand, a large number of significant differences were observed between the two shorter stay groups and the two longer stay groups.

The shorter stay groups were older, contained a significantly smaller number of single individuals and a significantly greater number of Blacks (significantly smaller number of Whites). A greater proportion of the shorter stay groups used heroin and a lesser proportion reported using marijuana as their principal drug. The shorter stay group also reported a greater or more frequent use of their principal drug (heroin, mostly) and a higher daily drug expense. The longer stay groups reported a higher rate of using secondary drugs. There was also a tendency for the longer stay group to report longer prison sentences, though the shorter stay group reported a higher proportion of arrests having occurred 2 or more years ago. Both the shortest and longest stay groups reported a significantly higher use of LSD.

The psychological test results showed lower MMPI paranoid and masculinity–femininity scale scores and lower introversion and depression scale scores for the shorter stay groups. The shorter stay groups also had significantly higher past time perspective scores and lower intelligence test scores. A set of tables reflecting the findings described above can be obtained from the senior author.

DISCUSSION

A variety of factors were probably responsible in causing differential length of stay. The results suggest that one of the factors responsible for shorter stays might have been pervasive involvement in a life style in which drug acquisition and use served as a central focus for daily activites. This type of addict might be expected to show a transitory desire but ostensibly a relative disinterest in eliminating his addiction. Staff employed in the detoxification ward observed that many individuals admitted to the unit openly expressed their desire to reduce their heroin habituation level, thereby hoping to attain the same "high" but with less money. The longer stay patients showed signs of more psychological discomfort, alienation from others, and dysphoria, while the shorter stay patients present themselves as much more integrated.

The results of this study were very likely influenced by the environment of the treatment facility and its location. The ward itself was often overcrowded, and individual attention was often difficult to obtain. The treatment facility was located some distance from the patients' homes, and it was noted that there was a tendency for the nonsingle drug addicts to leave earlier. In addition, the longer term rehabilitation programs available espoused philosophies which appeared to be directly contradictory to the life styles of most of the addicts admitted to the detoxification wards. The treatment programs, moreover, attempted to select very promising persons and to screen out those whom they predicted might be difficult to manage. The social and institutional factors identified above militated for longer stay only among those addicts who were either severely disturbed or very desperately concerned in eliminating their addiction.

The problem of length of stay in voluntary drug treatment programs is fairly widespread and costly, since early terminators, while incurring financial burden for the treating organization, fail to remain in the treatment environment long enough to alter the problem behavior. The study shows the presence of both social and demographic as well as psychological test differences among the length of stay groups. Closer scrutiny of such multileveled characteristics can potentially yield answers and approaches to drug treatment centers, administrators, and decision makers in order to cope with this problem. Further research, however, should include a wider range of psychological variables. The study of the relation between psychological types and length of stay may also yield fruitful results.

The present study points out a problem which we suspect is relatively prevalent among drug treatment programs, namely, that available drug treatment programs attract a small minority and conversely screen out the majority of drug addicts. The paradoxical consequence of this type of institutional behavior is the denial or unavailability of definitive treatment to those persons who cause the greatest problems to society. Development of programs located closer to the community and based on a variety of treatment programs, both psychological and chemical, seems indicated.

SUMMARY

Two hundred and one randomly selected admissions to a rural state hospital drug detoxification ward were interviewed and given psychological tests. Interview and psychological variables thus obtained were related to length of stay in the hospital. Results showed that length of stay was related to a number of demographic variables, amount and pattern of drug use, and personality and intelligence test scores. Ramifications of the results to further research and development of drug abuse treatment programs were discussed.

ACKNOWLEDGMENTS

This research was supported in part by the grant MH 17647 from the National Institute of Mental Health of the U.S. Public Health Service.

Our appreciation is expressed to Kathleen Sherman for her invaluable assistance in this research.

REFERENCES

CUMMINGS, R.J., and MCGARRAUGH, M. Report on services relating to drug abuse. *In a Final Report to the Hennepin County Task Force on Alcoholism and Inebriety*. Minneapolis, Minnesota, Hennepin County: Copeland Associates, 1972.

DELEON, G., HOLLAND, S., and ROSENTHAL, M.S. Phoenix House: Criminal activity of dropouts. *J. Amer. Med. Assoc.* 222: 686–689, 1972.

EDUCATIONAL TESTING SERVICE. *Extended Range Vocabulary Test-V-3*. Princeton, New Jersey: Educational Testing Service, 1962a.

EDUCATIONAL TESTING SERVICE. *Hidden Patterns Test CF-2*. Princeton, New Jersey: Educational Testing Service, 1972b.

GOUGH, H.G. *Manual for the California Psychological Inventory*. Palo Alto, California: Consulting Psychologists Press, 1957.

HATHAWAY, S.R., and MCKINLEY, J.C. *The Minnesota Multiphasic Personality Inventory Manual,* rev. ed. New York: Psychological Corp. 1951.

O'MALLEY, J.E., ANDERSON, W.H., and LAZARE, A. Failure of outpatient treatment of drug abuse I. Heroin. *Amer. J. Psychiat.* 128: 865–868, 1972.

STEIN, K.B. The TSC Scales: The outcome of a cluster analysis of the 550 MMPI items. In P. McReynold (ed.) *Advances in Psychological Assessment*. Palo Alto, California: Science and Behavioral Press, 1968.

STEIN, K.B., and CRAIK, K.H. Relationship between motoric and ideational activity preference and time perspective in neurotics and schizophrenics. *J. Consult. Psychol.* 29: 460–467, 1965.

STEIN, K.B., and LENROW, P. Expressive styles and their measurement. *J. Personality Social Psychol.* 16: 656–664, 1970.

STEIN, K.B., and ROZYNKO, V. Personality patterns of drug abusers. Manuscript, 1973.

The International Journal of the Addictions, 9(6), pp. 879–883, 1974

Illicit Drug Use by College Students: Three-Year Trends, 1970–1972

Douglas P. Ferraro, Ph.D.

David K. Billings, B.A.

Department of Psychology
University of New Mexico
Albuquerque, New Mexico

We have previously reported the 3-year trends in marijuana use among college students at a large Southwestern state university (Ferraro and Billings, 1974). Between 1970 and 1972 there were two significant trends in marijuana use which are worthy of special note. First, the student's initial use of marijuana occurred at a younger age. Second, an increasing number of students were using marijuana. However, the rate at which marijuana use was increasing appeared to be diminishing between 1971 and 1972 as compared to the preceding 2-year period. We now report similar 3-year trends in the illicit use of hallucinogens, stimulants, barbiturate-sedatives, and narcotics for the same student population.

METHOD

Shortly after commencement of the fall semester for the years 1970–1972, a three-part, 51–item, multiple-choice questionnaire was group administered to students attending introductory courses at the University of New Mexico. The survey method used has been described previously along with the results for Parts I and III of the survey which pertained to general background variables of the student and to the use of marijuana (Ferraro and Billings, 1974). This report presents data from Part II of the survey which was concerned with the illicit use of psychotropic drugs excluding marijuana. More explicitly, for each of the hallucinogenic, stimulant, barbiturate-sedative, and narcotic drug classes, students were asked whether they had ever used a drug not prescribed by a physician and if so, how often they had used the drug and when they had first used the drug.* The overall data sample was the same as used in our prior report on marihuana except that students who had not responded consistently on Part II of the survey were eliminated from further study. Consequently, the sizes of the student samples for the years 1970–1972 were reduced by 302, 347, and 345 students, respectively. The final sample sizes for the 3 years were 2,744, 2,409, and 2,787.

RESULTS

Trends in General Use of Illicit Drugs

The precentage of students who had ever illicitly used a psychotropic drug is presented by year for each drug class in the left side of Table 1. As expected in a college student population, hallucinogens and stimulants were used by more students than were barbiturates and narcotics. However, for each drug class there was a consistent increase in the percentage of drug users across the 3 survey years. A standard chi-square test of independence indicated that these upward trends in illicit drug use were significant ($p <$ .05, $df = 2$) across the 3 years for each drug class. The respective χ^2 values were: hallucinogens, 35.70; stimulants, 24.74; barbiturates, 31.39; narcotics, 56.14.

In our previous marijuana study we observed that the rate of increase in marijuana use had diminished between 1971 and 1972 as compared to the preceding 2-year period. Similar trends in general use of illicit drugs are suggested in the right side of Table 1 which presents the percentage of possible increase that actually occurred between successive years of the survey. This measure is a direct indicant of the rate of change in drug use. As it

* A copy of the questionnaire used may be obtained by writing to Dr. Ferraro at the address given in the Acknowledgments.

Table 1
Percentage of College Students Who Had Ever used Illicit Drugs and Percentage of Possible Change in Illicit Drug Use for Each Survey Year

Drug	Percentage use			Percentage change	
	1970	1971	1972	1970–1971	1971–1972
Hallucinogen	24.0	29.8	30.8	7.6	1.4
Stimulant	21.9	26.8	27.2	6.3	.5
Barbiturate	13.5	17.9	18.8	5.1	1.1
Narcotic	11.9	18.8	18.0	7.8	−1.0

may be seen from Table 1, a sizeable increase in drug use occurred between 1970 and 1971 for all drug classes with little further change in the rate of drug taking being observed between the subsequent two years. As a point of reference, the comparable percentage change scores for marijuana were 18.7% for 1970–1971 and 11.4% for 1971–1972.

Trends in Frequency of Illicit Drug Use

In order to avoid the confounding which would occur if students were surveyed in more than one year of the study, analysis of the trends in the frequency of using a particular drug were limited to those freshmen in each year's sample who had used the drug at least once. The resulting sample sizes across the 3 years for the separate drug classes were: hallucinogens, 923; stimulants, 762; barbiturates, 587; narcotics, 544 freshman students.

No significant trends in the frequency of drug use were obtained for the freshman students during the 3 survey years. Accordingly, the total number of drug experiences were averaged across the 3 years for presentation in Table 2. These data show that not only were hallucinogens and stimulants used by more college students, but they were also used a larger number of times than were barbiturates and narcotics. It might be noted, however, that all drug classes contained a sizeable portion of students who had used the drug more than 30 times. Most mentionable in this regard is that over 10% of the narcotic using freshman had had at least 30 illicit experiences with narcotics.

Trends in First Use of Illicit Drugs

In each year of the survey, the first use of an illicit drug of any class occurred before the college years for over 50% of the drug-using students.

Table 2

Total Number of Illicit Drug Experiences for Those College Freshmen Who Had Ever Used the Drug Given in Percentages for the Three Survey Years

	Number of drug experiences				
Drug	1	2–4	5–14	15–30	>30
Hallucinogen	16.4	21.7	23.8	15.0	23.1
Stimulant	15.0	23.0	25.7	11.8	24.5
Barbiturate	19.9	34.4	23.7	8.8	13.1
Narcotic	25.2	36.6	20.2	7.2	10.8

Table 3

Percentage of Illicit Drug Users Who First Used the Drug in Junior High School, Senior High School, or Undergraduate College for Each Survey Year

Drug	Grade	1970	1971	1972
Hallucinogen	Jr. High	3.3	4.3	6.9
	Sr. High	48.5	52.4	52.2
	College	48.2	43.3	40.9
Stimulant	Jr. High	5.1	6.5	9.9
	Sr. High	46.1	48.4	51.0
	College	48.8	45.1	39.1
Barbiturate	Jr. High	9.6	14.6	12.2
	Sr. High	54.0	54.2	59.1
	College	36.4	31.3	28.7
Narcotic	Jr. High	6.1	4.2	6.1
	Sr. High	50.0	41.7	52.3
	College	43.9	54.1	41.6

Table 3 further shows that there was a consistent increase across the 3 survey years in the incidence of first illicit drug use during both the junior high and senior high school grades. A standard chi-square test of independence indicated that these 3-year trends toward earlier drug use were statistically significant ($p < .05$) for each drug class except the barbiturates. The respective χ^2 values with four degrees of freedom were: hallucinogens, 15.84; stimulants, 19.34; barbiturates, 9.24; and narcotics, 15.86. Consistent with these trends, and of particular interest, is the general observation that a larger proportion of precollege users of illicit drugs were drawn from the junior high school grades across the 3-year period surveyed.

SUMMARY

The 3-year trends in illicit use of hallucinogens, stimulants, barbiturates, and narcotics by college students at the University of New Mexico closely paralleled the trends in marijuana use previously reported for these same students. Not only had an increasing number of students ever used an ilicit drug, but they had done so at an earlier age in each succeeding year of the survey. The rate of increase in illicit drug use was considerably greater between 1970 and 1971 than it was between 1971 and 1972. Indeed, the small changes observed between these latter 2 years indicate that illicit drug use might be stabilizing, or perhaps even tending toward a future downturn, among the college student population. However, since not all students can be expected eventually to use an illicit drug, some caution must be exercised in interpreting these latter trends. It may be that the apparent stability in the percentage of new users of illicit drugs harbors the fact that the proportion of potential drug users who have not yet used an illicit drug has been decreasing over the years rather than reflecting a decreasing student interest in illicit drug use.

ACKNOWLEDGMENTS

Research supported, in part, by Drug Resources for University Groups and Department of Psychology, University of New Mexico. The authors thank Marsha Summers and James Trost for their help in collecting the data and Elka Grisham for her preparation of the manuscript. Reprints may be obtained from Dr. Douglas P. Ferraro, 176 Psychology Hall, University of New Mexico, Albuquerque, N. M. 87131.

REFERENCE

FERRARO, D.P., and BILLINGS, D.K. Marihuana use by college students: Three-year trends, 1970–1972. *Intern. J. Addictions* 9: 321, 1974.

The International Journal of the Addictions, 9(6), pp. 885–890, 1974

Research Note

Sampling Technique for Medically Significant Drug Abuse

P. H. Blachly, M.D.

B. J. Blachly, R.N., M.S.

University of Oregon Medical School
Portland, Oregon

Although there are many reports of drug habits of students, there has been little information regarding how much of drug abuse is medically significant. Deaths from overdose provide data from extreme cases and are comparatively rare as opposed to admissions to emergency rooms. Further, some drugs of abuse such as marijuana and LSD do not in themselves cause death. One practical and measurable indication of significance is whether drug use is the direct or indirect cause of admission to a hospital.

With the assistance of the administrators and medical record librarians of several major hospitals in Portland and Salem, we sampled records at regular intervals for the 5 years, 1968 through 1972. These hospitals handle the vast majority of all hospitalizations in this area. All of the records for admissions to the emergency rooms of these hospitals were sampled for the first week in January, April, July, and October for the years 1968–1972. Every emergency room admission note was read, and any note in the chart indicating that the reason for admission was directly or indirectly related to drugs or alcohol was recorded as was the name of the drug when indicated. In addition, data was obtained for all admissions for drug abuse to the state hospital which serves this area. If more than one drug was indicated as a cause of admission, both drugs were listed so as to provide a pattern of the popularity of each drug. In approximately 15% of cases, more than one drug was used.

In the material from the private hospitals there are two possible sources of error. First, we have reason to believe that private physicians and private hospitals are more likely to underreport drug abuse as a reason for admission. Second, the small private hospitals tend to have fewer admissions so that there will be increased variability from one sampling period to another.

RESULTS AND DISCUSSION

Figure 1 indicates emergency room admissions due to alcohol and drugs to general hospitals. Inspection reveals that while alcohol is a more frequent cause for admission to Multnomah Hospital than drugs, the other hospitals' admissions are now about the same for drug misuse as for alcohol abuse. Multnomah Hospital and Emanuel Hospital get the bulk of admissions for drug and alcohol abuse in Multnomah County. Between 5 and 10% of admissions to the emergency room at Multnomah Hospital are directly related to drug or alcohol abuse.

Overall, medically significant drug abuse appeared to hit a peak in late 1970 and 1971 and appears to be less in 1972. This decrease is most marked for opiates and hallucinogens. Use of sedatives of the barbiturate type may be decreasing very slightly. Amphetamines may just be beginning to taper off.

The drugs labeled as "other" include a wide variety of medications, often psychotropic drugs such as antipsychotics and antidepressants prescribed by physicians. Their misuse may be increasing.

Inspection of Fig. 2, which names the drugs causing admission to Dammasch State Hospital, reveals that the peak for heroin was in 1970 and 1971 and likewise for other opiates, amphetamines, and LSD. (In this chart each square equals one patient and each column is a month, so that in this case all patients are recorded as opposed to the sampling procedure used at the general hospitals.) We would expect in time, as the use of methadone increases and heroin decreases, that there will be an increase in "opiates (other)."

The use of barbiturates seems to be unchanged or minimally decreasing, but this is more than compensated by other sedatives such as glutethamide, ethchlorvynol, and methaqualone. Volatile solvents such as glue account for very few admissions although there appeared to be some slight increase

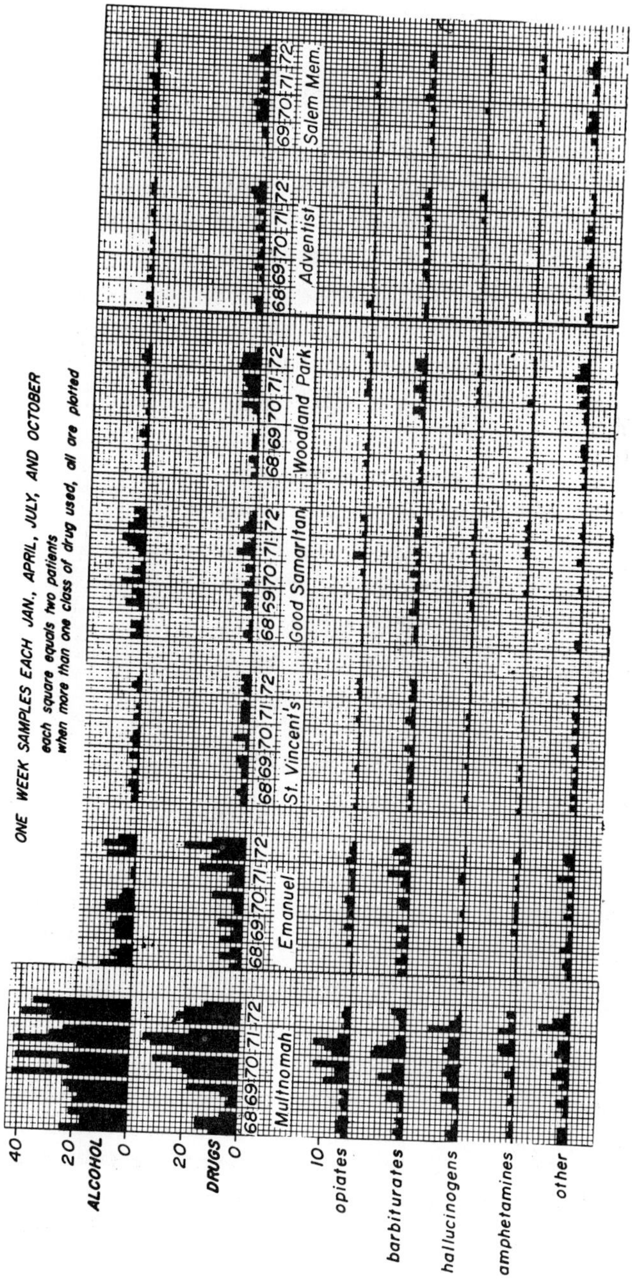

Fig. 1. Emergency room admissions due to alcohol and drugs.

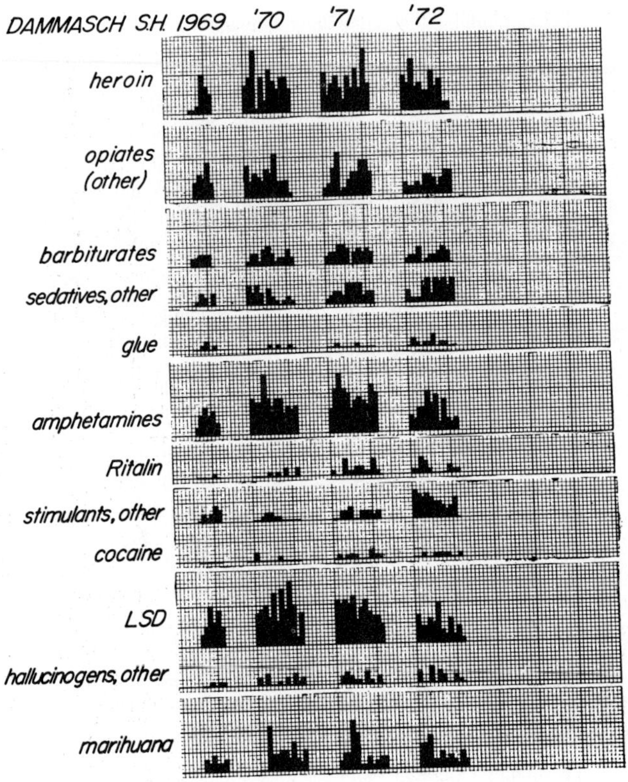

Fig. 2. Drugs named as cause of admission.

in 1972. Abuse of the stimulant methylphenidate had quite a fad, particularly among the Black community in 1970 and 1971, and it appears that this may be somewhat subsiding. Other stimulants, however, such as methamphetamine and desoxyephedrine, have become more popular. Whereas cocaine was rarely used in this community a few years ago, it seems to be gradually increasing.

Because the results of chemical analysis indicate that drugs purported to be mescaline and peyote are in fact LSD, the values for LSD and hallucinogens (other) should likely be combined. Nevertheless, it is encouraging to see that these drugs are less frequently the cause of admission than a year or two ago. The figures for marijuana are probably not significant, and it is very rare that marijuana would be a sole cause for admission.

The figures from Dammasch State Hospital and the general medical hospitals are generally consistent. They suggest that medically significant consequences of illicit drug abuse are no longer increasing, and in fact are probably decreasing with the peak of the disturbance having occurred in late 1970 and 1971.

Possible explanations for the decrease include the following.

1. The fad of drug use is no longer as attractive. (Campus reports suggest that college students are less interested in drugs.)
2. Drug users have learned to control their drug use so that it less frequently gives rise to hospitalization.
3. There has been no waiting list for acceptance into methadone treatment since late 1971.
4. Physicians are being more cautious in prescribing drugs with potential for abuse. This may be in part due to stricter drug control laws.
5. Law enforcement efforts may be more effective in curtailing availability of drugs.

We conclude that this method of sampling medically significant drug abuse is efficient, inexpensive, and gives a sample of trends of drug abuse. Methods of sampling that depend upon voluntary reporting from emergency rooms by clerks, whose main job is elsewhere, are fraught with inaccuracies and subjective variation. A combination of data from just Multnomah, Emanuel, and Dammasch Hospitals will adequately sample trends for this area.

SUMMARY

A procedure for the determination of the extent of medically significant drug abuse in a community was developed. All emergency room records for records for seven major hospitals in the area were read by one person for 1 week at quarterly intervals from 1968 until 1972. Similar information was obtained for all admissions to the state hospital serving this cachement area. Data reveal that overall drug use admissions reached a peak in 1971. The biggest decrease has been in LSD. Heroin has been decreasing, although less markedly. Barbiturates and other sedatives are unchanged, and amphetamines may just be beginning to decrease. Cocaine use, while small, has had a slight rise.

ACKNOWLEDGMENT

Supported in part by a grant from the Medical Research Foundation of Oregon.

The International Journal of the Addictions, 9(6), pp. 891–898, 1974

Research Note

Opiates, Amphetamines, Alcohol: A Comparative Study of American Soldiers*

Donald R. Rardin, Ph.D.

Thomas R. Lawson, M.S.W.

David J. Kruzich, M.S.W.

130th General Hospital
Medical Service Corps

INTRODUCTION

A questionnaire study was conducted in September 1971 by two of the present authors (Rardin, Lawson, and Rush, 1973). Individuals were placed into groups according to their drug habits, and it was suggested that the drug habits are reflective of a person's socialization. The present study extends to previous research by comparing individuals who primarily use one of the following drugs: opiates, amphetamines, alcohol. The basic purpose of this study is to obtain information about the relationships between individuals and their choice of drugs. Within this framework, the hypothesis

* Presented under the title "Personalities of Drug Abusers in the U.S. Army Europe" at the 4th International Institute on the Prevention and Treatment of Drug Abuse, Belgrade Yugoslavia, June 1973.

is that those who choose alcohol will be the least deviant and those who choose amphetamines will be the most deviant compared to a control group.

The term "primary drug used" is important as very few individuals use only one drug. As Kales (1969) has shown, several drugs are frequently abused at any given time, and the individual who is dependent upon a single drug is becoming a rare entity. Perhaps as Winick (1957) states, "In each case the drug fulfills a specific function in the personality economy in the individual, and it is this function which determines how difficult it will be for the individual addict to shed his drug." If the pattern of use serves to fulfill inner needs, the expectation would be that different drugs would serve different needs.

METHOD

Subjects

Four groups of 20 subjects were selected for this study. Three of these groups consisted of individuals seeking the aid of the "Getting Straight" drug rehabilitation center. This facility is an Army center with voluntary admission. Based on their choice of drugs, subjects were placed into the alcohol, opiate, or amphetamine groups. The control group was randomly selected.

Procedures

All participants were given the MMPI, questionnaires, and the Shipley-Hartford Scale of Living Test. The opiate, alcohol, and amphetamine groups were also given individual structured interviews. Further, as clients go through the rehabilitation program they are rated by the staff and by fellow clients on rating scales concerning peer relations, staff relations, work performance, and prognosis of becoming drug free.

RESULTS

Table 1 gives a current overview of the four groups. Age differences were partially controlled by the elimination of the oldest alcohol users. The control and alcohol groups were the most apt to marry and have children, and the amphetamine group the least. The IQ averages for all groups of

Table 1
Descriptive Statistics of the Subject's Current Status

	Control group	Alcohol group	Opiate group	Amphetamine group
1. Age	20.5	25.9	20.2	21.7
2. Time in service	20.4	65.3	26.9	23.9
3. Rank	3.4	4.2	3.3	3.2
4. Married	7	13	4	2
5. Children	8	14	2	1
6. Shipley-Hartford	98	102	108	104

subjects as estimated by the Shipley-Hartford are in the average range of intelligence.

Drug Use

Both the amount and variety of drugs used by the alcohol and control groups are much less than the opiate and amphetamine groups, with use by the control subjects being greater than the alcohol group (Table 2). Only six of the opiate group report frequent use of amphetamines while in the service, and only one reported frequent amphetamine use before being

Table 2
Drug Use Patterns[a]

Type of drug	Drugs used currently	Drugs used before army	Drugs now used frequently	Drugs used frequently before army
Amphetamines	Am Op	Am Op	Am Op	Am
Barbiturates	Am Op	Am Op		
Hallucinogins	Am Op	Am Op	Am	Am
Marijuana	Am Op Co	Am Op Co	Am Op Co	Am Op Co
Glue or Gas		Am	Op	
Opiates	Am Op	Op		
Cocaine	Op			
Alcohol	Am Op Al Co	Am Op Al Co	Al Co	Am Op Al Co

[a] Am = Amphetamine group; Op = opiate group; Al = alcohol group; Co = control group. Marked categories indicate five or more people in the designated drug group so responded to the questionnaire. For example, in row 1 (amphetamines) and column 1 (drugs used currently), the letters Am Op indicate that at least five individuals in the amphetamine and opiate groups currently use amphetamines.

in the Army. The amphetamine group reports considerably more use of hallucinogens.

Factors Influencing Use

The alcohol group was most apt to report parental use of drugs, primarily alcohol, and the control the least parental use. Similarly, parents of the alcohol group were most apt to advise, "Alcohol is OK but you shouldn't use other drugs because they are illegal." The opiate and amphetamine groups were, compared to the other groups, more apt to report that "Parents never discussed drugs with them." The control group was more apt to state that their parents definitely opposed any drug use.

Reasons given for use of drugs are listed in Table 3. The most frequent response, especially for the amphetamine group, concerned "escape." Interpersonal factors such as "gets people together" or "helps to make friends" were the least frequent. The alcohol and control groups were more apt to express feelings of inadequacy as reasons, and the opiate group most frequently listed boredom. The control group was less apt to list harassment as a reason.

Personal History

Table 4 compares the groups on the basis of family, authority, and school interactions. The amphetamine group reported the most conflict within their families. On measures dealing with authority situations, the

Table 3
Reasons for Using Drugs. Each Individual was Requested to List the Three Most Important Reasons for Using Drugs. There were 24 Choices, Three for each Reason

	Group			
Reason	Control	Alcohol	Opiate	Amphetamine
1. Intellectual	6	9	6	5
2. Harassment	2	8	12	9
3. Boredom	9	6	15	8
4. Pleasure	12	11	9	7
5. Friendship	4	1	1	4
6. Helplessness	8	6	1	2
7. Depression	3	5	4	5
8. Escape	11	11	12	24

Table 4
Family, School and Authority Conflicts[a]

		Group			
		Control	Alcohol	Opiate	Amphetamine
Family conflict	Separation or divorce	4	3	1½	1½
	Conflict with father	4	1	2	3
	Conflict with mother	4	2	3	1
	Conflict with siblings	[b]	3	2	1
	Siblings use drugs	[b]	3	1½	1½
School conflict	Years of education	3	4	1	2
	Expulsions or suspensions	4	3	1½	1½
	Poor grades	[b]	2	1	3
Authority conflict	Conflict—civilian boss	[b]	3	1	2
	Conflict—army boss	4	2	1	2
	Civilian arrests	[b]	3	1	2
	Article 15s or court martials	4	2	3	1
	Discipline action pending	4	3	1	2

[a] A rank of 1 indicates that that group reported the most conflict for that particular category.
[b] This information is not available.

opiate group reported the most difficulty. Again, when queried about school performance, the opiate group reported the most difficulty. The control group exhibited the least difficutly in these areas.

Personality Testing

The most significant scores on the MMPI are on scales 2, 4, 7, 8, and an auxiliary anxiety scale (Fig. 1). The scores for scale 2 are elevated for all groups. This scale is seen as an indicator of current mood, and the high scores indicate all groups are experiencing discomfort in their current

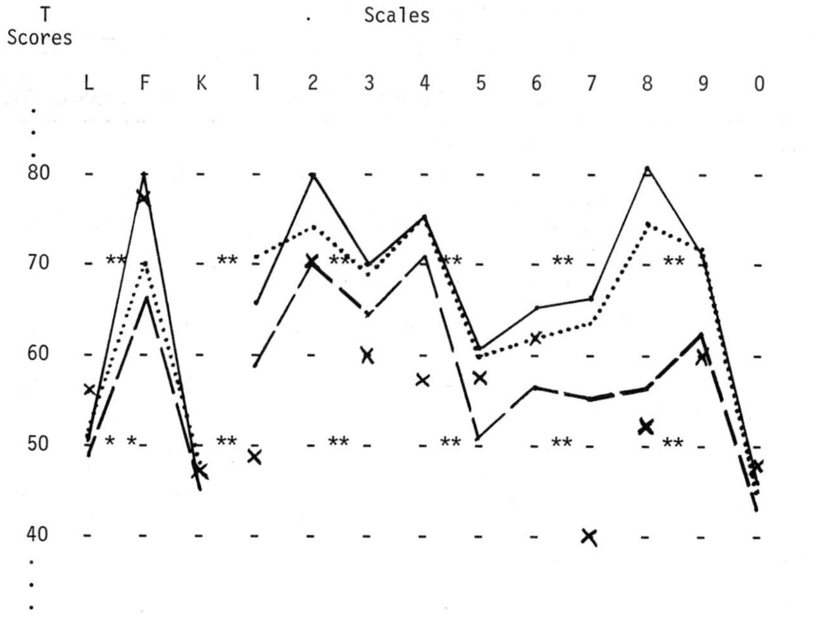

Fig. 1. MMPI results for (—) amphetamine group, (· · ·) opiate group, (- -) alcohol group, and (×) control group.

circumstances; possibly apathy, hopelessness, etc. All but the control group score high on scale 4. This scale is reflective of disidentification, social alienation, and anger at authority. Scale 7 and the auxiliary anxiety measure (Dahlstrom, 1960) all indicate that the amphetamine group is currently experiencing the most anxiety. The opiate, alcohol, and control groups follow in descending order. The amphetamine group also had the highest scores on scale 8 (ego disintegration, schizoid mentation, and alienation), followed again in descending order by the opiate, alcohol, and control groups. These differences are small and are primarily matters of degree, and the similarities across drug using groups are striking. An indication of the similarity of personality profiles is demonstrated by the results of a scale designed specifically to indicate alcoholism. The three drug groups all have elevated scores with the amphetamine group highest, followed in order by the opiate and alcohol groups.

Staff and Client Ratings

The staff at the rehabilitation center rated the individual clients on work performance, peer relations, staff relations, and prognosis for becoming drug free. The opiate group was rated the lowest and the alcohol group the highest. When clients rated themselves, the average rating was higher but the order of the group averages was the same.

DISCUSSION

The data for this study is wide ranging and from a small select sample of drug using individuals. There is some support for the hypothesis that people choose a particular drug because of personality factors. On nearly every indicie the control group compares favorably to the drug groups and, similarly, the alcohol group compares favorably to the opiate and amphetamine groups. The differences between the opiate and amphetamine groups are less obvious. Personality testing indicates that the amphetamine group experiences more anxiety and less coping ability than any of the other groups. The family histories indicate that there is also more family difficulty reported by the subjects in the amphetamine group. Emotionally, the amphetamine group appears less stable than the other groups. On the other hand, the opiate group appears to have greater conflict with schools and authorities. The staff and their peers at the rehabilitation center rate the opiate group the lowest. One post hoc explanation for these differences would be that while both groups exhibit social deviance and alienation, the opiate group experiences less anxiety (Fig. 1 and Table 4). The amphetamine group appears to manifest greater emotional pathology while the opiate group appears more similar to a character disorder designation.

This discussion has emphasized the differences between groups, but all of the drug using groups have experienced considerable difficulties in the areas explored. The differences are primarily of degree. For example, the MMPI profiles are quite parallel, the families of all groups have had considerable conflict, and all groups are currently experiencing difficulty functioning in the Army. The attempt of the present study was to take a broad in-depth look at individuals who are using drugs and asking for help. As such, nearly all of the data analyses are post hoc and highly subject to experimenter bias. A further limitation is that of studying drug-dependent personnel in a situation where they are asking for help. In fact, large numbers of drug-dependent individuals from the same population contract hepatitis, are provided with information about the rehabilitation center, and none of these people choose to participate. Perhaps only one small, special segment of the drug population is represented in the present population.

SUMMARY

A large amount of data was collected from the following groups of 20 subjects; alcohol dependent, amphetamine dependent, opiate dependent, and a control group. The amphetamine group exhibited the greatest degree of emotional pathology although the three drug-dependent groups were striking in their similarities.

REFERENCES

DAHLSTROM, G.M., and WELSH, G.S. *An MMPI Handbook*. Minneapolis: Univ. Minnesota Press, 1960, p. 449.

KALES, A., HEUSER, G., and KALES, J.D. Drug dependency: Investigations of stimulants and depressants. *Ann. Int. Med.* 70: 591–614, March 1969.

RARDIN, D.R., LAWSON, T.R., and RUSH, J.A. Drugs used by American soldiers in Europe. *Social Work* 18: 34–41, January 1973.

WINICK, C. Narcotics addiction and its treatment. *Law and Contemporary Problems* 22: 14, September 1957.

The International Journal of the Addictions, 9(6), pp. 899–902, 1974

Research Note

Changes in Locus of Control in Heroin Addicts

Willy Henik

Bronx State Hospital
New York, New York

George Domino

Fordham University
New York, New York

Abstract

Heroin addicts participating in a methadone maintenance treatment program were administered the I-E scale during the first and ninth weeks of the program; a matched control group of addicts on a waiting list for the same program was also tested and retested. Upon retest, the experimental group showed a statistically significant increase in the direction of internality, while the control group did not give evidence of such an increase.

Man's efforts to master his environment have been a focal point of various personality theorists. Perhaps the most explicit statement and the clearest empirical application of this concept can be found in Rotter's (1954, 1966) social learning theory with its emphasis on expectancies for internal vs external control of reinforcement, i.e., the degree to which an individual perceives events in his life as being a consequence of his own actions and therefore under his personal control, or as being unrelated to his behavior and therefore beyond personal control. The internally oriented individual believes that reinforcements are contingent on such personal qualities as skill and competence, while the externally oriented individual believes that forces independent of his own behavior, such as chance or fate, control his reinforcements.

This dimension, operationalized through a 29 forced-choice item scale, has been related to many variables including psychiatric nosology (e.g., Harrow and Ferrante, 1969), but little evidence is available as to the degree to which changes in one's status can alter control expectancies. This question is the focus of the present investigation of changes in control expectancies of heroin addicts participating in a methadone maintenance treatment program.

SUBJECTS AND PROCEDURE

The *S*s of this study were 62 male patients participating in a methadone maintenance treatment program at the Narcotic Addiction Unit at Bronx State Hospital. This program is based on the pattern developed by Dole and Nyswander (1968); admission is on a voluntary basis, with court referrals and overtly psychotic individuals not accepted. In addition to its medical aspects (methadone blockade), the 6-week inpatient treatment consists of a comprehensive rehabilitation effort, with emphasis on group treatment and availability of individual services.

The experimental group consisted of 31 *S*s admitted to the program and fulfilling the following criteria: White, male, between 22 and 36 years of age, with at least 4 years of mainline heroin use, a minimum score of 15 on the Shipley-Hartford Vocabulary scale, and a score of 31 or below on the Good Impression scale of the California Psychological Inventory. The control group consisted of 31 *S*s fulfilling identical criteria, selected from the waiting list, whose probable date of admission into the program was between 2 and 4 months from the date of testing. Both groups were also equated on socioeconomic level, marital status, employment history, and criminal background.

Subjects in the experimental group were initially tested within 24 hr of their admission to the program, and retested 9 weeks later. Since the inpatient treatment program was of 6 weeks duration, each *S* had the opportunity to return and live in his community for 3 weeks so that he was not retested just prior to or following his discharge when anxiety may be expected to be high. Control *S*s were also tested twice, 9 weeks apart, but prior to their eventual admission into the program. To control for possible temporal effects, experimental and control *S*s were tested in an alternate but randomized sequence, with almost all experimental *S*s tested within the same week as their control counterparts.

RESULTS AND DISCUSSION

A significant decrease was predicted in the I-E scores of the experimental *S*s as compared to those of control *S*s. The evaluation of change was based on covariance analysis, with initial scores serving as the covariate. Since only two groups were compared, the covariance analysis results are presented as *t* values for the adjusted final scores. Means and standard deviations of initial and final scores, adjusted final means, and *t* values for initial and adjusted scores are presented in Table 1.

No significant difference was found between the initial means, but upon retest the experimental group showed an average decrease of 2.03 points while the control group mean increased .58—a statistically significant difference. The prediction that, as a result of the changed realities of life brought about by participation in a methadone program, heroin addicts would show a decrease in external orientation was fully supported.

Social learning theory states that the probability of occurrence of a certain behavior is a function of the individual's expectancy that such behavior will achieve an available reinforcement. Though desirous of a certain goal, the individual may believe that there is no behavior in his repertoire that will permit him to achieve that goal. In such a case, he will anticipate no contingency between any effort on his part and the end result of the situation.

The parallel to addiction is clear. The system of impotence in which the addict finds himself and the grave limitations within which he has to function contribute to the extinction of whatever expectations he may have had of achieving desired reinforcements. He may not even believe that there

Table 1

	Experimental (N = 31)		Control (N = 31)			
	Mean	SD	Mean	SD	t	p
Initial	9.29	3.87	8.97	4.36	0.30	ns
Final	7.26	3.89	9.55	4.02		
Adjusted	7.15		9.65		3.27	.01

are any behaviors in his repertoire that will enable him to achieve such goals. No past effort on his part led to success in stopping the use of heroin.

Whatever else a therapeutic program offers the addict, it does provide him with the means to break the vicious cycle of his past experience. This in turn may be assumed to affect his expectancy that his future behavior will enable him to achieve desired reinforcements. The newly found confidence in his abilities is reflected in the decrease of his external orientation.

The above is at present a matter of conjecture and needful of empirical investigation. Similarly, the stability of the manifested change is a matter requiring further research, especially to determine the extent to which such change reflects temporary overconfidence or a genuine alteration in control expectancies. Finally, the above results should neither be taken as supportive of the therapeutic efficacy of methadone maintenance nor as indicative of more basic alterations in behavior. There are other possible explanations which need be investigated before being ruled out.

REFERENCES

DOLE, V.P., and NYSWANDER, M. Successful treatment of 750 criminal addicts. In *Proceedings of the First National Conference on Methadone Treatment*. New York: The Rockefeller Univ., 1968.

HARROW, M., and FERRANTE, A. Locus of control in psychiatric patients. *J. Consult. Clin. Psychol.* 33: 582–589, 1969.

ROTTER, J.B. *Social Learning and Clinical Psychology*. Englewood Cliffs, New Jersey: Prentice-Hall, 1954.

ROTTER, J.B. Generalized expectancies for internal versus external control of reinforcement. *Psychol. Monographs* 80: (whole no. 609), 1966.

The International Journal of the Addictions, 9(6), pp. 903–907, 1974

Research Note

A Comparison of Drug Users and Nonusers on a Midwestern University Campus

R. B. Dick, Ph.D.*

L. T. Brown, Ph.D.

Department of Psychology
Oklahoma State University
Stillwater, Oklahoma

Concern with the increasing popularity of drug use and experimentation on American college campuses has resulted in a number of surveys aimed at determining the extent of use, characteristics distinguishing users from nonusers, reasons for use, and so on (e.g., Blum and Associates, 1969; Garfield, Boreing, and Smith, 1971; Greenwald and Leutgert, 1971; Grupp, McCain, and Schmitt, 1971). The first purpose of the present study was to extend the data on campus drug use by surveying a large university campus in a Midwestern state. Creation of yet another questionnaire was avoided, however, by employing the first part of a questionnaire used in a survey of an urban commuter campus by Greenwald and Leutgert (1971). Since the administration and content of the questionnaires in the two studies were

* Present address: National Institutes of Mental Health, Regional Office IV, Atlanta, Georgia. Both authors assume equal responsibility for this paper; order of authorship was determined solely by the flip of a coin.

similar, it was hoped that as a second purpose of the study a direct comparison of several aspects of drug use could be made between the commuter campus of a university located in a large Midwestern city and the residential campus of a university situated in a small Midwestern city.

METHOD

The Instrument

The survey instrument was a 56-item multiple-choice questionnaire incorporating the first 43 items of Greenwald and Luetgert's (1971) questionnaire (modified to allow for differences between the two campuses) and 13 items prepared by the first author. Nine of the latter items replaced Greenwald and Luetgert's question No. 38 (concerned with frequency of drug use) and asked for frequency of use of each of the following drugs or drug groups: alcohol, marijuana, LSD, other hallucinogens (mescaline, DMT, DET, STP, psyilocybin, nutmeg, etc.), amphetamines (Benzedrine, Dexedrine, Methedrine), opiates (morphine, heroin, opium, methadone), cocaine, barbiturates (phenobarbital, Amytal, Nembutal, Seconal, Pentothal), and "any other drugs not listed above." For each drug category the respondent was asked to check one of five alternatives: "Never," "1 time," "2–10 times," "More than 10 times," and "Average at least once per week."*

Sample and Administration

The survey was conducted during the spring semester, 1972, at a Midwestern land-grant university which will be referred to as Midwestern State University (MSU). MSU shares common characteristics with several other Midwestern universities with enrollments in the 15,000 to 25,000 range.

A representative sample of 400 students, representing slightly over 2% of the student body, was drawn in the following manner: Using the 1971–1972 enrollment summary, 48 (6 colleges × 4 classes × 2 sexes) undergraduate quotas, and five graduate quotas (areas of study—e.g., biological sciences) were determined. Guided by the size and nature of the 53 quotas, a random sample was made of departments within colleges, and then of courses within departments. Permission was sought from instructors to enter the selected classes and distribute the questionnaires. (Instructor cooperation was a gratifying 100%.) That participation was voluntary, and

* A copy of the questionnaire may be obtained by writing the second author.

anonymity was stressed in a short talk given prior to handing out the questionnaires. One of the authors was present in each class surveyed to ensure that a uniform survey procedure was used. In cases where class enrollments exceeded the assigned quotas, a table of random numbers was used to determine which questionnaires should be retained and which dropped.

RESULTS

Statistical decisions were made using the standard chi-square test for contingency tables. The .05 level of significance was used.

Following Greenwald and Leutgert (1971), designation of students as drug users or nonusers was based on reported use of marijuana. Although the questionnaires divided frequency of marijuana use into five categories (see above), the requirement of the chi-square test that the expected *N* per cell be 5 or greater made it necessary to collapse the number of categories to at least 3: nonuser, minimal user (1 to 10 times), and regular user (more than 10 times). Collapsing the number of categories to 2 (nonusers vs users) was avoided whenever possible because of the authors' desire to distinguish between students using marijuana on only one or a few occasions and those using the drug on a more or less regular basis.*

Drug Experience

Excluding alcohol, 40% (160) of the MSU students reported drug use on at least one occasion. The drug experience of nearly all of these (38.5% of sample) consisted of, or included, marijuana. Relatively few students reported the use of drugs other than alcohol and marijuana; the amphetamines were the third most popular drug category, with use reported by 16.3% of the sample.

Marijuana Use on Two Campuses

Four general sets of conclusions emerge from a comparison of the results of the present survey with those of Greenwald and Leutgert (1971).

* Data summary tables, results of statistical analyses, and a detailed 14-page description and discussion of the results may be obtained by writing the second author. The following paragraphs serve only to note the general incidence of drug experience reported by MSU students and to summarize briefly a comparison of the present data with those of Greenwald and Leutgert (1971).

1. Probably reflecting the lapse of 4 years between the two surveys (1968–1972), MSU students report a higher incidence of marijuana use than University of Illinois at Chicago Circle (UICC) students (nearly 40% vs 24%). There is also evidence that over this 4-year period drug use increased among younger students: While UICC students in the 21 and above age range reported the highest incidence of drug use, MSU drug use is as prevalent among younger as older students. Of further relevance, MSU students reported 18 as the median age of first drug use (other than alcohol), 58% of MSU's regular users indicate that they have been using drugs for 2 or more years, and drug use is unrelated to number of semesters completed.

2. While drug use among UICC students was found to be unrelated to academic performance, use among MSU students tends to be linked with poorer grades. Furthermore, sex was unrelated to drug use among UICC students; in contrast, drug use on the MSU campus is more widespread among men than women. The latter finding may reflect a regional difference in attitudes toward drug use, and is not inconsistent with the traditionally greater freedom of men in less populated areas of the United States to consume alcohol and engage in other "venturesome" activities.

3. Drug users on both campuses tend to come from wealthier homes than nonusers; it appears, however, that the wealth of the father of the UICC user is more closely related to educational achievement, while that of the father of the MSU user is more closely linked with occupational status. A relatively high percentage of MSU users (31.0 and 46.3% of minimal and regular users, respectively) have fathers employed in occupations described as "Business and Sales," occupations which may not require high levels of academic achievement but which may nevertheless be high-salaried. In brief, the family background of the MSU drug user may be described as suburban middle or upper-middle class.

4. Finally, in contrast to the UICC drug user, the MSU user shows little evidence of independence from or rebellion against his family. The MSU user is as likely as the nonuser (a) to live in university or Greek housing (rather than private housing), (b) to regard himself as still living with his parents, (c) to consider his relationship with his parents as "harmonious," and (d) to rely on his parents for his income. Like the UICC user, he indicates relatively little interest in organized religion, but this appears to be the only evidence (along with his drug experience) that he may have turned his back on the traditional values of his middle-class background.

The MSU user, like his UICC counterpart, is most likely in absolute terms to be an Arts and Sciences student, but in relative terms he is just as likely to be pursuing a career in business or engineering. When combined with the data on economic background, then, these findings suggest that, unlike UICC students, MSU students who report drug experience continue to hold pretty much the same middle- and upper-middle-class values and goals as their parents.

REFERENCES

BLUM, R.H., and Associates. *Students and Drugs.* San Francisco: Jossey-Bass, 1969.

GARFIELD, E.F., BOREING, M.L., and SMITH, J.P. Marijuana use on a campus: Spring, 1969. *Intern. J. Addictions* 6(3): 487–491, 1971.

GREENWALD, B.S., and LEUTGERT, M.J. A comparison of drug users and nonusers on an urban commuter college campus. *Intern. J. Addictions* 6(1): 63–78, 1971.

GRUPP, S.E., MCCAIN, M.J., and SCHMITT, R.L. Marijuana use in a small college: A Midwest example. *Intern. J. Addictions* 6(3): 463–485, 1971.

The International Journal of the Addictions, 9(6), pp. 909–918, 1974

Research Note

The "Hang-Loose" Ethic and Drug Use Revisited*

George H. Wolkon, Ph.D.

Naomi Kantzer Jasso, Ph.D.

University of Southern California School of Medicine
Los Angeles, California

Sharon Gallagher, M.S.W.

Veterans Administration Hospital
Brentwood, California

Peter Cohn, M.S.W.

Westside Community Mental Health Center
San Francisco, California

Abstract

All the students in four elective classes in one high school reponded to a questionnaire concerning drug use, selected attitudes, and selected behaviors. There were few differences between drug users and nonusers in terms of the attitudes and behaviors

* This report is a much extended version of a project submitted in partial fulfillment of the requirements for the Master's degree at UCLA School of Social Welfare by the last two authors and Gail Schneider Nathanson under the direction of the first author.

measured. However, there were striking differences between the high school sample and youth who frequented a free clinic. The "hang-loose" ethic was much more apparent at the clinic. Implications are briefly discussed.

In attempts to elucidate the increased use of drugs among youth, diverse economic, political, psychological, and sociological explanations have emerged. Common to a great many of these interpretations is the association between drug use and a rejection of traditional values, attitudes and behaviors, and the generation gap. More specifically, it has been proposed that drug use is associated with adherence to a "hang-loose" ethic, an ethic which questions and rejects the traditions of conventional society (Simmons and Winogard, 1966; Miller, 1971). In a study of university students, Suchman (1968) concluded, "that the more the student embraces the 'hang-loose' ethic, the more frequently will he make use of marijuana."

The association between a "hang-loose" ethic and drug use has not been examined as extensively for high school age youth. There are indications, however, that the association does exist in the United States (Wechsler and Thum, 1971; Tec, 1972) and in Canada (Smart and Fejer, 1971).

The purpose of the present study is to test Suchman's (1968) hypothesis that "the more the student embraces the 'hang-loose' ethic (as opposed to the so-called 'Protestant Ethic') the more frequently he will make use of drugs" with a high school sample.

METHOD

The study was conducted in a high school in a developing suburban area of Los Angeles. A questionnaire eliciting background information, drug use information, and attitudes and behaviors was completed by all 74 students attending four classes on the day of the questionnaire administration. Two of the classes were an elective course available to all juniors and seniors. The other two classes were an elective course for students in the top 15% academically. Anonymity was assured. This sample may not be truly representative of high school youth; however, it is a useful one given the barriers to systematic data collection (Richards and Carrol, 1970).

The sample, composed of 33 males and 41 females, have a mean age of 16.8, are all caucasian, and are from the upper-middle class with 59% reporting an annual family income over $15,000. The reported religious distribution is Protestant (43%), followed by Catholic (30%), Jewish (10%), and other (17%).

FINDINGS

Drug Use. Forty-seven percent of the students reported using at least one drug within the last year. Most often used was marijuana, with 45% of the students reporting some use for the year. The second most commonly used drug was amphetamines (20%), followed by barbiturates (15%), LSD or mescaline (15%), opiates (9%), and speed (7%).* These percentages are consistent with other surveys (Brown, 1971; San Mateo County, 1970).

Although the prevalence of any drug use is high, the frequency of use is not high. Although 45% of our sample had used marijuana in the preceding year, 18% experimented once or twice, 12% used it once or twice a month, 14% used it once or twice a week, and only one person made use of marijuana about every day. Thus 27% of the sample used marijuana at least once or twice a month. This figure is comparable with the San Mateo report. Of the other drugs surveyed, 4 students (5%) reported using a drug once or twice a week, and only 3 students (4%) said they used a drug other than marijuana daily.

Drug User Types. Three drug user types are identified based on the reported frequency of drug use with reference to marijuana: (1) nonusers of any drug ($N = 39$), (2) users of marijuana only ($N = 16$), and (3) users of marijuana along with drugs ($N = 19$).†

Drug Use and Background Characteristics. No statistically significant relationships were found between the categories of drug users and age, sex, income, and religion.

Drug Use and Academic Achievement. The two types of classes, the

* The questionnaire included a separate section regarding the use of speed because of its highly publicized dangerous affects. All subjects who reported use of speed reported the same use of amphetamines. Ten subjects reporting use of amphetamines did not report using speed.

† This category contains two students who used other drugs only. Unfortunately, frequency of drug use is not evident in this typology. Frequency and type of drug could not be taken into account simultaneously because of the small number of students. However, preliminary analysis indicated that basically the same results to be reported here were obtained using only the frequency typology.

academically heterogeneous elective class and the homogeneous bright class were compared on drug use. A significantly greater number of heterogeneous students than bright students used marijuana along with other drugs (38% vs 12%). Self-reported grade point average of the heterogeneous students was similarly related to drug use but was not statistically significant.

Drug Use, Alcoholic Beverages, and Cigarettes. Fifty-eight percent of the students reported any drinking of beer, 66% for wine, and 37% for hard liquor. Only the use of hard liquor was associated with the drug use types. Almost 3 times as many "once in a while" drinkers of hard liquor used marijuana along with other drugs than did "never" drinkers (44% vs 15%). It was felt that the drinking of hard liquor might be associated with adherence to the "hang-loose" ethic. The data analysis, however, did not confirm it.

Thirty percent of the students report smoking at least once in a while, and there are more regular smokers (19%) than regular drinkers (beer, 8%; wine, 5%; hard liquor, 0%). Fifty-nine percent of those students who do any smoking of cigarettes used marijuana along with other drugs as compared to 12% of those who report no smoking.

Comparing the drinking of hard liquor for the drug-use types, 63% of the youth using marijuana along with other drugs reported use of hard liquor, as compared to 44% of the marijuana only users and 21% of the nondrug users. With regard to cigarette smoking, 68% of those people using marijuana along with other drugs smoke at least once in a while, as compared to 38% of those who use marijuana only and 8% of the nondrug users. These findings are consistent with the findings of national surveys (Josephson et al., 1971; National Commission, 1972); but inconsistent with Suchman (1968).

Behavioral and Attitudinal Indicators of the "Hang-Loose" Ethic. The specific findings in Table 1 indicate that the behaviors related to drug use were nonactivist type behaviors (plans after high school and membership in organizations) while activist behaviors (demonstrations and marches) were not related to drug use.

Attitudinal Indicators of the "Hang-Loose" Ethic. Attitudinal adherence to the "hang-loose" ethic was measured by seven attitudes listed in Table 2. No reliable relationships were obtained between any of the attitudes and drug use.

Table 1
Association between Behavioral Measures of "Hang-Loose" Ethic and Drug Use for High School Sample

		% Using marijuana along with other drugs	χ^2 ($df = 2$)
1. Plans after high school	College only plan:	19	7.67*
	Other plan, or more than 1 plan:	53	
2. Belongs to school organization	Yes:	14	9.19**
	No:	40	
3. Belongs to nonschool organization	Yes:	7	9.24***
	No:	39	
4. Participated in an antiwar activity	Yes:	41	2.78
	No:	21	
5. Participated in a demonstration or protest march	Yes:	25	1.24
	No:	26	
6. Grade average	"B" or more:	18	2.63
	"B −" or less:	33	
7. Cooperation marks	Mostly E:	20	1.13
	Mostly S or U:	30	
8. Work habits marks	Mostly E:	22	.62
	Mostly S or U:	27	
9. Times in detention	Never:	19	4.77
	Once or more:	30	

* $p < .05$. ** $p < .02$. *** $p < .01$.

Table 2
Comparison of Clinic and High School for Attitudinal Measures of the "Hang-Loose" Ethic

	Clinic, %	High school, %	χ^2 ($df = 1$)
High rejection of school authority	63	35	10.22*
High rejection of law (from Thurstone, 1931)	77	54	7.18*
High anomie (Srole, 1956)	71	40	12.55**
Low control of fate (Coleman et al., 1966)	49	24	9.38*
Highly hassled by parents	66	39	9.79*
High disagreement with parents	61	28	14.32**
Liberal social attitude (from Kerlinger, cited in Shaw and Wright, 1967.	63	48	2.85

* $p < .01$. ** $p < .001$.

Free Clinic Youth and the "Hang-Loose" Ethic. Except for the behavioral measures of plans after high school and participation in formal activities, there was no statistically significant association between attachment to a "hang-loose" ethic and drug use for the high school sample. In addition, the students tend to have attitudes that are not generally in contradiction to traditional values. The question arises, then, as to whether the "hang-loose" ethic is not more common for high school age youth believed to be out of the mainstream of traditional society.

The same attitudinal and behavioral data were obtained from a sample of 75 high school age youth attending a Los Angeles urban free clinic (Jasso and Wolkon, 1973).

The clinic youth present strikingly higher frequency of drug use than the high school. Indeed, the light users in the clinic used drugs more often than the heavy users in the high school. For this reason, clinic and high school attitudes could not be compared controlling for drug-use types. Thus the total clinc sample is compared with the total high school sample.

Table 2 presents the results for the attitudinal comparisons between the clinic and high school youth. For each measure, except one, the clinc youth more often embrace the "hang-loose" ethic than the high school sample.

Further, in response to the question, "Do you feel close to your parents?", 56% of the clinc sample and 15% of the high school sample responded negatively.

The clinic youth also adhere to the "hang-loose" ethic relatively more often than the high school youth as measured by the behavioral indicators except for grades in school (Table 3).

First Experience with Drugs. The clinic youth reported first trying drugs about a year younger than the high school youth (13.9 vs 14.8). The two groups did not differ significantly, however, for the first drug tried. Sixty-eight percent of the clinic and 76% of the high school started with marijuana.

Should Drugs be Legalized? The results (Table 4) indicate that the clinic youth significantly more often than the high school feel that drugs should be legalized for everyone. The rank order of legality of drugs was the same for the high school and clinic groups.

The publicity given the dangerous affects of speed as compared to amphetamines in general is manifested in the greater percentage of respondents who think speed should be illegal as compared to amphetamines (high school $\chi^2 = 8.08$, $p < .01$; clinic $\chi^2 = 9.19$, $p < .01$).

Table 3
Comparison of Clinic and High School for Behavioral Measures of "Hang-Loose" Ethic

	Clinic, %	High school, %	χ^2 ($df = 1$)
1. Plan after high school is not college, or more than one plan	69	22	31.61***
2. Does *not* belong to school organizations	81	49	15.00***
3. Does *not* belong to nonschool organizations	80	60	5.98*
4. Participated in an antiwar activity	51	23	11.11***
5. Participated in a demonstration or protest march	56	16	23.82***
6. Grade average, "B −" or less	57	49	0.55
7. Cooperation marks mostly S or U	64	51	1.82
8. Work habits marks mostly S or U	66	68	0.003
9. In detention six or more times	30	7	14.58***
10. Referred to social adjustment or opportunity room once or more	35	3	22.14***
11. Suspended once or more	36	12	10.61**
12. Opportunity transferred once or more	25	3	11.01***
13. Expelled once or more	20	1	11.84***

[a] $df = 2$.
* $p < .02$.
** $p < .01$.
*** $p < .001$.

DISCUSSION

The majority of the high school sample who used drugs were not heavy users and can more accurately be described as experimenters or infrequent users. The high school sample tend to have similar attitudes which are not generally in contrast to traditional values. The youth appear similar to the majority of youthful drug users in the United States (National Commission, 1972). "These experimenters are characteristically quite conventional and practically indistinguishable from the non-user in terms of life style, activities, social integration and vocational or academic performance." For an opposing point of view see Rollins and Holden (1972).

The high school sample not only used drugs less often than youth who attended a free clinic, but also differed from them in both attitudes and behaviors. The clinic youth adhered more to the "hang-loose" ethic than did

Table 4
Legalization of Drugs for Clinic and High School Sample

		Clinic, %	High school, %	χ^2 ($df = 2$)
Marijuana	Illegal	8	46	32.61*
	Legal for adults	19	25	
	Legal for everyone	73	29	
LSD, mescaline	Illegal	55	96	32.97*
	Legal for adults	25	3	
	Legal for everyone	20	1	
Amphetamines	Illegal	41	81	24.78*
	Legal for adults	30	11	
	Legal for everyone	30	7	
Speed	Illegal	68	98	22.39*
	Legal for adults	17	1	
	Legal for everyone	15	1	
Downers	Illegal	48	82	17.85*
	Legal for adults	30	11	
	Legal for everyone	22	7	
Opiates	Illegal	79	99	12.01[a]
	Legal for adults	21	1	

[a] $df = 1$. The category "legal for everyone" was dropped from the analysis because too few people checked it.
* $p < .001$.

the high school youth. In short, the clinic youth are more typical of the stereotyped drug user because of their tendency to reject the traditions of conventional society.

The data presented indicate that the stereotypes of the "hang-loose hippie" and the "rebellious recalcitrant" are no longer, if they ever were, appropriate to the typical high school drug user. A substantial if not major portion of youthful drug users are not otherwise deviant from or threatening to establishment values. As the lack of threat to the establishment is recognized by the public, attempts to control the individual's use of drugs will most likely change from legal repressive methods directed to the individual user to other types of voluntary social influence methods. Their focus will be on social values and, when information is available, on the medical and health implications of taking and even experimenting with particular drugs.

The attitudes and life style of those youth who frequent the free clinic do conform to the stereotypes that frighten the establishment. Thus the question that must be addressed is how to prevent the drug experimenters and light users in the high schools from changing their life style and attitudes, and how to prevent them from increasing their use of drugs. The data presented here do not allow specific suggestions but do allow some general areas to be explored further; namely, the relationship of the adolescent with his parents and the relationship of the adolescent with his school prior to the youth's alienation.

REFERENCES

BROWN, M. *Stability and Change in Drug Use Patterns Among High School Students.* Fullerton, California: Center for Governmental Studies, California State College, 1971 (offset).

COLEMAN, J., CAMPBELL, E., HOBSON, C., McPARTLAND, J., MOOD, A., WEINFIELD F., and YORK, P. *Equality of Educational Opportunity.* Washington D.C.: United States Government Printing Office, 1966.

JASSO, N.K., and WOLKON, G.H. "Drug use, attitudes and behavior of youth in an urban free clinic." Presented at the Western Psychological Association Convention, April 1973.

JOSEPHSON, E., HABERMAN, P., ZANES, A., and ELINSON, J. Adolescent marijuana use: report on a national survey. Newark, New Jersey: Unpublished paper presented, First International Conference on Student Drug Surveys, College of Medicine and Dentistry of New Jersey.

MILLER, H., On hanging loose and loving: the dilemma of present youth. *J. Social Issues* **27**(3): 35–46, 1971.

NATIONAL COMMISSION OF MARIHUANA AND DRUG ABUSE. *Marijuana, A Signal of Misunderstanding.* New York: The New American Library, 1972.

RICHARDS, L.G., and CARROL, E.E. Illicit drug use and addiction in the United States. *Public Health Rep.* 83(December): 1035–1041, 1970.

ROLLINS, J.H., and HOLDEN, R.H. "Adolescent drug use and the alienation syndrome." Paper presented at the American Psychological Association Convention, 1972.

SAN MATEO COUNTY DEPARTMENT OF PUBLIC HEALTH AND WELFARE. *Five Mind Altering Drugs (Plus One).* San Mateo: The Research and Statistics Section, 1970.

SHAW, M.E., and WRIGHT, J.M. *Scales for the Measurement of Attitudes.* New York: McGraw-Hill, 1967, pp. 322–323.

SIMMONS, J.L., and WINOGARD, B. *It's Happening: A Portrait of the Youth Scene Today.* Santa Barbara, California: Marc-Laird Publication, 1966.

SMART, R.G., and FEJER, D. Recent trends in illicit drug use among adolescents. Toronto: *Bi-monthly J. Dept. Nat. Health Welfare, Ottawa, Canada.* Supplement 68(May–August): 13 pp., 1971.

SROLE, L. Social integration and certain corollaries. *Amer. Sociol. Rev.* 21(October): 709–716, 1956.

SUCHMAN, E.A. A "hang-loose" ethic and the spirit of drug use. *J. Health Social Behavior.* 9(June): 146–155, 1968.

TEC, N. Some aspects of high school status and differential involvement with marijuana: a study of suburban teenagers. *Adolescence,* 7(Spring): 1–28, 1972.

THURSTONE, L.L. (ed.). *The Measurement of Social Attitudes*. Chicago: Univ. of Chicago Press, 1931.

WECHSLER, H., and THUM, D. The social context of drug use. *New York Law J., Special Edition of Drugs*. pp. 30–31, December 1971.

The International Journal of the Addictions, 9(6), pp. 919–930, 1974

Cumulative Index, International Journal of the Addictions, Volume 9

SECTION 1, AUTHOR–TITLE LIST

Issue No.	Page	Author	Title
9:1	1	Herbert H. Blumberg S. Daryl Cohen B. Elizabeth Dronfield Elizabeth A. Mordecai J. Colin Roberts David Hawks	British Opiate Users: I. People Approaching London Drug Treatment Centres
	25	Michael Rohrbaugh Gerald Eads Samuel Press	Effects of the Vietnam Experience on Subsequent Drug Use Among Servicemen
	41	Harvey L. Ruben	Rehabilitation of Drug and Alcohol Abusers in the U.S. Army
	57	Roderick S. Carman	Values, Expectations, and Drug Use Among High School Students in a Rural Community
	81	Stanley Einstein	Drug Abuse Training and Education: The Physician
	101	Gary Fisher Allan Steckler	Psychological Effects, Personality and Behavioral Changes Attributed to Marihuana Use
	127	Jerome S. Miller John Sensenig Jonathan S. Raymond	Value Structure as a Predictor of Type of Discharge Among Residential Addicts
	137	Allen Frances	A Comprehensive Military Drug and Alcohol Program
	145	A. E. Raynes C. Climent V. D. Patch F. Ervin	Factors Related to Imprisonment in Female Heroin Addicts

	151	Dan Arnon Marc H. Kleinman Benjamin Kissin	Psychological Differentiation in Heroin Addicts
	161	Thomas J. Cox Bill Longwell	Reliability of Interview Data Concerning Current Heroin Use from Heroin Addicts on Methadone
	167	Harry Silsby Forest S. Tennant, Jr.	Short-Term, Ambulatory Detoxification of Opiate Addicts Using Methadone
9:2	171	Arthur Falek	Chemical Mutagenesis and Drugs of Abuse in Man—A Current View of the Problem
	185	Paul C. Whitehead	Multidrug Use: Supplementary Perspectives
	205	Herbert H. Blumberg S. Daryl Cohen B. Elizabeth Dronfield Elizabeth A. Mordecai J. Colin Roberts David Hawks	British Opiate Users: II. Differences between Those Given an Opiate Script and Those Not Given One
	221	Thomas Henchy Byron Eckerson Jesse L. Paez	The Relationship between Age and/or Negative Experiences and Success on a Methadone Maintenance Program
	229	Raymond A. Lloyd Richard N. Katon Robert L. Dupont	Evolution of a Treatment Approach for Young Heroin Addicts. Comparison of Three Treatment Modalities
	241	Betty Crowther	The College Opiate User
	255	Arthur G. Cryns	Personality Characteristics of Heroin Addicts in a Methadone Treatment Program: An Exploratory Study
	267	Joseph Powell Stokes	Personality Traits and Attitudes and Their Relationship to Student Drug Using Behavior
	289	Richard S. Campbell Jeffrey B. Freeland	Patterns of Drug Abuse
	301	D. Dwayne Simpson S. B. Sells	Patterns of Multiple Drug Abuse: 1969–1971
	315	Carolyn A. Eldred Barry S. Brown Cynthia Mahabir	Heroin Addict Clients' Description of Their Families of Origin
	321	Douglas P. Ferraro David K. Billings	Marihuana Use by College Students: Three-Year Trends, 1970–1972
	329	Robert Bloom J. Ray Hays G. Michael Winburn	Marijuana Use in Urban Secondary Schools: A Three-Year Comparison

	337	Patricia B. Sutker Albert N. Allain Charles E. Moan	Addict Attitudes toward Methadone Maintenance: A Preliminary Report
	345	Carlos E. Climent Anthony Raynes Ann Rollins Robert Plutchik	Epidemiological Studies of Female Prisoners. II: Biological, Psychological, and Social Correlates of Drug Addiction
	351	Charles R. Lett C. Robert Ingram, Jr.	Progression Time to Narcotic Use in a Southwestern Addict Population
9:3	355	Raymond M. Costello Sandra Lee Schneider	Mortality in an Alcoholic Cohort
	365	David E. Raskin	International Issues in Drug Abuse
	373	Reginald G. Smart Paul C. Whitehead	The Uses of an Epidemiology of Drug Use: The Canadian Scene
	389	John A. Ewing	Behavioral Approaches for Problems with Alcohol
	401	Albert S. Carlin Robin Dee Post	Drug Use and Achievement
	411	Barry M. Maletzky	Assisted Covert Sensitization for Drug Abuse
	431	Kenneth B. Stein Vitali Rozynko	Psychological and Social Variables and Personality Patterns of Drug Abusers
	447	G. J. Steinfeld E. A. Rautio A. H. Rice M. J. Egan	Group Covert Sensitization with Narcotic Addicts (Further Comments)
	465	Don Wallace Darlene Hiner	Some Descriptive Measures on 100 Consecutive VA Hospital Drug Abuse Admissions
	475	Bernard Segal	Drug Use and Fantasy Processes: Criterion for Prediction of Potential Users
	481	Elizabeth E. Force Jack W. Millar	An Epidemioligical and Ecological Study of Risk Factors for Narcotics Overdose: I. Retrospective Study of Psychosocial Factors
	489	Jorge A. Viamontes Barbara J. Powell	Demographic Characteristics of Black and White Male Alcoholics
9:4	495	Marvin Green Carl Zelson Hans Behrendt	Sweating Function in the Heroin Withdrawal Syndrome of Neonates
	503	Keith W. Jacobs	Asthmador: A Legal Hallucinogen
	513	William I. Barton	Narcotics-Related Deaths Decrease in 1972 from the Number of Narcotics-Related Deaths in 1971

	531	Jens J. B. Winsløw	Drug Use and Social Integration
	541	Russel N. Cassel Gail Zander	Teach Me What I Want to Know About Drugs for Junior High School Students
	569	Jerry L. Strimbu O. Suthern Sims, Jr.	A University System Drug Profile
	585	William Warren Garitano Ruth E. Ronall	Concepts of Life Style in the Treatment of Alcoholism
	593	William W. Van Stone	Treating the Drug-Dependent Veteran—Perspectives from a Veterans Administration Hospital
	605	John C. LaRosa Stephen H. Lipsius Judith H. LaRosa	Experiences with a Combination of Group Therapy and Methadone Maintenance in the Treatment of Heroin Addiction
9:5	619	William S. Arnon Douglas Daily	Short- and Long-Term Therapeutic Communities: A Follow-Up and Cost Effectiveness Comparison
	637	Michael Peretz Frederick B. Glaser	Value Change in Drug Education: The Role of Encounter Groups
	653	Mark H. Greene Napoleon Turner, Jr. Robert L. DuPont	Amphetamines in the District of Columbia. III. Central Nervous System Stimulant Abuse in a Population of Narcotics Addicts in Treatment, with an Emphasis on Phenmetrazine
	663	Albert A. Kurland Thomas E. Hanlon O. Lee McCabe	Naloxone and the Narcotic Abuser: A Controlled Study of Partial Blockade
	673	James H. Williams Alan VanLewen Tessa Breen	Evaluation of a 6-Day Course in Alcoholism Education and Orientation
	701	George S. Snyderman	Rehabilitating the Ex-Offender, Ex-Addict
	719	Richard S. Campbell Jeffrey B. Freeland	The Hippie Turns Junkie: The Emergence of a Type
	731	O. Lee McCabe Albert A. Kurland Dorothy Sullivan	A Study of Methadone Failures in an Abstinence Program
	741	Henry S. G. Cutter Albert Samaraweera Richard A. Fish Louis Morris Repton Merritt	Emotional Openness and Mood Change in Marathon Group Psychotherapy

	749	Fred Streit Donald L. Halsted Pietro J. Pascale	Differences among Youthful Users and Non-Users of Drugs Based on Their Perceptions of Parental Behavior
	757	Frederick W. Obitz Kimberly Cooper Donald C. Madeiros	General and Specific Perceived Locus of Control in Heroin Addicts
9:6	761	Paul W. Haberman Michael M. Baden	Drinking, Drugs, and Death
	775	Barry M. Maletzky	Addiction to Propoxyphene (Darvon): A Second Look
	785	K. L. Lu	The Indexing and Analysis of Drug Indulgence
	805	Walter V. Collier Yasser A. Hijazi	A Follow-Up Study of Former Residents of Daytop Village, Inc.
	827	Thomas J. Prendergast, Jr.	Family Characteristics Associated with Marijuana Use Among Adolescents
	841	S. Creel R. Berkson J. Reilly P. Butler B. Walker L. Carrozza J. Morrison R. O'Connell V. Patch	Counseling Utilization Related to Dose Reduction in Methadone Maintenance
	851	Lee H. Bowker	Student Drug Use and the Perceived Peer Drug Environment
	863	Roy Stern N. B. Edwards Furey A. Lerro	Methadone on Demand as a Heroin Detoxification Procedure
	873	Vitali V. Rozynko Kenneth B. Stein	Social and Psychological Factors Associated with Length of Stay in a Drug Treatment Facility
	879	Douglas P. Ferraro David K. Billings	Illict Drug Use by College Students: Three-Year Trends, 1970–1972
	885	P. H. Blachly B. J. Blachly	Sampling Technique for Medically Significant Drug Abuse
	891	Ronald R. Rardin Thomas R. Lawson David J. Kruzich	Opiates, Amphetamines, Alcohol: A Comparative Study of American Soldiers
	899	William Henik George Domino	Changes in Locus of Control in Heroin Addicts
	903	R. B. Dick L. T. Brown	A Comparison of Drug Users and Nonusers on a Midwestern University Campus

909 George H. Wolkon, Naomi Kantzer Jasso, Sharon Gallagher, Peter Cohn — The "Hang-Loose" Ethic and Drug Use Revisited

SECTION 2, SUBJECT INDEX

This subject index follows the format of the National Library of Medicine's *Index Medicus*. Headings have been added.

Entries take this form: Volume and number, senior author, first page of article. For example, 9:5 McCabe (731) refers to O. Lee McCabe, Albert A. Kurland, and Dorothy Sullivan's "A Study of Methadone Failures in an Abstinence Program," found in issue 5 of this volume, beginning on page 731. From this section of the index, reference may be made to Section 1 for the full title and authors of a particular article.

All original contributions to *The International Journal of the Addictions*, Volume 9, are indexed. Book reviews and communications are not included.

ABSTINENCE
9:5 McCabe (731)
ACHIEVEMENT AND DRUG USE
9:3 Carlin (401)
ADDICTIONS—DEFINITIONS
9:1 Einstein (81)
ADDICTS
see under category:
HEROIN USERS, etc.
ADDICTS ATTITUDES TOWARD TREATMENT
9:1 Blumberg (1)
9:2 Sutker (337)
9:5 McCabe (731)
9:6 Rozynko (873)
ADOLESCENT DRUG USERS
9:2 Lloyd (229)
9:6 Prendergast (827)
AGE AND DRUG USE
9:2 Crowther (241)
AGE AND TREATMENT OUTCOME
9:2 Henchy (221)
ALCOHOL–NARCOTIC POSTMORTEM FINDINGS
9:6 Haberman (761)
ALCOHOLISM
9:3 Ewing (389)
9:3 Viamontes (489)
9:5 Williams (673)
ALCOHOLISM—MILITARY
9:1 Ruben (41)
ALCOHOLISM—PHYSIOLOGICAL EFFECTS
9:3 Costello (355)
ALCOHOLISM—PSYCHOLOGICAL FACTORS
9:4 Garitano (585)
AMPHETAMINE USE
9:5 Greene (653)
ANTAGONISTS
see DRUG ANTAGONISTS
ARMY TREATMENT PROGRAMS
see REHABILITATION—U.S. ARMY PROGRAMS; V.A. DRUG TREATMENT PROGRAMS
ASTHMADOR
9:4 Jacobs (503)
BEHAVIOR
9:1 Fisher (101)
9:3 Carlin (401)
9:5 Obitz (757)
see also VALUE ANALYSIS
BEHAVIOR—ALCOHOLICS
9:4 Garitano (585)
BEHAVIOR THERAPY
9:3 Maletzky (411)

9:3 Steinfeld (447)
9:5 Cutter (741)
BEHAVIOR THERAPY—ALCOHOLISM
9:3 Ewing (389)
CANNABIS USERS
9:1 Fisher (101)
9:2 Ferraro (321)
9:2 Bloom (329)
9:3 Segal (475)
9:6 Prendergast (827)
9:6 Ferraro (879)
CASE STUDIES—ASTHMADOR USE
9:4 Jacobs (503)
CASE STUDIES—DARVON
9:6 Maletzky (775)
CHROMOSOMES—MUTAGENIC, TERATOGENIC, AND CARCINOGENIC DAMAGE BY DRUGS
9:2 Falek (171)
CLINICAL FINDINGS ON DRUG ABUSE
9:6 Blachly (885)
CLINICAL PROCEDURES IN DRUG CELL DAMAGE STUDIES
9:2 Falek (171)
CONDITIONING
see THERAPY—CONDITIONING; COVERT SENSITIZATION
COST EFFECTIVENESS OF DRUG TREATMENT
9:5 Arnon (619)
COUNSELING IN DRUG TREATMENT
9:6 Creel (841)
COVERT SENSITIZATION
9:3 Maletsky (411)
9:3 Steinfeld (447)
CRIME–DRUG RELATIONSHIPS
9:5 Arnon (619)
9:5 Snyderman (701)
DARVON MISUSE
9:6 Maletzky (775)
DAYTOP VILLAGE
9:6 Collier (805)
DEATH
see MORTALITY
DEMOGRAPHIC VARIABLES—ALCOHOLISM
9:3 Viamontes (489)
DEMOGRAPHIC VARIABLES—CANNABIS USE
9:1 Fisher (101)
DEMOGRAPHIC VARIABLES—DRUG USE
9:2 Blumberg (205)
9:3 Wallace (465)
9:4 Strimbu (569)
DEMOGRAPHIC VARIABLES—WOMEN HEROIN USERS
9:1 Raynes (145)
DEMOGRAPHIC VARIABLES—NARCOTIC-RELATED DEATHS
9:4 Barton (513)
DEMOGRAPHIC VARIABLES—OPIATE USE
9:1 Blumberg (1)
DETOXIFICATION
9:6 Stern (863)
9:6 Rozynko (873)
DETOXIFICATION—METHADONE
9:1 Silsby (167)
9:2 Lloyd (229)
DOSAGE
see METHADONE—DOSAGE
DRUG ANTAGONISTS
9:5 Kurland (663)
DRUG AND NARCOTIC CONTROL—DARVON
9:6 Maletzky (775)
DRUG AND NARCOTIC CONTROL—INTERNATIONAL
9:3 Raskin (365)
DRUG USE—BRITAIN
9:1 Blumberg (1)
9:2 Blumberg (205)
DRUG USE—CANADA
9:2 Whitehead (185)
9:3 Smart (373)
DRUG USE—DENMARK
9:4 Winsløw (531)
DRUG USE—DISTRICT OF COLUMBIA
9:3 Force (481)
9:4 LaRosa (605)
9:5 Greene (653)

DRUG USE—EASTERN U.S.
9:2 Cryns (255)
DRUG USE—MID-ATLANTIC U.S.
9:5 Streit (749)
DRUG USE—MIDWEST U.S.
9:6 Dick (903)
DRUG USE—RURAL U.S.
9:1 Carman (57)
DRUG USE—SOUTHEAST ASIA
9:1 Rohrbaugh (25)
DRUG USE—SOUTHERN U.S.
9:2 Sutker (337)
9:3 Segal (475)
9:4 Strimbu (569)
9:6 Prendergast (827)
DRUG USE—SOUTHWEST U.S.
9:2 Ferraro (321)
9:2 Lett (351)
9:3 Wallace (465)
9:6 Ferraro (879)
DRUG USE—URBAN U.S.
9:2 Bloom (329)
DRUG USE—WESTERN U.S.
9:6 Blachly (885)
9:6 Wolkon (909)
DRUG USE—MILITARY
9:1 Rohrbaugh (25)
9:1 Ruben (41)
9:1 Silsby (167)
9:4 Van Stone (593)
9:6 Rardin (891)
DRUG USE PATTERNS
9:1 Fisher (101)
9:2 Whitehead (185)
9:2 Campbell (289)
9:2 Simpson (301)
9:2 Lett (351)
9:4 Strimbu (569)
9:5 Campbell (719)
9:6 Lu (785)
9:6 Rardin (891)
DRUG USE—PHYSIOLOGICAL EFFECTS
9:2 Falik (171)
9:4 Green (495)
9:4 Jacobs (503)
9:6 Blachly (885)
DRUG USE—PSYCHOLOGICAL EFFECTS
9:1 Fisher (101)
DRUG USE—PSYCHOLOGICAL FACTORS
9:1 Fisher (101)
9:1 Miller (127)
9:1 Arnon (151)
9:2 Stokes (267)
9:3 Carlin (401)
9:3 Stein (431)
9:3 Wallace (465)
9:3 Segal (475)
9:5 Streit (749)
9:5 Obitz (757)
EDUCATION—ALCOHOLISM TREATMENT
9:5 Williams (673)
EDUCATION—DRUG USE
9:1 Einstein (81)
9:4 Cassel (541)
9:5 Peretz (637)
EPIDEMIOLOGY OF DRUG USE
9:1 Rohrbaugh (25)
9:2 Climent (345)
9:3 Smart (373)
9:3 Force (481)
9:4 Winsløw (531)
9:6 Ferraro (879)
FAMILY
9:2 Eldred (315)
9:5 Streit (749)
9:6 Prendergast (827)
FOLLOW-UP OF DAYTOP RESIDENTS
9:6 Collier (805)
HALLUCINOGENS—ALKALOID
9:4 Jacobs (503)
HASHISH USERS
9:4 Winsløw (531)
HEROIN USERS
9:1 Arnon (151)
9:1 Cox (161)
9:2 Lloyd (229)
9:2 Cryns (255)
9:2 Eldred (315)
9:4 LaRosa (605)
9:5 Obitz (757)
9:6 Creel (841)
9:6 Henik (899)
HEROIN USERS—WOMEN

9:1 Raynes (145)
9:2 Climent (345)
HEROIN WITHDRAWAL SYNDROME
9:4 Green (495)
HIGH SCHOOL DRUG USERS
see STUDENT DRUG USE; ADOLESCENT DRUG USERS
HIPPIE—JUNKIE
9:5 Campbell (719)
HOSPITALS
9:3 Wallace (465)
9:6 Blachly (885)
see also V.A. DRUG TREATMENT PROGRAMS
INDEX OF RATE AND TYPE OF DRUG USE
9:6 Lu (785)
INPATIENT TREATMENT
see TREATMENT PROGRAMS
INTERNATIONAL ISSUES IN DRUG CONTROL
9:3 Raskin (365)
"LIFE STYLE" OF ALCOHOLICS
9:4 Garitano (585)
LSD
9:5 Campbell (719)
MAINTENANCE PROGRAMS—METHADONE
9:1 Cox (161)
9:2 Henchy (221)
9:2 Cryns (255)
9:2 Sutker (337)
9:4 LaRosa (605)
9:6 Creel (841)
MAINTENANCE PROGRAMS—OPIATE
9:2 Blumberg (205)
MARIJUANA
see CANNABIS
MEDICALLY SIGNIFICANT DRUG ABUSE
9:6 Blachly (885)
METHADONE—DOSAGE
9:6 Creel (841)
METHADONE—SELF-ADMINISTRATION
9:6 Stern (863)
MOOD CHANGE IN DRUG-DEPENDENT PERSONS
9:5 Cutter (741)
MORTALITY—ALCOHOLICS
9:3 Costello (355)
9:6 Haberman (761)
MORTALITY—DRUG USERS
9:6 Haberman (761)
MORTALITY—NARCOTIC USERS
9:4 Barton (513)
MULTIDRUG USE
9:2 Whitehead (185)
9:2 Simpson (301)
MULTIMODALITY TREATMENT
see TREATMENT PROGRAMS
MUTAGENESIS—CHEMICAL
9:2 Falek (171)
NALOXONE
9:5 Kurland (663)
NARCOTIC-ALCOHOL POSTMORTEM FINDINGS
9:6 Haberman (761)
NARCOTIC USERS
9:2 Campbell (289)
9:3 Steinfeld (447)
9:3 Force (481)
9:5 Greene (653)
9:5 Kurland (663)
NEONATES OF HEROIN-ADDICTED MOTHERS
9:4 Greene (495)
NIMH STUDIES
9:2 Campbell (289)
9:2 Simpson (301)
OPIATE USERS
9:1 Blumberg (1)
9:1 Rohrbaugh (25)
9:1 Silsby (167)
9:2 Blumberg (205)
9:2 Crowther (241)
OVERDOSE—ADDICTS ATTITUDES
9:3 Force (481)
OVERDOSE—NARCOTIC
9:4 Barton (513)
PEER INFLUENCE IN DRUG USE
9:6 Bowker (851)
PERSONALITY ASSESSMENT
9:2 Cryns (255)
9:2 Stokes (267)
9:3 Stein (431)

9:3 Wallace (465)
9:6 Rardin (891)
9:6 Henik (899)
PHENMETRAZINE
9:5 Greene (653)
PHYSICAL EFECTS OF DRUG USE
see DRUG USE—PHYSIOLOGICAL EFFECTS
PHYSICIANS IN DRUG ABUSE TREATMENT
9:1 Einstein (81)
PRISONS
9:2 Climent (345)
9:5 Snyderman (701)
PRISONS—FEMALE HEROIN USERS
9:1 Raynes (145)
PROGRESSION TIME TO NARCOTIC USE
9:2 LETT (351)
PROPOXYPHENE
see DARVON
PSYCHOLOGICAL EFFECTS OF DRUG USE
see DRUG USE—PSYCHOLOGICAL EFFECTS
PSYCHOTOGEN USERS
9:5 Campbell (719)
QUESTIONNAIRES
9:1 Carman (57)
9:3 Steinfeld (447)
9:4 Cassel (541)
RECIDIVISM
9:1 Silsby (167)
9:5 Snyderman (701)
9:6 Collier (805)
REHABILITATION
9:5 Snyderman (701)
REHABILITATION—U.S. ARMY PROGRAMS
9:1 Ruben (41)
9:1 Frances (137)
RESEARCH INSTRUMENTS—ADJECTIVE CHECK LIST DATA
9:2 Eldred (315)
RESEARCH INSTRUMENTS—COMPUTERIZED
9:4 Cassel (541)
RESEARCH INSTRUMENTS—DEVELOPMENT OF FACTOR ANALYSIS IN DRUG USE
9:2 Stokes (267)
RESEARCH INSTRUMENTS—EGO DEVELOPMENT SCALE
9:4 Cassel (541)
RESEARCH INSTRUMENTS—EPIDEMIOLOGICAL
9:3 Smart (373)
RESEARCH INSTRUMENTS—FUTURE AND PAST TIME PERSPECTIVE TEST
9:3 Stein (431)
RESEARCH INSTRUMENTS—I–E DATA
9:4 Cassel (541)
9:5 Obitz (757)
9:6 Henik (899)
RESEARCH INSTRUMENTS—INDEX OF RATE AND TYPE OF DRUG USE
9:6 Lu (785)
RESEARCH INSTRUMENTS—MIST
9:3 Stein (431)
RESEARCH INSTRUMENTS—MMPI DATA
9:3 Stein (431)
9:6 Rardin (891)
RESEARCH INSTRUMENTS—NIMH–TCU DRUG ABUSE REPORTING PROGRAM DATA
9:2 Simpson (301)
RESEARCH INSTRUMENTS—PERSONAL ORIENTATION INVENTORY DATA
9:2 Cryns (255)
RESEARCH INSTRUMENTS—POMS
9:5 Cutter (741)
RESEARCH INSTRUMENTS—RELIABILITY OF INTERVIEWS
9:1 Cox (161)
RESEARCH INSTRUMENTS—ROD AND FRAME TEST DATA
9:1 Arnon (151)
RESEARCH INSTRUMENTS—ROTTER'S SOCIAL LEARNING

THEORY OF PERSONALITY DATA
9:1 Carman (57)
RESEARCH INSTRUMENTS—(SO)–CPI
9:3 Stein (431)
RESEARCH INSTRUMENTS—TSC
9:3 Stein (431)
RETENTION RATES
9:1 Miller (127)
9:2 Henchy (221)
9:5 Arnon (619)
9:5 Kurland (663)
9:5 McCabe (731)
9:6 Rozynko (873)
SENSITIZATION
see COVERT SENSITIZATION
SEX DIFFERENCES IN DRUG USE
9:1 Arnon (151)
9:2 Lett (351)
9:6 Lu (785)
9:6 Bowker (851)
SOCIAL INTEGRATION AND DRUG USE
9:4 Winsløw (531)
SOCIETY AND DRUG USE
9:1 Rohrbaugh (25)
9:1 Einstein (81)
SOCIOECONOMIC FACTORS IN CANNABIS USE
9:2 Bloom (329)
SOCIOECONOMIC FACTORS IN DRUG USE
9:1 Carman (57)
9:2 Crowther (241)
9:2 Bloom (329)
9:3 Stein (431)
STAFF
see TREATMENT FACILITIES—STAFF
STUDENT DRUG USE
9:1 Carman (57)
9:2 Crowther (241)
9:2 Stokes (267)
9:2 Ferraro (321)
9:2 Bloom (329)
9:3 Segal (475)
9:4 Winsløw (531)
9:4 Cassel (541)
9:4 Strimbu (569)
9:5 Streit (749)
9:6 Bowker (851)
9:6 Ferraro (879)
9:6 Dick (903)
9:6 Wolkon (909)
THERAPUETIC APPROACHES—COMPARISONS
9:3 Lloyd (229)
9:5 Arnon (619)
THERAPEUTIC COMMUNITIES—COST COMPARISONS
9:5 Arnon (619)
THERAPY—CONDITIONING
9:3 Maletzky (411)
9:3 Steinfeld (447)
see also COVERT SENSITIZATION
THERAPY—GROUP
9:4 LaRosa (605)
9:5 Peretz (637)
9:5 Cutter (741)
TREATMENT EVALUATION
9:1 Ruben (41)
9:1 Miller (127)
9:6 Collier (805)
9:6 Rozynko (873)
TREATMENT EVALUATION—METHADONE
9:5 McCabe (731)
TREATMENT FACILITIES—DEVELOPMENT AND ORGANIZATION
9:1 Ruben (41)
9:1 Einstein (81)
9:1 Frances (137)
9:2 Lloyd (229)
9:4 Van Stone (593)
9:5 Williams (673)
9:5 Snyderman (701)
TREATMENT FACILITIES—STAFF
9:5 Peretz (637)
9:5 Williams (673)
9:6 Stern (863)
TREATMENT PROGRAMS—ALCOHOLISM
9:3 Ewing (389)
9:4 Garitano (585)
TREATMENT PROGRAMS—INPATIENT
9:1 Miller (127)
9:6 Stern (863)

TREATMENT PROGRAMS—MULTIMODALITY
9:1 Frances (137)
9:2 Lloyd (229)
9:4 Van Stone (593)
9:4 LaRosa (605)
see also REHABILITATION—U.S. ARMY PROGRAMS; V.A. TREATMENT PROGRAMS
UN ROLE IN DRUG CONTROL
9:3 Raskin (365)
V.A. DRUG TREATMENT PROGRAMS
9:3 Wallace (465)
9:4 Van Stone (593)
VALERIC ACID—COVERT SENSITIZER
9:3 Maletzky (411)
VALUE ANALYSIS OF DRUG USERS
9:1 Carman (57)
9:1 Miller (127)
9:3 Carlin (401)
9:5 Peretz (637)
VALUE ANALYSIS—"HANG LOOSE" ETHIC
9:6 Wolkon (909)
WITHDRAWAL SYNDROME—HEROIN NEONATES
9:4 Green (495)

CLINICAL TOXICOLOGY

Volume 7 Number 5 1974

CONTENTS OF THIS ISSUE

J. H. WILLS, F. COULSTON, E. S. HARRIS, E. W. MC CHESNEY, J. C. RUSSELL, AND D. M. SERRONE: Inhalation of Aerosolized Ethylene Glycol by Man 463

JACK E. WALLACE, KENNETH BLUM, AND JASBIR M. SINGH: Determination of Drugs in Biologic Specimens—A Review. 477

GEORGE CLAUS: Environmental Carcinogens: Is There a Threshold of Exposure?. 497

M. M. KAPLAN, D. C. REGISTER, A. H. BIERMAN, AND R. L. RISACHER: A Nonfatal Case of Intentional Scopolamine Poisoning 509

RONALD B. STEWART, MARGARET FORGNONE, FRANKLIN E. MAY, JANE FORBES, AND LEIGHTON E. CLUFF: Epidemiology of Acute Drug Intoxications: Patient Characteristics, Drugs, and Medical Complications. 513

J. T. SOBOTA AND W. L. LUMMIS: Absence of Drug Abuse in Prisoners in a Major Correctional Institution. 531

CLINICAL TOXICOLOGIST'S NOTEBOOK: COCAINE 541

NEWS ITEMS 545

A complimentary copy will be sent on request

Contributions to This Journal Are Published Free of Charge

MARCEL DEKKER, INC., New York

A Statement of Purpose

INSTITUTE FOR THE STUDY OF DRUG MISUSE, Inc.

The Institute for the Study of Drug Misuse, Inc. (formerly the Institute for the Study of Drug Addiction) was established in 1965 as an international organization to develop clear channels of communication and to encourage research in the field of drug abuse. To fulfill its goals, the Institute participates in research, professional training, and education. In addition, it serves as a consulting agency in the establishment of treatment programs in the United States and abroad. As professional, government, and lay concern increases in the field of drug abuse, the Institute has been called upon to serve as a resource agency for the dissemination of scientific materials through the press, television, radio, and other media.

In order to achieve its purposes, the Institute for the Study of Drug Misuse:

Sponsors the INTERNATIONAL JOURNAL OF THE ADDICTIONS, published by Marcel Dekker, Inc.

Sponsors national and international conferences and workshops in cooperation with universities, medical teaching centers, governmental agencies, and private industry.

Sponsors a lecture series "The Use and Misuse of Drugs and Alcohol," for professionals and interested lay people.

Sponsors international awards for significant research reports focusing upon various aspects of drug abuse.

The expanding programs of the Institute have been dictated by the present crisis in drug abuse. It is apparent that in the United States and in the world at large, certain social forces are at work which have magnified the scope of the problem. In order to insure that the Institute reaches the broadest group of interested individuals, it has become necessary to establish several categories of membership.

Membership in the Institute for the Study of Drug Misuse is tax exempt.

For membership information, write:

Institute for the Study of Drug Misuse, Inc.
111 Fifth Avenue
New York, N.Y. 10003

INFORMATION FOR AUTHORS SUBMITTING MANUSCRIPTS

Send a clear double-spaced typewritten original and two duplicate copies to the Editor, *International Journal of the Addictions*, Institute for the Study of Drug Misuse, Inc., 111 Fifth Avenue, New York, N.Y. 10003. DOUBLE-SPACE the entire manuscript; do not use single spacing anywhere.

Include authors' academic degrees and present affiliation. If applicable, cite auspices under which work being reported was done. Specify address to which requests for reprints should be sent.

Begin your TITLE with a word useful in indexing. Put news of your finding or a statement of the problem first. Major and minor headings may be used in the text; indicate major headings by typing in capitals. Provide a 100-word SUMMARY at the end.

Use METRIC UNITS of measure. If measurements were made in English units, give metric equivalents.

Cite all TABLES and FIGURES in the text. Tables should have titles, and figures should have brief legends. In tables, give each column a heading. Indicate units of measure in parentheses in the heading for each column. Do not use vertical rules. Do not use horizontal rules other than those in the heading and at the bottom. Submit PHOTOGRAPHS as glossy prints, untrimmed and unmounted; identify each with pencil lightly on the back and indicate top.

ARTWORK will not be returned unless specifically requested, and will be disposed of three months after publication.

REFERENCES in the text should be enclosed in parentheses and include the author's surname and the date of the item cited. Keep footnotes to a minimum.

The BIBLIOGRAPHY (double-spaced) should be given at the end of the article in alphabetical order. Journal references should include authors, title, name of journal abbreviated according to *Chemical Abstracts List of Periodicals,* inclusive page numbers, and date. Book references should include authors, title, place of publication, publisher, and date.

THE INTERNATIONAL JOURNAL OF THE ADDICTIONS

Published by Marcel Dekker, Inc., New York
Sponsored by The Institute for the Study of Drug Misuse, Inc., New York

THE INTERNATIONAL JOURNAL OF THE ADDICTIONS

Volume 9 Number 6 1974

CONTENTS

Drinking, Drugs, and Death: Paul W. Haberman and Michael M. Baden ... 761
Addiction to Propoxyphene (Darvon): A Second Look: Barry M. Maletzky ... 775
The Indexing and Analysis of Drug Indulgence: K. H. Lu ... 785
A Follow-up Study of Former Residents of a Therapeutic Community: Walter V. Collier and Yasser A. Hijazi ... 805
Family Characteristics Associated with Marijuana Use among Adolescents: Thomas J. Prendergast ... 827
Counseling Utilization Related to Dose Reduction in Methadone Maintenance: S. Creel, R. Berkson, J. Reilly, P. Butler, B. Walker, L. Carrozza, J. Morrison, R. O'Connell, and V. Patch ... 841
Student Drug Use and the Perceived Peer Drug Environment: Lee H. Bowker ... 851
Methadone on Demand as a Heroin Detoxification Procedure: Roy Stern, N. B. Edwards, and Furey A. Lerro ... 863
Social and Psychological Factors Associated with Length of Stay in a Drug Treatment Facility: Vitali V. Rozynko and Kenneth B. Stein ... 873
Illicit Drug Use by College Students: Three-Year Trends, 1970–1972: Douglas P. Ferraro and David K. Billings ... 879

Research Notes

Sampling Technique for Medically Significant Drug Abuse: P. H. Blachly and B. J. Blachly ... 885
Opiates, Amphetamines, Alcohol: A Comparative Study of American Soldiers: Donald R. Rardin, Thomas R. Lawson, and David J. Kruzich ... 891
Changes in Locus of Control in Heroin Addicts: Willy Henik and George Domino ... 899
A Comparison of Drug Users and Nonusers on a Midwestern University Campus: R. B. Dick and L. T. Brown ... 903
The "Hang-Loose" Ethic and Drug Use Revisited: George H. Woikon, Naomi Kantzer Jasso, Sharon Gallagher, and Peter Cohn ... 909

Index to Volume 9 ... 919

Cover Illustration: "Here three parts of the business is left for me to do, and the fourth left unfinished, while you do nothing but soak with the guests all day long," by Edmund J. Sullivan, for Oliver Goldsmith's "The Vicar of Wakefield," 18th century. Courtesy of the Picture Collection, The Branch Libraries, New York Public Library

MARCEL DEKKER, INC., New York